ICG Fluorescence Imaging and Navigation Surgery

Mitsuo Kusano • Norihiro Kokudo •
Masakazu Toi • Masaki Kaibori
Editors

ICG Fluorescence Imaging and Navigation Surgery

Springer

Editors
Mitsuo Kusano
Department of Surgery
Seiwa Memorial Hospital
Sapporo
Hokkaido
Japan

Norihiro Kokudo
Hepato-Biliary-Pancreatic Surgery Division
Artificial Organ and Transplantation Division
Department of Surgery
Graduate School of Medicine
University of Tokyo
Tokyo
Japan

Masakazu Toi
Department of Breast Surgery
Graduate School of Medicine
Kyoto University
Kyoto
Japan

Masaki Kaibori
Department of Surgery
Hirakata Hospital
Kansai Medical University
Hirakata
Japan

ISBN 978-4-431-55527-8 ISBN 978-4-431-55528-5 (eBook)
DOI 10.1007/978-4-431-55528-5

Library of Congress Control Number: 2016932391

Springer Tokyo Heidelberg New York Dordrecht London

Printed on acid-free paper

Springer Japan KK is part of Springer Science+Business Media (www.springer.com)

Foreword

Professor Mitsuo Kusano, a former professor in the Department of Surgery, Showa University, and a former president of the Kushiro Rosai Hospital, has published this remarkable book, *ICG Fluorescence Imaging and Navigation Surgery*. His work has been supported and assisted proactively by the co-editors Professor Norihiro Kokudo, in the Department of Hepato-Biliary-Pancreatic Surgery, Tokyo University; Professor Masakazu Toi, in the Department of Breast Surgery, Kyoto University Hospital; and Associate Professor Masaki Kaibori, in the Department of Surgery, Kansai Medical University. This book reports updated information on some of the most widely investigated indocyanine green (ICG) fluorescence methods.

As a member of the Japan Surgical Society and the Japan Surgical Association, Professor Kusano, the chief editor of the book, is well known for being one of the most energetic surgeons in his field, as well as for his gentle nature. He graduated from the School of Medicine, Hokkaido University, Japan, in 1970. After his residency in surgery, he spent more than 18 years in the Department of Surgery, Asahikawa Medical University, Japan. During that time as an associate professor, he already had been recognized as one of the most skilled surgeons. He was also interested in surgical research such as for liver cirrhosis, hepatocyte function, hepatocytes, and islet cell transplantation. After moving to the Department of Surgery, Showa University, as professor and chairman in 1993, he built upon his achievements and distinguished himself in the field of hepato-biliary-pancreatic surgery. Establishing a way to carry out safe and appropriate surgery, Professor Kusano devoted his attention to ICG as a contrast medium for a new method of imaging which was obtained after the emission of LED in addition to a test drug to evaluate liver function. He has contributed many studies of sentinel node navigation surgery in the field of gastroenterological and breast surgery.

This book is a collection of recent developments in ICG fluorescence. One of the most valuable aspects of the book is its detailed description of ICG, elucidating the basic nature of ICG fluorescence, the characteristics of photodynamic detection methods, and its applications for surgery. Interestingly, intraoperative ICG angiography and lymphography in addition to sentinel node navigation surgery in various areas, including the brain, head and neck, breast, gastrointestinal, hepato-biliary-pancreatic, and pediatric surgery, are described here.

Fulfilling Professor Kusano's dream, safe and appropriate therapy using ICG fluorescence can be provided to patients in various surgical fields and then the established technology can spread from Japan to the rest of the world. I hope this book will provide useful information to both the readers and their patients in applying this advanced technology using ICG fluorescence.

Department of Gastroenterological Surgery I
Hokkaido University
Sapporo, Japan
July 14, 2015

Akinobu Taketomi

Preface

It is our great pleasure to publish *ICG Fluorescence Imaging and Navigation Surgery*, a book comprising 43 chapters in which the latest information from basic and clinical research of indocyanine green (ICG) fluorescence surgery are described. The reader may be surprised to learn that ICG fluorescence imaging has been employed in so many clinical fields.

First, we express our sincere appreciation to all authors and staff who contributed to the publication of this book.

The basic study of ICG fluorescence imaging began in the 1970s. It was then applied in the ophthalmic field, and in the 2000s it started being used in breast cancer surgery to detect sentinel nodes. Its application to the digestive system started from 2006, demonstrating the detection of sentinel lymph nodes of stomach and colon cancers.

In recent years, it has come to be widely applied in various clinical fields. First, it can be used as a contrast agent not only for cerebral and coronary angiography but also for lymphangiography and cholangiography. Second, the usefulness of this method has been recognized in hepatic surgery, such as the tattooing of hepatic segments and the detection of liver tumors. The assessment of the vascularity of skin grafts by ICG fluorescence is one of its attractive applications in plastic surgery. In this book, many other useful and promising ICG fluorescence approaches are described.

ICG has been used as a vital dye to measure the circulating blood volume and as a diagnostic test reagent to evaluate liver function tests. Several decades have passed since it was discovered that ICG possessed the characteristic property to generate a fluorescence following conjugation with plasma protein. But the mechanism of the fluorescence-quenching phenomenon and the generation of ICG fluorescence in response to other substances such as methanol and ethanol have not been fully elucidated.

In recent years, the ICG fluorescent endoscope for thoracoscopic and laparoscopic surgery has been developed, enabling sentinel node navigation surgery in gastrointestinal tract cancers. We are convinced that endoscopic surgery when combined with ICG fluorescent imaging provides a more powerful approach for minimally invasive surgery.

We wish to express many thanks again to all authors for their great contribution to the publication of this important book that accelerates not only research of fluorescence imaging but also ICG fluorescent-navigated surgery.

Sapporo, Japan Mitsu Kusano
Tokyo, Japan Norihiro Kokudo
Kyoto, Japan Masakazu Toi
Hirakata, Japan Masaki Kaibori

Contents

Part I
Basis of ICG Fluorescence Method

Chapter 1
Photodynamic Characteristics of ICG Fluorescence Imaging

Mitsuharu Miwa

Abstract A recently developed ICG fluorescence imaging technique (termed ICG fluorescence method) has shown promise in clinical imaging. The ICG fluorescence method is suitable for use as an intraoperative diagnostic tool and has been applied to many clinical fields including breast cancer sentinel lymph navigation surgery, coronary artery bypass grafting, brain surgery, plastic surgery, and digestive surgery, owing to its safety (nonradioactive tracer), small size, light weight, and reasonable instrumentation costs. In this section, the optical characteristics and important considerations for ICG are described.

Keywords Indocyanine green (ICG) • Near infrared • Fluorescence

1.1 Indocyanine Green (ICG)

Indocyanine green (ICG) is a water-soluble compound that has been clinically approved in many countries for over 50 years for use in medical diagnostics, including determining cardiac output, hepatic function, and liver blood flow. The molecular formula of ICG is shown in Fig. 1.1, with a molecular weight of 755. When ICG is injected into human tissues, it immediately binds tightly to blood plasma. The majority of injected ICG is accumulated by hepatic parenchymal cells and is then excreted from hepatic cells into bile juice without being metabolized. The typical medical applications of ICG include hepatic function and liver blood flow diagnostics, which use measurement of optical absorption functions. ICG exhibits well-established fluorescence properties, and the fluorescence characteristics are commonly used for diagnostic retina or choroid imaging in the field of ophthalmology [1]. The peak optical absorption wavelength of ICG is approximately 800 nm, with peak fluorescence wavelengths of approximately 840 nm in the blood. These near-infrared wavelengths are able to penetrate deeper into human tissue compared with visible wavelength fluorescence compounds such as fluorescein.

M. Miwa (✉)
Hamamatsu Photonics K.K. Development Center, 5000 Hirakuchi, Hamakita-ku, Hamamatsu, Shizuoka 434-8601, Japan
e-mail: miwa@crl.hpk.co.jp

M. Kusano et al. (eds.), *ICG Fluorescence Imaging and Navigation Surgery*,
DOI 10.1007/978-4-431-55528-5_1

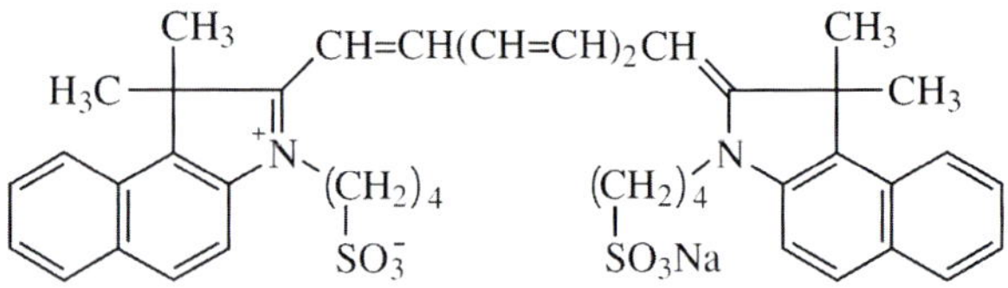

Fig. 1.1 Molecular formula of ICG

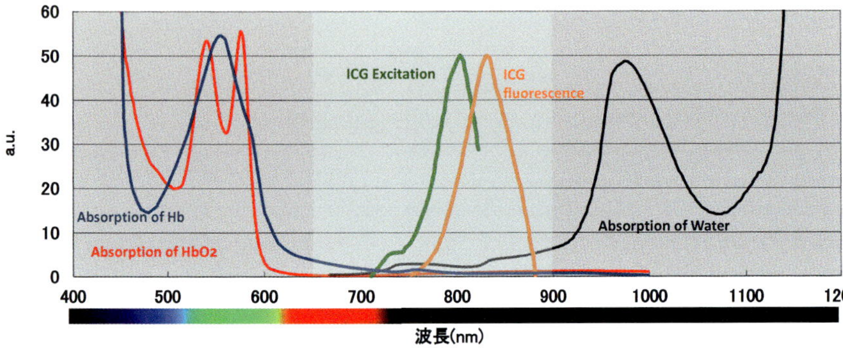

Fig. 1.2 Optical characteristics of ICG and absorption spectra of hemoglobin and water

1.2 Optical Characteristics of ICG

The optical characteristics of ICG is shown in Fig. 1.2.

The peak optical absorption wavelength of ICG is approximately 800 nm, with a fluorescence wavelength of approximately 810 nm in water and 840 nm in the blood. These wavelengths cannot be observed by the naked eye, while the use of video camera with high sensitivity in the near-infrared wavelength is used for measuring ICG fluorescence. The use of optical technology in the near-infrared wavelength for tissue measurement of ICG is advantageous as it can avoid the influence of autofluorescence and allow measurement of relatively deep tissues. The limitation of depth observation in human tissues is strongly related to the wavelength. For tissue measurement, hemoglobin and water are the main absorbance molecules. The optical absorption spectra of hemoglobin and water are also shown in Fig. 1.2. Hemoglobin strongly absorbs light at wavelengths shorter than 650 nm, while water absorbs light at wavelengths longer than 900 nm. The wavelength between 650 and 900 nm, termed the "optical window," has a high transparency because of low light absorbance by hemoglobin and water. The peak excitation and emission wavelengths of ICG are 800 nm and 840 nm in the blood, respectively, which are both within the optical window. Thus, the ICG fluorescence method can be used to provide angiographic assessment of blood vessels or lymphatic vessels located relatively deep (up to 10 mm) in tissue. With respect to image quality for tissue measurement, it is necessary to consider both light absorption and scattering. In particular, adipose tissue has low optical absorption but very high scattering characteristics, which results in blurring of the fluorescent image.

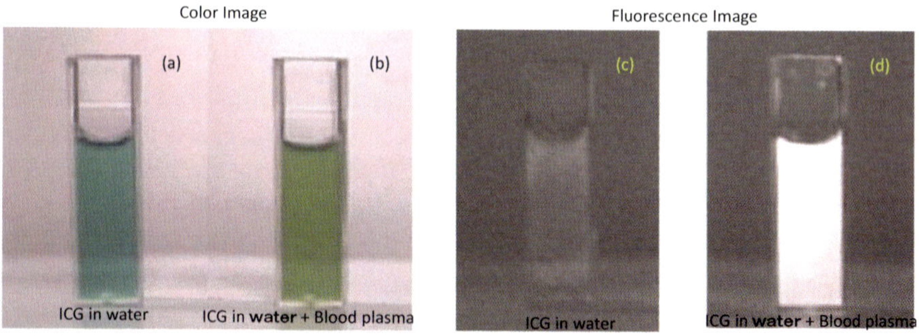

Fig. 1.3 ICG diluted by water (*left*) and ICG diluted by water with blood plasma (*right*). Color Image: (**a**) ICG in water, (**b**) ICG in water + Blood plasma. Fluorescence Image: (**c**) ICG in water, (**d**) ICG in water + Blood plasma

1.3 How ICG Generates Fluorescence

The color images (Fig. 1.3, left panel) and fluorescence images (Fig. 1.3, right panel) under conditions of ICG diluted by water (Fig. 1.3, left image) and addition of a small amount of blood plasma (Fig. 1.3, right image) are presented. ICG that has just been diluted by water exhibits an unstable and relatively weak fluorescence intensity (Fig. 1.3c). However, the fluorescence intensity increases when blood plasma is added to the ICG solution (Fig. 1.3d). A similar phenomenon occurs in human tissues, whereby an injected ICG solution immediately combines with blood plasma to generate strong fluorescence. Although ICG was originally considered to combine with albumin, it was more recently reported to predominantly bind to alpha-1 lipoprotein [2]. Yoneya et al. also demonstrated that ICG fluorescence is generated by high-density lipoprotein (HDL) and low-density lipoprotein (LDL) from blood plasma using electrophoresis and suggested that HDL is the major component involved in ICG fluorescence [3]. ICG fluorescence is also induced by dimethyl sulfoxide (DMSO), methanol (CH_3OH), and ethanol (C_2H_6O) [4], which are easier to use than lipoprotein for creating an ICG fluorescence phantom.

1.4 Considerations of the ICG Fluorescence Method

1.4.1 Toxicity

ICG exhibits a low toxicity with few side effects (36 out of 21,278 cases; 0.17 %), which include shock symptoms (0.02 %), nausea (0.08 %), angialgia (0.04 %), and fever (0.02 %). ICG should be used carefully in elder subjects with decreased physiological function, as well as in pregnant and lactating women [5].

1.4.2 *Concentration and Dose of ICG Injection for Fluorescence Imaging*

The typical concentration and dose of ICG injection for a diagnostic liver function test using the light absorption properties of ICG are 5 mg/ml and 0.5 mg/kg, respectively. However, for ICG fluorescence imaging, much lower concentrations and doses are recommended for improved fluorescence efficiency and to avoid the quenching effect. The concentration and total dose of ICG injection vary with the application. For example, 2.5 mg/ml concentration and approximately 0.5–1.0 ml ICG are typically used for breast cancer sentinel lymph node (SLN) navigation surgery, although there is some evidence of improved SLN detection rate with concentrations $\leq$0.5 mg/ml.

1.4.3 *Quenching Effect*

The fluorescence intensity of ICG does not always correspond to its concentration. In the case of fluorescence imaging, the fluorescence intensity of ICG is almost linearly increased with concentration within a low concentration range, while the fluorescence intensity then peaks and subsequently decreases at higher concentrations, a phenomenon termed the "quenching effect." ICG acts as a fluorescent substance as well as an optical absorber. When the ICG concentration is too high, ICG will absorb the fluorescence light itself, which is the main cause of quenching. The fluorescence intensity at two different concentrations of ICG/ethanol solution is shown in Fig. 1.4 (color image, Fig. 1.4a, b; fluorescence image, Fig. 1.4c, d). Although the concentration of the left solution is 25 mg/5 ml (25 mg ICG diluted by 5 ml ethanol), while the right solution is 25 mg/1000 ml solution, the light excitation intensities are the same. Thus, a very high-concentration ICG solution shows lower fluorescence intensity, while a low-concentration ICG solution shows

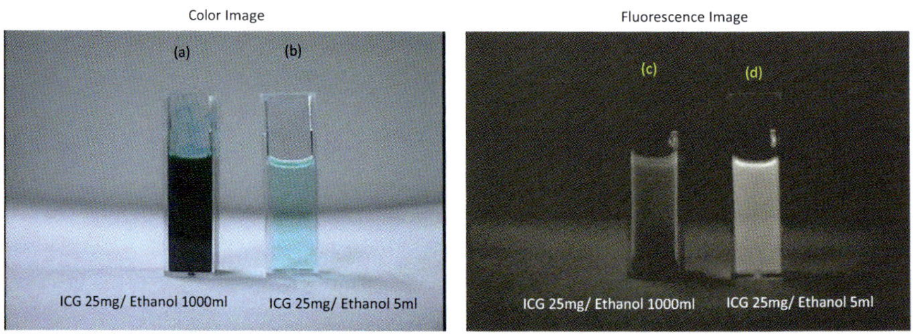

Fig. 1.4 Quenching effect. Color Image: (**a**) ICG 25 mg/ Ethanol 5ml, (**b**) ICG 25 mg/Ethanol 1000ml. Fluorescence Image: (**c**) ICG 25 mg/Ethanol 5ml, (**d**) ICG 25 mg/Ethanol 1000ml

higher fluorescence intensity. Clinically, a very dark ICG color-stained lymph node with very low fluorescence intensity due to quenching is rarely observed.

References

1. Flower RW (1993) Extraction of choriocapillaris hemodynamic data from ICG fluorescence angiogram. Investig Ophthalmol Visual Sci 34(9)
2. Baker KJ (1966) Binding of sulfobromophthalein (BSP) sodium and indocyanine green (ICG) by plasma alpha-1 lipoproteins. Proc Soc Exp Biol Med 122:957–963
3. Shin Yoneya, Tamiya Saito, Yoshiko Komatsu et al (1998) Binding properties of indocyanine green in human blood. IOVS 39(7)
4. Benson RC, Kues HA (1978) Fluorescence properties of indocyanine green as related to angiography. Phys Med Biol 23(1):159–163
5. Daiichi Sankyo, Instruction Manual of Diagnogreen

Chapter 2
Indocyanine Green Fluorescence Properties

Seiji Ohtsubo and Mitsuo Kusano

Abstract The properties of indocyanine green (ICG) enable the observation of fluorescence images with a photodynamic eye (PDE) system after ICG is injected into a subject locally or intravenously. Over the last decade, many clinical applications using an ICG approach have been introduced, e.g., the detection of sentinel nodes in breast cancer and melanoma and the use of ICG as the contrast medium in cerebral angiography. However, an insufficient amount of basic research on the fluorescence properties of ICG has been done. In the present study, we first sought to identify the optimal ICG concentration that provides the maximum brightness fluorescence, in an in vitro experiment. The ICG solution used was 2.5 mg/10 mL of distilled water (original ICG solution). For additional diluted ICG solutions, we used physiological saline (saline) and distilled water. The results did not reveal the optimal concentration ratio of ICG and diluted solutions for obtaining the maximum fluorescence and intensity in each respective solution. In the next experiment, we added bovine albumin (2 g/dL) to each diluted solution. We then evaluated the appropriate dilution ratio of bovine albumin solution and ICG solution, and the maximum brightness of the ICG fluorescence was observed using the dilution of ICG solution to approx. 90-fold from 100-fold. In another experiment, the maximum intensity of ICG fluorescence was present in approx. 90-fold-diluted ICG solution in plasma. We further assessed the characteristics of ICG fluorescence in various conditions of temperature, pH, and light/dark. We observed no remarkable changes of ICG fluorescence intensity from 10 to 50 °C. Additionally, the ICG fluorescence was affected by the acid or alkali status and was preserved under the cold/dark condition.

Keywords Indocyanine green • Fluorescence properties • Basic research

S. Ohtsubo (✉)
Department of Oral and Maxillofacial Surgery, Japan Labor Health & Welfare Organization, Kushiro Rosai Hospital, 13-23, Nakazono-cho, Kushiro, Hokkaido 085-8533, Japan
e-mail: s-ohtsubo@kushiroh.rofuku.go.jp

M. Kusano
Department of Surgery, Seiwa Memorial Hospital, 1-5-1-1, Kotoni, Nishi-ku, Sapporo, Hokkaido 063-0811, Japan

M. Kusano et al. (eds.), *ICG Fluorescence Imaging and Navigation Surgery*,
DOI 10.1007/978-4-431-55528-5_2

2.1 Introduction

The liver function test agent indocyanine green (ICG) is known to emit fluorescence at 845 nm [1], and ICG fluorescence imaging methods have been widely used in the clinical fields to evaluate vascular and lymphatic systems [2–5]. The fluorescence images produced with ICG cannot be observed without using an ICG fluorescence near-infrared camera. We have used 25-mg ICG diluted with 10 mL of distilled water in our studies, but the fluorescence intensity of ICG changes with variations in the ICG concentration, temperature, and pH conditions. As the fluorescence properties of ICG have not been carefully evaluated, we carried out a series of experiments to elucidate the characteristic properties of ICG fluorescence.

2.2 Materials and Methods

2.2.1 Experimental Protocol

In our observations of ICG fluorescence intensity, we used the observation platform of a PDE camera (Photo Dynamic Eye [PDE], Hamamatsu Photonics, Iwata, Japan) fixed 50 mm away from the samples (Fig. 2.1).

1. The evaluation of the ICG fluorescence intensity (FI) in various concentrations of ICG solutions

We prepared the original ICG solution (25 mg, with 10-mL distilled water), with saline, with distilled water, and with plasma. We used filter paper (0.6 mm thick, 6-mm dia.) to which 20 μL of ICG solution was instilled (Fig. 2.1). We prepared ICG solutions with the following concentration ratios: 2, 4, 8, 16, 32, 64, 128, 256, 512, 1,024, and 2,048 times (Fig. 2.2). The FI of the saline and distilled water after adding the 2.0 g/dL bovine albumin was used throughout the experiment.

We evaluated the histogram of each sample using image analysis software after the histogram was captured by a personal computer. We also examined the absorbance of the ICG solutions by spectrophotometry.

2. The fluorescence properties of ICG under changes of temperature, pH, and light conditions

Based on the results of a preliminary experiment (data not shown), we used ICG solution diluted by 100 times the original ICG solution with 2 g/dL bovine albumin. First, under the same imaging conditions, we evaluated the FI with variations in temperature, pH status, and the light/dark condition as follows: (a) at room temperature (RT) under light from a fluorescent lamp for 24 h (the RT/light condition), (b) at RT in a completely dark darkroom (the RT/dark condition), (c) at 4 °C under fluorescent lamp light for 24 h (cold/light condition), and (d) at 4 °C in the

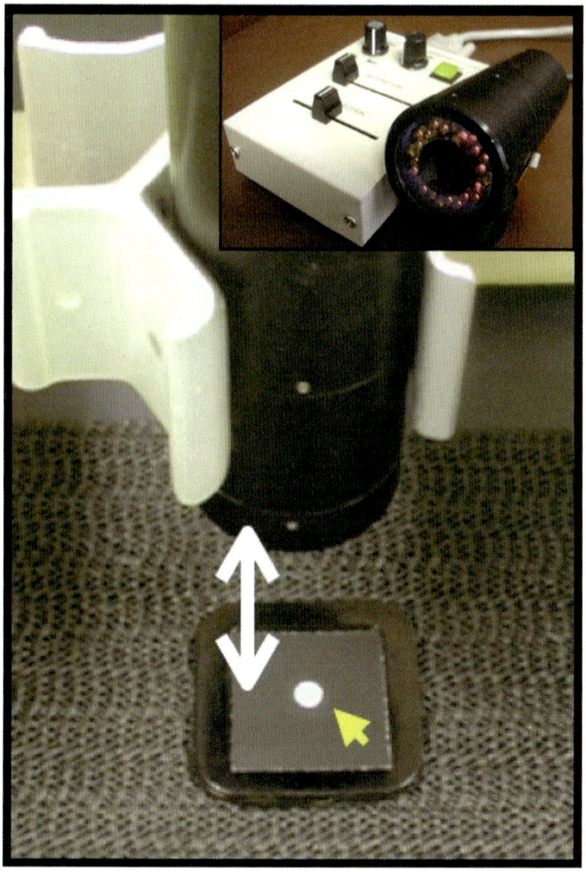

Fig. 2.1 The PDE camera was fixed 50 mm away from the sample (*white arrows*). *Yellow arrowhead*: the filter paper (0.6 mm thick, 6-mm dia.) to which 20 μL of ICG solution was instilled

darkroom (cold/dark condition). We assessed the FI in each condition up to 56 days at 7-day intervals.

We next examined the FI of the samples at the same concentrations from 10 to 50 °C. Lastly, we examined the FI of samples at the same concentrations from pH 3.0 to pH 11.0.

Four samples in each experimental group were prepared under the same condition, and the average FI value of the four samples was evaluated throughout the experiment.

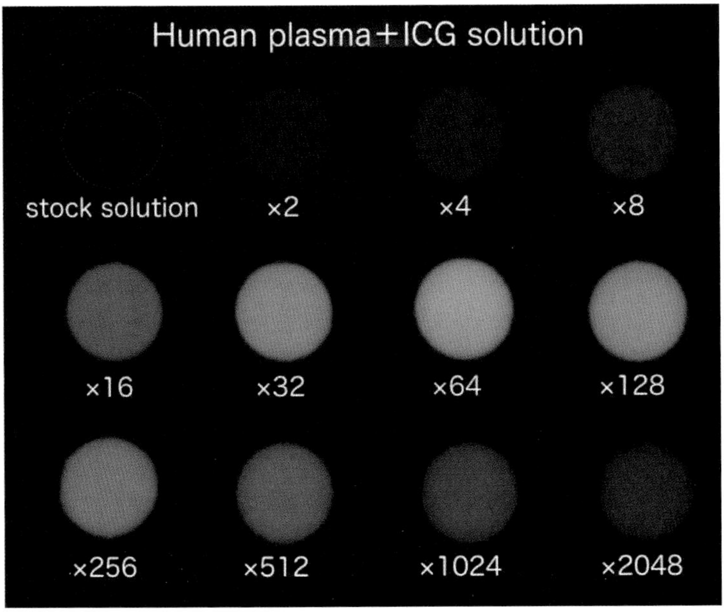

Fig. 2.2 ICG solutions with concentration ratios (human plasma)

2.2.2 Preliminary Study of the Clinical Applications of Fluorescence Imaging Using the Optimal Concentration of ICG Solution

Based on the results of the above experiments, we examined the ICG FI after a subcutaneous injection of 0.4 mL of a 100-fold dilution of the original ICG solution into the palm side of the forearm of a consenting breast cancer patient with lymphedema. We also injected the ICG original solution into the back of the hand on the same side.

2.3 Results

Our measurements of the absorbance provided by the various dilution series, saline, distilled water, and plasma dilution showed the correct hyperbolic pattern, which demonstrated that the ICG diluting procedure in this experiment was acceptable (Fig. 2.3). We were able to observe the ICG fluorescence in both saline and distilled water, although these samples showed very low fluorescence intensity compared to that of the plasma (Fig. 2.4). The maximum FI of the plasma was in the vicinity of the original ICG solution diluted 80-fold from 90-fold (Fig. 2.5).

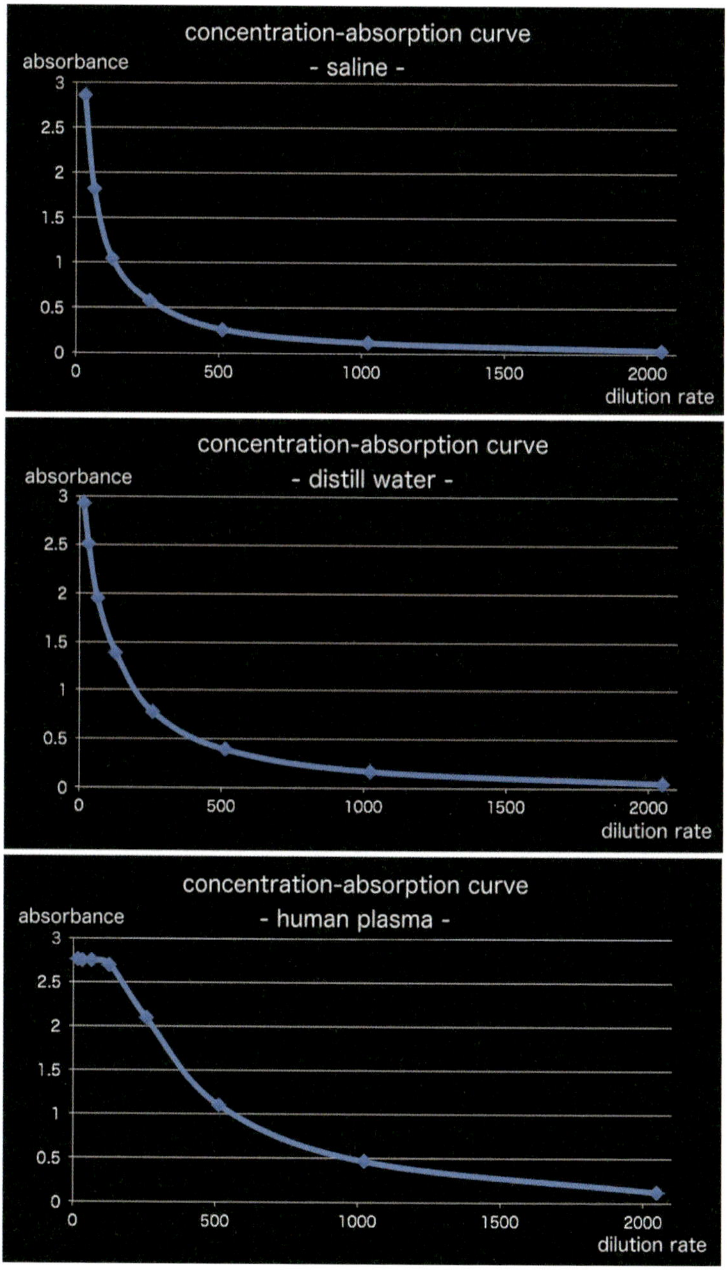

Fig. 2.3 Concentration-absorption curves for saline, distilled water, and human plasma

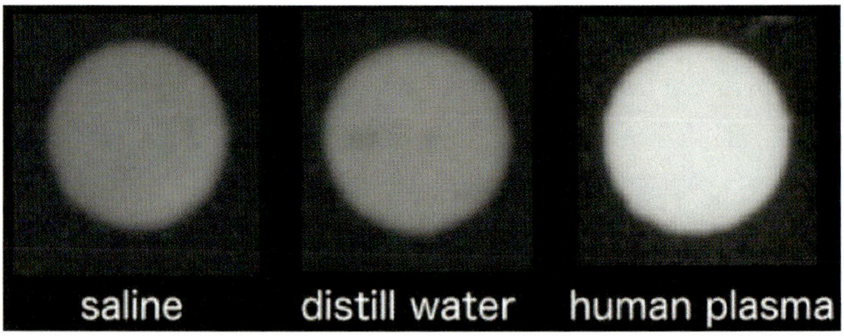

Fig. 2.4 ICG fluorescence images of the same intensity (32× dilution)

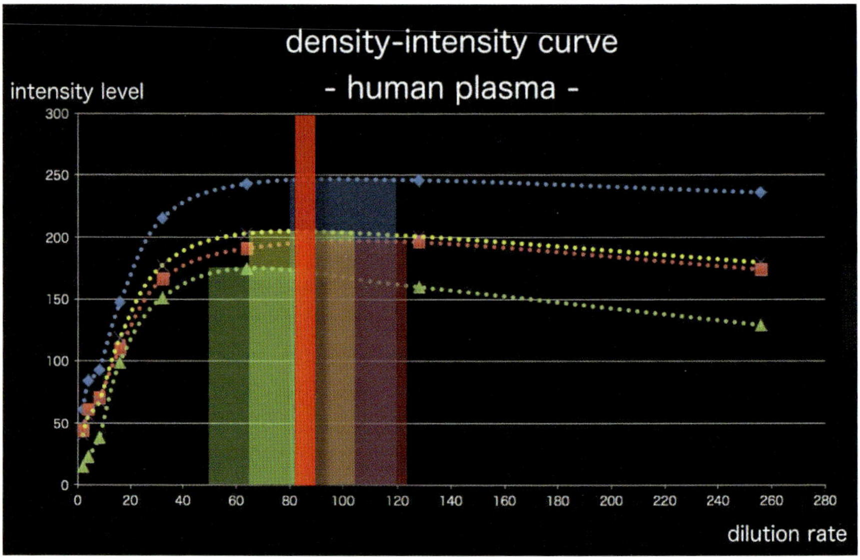

Fig. 2.5 Density-intensity curve of human plasma. The maximum FI of the plasma was in the vicinity of the original ICG solution diluted 80-fold from 90-fold (*red bar*)

However, in saline and in distilled water, there were variations in the FI, and it was not clear what the appropriate ICG concentration was for maximum brightness (Fig. 2.6). We therefore added bovine albumin (2 g/dL) to the original ICG solution. We were then able to obtain the maximum brightness in the vicinity of the original ICG solution diluted 90-fold from 100-fold ICG solution. The FI of the plasma was not changed by adding bovine albumin (Fig. 2.7).

With the subcutaneous injection of a 100-fold dilution of the original ICG solution in a breast cancer patient with postoperative lymphedema, the FI did not decline (Fig. 2.8).

The time-dependent change of ICG fluorescence intensity is shown (Fig. 2.9). The FI at 7 days in the RT/light condition was attenuated by 80 %. In an additional

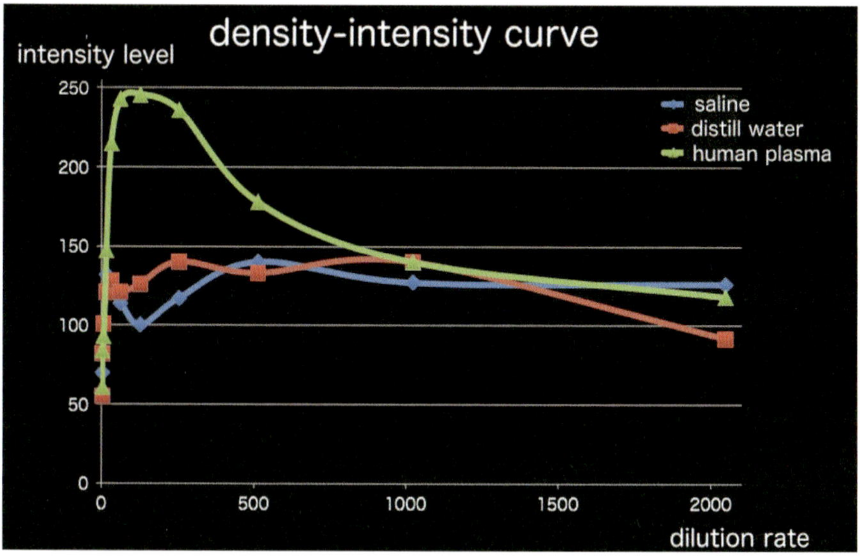

Fig. 2.6 Density-intensity curves of three samples. In the saline and distilled water, it was not clear what the appropriate ICG concentration was for maximum brightness (*red* and *blue lines*)

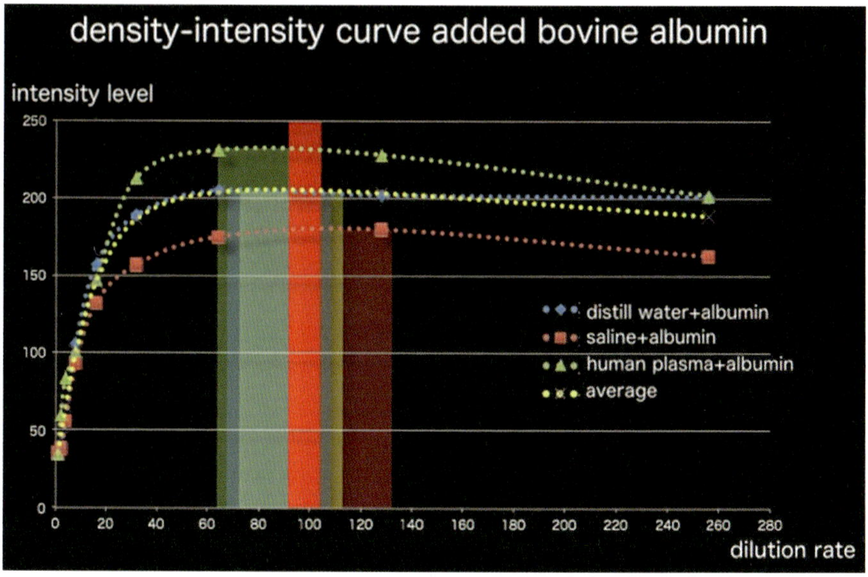

Fig. 2.7 Density-intensity curve of three samples with added bovine albumin. The maximum brightness was in the vicinity of the original ICG solution diluted 90-fold from 100-fold ICG solution (*red bar*)

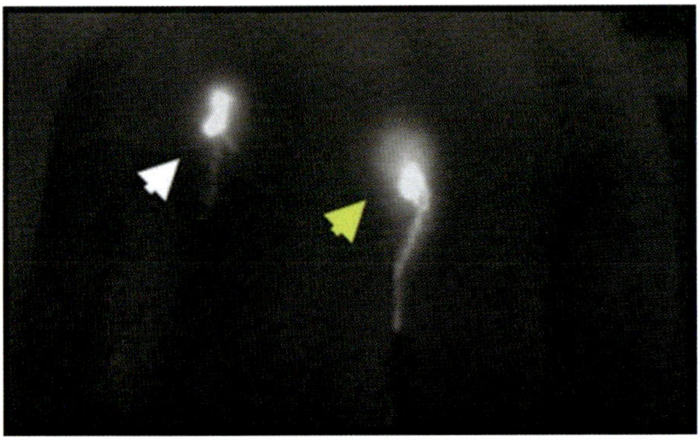

Fig. 2.8 ICG fluorescence intensity. *White arrowhead*: the fluorescence of the ICG original solution. *Yellow arrowhead*: the fluorescence of the 100-fold-diluted ICG original solution

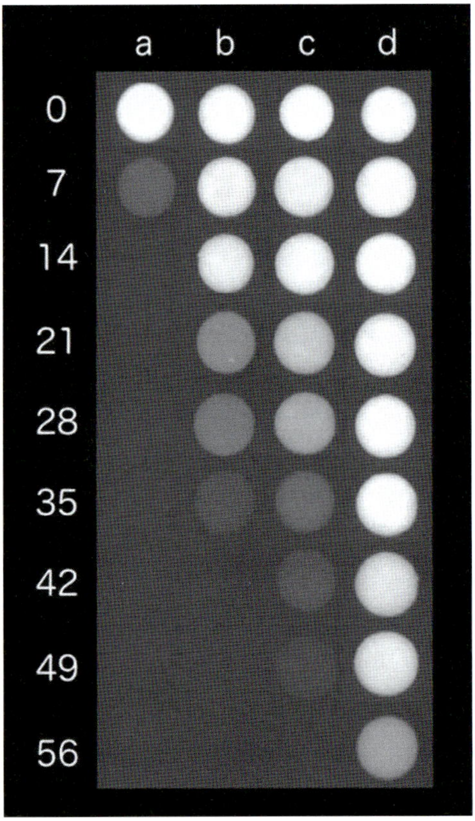

Fig. 2.9 Time-dependent changes of ICG fluorescence images. (**a**): At room temperature under light from a fluorescent lamp for 24 h (RT/light). (**b**): At room temperature in a completely dark darkroom (RT/dark). (**c**): At 4 °C under fluorescent lamp light for 24 h (cold/light). (**d**): At 4 °C in the darkroom (cold/dark)

experiment, the FI was linearly attenuated (Fig. 2.10). In the RT/dark and the cold/light conditions, the attenuation of FI was observed from day 14. The attenuation rate reached 50 % in the RT/dark condition around day 21, and in the cold/light

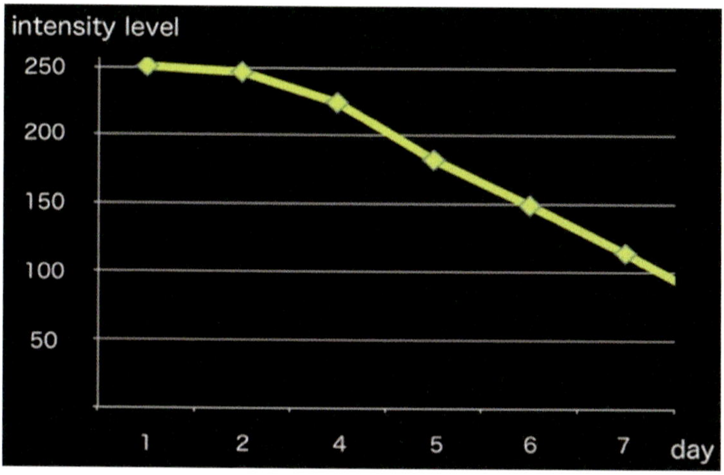

Fig. 2.10 Fluorescence intensity at 7 days in the RT/light condition

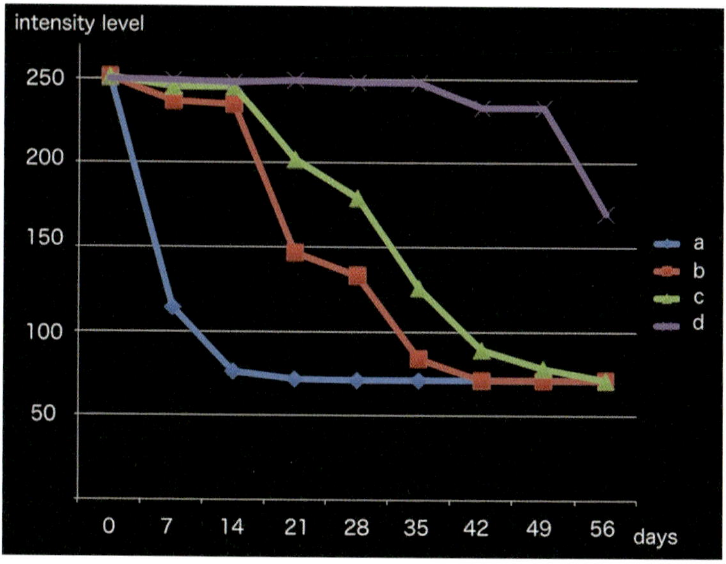

Fig. 2.11 Time-dependent changes in the ICG fluorescence intensity level. (**a**): RT/light. (**b**): RT/dark. (**c**): Cold/light. (**d**): Cold/dark

condition, it did so by about day 28. The FI decayed from day 35 in the cold/dark conditions. At day 56, the attenuation rate was less than 50 % in the cold/dark conditions (Fig. 2.11).

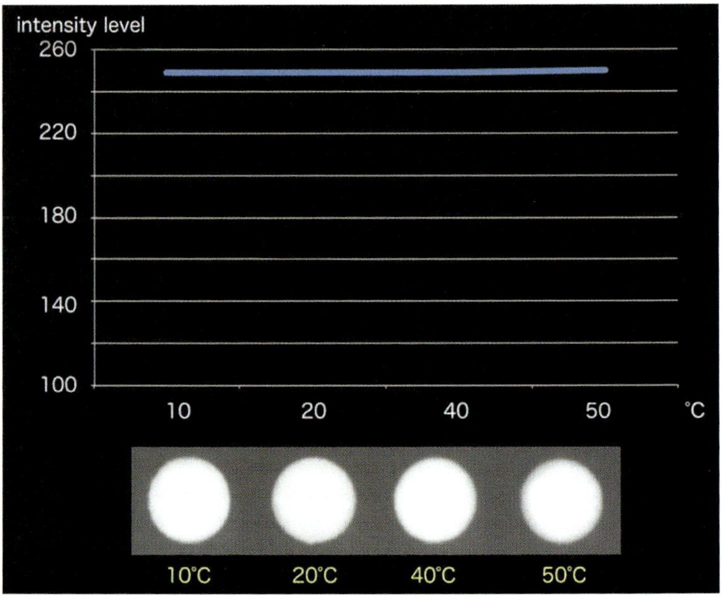

Fig. 2.12 Fluorescence intensity in accord with the temperature (from 10 °C to 50 °C)

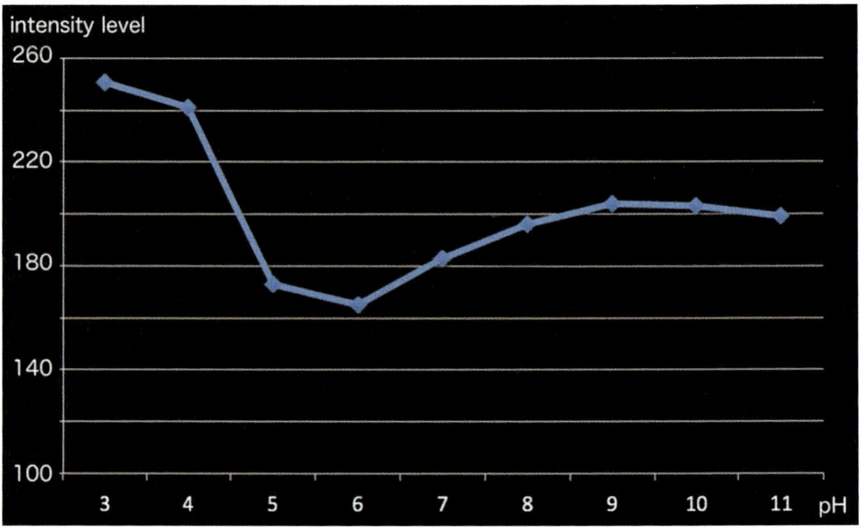

Fig. 2.13 Fluorescence intensity and pH (from pH 3.0 to pH 11.0)

We show the FI in temperature and brightness changes in Fig. 2.12. No notable change in FI was observed with the different temperature conditions (Fig. 2.12). Regarding the pH conditions, we found that the FI was affected by the acid versus alkali status of a dilute solution (Fig. 2.13).

2.4 Discussion

ICG fluorescence navigation surgery has been widely used [2–5], but varying amounts of ICG and concentrations of ICG solution for local and intravenous injections have been used in different clinical fields, and the optimal parameters for the use of ICG have not been established. ICG solution made of 25 mg of ICG dissolved in distilled water has been used conventionally for intravenous or subcutaneous injections, whereas in the ophthalmic field, 3 mL of 25 mg of ICG dissolved in distilled water has been used. The lack of basic research regarding the use of ICG needed to be addressed, and thus, in the present study, we attempted to elucidate the characteristic properties of ICG solution [6–8]. We prepared samples of ICG solution with different concentrations to identify the best concentration(s) for producing the strongest ICG intensity.

It is known that that ICG in itself does not possess the property of emitting fluorescence without coupling with albumin or α- or β-lipoprotein [6]. However, we observed the fluorescence of saline and that of distilled water itself even though the FI was rather poor (Fig. 2.4). In addition, the FI values were not constant, and we thus did not identify the appropriate ICG concentration or solution that produces the strongest FI (Fig. 2.6).

The reasons why the present results were obtained are not yet known. Prior studies and drug information inserts [9] including explanations such as "this drug is unstable in the solution state, and rapidly stabilized by the photochemical reaction after being combined with serum protein" [9, 10] provide a clue; ICG solution is apparently unstable when combined with saline or distilled water alone. It seems that bovine albumin should be added to the ICG in a diluted solution of saline or distilled water to obtain the maximum brightness. In the present study, the ICG original solution diluted 100-fold from 90-fold provided the highest FI (Fig. 2.7). When a similar dilution procedure is used in vivo, the highest ICG FI could be obtained. In our preliminary clinical trial using an injection into the palm of lymphedema patients, there was no difference in FI values between the ICG original solution and the 100-fold-diluted solution (Fig. 2.8).

Our search for the optimal concentration for the highest ICG fluorescence intensity in plasma, with or without bovine albumin added, showed the maximum ICG fluorescence intensity when the stock solution was diluted 90-fold from an 80-fold solution (Fig. 2.5). Therefore, by using the concentration diluted 90-fold from 80-fold stock solution in the blood vessels, higher ICG fluorescence intensity should be observable.

Our experiments also revealed that differences in temperature and pH affect ICG's fluorescence intensity and confirmed that the FI is strongly affected by the presence/absence of light (Figs. 2.9, 2.12, and 2.13). Observations of resected tissues using ICG fluorescence should be the focus of future studies. Our present findings suggest that when using ICG to evaluate resected tissues, it is better to use dark and cold conditions, which can maintain the ICG fluorescence brightness.

Our results also confirmed that the ICG fluorescence declines with time and that it is affected by the acid and alkali status of a dilute solution (Fig. 2.13). Sites of inflammation in vivo tend to be acidic, whereas pus tends to be alkaline. It may be possible to obtain sufficient ICG fluorescence images even at low concentrations for such tissue or pus materials. Since there is little basic research on ICG, we introduced an empirical approach in an attempt to identify the best ICG concentrations for clinical use. We found that by controlling the concentration of ICG, the amount of the injection of ICG solution, and the light/dark and pH conditions, it is possible to obtain useful information based on ICG fluorescence.

We also examined the FI of distilled water and physiological saline. Distilled water and physiological saline were confirmed to emit ICG fluorescence. Although we were unable to identify the optimal concentration providing the highest ICG fluorescence intensity, we found that with distilled water and with physiological saline solution with added albumin, the FI was higher in the vicinity of the original solution following 90–100-fold dilution. Regardless of the presence or absence of albumin in the plasma, the FI was higher in the vicinity of the original solution following 80–90-fold dilution. The ICG was strongly affected by the light and by the acid/alkali status, without being affected by temperature.

References

1. Benson RC, Kunes HA (1978) Fluorescence properties of indocyanine green as related to angiography. Phys Med Biol 23(1):159–63
2. Novotny HR, Alvis D (1960) A method of photographing fluorescence in circulating blood of the human eye. Tech Doc Rep SAMTDR USAF Sch Aerosp Med 60–82:1–4
3. Raabe A, Nakaji P, Beck J et al (2005) Prospective evaluation of surgical microscope-integrated intraoperative near-infrared indocyanine green videoangiography during aneurysm surgery. J Neurosurg 103(6):982–9
4. Motomura K, Inaji H, Komoike Y et al (1999) Sentinel node biopsy guided by indocyanine green dye in breast cancer patients. Jpn J Clin Oncol 29(12):604–7
5. Ogata F, Narushima M, Mihara M et al (2007) Intraoperative lymphography using indocyanine green dye for near-infrared fluorescence labeling in lymphedema. Ann Plast Surg 59(2):180–4
6. Baker KJ (1966) Binding of sulfobromophthalein (BSP) sodium and indocyanine green (ICG) by plasma alpha-1 lipoproteins. Proc Soc Exp Biol Med 122(4):957–63
7. Sakatani K, Kashiwasake-Jibu M, Taka Y et al (1997) Noninvasive optical imaging of the subarachnoid space and cerebrospinal fluid pathways based on near-infrared fluorescence. J Neurosurg 87(5):738–45
8. Yoneya S1, Saito T, Komatsu Y et al (1998) Binding properties of indocyanine green in human blood. Invest Ophthalmol Vis Sci 39(7):1286–1290
9. ICG Package insert: Packager: Novadaq Technologies Inc. NDC Code(s): 66259-424-01. Accessed Jan 2015 at: http://dailymed.nlm.nih.gov/dailymed/drugInfo.cfm?setid=f653f4c4-000b-409b-8f03-a7ae2243aee4
10. Fox IJ, Wood EH (1960) Indocyanine green: physical and physiologic properties. Proc Staff Meet Mayo Clin 35:732–44

Chapter 3
Characteristics of the Photodynamic Eye Camera

Takahiro Shikayama

Abstract We developed near-infrared fluorescence imaging system for indocyanine green (ICG) as optical enhancer and tried to use the system for evaluation purpose of blood and/or lymphatic vessel observation during the operation. The excitation wavelength of ICG is in the near-infrared wavelength between 750 and 810 nm, and the fluorescence occurs maximum wavelength at 845 nm in plasma.

The near-infrared fluorescence imaging system Photodynamic Eye (pde-neo, Hamamatsu Photonics, Hamamatsu, Japan) is equipped with light emitting diode (LED) that emits near-infrared wavelength of 760 nm as excite light and a charge-coupled device (CCD) as image detector with an optical high-pass filter in front of CCD so that fluorescence signal can be detected efficiently. This system consists of the camera unit, controller which operates the camera unit, and remote controller which controls the LED intensity, video gain, and offset. The fluorescence image is sent to a digital video processor to be displayed on a TV monitor in real time.

The features of the system are safe (X-ray radgiation-free), compact size, real time, user-friendly, and cost-effective. It's verified that the system is applicable to various applications and promising technique for intraoperative diagnosis.

Keywords Near-infrared fluorescence • Fluorescence imaging • Indocyanine green • Intraoperative imaging

3.1 History of Development of the pde-neo

Medical imaging technologies such as PET using a radiation tracer, X-rays CT using radiation, MRI using a nuclear magnetic resonance phenomenon, and ultrasonic wave CT using an ultrasonic wave are key methods for assessment of human tissues. By contrast, imaging technologies using light are not as well developed as they exhibit strong scattering and absorption problems in living tissue.

T. Shikayama (✉)
Hamamatsu Photonics KK, 5000, Hirakuchi, Hamakita-ku, Hamamatsu, Shizuoka 434-8601, Japan
e-mail: shika@crl.hpk.co.jp

M. Kusano et al. (eds.), *ICG Fluorescence Imaging and Navigation Surgery*,
DOI 10.1007/978-4-431-55528-5_3

Nevertheless, recent studies on the behavior of light in the living body have developed a technique termed light CT. Fluorescence imaging using the contrast media of light is a widely used optical imaging technique. Herein, we provide a description of near-infrared fluorescence imaging equipment that uses ICG for measurement of the contrast media of light.

Hemoglobin and water are the principal optical absorption molecules in the living body. Hemoglobin has strong absorption of wavelengths of visible light less than 600 nm, while water has strong absorption against wavelengths greater than 900 nm. Thus, it was generally considered that the permeability of light in the living body tissue is poor. However, near-infrared wavelength light (600–900 nm; "optical window") can be transmitted to relatively deep tissues, as the absorption of hemoglobin or water is low. Therefore, near-infrared light has been developed as an imaging technique for safe and noninvasive tissue diagnosis in humans. For example, if near-infrared light is illuminated within a living body, comparatively thin parts will be visualized, including the palm and deeper structures such as blood vessels; as near-infrared light is absorbed by intravascular hemoglobin, selective imaging of parts of blood vessels is possible.

Although the absorption of water and hemoglobin is small and near-infrared wavelength light has a comparatively high permeability in living tissues, degradation of image quality occurs due to light scattering. As such, prior to near-infrared imaging, fluorescent and luminescent materials can be injected and detected for initial tissue imaging. For example, a near-infrared fluorescence imaging instrument using a fluorescent material was used recently reported to improve the sensitivity and the signal-to-noise ratio of imaging sensors such as charge-coupled device (CCD) and complementary metal oxide semiconductor (CMOS). Near-infrared fluorescence imaging is safe (no radiation) and simple and provides real-time data, and large and expensive equipments including PET, X-ray CT, and MRI are not required.

3.2 The Basic Configuration of pde-neo

An infrared observation camera system, Photodynamic Eye (*pde*-neo or PDE; Hamamatsu Photonics K.K., Japan) has been developed for clinical near-infrared fluorescence imaging (Fig. 3.1). The basic configuration of *pde*-neo consists of a camera unit and an image processing controller (Fig. 3.2). The system is connected with a camera cable for exclusive use, and the image output is displayed on an external monitor. The basic specification of *pde*-neo is shown in Table 3.1.

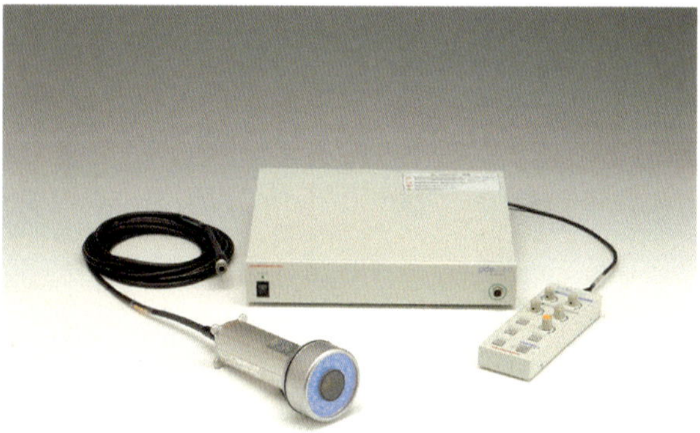

Fig. 3.1 The appearance picture of the infrared observation camera system Photodynamic Eye (pde-neo)

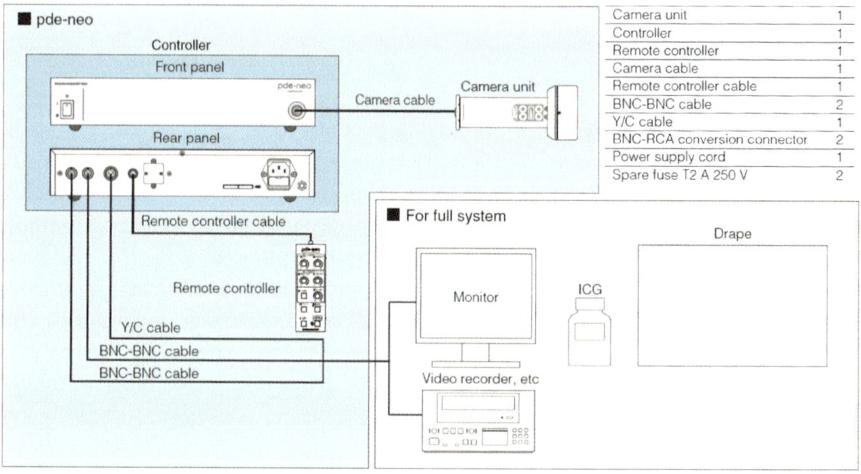

Fig. 3.2 Basic composition of pde-neo

Table 3.1 Basic specification

Camera unit		Sensor: solid-state image sensing device
		White LED and infrared auxiliary lighting function
		Hand operation function
		Contrast enhancement function, auxiliary lighting intensity control
Controller		Contrast enhancement function
Video output		2ch (BNC), 1ch (Y/C)
Outside dimension	Camera unit	About 80 × 182 × 80 mm (W × D × H)
	Controller	About 322 × 283 × 55 mm (W × D × H)
Mass	Camera unit	About 0.5 kg
	Controller	About 2.6 kg

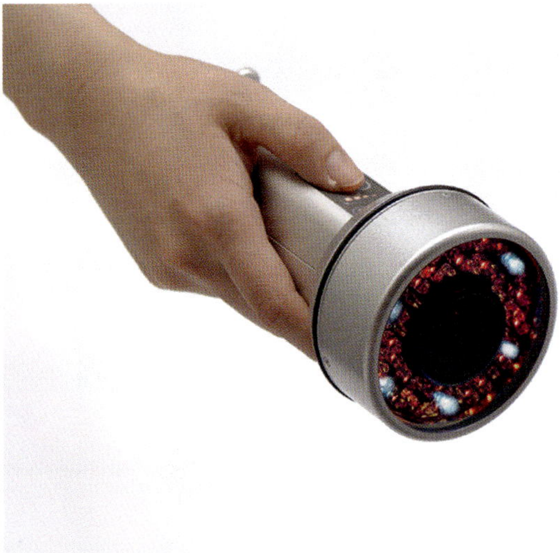

Fig. 3.3 Camera unit of pde-neo

3.3 Camera Unit

The camera unit is small, lightweight, and handheld (Fig. 3.3). Near-infrared wavelength excitation light of an LED (IEC class 1) is located at the front of the unit to provide an infrared auxiliary lighting function. A white LED is also attached for general lighting. The CCD camera has sensitivity in the visible to near-infrared wavelength domain, and the camera lens and optimal filter are built into a camera unit. Four switches on the camera unit allow handheld control over the infrared LED, white LED, and color image/fluorescence imaging. Connection of a remote control device (Fig. 3.4) allows control over infrared LED, white LED, selection of color image/fluorescence image, control of color display, contrast, and brightness, and equipment setup. Focus control is provided by turning the camera head.

3.4 Controller Part

The controller of the *pde*-neo provides contrast enhancement function. The image output of the *pde*-neo is an NTSC signal, and two BNC terminals and one S-connector allow output to multiple external input devices, as well as one monitor or multiple handy cams or HDD recorders to save dynamic images. The contrast enhancement function provides brightness and contrast control. Contrast is the difference between intensity of the white and black parts on a screen. An increase in contrast will increase the brightness of the white display on the screen, although it is important for the luminance of the black part of the image not to change. It is the feature that the difference of control of intensity is emphasized. As brightness reflects signal intensity, it also reflects the degree of luminance of the whole screen

Fig. 3.4 Remote controller of pde-neo

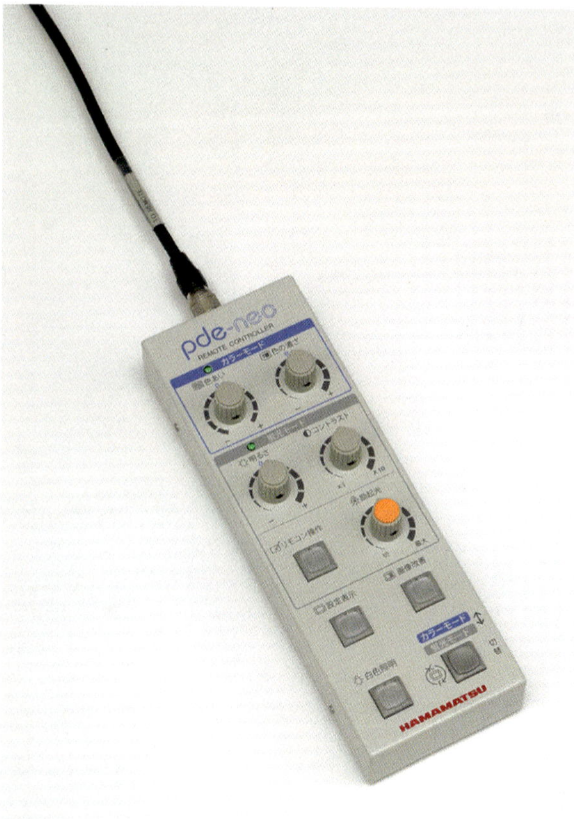

display. If intensity is raised, the increase of luminance of the whole display will result in an increase in brightness of the white part, although the luminance of the black part is also increased.

3.5 User Directions for the pde-neo

Pde-neo can image the fluorescence of ICG, a near-infrared fluorescence reagent. Fluorescence is a phenomenon involving emission of light of a wavelength other than the excitation wavelength. The directions for *pde*-neo are described in Fig. 3.5. First, the fluorescence reagent ICG is injected into the tissue for observation. Next, the target for observation is imaged by the camera unit of *pde*-neo using the near-infrared LED. A fluorescence reagent is then excited by the near-infrared LED, resulting in emission of light with a wavelength of approximately 845 nm [1]. The reflected light is detected and imaged by *pde*-neo on the body surface.

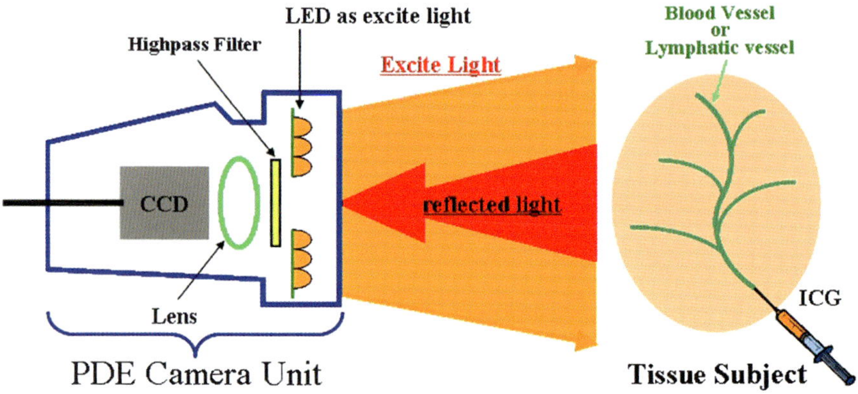

Fig. 3.5 Schematic view of the directions for PDE

Using *pde*-neo, fluorescence imaging can be assessed in real time after injection, to a depth of approximately 10–15 mm, depending on the tissues to be imaged.

There are a number of important considerations for measurement of fluorescence, including the light volume in which near-infrared LED emits. When the target for observation (e.g., a lymph vessel and lymph node) is covered with fat or other tissues, an image may blur due to the effect of scattering. By performing a skin incision over the tissue to be imaged, the scattering effects can be reduced and the fluorescence intensity increased. When the fluorescence intensity is too high, the distinction of a lymph vessel and lymph node becomes difficult due to image saturation. Thus, improved imaging can be obtained by reducing the fluorescence intensity and adjusting the light volume by lowering the light volume of the LED, before and after performing the skin incision.

There are two important considerations when using the *pde*-neo in an operating room. First, the camera unit of *pde*-neo cannot be sterilized by gaseous or plasma sterilization. Therefore, when using it in a clean area, a sterilized surgical drape is used. Surgical light is also an important consideration. The wavelength of the light of a surgical light (as well as halogen light or xenon light) contains a near-infrared wavelength far stronger than the fluorescence of ICG. Thus, the surgical light needs to be turned off at the time of fluorescence observation. As fluorescent light produces only minimal near-infrared light, it does not have a strong effect on image observation.

An example of angiography using ICG and PDE in the rat is shown in Fig. 3.6. The visible observation image using the common camera is shown in Fig. 3.6a. The fluorescence observation image using PDE is shown in Fig. 3.6b. ICG at 0.1–0.2 cc volumes are injected into the rat tail vein. Although we cannot identify the green ICG on the visible observation image, the ICG fluorescence image of the blood vessel is clearly identified using PDE.

In summary, pde-neo and PDE are near-infrared fluorescence imaging systems that allow noninvasive visualization of a blood vessel or a lymph vessel in real time

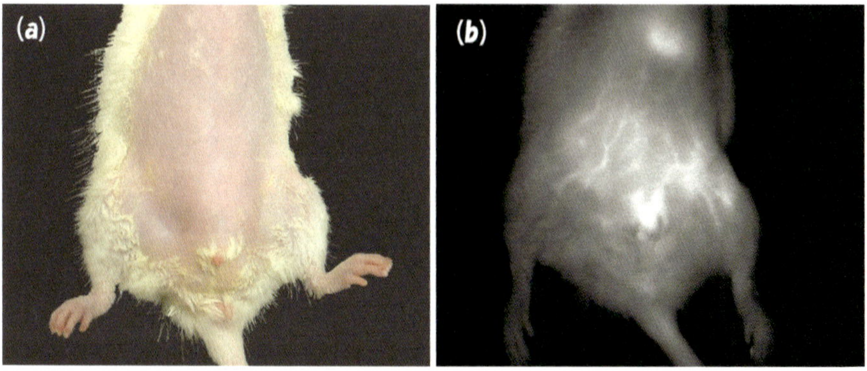

Fig. 3.6 Angiography of a rat. (**a**) The visible observation image using a common camera. (**b**) The fluorescence image using PDE

from the body surface, by imaging infrared fluorescence from the fluorescence reagent injected into the body. Near-infrared fluorescence imaging by pde-neo was originally used for sentinel lymph node biopsy in breast cancer [2]. However, there is now increasing application to cardiovascular surgery, cerebral blood vessel surgery [3], plastic surgery [4], and digestive organ surgery [5, 6].

References

1. Benson RC, Kues HA (1978) Fluorescence properties of indocyanine green as related to angiography. Phys Med Biol 23:159–163
2. Kitai T, Inomoto T, Miwa M et al (2005) Fluorescence navigation with indocyanine green for detecting sentinel lymph nodes in breast cancer. Breast Cancer 12(3):211–215
3. Awano T, Sakatani K, Yokose N et al (2010) EC-IC bypass function in Moyamoya disease and non-Moyamoya ischemic stroke evaluated by intraoperative indocyanine green fluorescence angiography. Adv Exp Med Biol 662:519–524
4. Azuma R, Morimoto Y, Masumoto K et al (2008) Detection of skin perforators by indocyanine green fluorescence nearly infrared angiography. Plast Reconstr Surg 122(4):1062–1067
5. Miyashiro I, Miyoshi N, Hiratsuka M et al (2008) Detection of sentinel node in gastric cancer surgery by indocyanine green fluorescence imaging: comparison with infrared imaging. Ann Surg Oncol 15(6):1640–1643
6. Kai K, Satoh S, Watanabe T, Endo Y (2010) Evaluation of cholecystic venous flow using indocyanine green fluorescence angiography. J Hepatobiliary Pancreat Sci 17(2):147–151

Part II
Neurosurgery

Chapter 4
ICG Videoangiography in Neurosurgical Procedures

Yoshiaki Kumon, Hideaki Watanabe, Shiro Ohue, and Takanori Ohnishi

Abstract Indocyanine green videoangiography (ICG-VAG) has recently been used for neurosurgical procedures, and its usefulness and drawbacks were evaluated. ICG-VAG showed blood flow in the vessels as the hemodynamic change of ICG fluorescence intensity. In clipping cerebral aneurysms, preservation of blood flow in the parent and perforating arteries and occlusion of the aneurysm were recognized. In bypass surgery, the patency of blood flow from the graft was observed. In carotid endarterectomy, the precise stenosis area or residual stenosis was observed before or after surgery. In removal of arteriovenous malformation, the feeding arteries, draining veins, and the nidus were clearly demonstrated. In tumor surgery, tumor-related vessels, normal brain parenchyma vessels, bridging veins, and tumor margin infiltration were observed. These findings obtained using ICG-VAG were useful to achieve these surgeries safely and completely without complications associated with the use of ICG-VAG.

Recently, the semiquantitative flow measurement using the analysis software such as FLOW 800 was used for bypass, vascular malformation, and acute stroke surgery. Endoscopic ICG-VAG was applied in aneurysm clipping and pituitary adenoma surgery.

Although there are some drawbacks associated with the use of ICG-VAG such as the presence of blind spots and the difficulty with true quantitative blood flow analysis, it is a useful intraoperative examination because of its safety and convenience.

Keywords Indocyanine green videoangiography • Neurosurgical procedure • Cerebral blood flow

---

Y. Kumon, M.D., Ph.D. (✉)
Division of Neurosurgery, Department of Regeneration of Community Medicine, Ehime University Graduate School of Medicine, Shitsukawa, Toon, Ehime 791-0295, Japan
e-mail: ykumon@m.ehime-u.ac.jp

H. Watanabe, M.D., Ph.D. • S. Ohue, M.D., Ph.D. • T. Ohnishi, M.D., Ph.D.
Department of Neurosurgery, Ehime University Graduate School of Medicine, Shitsukawa, Toon, Ehime 791-0295, Japan

M. Kusano et al. (eds.), *ICG Fluorescence Imaging and Navigation Surgery*,
DOI 10.1007/978-4-431-55528-5_4

4.1 Introduction

Indocyanine green (ICG) is a dark green-blue-colored, water-soluble compound with a molecular weight of 774.96. In the body, ICG combined with lipoprotein in the blood is transported to liver, and it is absorbed into liver cells and excreted into the bile without metabolism. ICG has been used to examine liver cell function. Since ICG is a fluorescent material emitting fluorescence [1], it has been used for angiography of the retina and choroid in the field of ophthalmology [2, 3].

The fluorescent material is stimulated by absorption of specific wavelength light, and it emits energy as fluorescence while returning from the stimulated state to the resting condition. In ICG, the wavelength of the stimulating light is 790–805 nm and that of fluorescence is 835 nm [4]. Both waves are infrared and difficult to observe by the naked eye. Thus, a camera capable of detecting infrared radiation is necessary for fluorescent imaging. ICG florescence imaging becomes possible by a system in which the camera irradiates infrared radiation with a specific wavelength and detects the ICG fluorescent wavelength. The development of ICG observing systems has led to its application in other medical fields. It has been used intraoperatively for cerebral angiography in neurosurgery [5, 6], coronary angiography in heart surgery [7], neck angiography in neck surgery [8], and visualization of lymph nodes in cancer surgery [9, 10]. Although usual intraoperative angiography has some complications such as embolic events, ICG-videoangiography (ICG-VAG) can be done easily with intravenous injection of ICG, in a short time, and without leaving the operative field. This method may further develop and its use will be expanded.

We are using this method for neurosurgical procedures such as cerebrovascular surgeries and tumor surgeries. Therefore, we present our experience and review literatures concerning this method. Its usefulness and drawbacks in these neurosurgical procedures were evaluated.

4.2 Patients and Methods (Experience in our Hospital)

Using ICG-VAG, aneurysmal clipping surgery (77 cases), bypass surgery (14 cases), carotid endarterectomy (35 cases), surgery for vascular malformation (6 cases), and removal of brain tumor (13 cases) have been performed in our hospital. One ampoule of ICG (25 mg) was diluted with 5 mL of vaporized water, and 2.5–25 mg were injected intravenously and flushed with 10-mL saline. The intensity of light in the operating room was then reduced for observation of ICG fluorescence with the monitor camera. ICG fluorescence cannot be observed by naked eye observation; it can be seen only on the monitor. One examination usually requires 5 mg of ICG, and one surgical procedure usually requires up to 25 mg of ICG. After ICG intravenous injection, ICG fluorescence can be observed 15–20 s later in the intracranial arteries and 30–40 s later in the veins. The intensity of fluorescence usually reaches its peak at 50–60 s and then decreases, so that fluorescence disappears 10 min after injection. We usually observed ICG fluorescence in the vessels for 2 min after injection; no side effects occurred due to ICG-VAG.

In the present study, two types of microscope-integrated ICG-VAG (Zeiss and Leica) were used.

4.3 Results and Discussion

4.3.1 ICG-VAG for Clipping Cerebral Aneurysm

The purpose of clipping the neck of a cerebral aneurysm is to occlude the aneurysm neck without stenosis or occlusion of the parent arteries and perforating arteries. However, it has been reported that, after clipping surgery, a neck remnant could be seen in 4–19 % of cases, and occlusion of parent arteries and/or perforating arteries was observed in 0.3–12 % of cases [11–16]. Therefore, it may be necessary to improve surgical technique and to monitor these findings during surgery. Although the precise examination for this purpose is cerebral angiography, this examination takes time and has various side effects, such as embolic events [17–19]. Recently, Doppler ultrasound imaging and endoscopy have been used for intraoperative monitoring [20–22], but it is difficult to detect a neck remnant and flow disturbances of fine arteries such as perforating arteries with Doppler ultrasound, and endoscopy has difficulties in that there is a blind area, and intravascular blood flow is hard to recognize. Therefore, ICG-VAG was found to be a useful examination instead of cerebral angiography [6, 23–26], following the report by Raabe et al. in 2003 [5]. Especially for preservation of perforating arteries, ICG-VAG is superior to conventional cerebral angiography.

ICG-VAG, as well as Doppler ultrasound and endoscopy, was performed for 77 cases (87 aneurysms) in our hospital. There are several important points for this examination. (1) The operative field should be clean, because cotton and blood disturbed the observation of ICG fluorescence. (2) The magnification rate should be controlled, and it has been reported that 6–8 X is appropriate. Usually, ICG-VAG was done before and after clipping a cerebral aneurysm and added if necessary for each case. Before clipping, the anatomical relationship between the aneurysm neck and the parent or perforating arteries was observed. Fine arteries from the anterior and posterior communicating arteries of 0.2 mm in diameter could be observed using ICG-VAG, as well as the anterior choroidal artery, Heubner's artery, and the posterior communicating artery (Fig. 4.1a–d). However, it is important to note that calcified and/or sclerotic arteries decrease the intensity of ICG fluorescence on the monitor (Fig. 4.1e, f). After clipping, ICG-VAG was done following Doppler ultrasound and endoscopic observation. Several points should be observed, such as (1) occlusion of the aneurysm (no recognition of ICG fluorescence in the

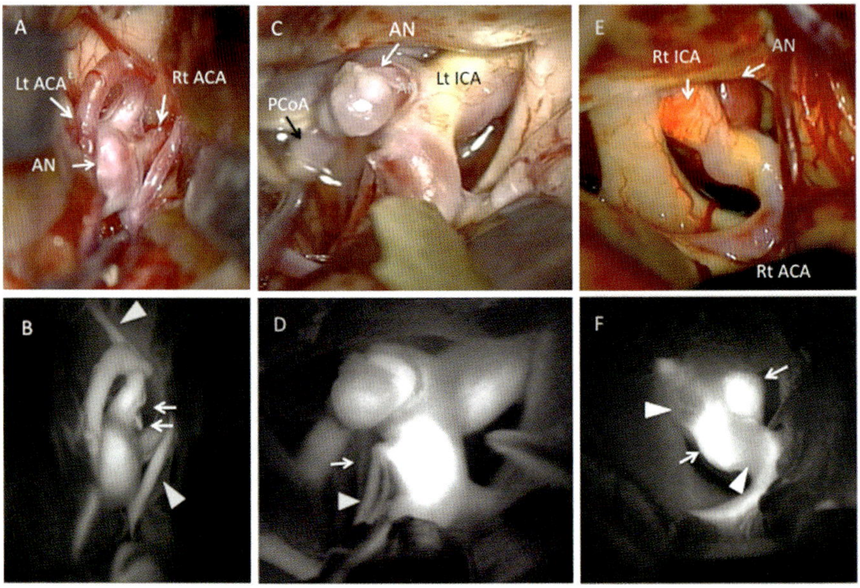

Fig. 4.1 Operative findings of an anterior communicating artery (ACoA) aneurysm, a left internal carotid artery (ICA)–posterior communicating artery (PCoA) aneurysm, and a right ICA–PCoA aneurysm. (**a**) Operative view through the microscope of an ACoA aneurysm via the interhemispheric approach. (**b**) ICG-VAG image during ACoA aneurysm surgery via the interhemispheric approach. Fine perforating arteries from the anterior cerebral artery (ACA) (arrows), as well as Heubner's arteries (*arrowheads*), can be observed. (**c**) Operative view through the microscope of a left ICA–PCoA aneurysm via the left pterional approach. (**d**) ICG-VAG image during left ICA–PCoA aneurysm surgery via the left pterional approach. Fine perforating arteries from the PCoA (*arrow*) and anterior choroidal artery (*arrowhead*) can be observed. (**e**) Operative view through the microscope of a right ICA–PCoA aneurysm via the right pterional approach. (**f**): ICG-VAG image shows poor blood flow at the sclerotic portion of the ICA (*arrowheads*) and good blood flow at the aneurysm and ICA with a normal wall (*arrows*)

aneurysm), (2) no occlusion of perforating arteries, (3) no aneurysm neck remnant, and (4) no stenosis of parent arteries. The compression of the vascular structure using a suction tip or a micro-sonde and change of the microscope angle are sometimes necessary for observation of microscopic dead field behind the parent artery, aneurysm, and clip.

In addition to these points, change of flow velocity during ICG-VAG should be mentioned. One case showed decreased fluorescence intensity at the parent artery (internal carotid artery) proximal to the aneurysm after clipping (Fig. 4.2b, c). The flow velocity of ICG fluorescence at this artery and the ophthalmic artery became normal after clip reapplication (Fig. 4.2d, e).

Furthermore, ICG fluorescence remains observed in the vessels (especially in the veins); an interval more than 5 min may usually be necessary for repeated examinations. When the clip was reapplied in a short time after a first incomplete clipping procedure, ICG fluorescence remained in the aneurysm. In this situation,

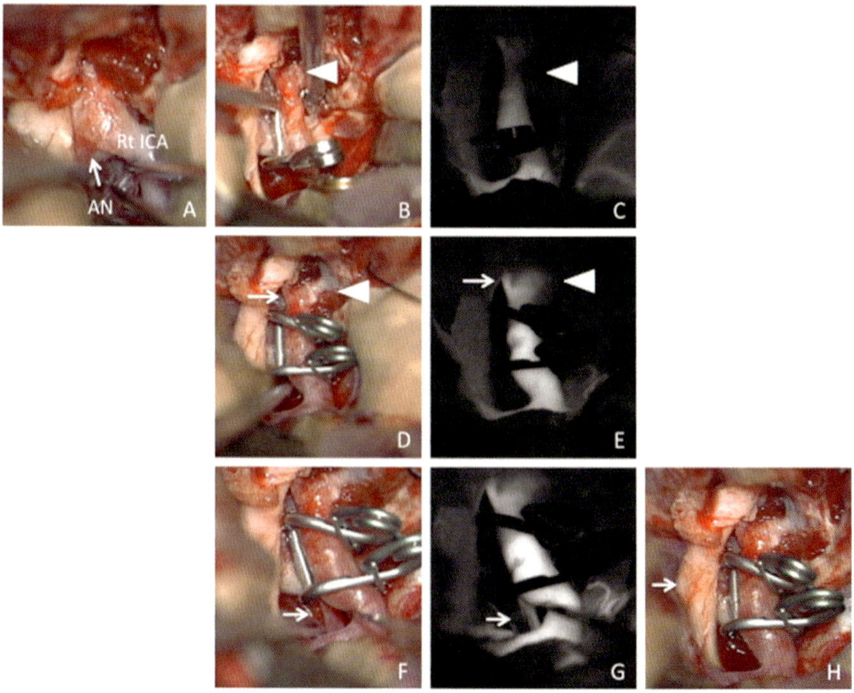

Fig. 4.2 Operative findings of right ICA–ophthalmic artery (OphA) aneurysm surgery via the right pterional approach.
(**a**) Operative view through the microscope shows an aneurysm located under the right optic nerve (*arrow*). (**b**) Operative view through the microscope after first clipping aneurysm using one fenestrated clip is suspected the stenosis of ICA (*arrowhead*). (**c**) ICG-VAG image after first clipping aneurysm shows decreased ICG fluorescence intensity in the ICA proximal to the aneurysm (*arrowhead*) due to stenosis of this artery. (**d**) Operative view through the microscope after reapplication using two fenestrated clips to reduce ICA stenosis (*arrowhead*). (**e**) ICG-VAG image after reapplication shows good intensity of ICG fluorescence in ICA (*arrowhead*) and OphA (*arrow*). (**f**) Operative view through the microscope after clip reapplication shows preservation of perforating arteries (*arrow*). (**g**) ICG-VAG image shows good intensity of ICG fluorescence in the perforating arteries from PCoA (*arrow*). (**h**) Operative view through the microscope after puncture of aneurysm shows decompression of optic nerve (*arrow*) by aneurysm

it is important to observe whether intensity of ICG fluorescence in the aneurysm increases for 3 min after injection. The duration of examination needs to be considered, because it has been reported that brain temperature increased during observation using ICG-VAG [27]. The Zeiss microscope system stops automatically after 5 min of usage.

Since ICG-VAG is easy and safe for neurosurgical procedures with a microscope, it has become the routine examination for clipping cerebral aneurysms. However, surgical complications have been reported even though ICG-VAG was done [23, 24, 26]. Dashti et al. reported that a neck remnant was recognized in 6 % of surgeries, especially for anterior communicating artery aneurysms, and parent artery stenosis and occlusion of the perforating artery were observed in 6 % of surgeries, especially for middle cerebral artery aneurysms [28]. Roessler et al. reported that the postoperative angiography demonstrated unexpected residual aneurysms in 9.1 % of successful ICG-VAG-guided clip applications [29]. In the present study, perforating artery infarction was observed in 5 cases with a middle cerebral artery aneurysm and one case with anterior communicating artery aneurysm. Among them, one case showed transient hemiparesis, and others were asymptomatic fortunately. Because a blind field such as behind the clip may exist even with ICG-VAG, Doppler ultrasound, endoscopic observation, and electrophysiological monitoring should be added for safe and precise clipping surgery. Recently, the association of endoscopic ICG-VAG with microscopic ICG-VAG allowed a better observation of perforating arteries located deeply [30, 31].

4.3.2 ICG-VAG for Bypass Surgery

Extracranial (EC)–intracranial (IC) bypass surgery is performed for patients with hemodynamic atherosclerotic vascular lesion or moyamoya disease and patients with large or complex cerebral aneurysms that require proximal artery occlusion or trapping aneurysm. The intraoperative assessment of graft patency is essential for successful EC–IC bypass surgery. The usefulness of ICG-VAG for flow evaluation in bypass surgery has been reported [6, 32–34]. Woitzik et al. reported that this examination was useful for recognition of patency of anastomosis by comparing the findings of ICG-VAG with those of postoperative computed tomography angiography [6].

We performed ICG-VAG for 14 cases involving superficial temporal artery (STA) and middle cerebral artery (MCA) anastomosis. After the anastomosis, ICG-VAG was done to observe the patency of the anastomosis and blood flow from the STA to the anastomosed MCA, following Doppler ultrasound examination. The patency of the anastomosis observed on ICG-VAG was recognized also on postoperative cerebral angiography or computed tomography angiography. Although patency of the anastomosis can be recognized using Doppler ultrasound, ICG-VAG could show blood flow itself.

ICG-VAG demonstrated the flow from the STA 20 s after ICG injection (Fig. 4.3b), and the vessels of the brain surface were recognized 40 s later (Fig. 4.3c). In this case, the fine arterial network characteristic of moyamoya disease was observed clearly. Furthermore, in ICG-VAG for bypass surgery, cleaning the operative field is important, and surgicel applied on the anastomosed region for hemostasis is mentioned. We usually remove this surgicel before ICG-VAG, since a small amount of surgicel disturbs observation of ICG fluorescence at the anastomotic region.

Recently, a microscope-integrated software tool for instant color-coded visualization and analysis of the temporal distribution dynamics of the fluorescence ICG (FLOW 800) was created. Prinz et al. evaluated usefulness of FLOW 800 in

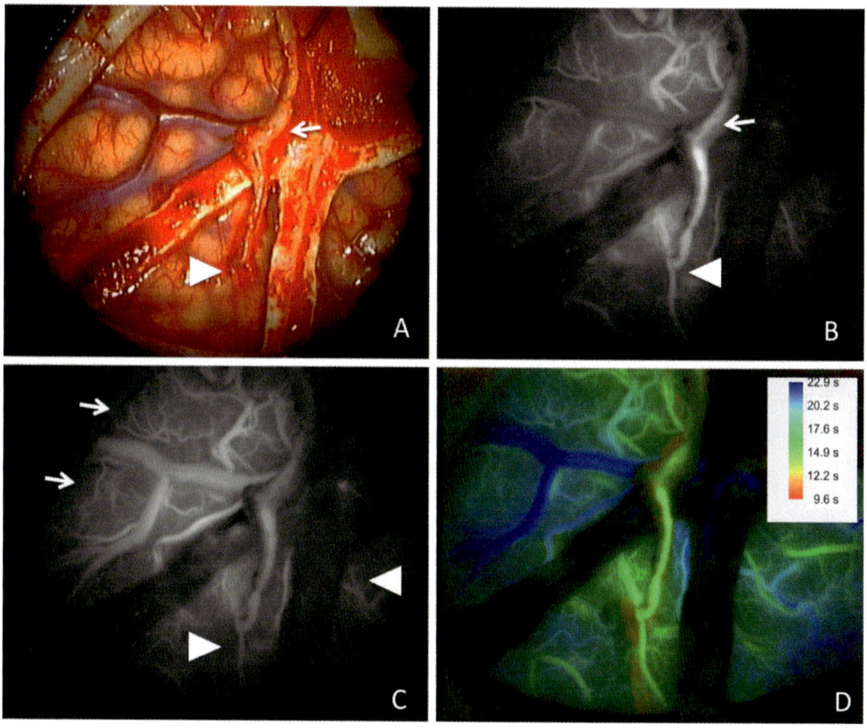

Fig. 4.3 Operative findings during bypass surgery for moyamoya disease.
(**a**) Operative view through the microscope after anastomosis of the left superficial temporal artery (STA) (*arrow*) and middle cerebral artery. (**b**) Image 20 s after ICG injection shows patency of the anastomosed portion (*arrowhead*) from STA (*arrow*). (**c**) Image 40 s after ICG injection shows blood flow from the STA (*arrowheads*) and from the collateral circulation (*arrows*). (**d**) Image by FLOW 800 shows the timing of fluorescence flow as a different color. The number means the time after the start of recording

30 cases undergoing bypass surgery and concluded that FLOW 800 may detect procedure-related hemodynamic changes within the microcirculation and macrocirculation but should not be used as a stand-alone tool for quantitative flow assessment [34]. Figure 4.3d shows our case using FLOW 800. The fast-flow area (area supplied by the bypass) was shown as yellow green, the medium speed flow area (area supplied by an intracerebral artery) was shown as light blue, and the show speed area (veins) was shown as blue.

4.3.3 ICG-VAG for Carotid Endarterectomy (CEA)

CEA is a safe and durable treatment that has been shown to prevent ipsilateral stroke. This procedure should be performed without cerebral embolism or residual

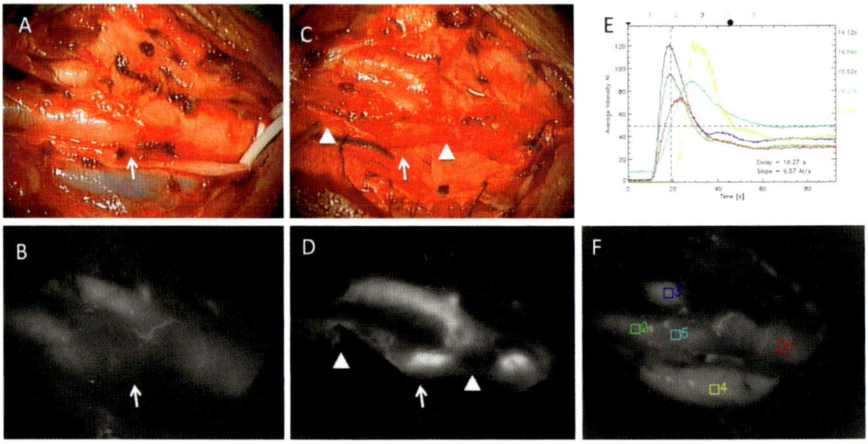

Fig. 4.4 Operative findings of carotid endarterectomy (CEA) for right carotid stenosis. (**a**) Operative views through the microscope before arteriotomy. (**b**) ICG-VAG image before the arteriotomy shows poor blood flow at the carotid bifurcation where the plaque is located (*arrow*). (**c**) Operative views through the microscope after CEA. (**d**) ICG-VAG image after CEA shows good intensity of ICG fluorescence at the carotid bifurcation (*arrow*), but the cotton and the blood obscured the fluorescence intensity in the artery (*arrowheads*). (**e**, **f**) Flow 800 analysis showing the time–intensity curves at the plotted areas demonstrates the improvement of blood flow at the area plaque located (plotted areas 2, *green*; 5, *light blue*)

plaque. The usefulness and limitations of ICG-VAG for CEA have been reported, and authors emphasized the importance of usage of a mixture of 12.5 mg of ICG and 5 ml of distilled water as a single injection to visualize ICA blood stream [35, 36].

We performed ICG-VAG for CEA in 35 surgeries. In early 10 surgeries, we injected 5 mg of ICG for one examination, and it was difficult to recognize the usefulness of ICG-VAG for this surgery. The reasons for this lack of usefulness were the thick wall of the carotid artery, sclerotic changes, calcified regions, vasa vasorum of the carotid artery, and difficulty of cleaning the operative field due to oozing blood. In later 25 surgeries, we injected 12.5 mg of ICG for one examination. Before arteriotomy, blood flow within the ICA was rapidly visualized with a latency of 10–20 s following ICG injection, followed by subsequent contrast enhancement of the venous system. Definitive lack of fluorescence was observed in some cases (Fig. 4.4a, b), although severe calcification of the plaque did not allow determination of the exact location of the stenosis. At the distal end, ICA patency was seen with no stenosis in many cases. At the end of surgery, the ICA was demonstrated to be patent by homogeneous enhancement, although the cotton and blood disturbed observation of ICG fluorescence (Fig. 4.4c, d). Image by FLOW 800 showed the time–intensity curves at the plotted areas, and it was useful to recognize the flow improvement after CEA (Fig. 4.4e, f).

4.3.4 *ICG-VAG for Vascular Malformations*

In surgery of arteriovenous malformations (AVMs), it is crucial to recognize the feeding arteries, nidus, and draining veins. ICG-VAG provides information about vessel architecture and patency by the difference in the timing of enhancement of these structures. The usefulness and limitations of ICG-VAG for AVM surgery have been reported [37–41]. This technique is useful for early identification of AVM arteries and veins, helping the surgeon to formulate and modify the operative strategy for attacking these formidable lesions. The information, which is provided within seconds of an injection, can potentially make surgery safer and faster, giving the surgeon more confidence in resecting AVM arteries while preserving draining veins. The major limitation of ICG-VAG is that it captures only what is visible within the field of the microscope. Consequently, ICG is frequently of limited use for deep-seated AVMs such as thalamic lesion. Although intraoperative digital subtraction angiography (DSA) remains the "gold standard" for evaluation of vascular flow in AVM surgery, ICG-VAG may decrease the need to perform DSA multiple times.

We performed ICG-VAG for cerebral AVMs in 2 surgeries. In the cryptic AVM hidden in the occipital sulcus, recognition of draining vein using ICG-VAG was useful to confirm the location of nidus (Fig. 4.5b, c, d). After removal of AVM (Fig. 4.5e), the draining vein was not shown on ICG-VAG image (Fig. 4.5f). These findings were confirmed using intraoperative DSA (Fig. 4.5a, g).

Faber et al. reported the usefulness of FLOW 800 in two patients with frontal or temporal AVMs [37]. They concluded that color-coded analytical ICG-VAG with FLOW 800 enabled intraoperative real-time analysis of arterial and venous vessel architecture and might increase the efficacy and safety of neurovascular surgery in a selected subset of superficial AVMs.

4.3.5 *ICG-VAG for Spinal Arteriovenous Fistula (AVF)*

In surgical treatment of spinal AVF, identification and complete interruption of fistulae are essential, but not always obvious during surgery. The reported advantages of ICG-VAG for this surgery are the identification of the fistulous site and confirmation of its obliteration during surgery [42–44]. The reported disadvantages are the increase of operating time and the limited visualization to the operating field with a need to fully expose the fistula [43, 44]. Intra-arterial ICG-VAG may localize the exact fistula portion by minimizing the influence of normal arterial vasculature simultaneously enhanced by conventional peripheral venous ICG injection [44].

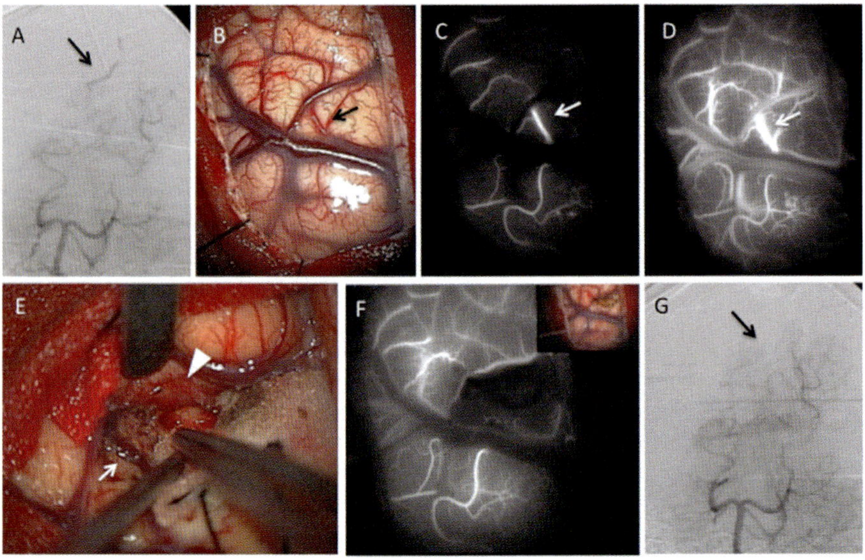

Fig. 4.5 Operative findings of arteriovenous malformation (AVM) hidden in the right occipital lobe sulcus. (**a**) Intraoperative vertebral angiography (VAG) shows early venous filling (*arrow*). (**b**) Operative view through microscope shows a draining vein as a red vein (*arrow*) at the right occipital cortex before removal. (**c, d**) ICG-VAG images before removal show early appearance of ICG fluorescence in this vessel (*arrow*). (**e**) Operative view through the microscope shows a feeder (*arrowhead*) and a drainer (*arrow*). (**f**) After removal, ICG-VAG image shows no early venous enhancement of ICG. (**g**) Intraoperative VAG shows disappearance of early venous filling recognized before surgery (*arrow*)

4.3.6 ICG-VAG for Cavernous Malformations (CMs)

The usefulness of ICG-VAG for removing CMs has been reported [45, 46]. Murakami et al. reported that ICG-VAG could directly visualize cerebral CMs and orbital cavernous angiomas, and it demonstrated slow and low perfusion within the lesions. They concluded that, by understanding the characteristic features of flow dynamics, the intraoperative ICG-VAG provides useful information for microsurgical resection of cerebral CMs [45]. Endo et al. examined the potential utility of ICG-VAG for the surgical treatment of intramedullary CMs in 8 cases. They concluded that ICG-VAG provided useful information with regard to the detection of lesion margins by demonstrating intramedullary CMs as avascular areas. In cases with venous anomalies, ICG-VAG contributed to safe and complete removal of the lesions by visualizing the venous structure. In extramedullary CMs, ICG-VAG demonstrated the characteristics of slow blood flow within cavernous malformations [46].

On the other hand, Niemela et al. commented that its clinical value for microsurgery of brain CM is very limited, since ICG-VAG does not help in finding the lesion. Furthermore, the extent of removal of a CM cannot by reliably estimated using ICG-VAG [47].

4.3.7 ICG-VAG for Tumors in the Central Nervous System

For tumor surgeries, ICG-VAG was used in the identification of tumor vessels, normal brain parenchyma vessels, bridging veins, and tumor margin [48–53].

Hemangioblastomas remain a surgical challenge due to their AVM-like vascular structure. Identification of the feeding arteries and draining veins, as well as tumor location, is crucial for en bloc tumor resection and cure during surgery. ICG-VAG could provide dynamic images of blood flow in the tumor and its related vessels under surgical view. The usefulness of ICG-VAG for resection of hemangioblastomas has been reported previously [48–50]. Tamura et al. reported the usefulness of this method in nine surgeries for patients with hemangioblastomas of the cerebellum, medulla oblongata, or spinal cord. They concluded that ICG-VAG was a safe and easy modality for confirming the vascular flow patterns in hemangioblastomas. In addition, ICG-VAG provided useful information for intracystic small lesions or lesions concealed under thin brain tissue in order to accomplish total resection of these tumors [48]. Hao et al. reported the limitations in their experience of 7 surgeries for spinal hemangioblastomas; one was partially removed, though 6 tumors were completely removed. The partially removed tumor was located deep in the spinal cord parenchyma, which did not take up fluorescent dye and was, therefore, not visualized by ICG-VAG. They concluded that the benefits of this technique might be limited for deep tumors and ventral tumors [50].

We used ICG-VAG for removing hemangioblastoma in the brain stem. Before removal, ICG-VAG could demonstrate the feeding arteries and draining veins, as well as tumor location, in the brain by differences in flow velocity of ICG fluorescence (Fig. 4.6a, b, c). Feeding arteries are recognized first, followed by tumor itself, and then finally draining veins. During the removal procedure, the feeding arteries and draining veins are coagulated and cut, and then the tumor is resected, according to the information provided by ICG-VAG, as well as preoperative angiography. Interpretation of these dynamic images of tumor blood flow was useful to discriminate the transit feeders from the true feeding artery and to decide which draining vein to preserve until the last stage of the procedure. After tumor removal, ICG-VAG images confirmed tumor elimination (Fig. 4.6d, e, f).

There are some reports concerning other brain tumor surgeries using ICG-VAG [51–53]. D'Avella et al. evaluated the usefulness for surgery of parasagittal meningiomas occluding the superior sagittal sinus in 5 cases. During this surgery, for a safe and radical resection, crucial issues are accurate preoperative radiological examination, preservation of functional veins during both dura opening and tumor dissection, and boundary identification of the invaded portions of the venous sinus. Using ICG-VAG, the venous collateral pathway was easily identified and preserved in all cases [51]. Ferroli et al. also reported that the recognition of flow

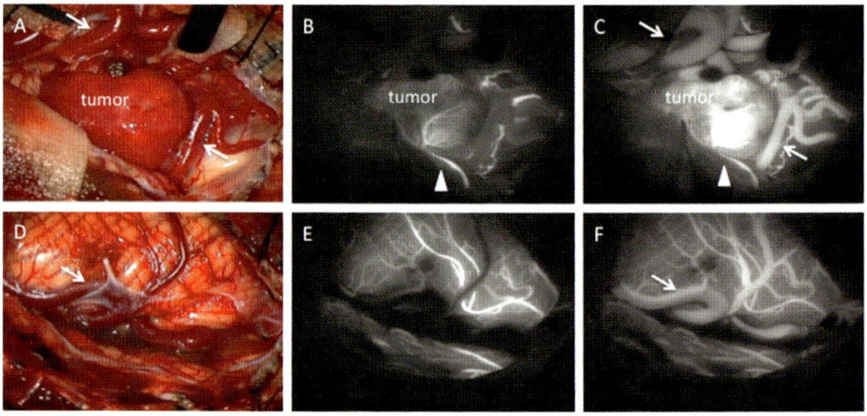

Fig. 4.6 Operative findings of brainstem hemangioblastoma via the midline suboccipital approach. (**a**) Operative view through the microscope shows red-colored tumor at the brainstem. (**b**, **c**) ICG-VAG images before tumor removal show feeding artery (*arrowheads*) and draining veins (*arrows*). (**d**) Operative view through the microscope shows total removal of the tumor. (**e**, **f**) ICG-VAG images after removal of the tumor show normal filling of ICG in the main draining vein (*arrow*)

pattern in the venous ICG-VAG might be useful to predict the presence of a safe collateral circulation for the veins that are at risk for intentional or unintentional damage during surgery [52]. Litvack et al. used ICG fluorescence endoscopy for pituitary tumor surgery in 16 patients and concluded that ICG fluorescence endoscopy showed promise as an intraoperative modality to visually distinguish pituitary tumors from normal tissue and to visually identify areas of dural invasion, thereby facilitating complete tumor resection and minimizing injury to surrounding structures [53].

4.4 Conclusion and Future Considerations

ICG-VAG is an easy and safe intraoperative angiography procedure, and it can demonstrate precise information about blood flow in neurosurgical procedures. This method has already become the standard intraoperative examination for vascular and tumor surgeries; therefore, some limitations should be heeded.

Recently, semiquantitative blood flow analysis using FLOW 800 has also come to be used for objective evaluation instead of subjective recognition of ICG fluorescence flow [34, 37]. This flow analysis could demonstrate brain hemodynamic changes during decompression craniectomy for malignant cerebral infarction and clipping for ruptured cerebral aneurysm and contribute to recognize the pathophysiology of human stroke or to predict the prognosis of patients [54, 55]. But flow images using this software should not be understood as a stand-alone tool for quantitative flow assessment [34]. In the future, true quantitative blood flow analysis using fluorescence angiography may become possible following studies coupled with thermal imaging [56], magnetic resonance imaging [57], and fluorescence molecular tomography [58].

References

1. Bensori RC, Kunes HA (1978) Fluorescence properties of indocyanine green as related to angiography. Phys Med Biol 23:159–163
2. Hayashi K, de Laey JJ (1985) Indocyanine green angiography of submacular choroidal vessels in the human eye. Ophthalmologica 190(1):20–9
3. Novotny HR, Alvis DL (1961) A method of photographing fluorescence in circulating blood in the human retina. Circulation 24:82–86
4. Dzurinko VL, Gurwood AS, Price JR (2004) Intravenous and indocyanine green angiography. Optometry 75(12):743–55
5. Raabe A, Beck J, Gerlach R et al (2003) Near-infrared indocyanine green video angiography: a new method for intraoperative assessment of vascular flow. Neurosurgery 52:132–139
6. Woitzik J, Horn P, Vajkoczy P et al (2005) Intraoperative control of extracranial-intracranial bypass patency by near-infrared indocyanine green videoangiography. J Neurosurg 102:692–698
7. Desai ND, Miwa S, Kodama D et al (2005) Improving the quality of coronary bypass surgery with intraoperative angiography: validation of a new technique. J Am Coll Cardiol 46:1521–5
8. Siedek V, Waggershauser T, Berghaus A et al (2009) Intraoperative monitoring of intraarterial paraganglioma embolization by indocyaningreen fluorescence angiography. Eur Arch Otorhinolaryngol 266(9):1449–54
9. Kitai T, Inomoto T, Miwa M et al (2005) Fluorescence navigation with indocyanine green for detecting sentinel lymph nodes in breast cancer. Breast Cancer 12(3):211–215
10. Kusano M, Tajima Y, Yamazaki K et al (2008) Sentinel node mapping guided by indocyanine green fluorescence imaging: a new method for sentinel node navigation surgery in gastrointestinal cancer. Dig Surg 25:103–108
11. Alexander T, Macdonald R, Weir B et al (1996) Intraoperative angiography in cerebral aneurysm surgery: a prospective study of 100 craniotomies. Neurosurgery 39:10–17
12. Drake C, Allcock J (1973) Postoperative angiography and the "slipped" clip. J Neurosurg 39:683–689
13. Macdonald R, Wallace M, Kestle J (1993) Role of angiography following aneurysm surgery. J Neurosurg 79:826–832
14. Proust F, Hannequin D, Langlois O et al (1995) Causes of morbidity and mortality after ruptured aneurysm surgery in a series of 230 patients. The importance of control angiography. Stroke 26:1553–1557
15. Rauzzino MJ, Quinn CM, Fisher WS (1998) Angiography after aneurysm surgery: indications for "selective" angiography. Surg Neurol 49:32–40
16. Suzuki J, Kwak R, Katakura R (1980) Review of incompletely occluded surgically treated cerebral aneurysms. Surg Neurol 13:306–310
17. Chiang V, Gailloud P, Murphy K et al (2002) Routine intraoperative angiography during aneurysm surgery. J Neurosurg 96:988–992
18. Katz J, Gologorsky Y, Tsiouris A et al (2006) Is routine intraoperative angiography in the surgical treatment of cerebral aneurysms justified? A consecutive series of 147 aneurysms. Neurosurgery 58:719–727
19. Klopfenstein J, Spetzler R, Kim L et al (2004) Comparison of routine and selective use of intraoperative angiography during aneurysm surgery: a prospective assessment. J Neurosurg 100:230–235

20. Amin-Hanjani S, Meglio G, Gatto R et al (2006) The utility of intraoperative blood flow measurement during aneurysm surgery using an ultrasonic perivascular flow probe. Neurosurgery 58:ONS 305–312
21. Bailes JE, Tantuwaya LS, Fukushima T et al (1997) Intraoperative microvascular Doppler sonography in aneurysm surgery. Neurosurgery 40:965–70
22. Zhao J, Wang Y, Zhao Y et al (2006) Neuroendoscope-assisted minimally invasive microsurgery for clipping intracranial aneurysms. Minim Invasive Neurosurg 49(6):335–41
23. Imizu S, Kato Y, Sangli A et al (2008) Assessment of incomplete clipping of aneurysms intraoperatively by a near-infrared indocyanine green-video angiography (Niicg-Va) integrated microscope. Minim Invasive Neurosurg 51:199–203
24. Oliveira M, Beck J, Seifert V et al (2007) Assessment of blood in perforating arteries during intraoperative near-infrared indocyanine green videoangiography. Neurosurgery 61(6 Suppl 3):1300–10
25. Raabe A, Nakaji P, Beck J et al (2005) Prospective evaluation of surgical microscope-integrated intraoperative near-infrared indocyanine green videoangiography during aneurysm surgery. J Neurosurg 103:982–989
26. Suzuki K, Kodama N, Sasaki T et al (2007) Confirmation of blood flow in perforating arteries using fluorescein cerebral angiography during aneurysm surgery. J Neurosurg 107:68–73
27. Keller E, Ishihara H, Nadler A et al (2002) Evaluation of brain toxicity following near infrared light exposure after indocyanine green dye injection. J Neurosci Methods 17(1):23–31
28. Dashti R, Laakso A, Niemelä M et al (2009) Microscope-integrated near-infrared indocyanine green videoangiography during surgery of intracranial aneurysms: the Helsinki experience. Surg Neurol 71(5):543–50
29. Roessler K, Krawagna M, Dorfler A et al (2014) Essentials in intraoperative indocyanine green videoangiography assessment for intracranial aneurysm surgery: conclusions from 295 consecutively clipped aneurysms and review of the literature. Neurosurg Focus 36, E7
30. Bruneau M, Appelboom G, Rynkowski M et al (2013) Endoscope-integrated I.C.G. technology: first application during intracranial aneurysm surgery. Neurosurg Rev 36:77–84
31. Nishiyama Y, Kinouchi H, Senbokuya N et al (2012) Endoscopic indocyanine green angiography in aneurysm surgery: an innovative method for intraoperative assessment of blood flow in vasculature hidden from microscopic view. J Neurosurg 117:302–8
32. Ferroli P, Ciceri E, Addis A et al (2008) Self-closing surgical clips for use in pericallosal artery-pericallosal artery side-to-side bypass. J Neurosurg 109(2):330–4
33. Peña-Tapia PG, Kemmling A, Czabanka M et al (2008) Identification of the optical cortical target point for extracranial-intracranial bypass surgery in patients with hemodynamic cerebrovascular insufficiency. J Neurosurg 108:655–661
34. Prinz V, Hecht N, Kato N et al (2014) FLOW 800 allows visualization of hemodynamic changes after extracranial-to-intracranial bypass surgery but not assessment of quantitative perfusion or flow. Neurosurgery 10(Suppl 2):231–9
35. Haga S, Nagata S, Uka A et al (2011) Near-infrared indocyanine green videoangiography for assessment of carotid endarterectomy. Acta Neurochir 153:1641–1644
36. Lee C-H, Jung YS, Yang H-J et al (2012) An innovative method for detecting surgical errors using indocyanine green angiography during carotid endarterectomy: a preliminary investigation. Acta Neurochir 154:67–73
37. Faber F, Thon K, Fesl G et al (2011) Enhanced analysis of intracerebral arteriovenous malformations by the intraoperative use of analytical indocyanine green videoangiography: technical note. Acta Neurochir 153:2181–2187
38. Hanggi D, Etminan N, Steiger H-J et al (2010) The impact of microscope-integrated intraoperative near-infrared indocyanine green videoangiography on surgery of arteriovenous malformations and dural arteriovenous fistulae. Neurosurgery 67:1094–1104

39. Killory BD, Nakaji P, Gonzales LF et al (2009) Prospective evaluation of surgical microscope-integrated intraoperative near-infrared indocyanine green angiography during cerebral arteriovenous malformation surgery. Neurosurgery 65:456–462
40. Takagi Y, Kikuta K, Nozaki K et al (2007) Detection of a residual nidus by surgical microscope-integrated intraoperative near-infrared indocyanine green videoangiography in a child with a cerebral arteriovenous malformation. J Neurosurg 107(5 Suppl):416–8
41. Zaidi HA, Abia AA, Nakaji P et al (2014) Indocyanine green angiography in the surgical management of cerebral arteriovenous malformations: lessons learned in 130 consecutive cases. Oper Neurosurg 10:246–251
42. Hanel RA, Nakaji P, Spetzler RF (2010) Use of microscope-integrated near-infrared indocyanine green videoangiography in the surgical treatment of spinal dural arteriovenous fistulae. Neurosurgery 66:978–85
43. Oh JK, Shin HC, Kim TY et al (2011) Intraoperative indocyanine green video-angiography. Spine 36:E1578–E1580
44. Horie N, So G, Debata A et al (2012) Intra-arterial indocyanine green angiography in the management of spinal arteriovenous fistulae. Spine 37:E264–267
45. Murakami K, Endo T, Tominaga T (2012) An analysis of flow dynamics in cerebral cavernous malformation and orbital cavernous angioma using indocyanine green videoangiography. Acta Neurochir 154:1169–1175
46. Endo T, Aizawa-Kohama M, Nagamatsu A et al (2013) Use of microscope-integrated near-infrared indocyanine green videoangiography in the surgical treatment of intramedullary cavernous malformations: report of 8 cases. J Neurosurg Spine 18:443–449
47. Niemela M, Kivelev J, Hernesniemi J (2012) The clinical value of indocyanine green angiography in the microsurgery of brain cavernomas is very limited. Acta Neurochir 154:1177–1178
48. Tamura Y, Hirota Y, Miyata S et al (2012) The use of intraoperative near-infrared indocyanine green videoangiography in the microscopic resection of hemangioblastomas. Acta Neurochir 154:1407–1412
49. Hojo M, Arakawa Y, Funaki T et al (2014) Usefulness of tumor blood flow imaging by intraoperative indocyanine green videoangiography in hemangioblastoma surgery. World Neurosurg 82(3/4):e495–e501
50. Hao S, Li D, Ma G et al (2013) Application of intraoperative indocyanine green videoangiography for resection of spinal cord hemangioblastoma: advantages and limitations. J Clin Neurosci 20:1269–1275
51. D'Avella E, Volpin F, Manara R et al (2013) Indocyanine green videoangiography (ICGV)-guided surgery of parasagittal meningiomas occluding the superior sagittal sinus (SSS). Acta Neurochir 155:415–420
52. Ferroli P, Acerbi F, Tringali G et al (2011) Venous sacrifice in neurosurgery: new insights from venous indocyanine green videoangiography. J Neurosurg 115:18–23
53. Litvack ZN, Zada G, Laws ER Jr (2012) Indocyanine green fluorescence endoscopy for visual differentiation of pituitary tumor from surrounding structures. J Neurosurg 116:935–941
54. Woitzik J, Peña-Tapia PG, Schneider UC et al (2006) Cortical perfusion measurement by indocyaninegreen videoangiography in patients undergoing hemicraniectomy for malignant stroke. Stroke 37:1549–1551
55. Schubert GA, Seiz-Rosenhagen M, Ortier M et al (2012) Cortical indocyanine green videography for quantification of acute hypoperfusion after subarachnoid hemorrhage: a feasibility study. Neurosurgery 71:ons260–267
56. Manley DM, Xiang B, Kupriyanov VV (2007) Visualization and grading of regional ischemia in pigs in vivo using near-infrared and thermal imaging. Can J Physiol Pharmacol 85 (3–4):382–95
57. Davis SC, Pogue BW, Springett R et al (2008) Magnetic resonance-coupled fluorescence tomography scanner for molecular imaging of tissue. Rev Sci Instrum 79(6):064302
58. Ntziachristos V, Tung CH, Bremer C et al (2002) Fluorescence molecular tomography resolves protease activity in vivo. Nat Med 8(7):757–60

Part III
Head and Neck Surgery

Chapter 5
ICG Fluorescent Image-Guided Surgery in Head and Neck Cancer

Junkichi Yokoyama and Shinich Ohba

Abstract Neck lymph node metastasis is the most significant prognostic factor of head and neck cancer; however, there remains debate as to the most effective treatment of clinical N0 neck metastasis. Sentinel lymph node (SLN) navigation surgery decreases morbidity associated with neck dissections and reduces the potential of recurrences. While radiocolloids have been previously used to detect SLN, disadvantages of radiocolloids are not only the lack of real-time intraoperative visual information but also the phenomena of "shine-through" radio-activity due to scattering from the primary site. This is especially problematic in cases of cancer located at the floor of the mouth. Additionally, radiocolloids may expose patients and medical staff to irradiation.

To negotiate these problems, ICG (indocyanine green) fluorescence imaging has been used for the detection of SLN, translymphatic chemotherapy, and intra-arterial chemotherapy in cases of head and neck cancer. The advantages of ICG fluorescence imaging include access to real-time intraoperative visual information and little affections of "shine through" even in cases of the floor of the mouth.

Keywords ICG (indocyanine green) fluorescence imaging • Sentinel lymph node (SLN) • Head and neck cancer • Translymphatic chemotherapy • Intra-arterial chemotherapy

5.1 Introduction

The sentinel lymph node (SLN) is defined as the lymph node that first receives lymphatic drainage from the primary cancer [1]. The SLN is thought to be the foremost possible micrometastatic site via lymphatic drainage from the primary

---

J. Yokoyama (✉)
Department of Otolaryngology Head and Neck Surgery, Juntendo University, Tokyo, Japan

Department of Otolaryngology Head and Neck Surgery, Moriyama Memorial Hospital, 7-12-7 Nishikasai, Edogawa-ku, Tokyo 134-0088, Japan
e-mail: jyokoya@juntendo.ac.jp

S. Ohba
Department of Otolaryngology Head and Neck Surgery, Juntendo University, Tokyo, Japan

M. Kusano et al. (eds.), *ICG Fluorescence Imaging and Navigation Surgery*,
DOI 10.1007/978-4-431-55528-5_5

cancer. Consequently, the pathological status of the SLN can be examined to predict the status of all regional lymph nodes. For this reason, if the SLN is recognized as being negative for cancer metastasis, unnecessary dissection can be avoided and a positive prognosis achieved. This SLN concept is well established in the treatment of patients with several types of solid carcinomas, such as melanoma and breast cancer [2–4]. The SLN concept has revolutionized surgical strategies and modern techniques benefit patients by preventing a range of complications associated with unnecessary prophylactic dissection in cases when the SLN is negative for cancer metastasis. Recently, this highly advantageous SLN concept has been applied to the examination of head and neck cancers [5, 6].

5.2 Sentinel Lymph Node (SLN) Navigation Surgery

In clinically negative neck (cN0) of oral cancer, 20 to 30 % of patients have occult nodal metastases [7]. Neck metastasis is the most significant prognostic factor in oral cancer. However, to date there is no effective noninvasive diagnostic modality for the identification of occult regional disease in patients with cN0. As a result, prophylactic neck dissection in patients with T1/T2 oral cancer with cN0 neck is the procedure typically conducted. This is a significant concern given that approximately 70 to 80 % of neck dissection specimens are found to be negative for regional metastatic disease. In addition, prophylactic neck dissection is associated with severe postoperative complications such as swallowing and shoulder dysfunction.

Due to the critical need for an accurate noninvasive diagnostic approach to cN0 neck, SLN navigation surgery has been applied to patients with oral cancer of the cN0 neck.

Paleri et al. [8] performed a meta-analysis on 19 of these studies in order to examine a larger combined body of data. They reviewed 367 patients, including 301 patients with oral cavity lesions, and found a 97.7 % sentinel node identification rate. The combined sensitivity of SLN biopsy was 92.6 % with a false-negative rate of 3 %. The pooled data provides compelling evidence that there is no statistical difference between SND (selective neck dissection) and SLN biopsy in terms of recurrence, disease-free survival, and mortality.

In 2004, Ross et al. [9] performed a prospective randomized study of 134 patients with T1/T2 oral cavity cancer. They randomized 79 patients to receive SLN biopsy alone and 55 patients to receive SLN biopsy plus elective neck dissection. Sentinel node detection rates were 93 %, and 42 (34 %) patients were upstaged as a result of SLN biopsy.

Overall sensitivity was 93 % with an average follow-up of 2 years. However, sensitivity for floor-of-mouth (FOM) lesions proved to be only 80 % due to "shine through," which was significantly lower than the results of other subsites in whose sensitivity was 100 %. Of those patients treated with SLN biopsy, only 3.8 % experienced recurrences of disease within 24 months. Those treated with SLN biopsy plus elective neck dissection recorded a 4 % false-negative rate. This study clearly demonstrates that SLN biopsy is as good as elective neck dissection with regard to identifying metastatic disease. However, the study also identified the FOM as a site prone to failure with SLN biopsy.

The obvious pitfall of SLN biopsy is its poor performance in identifying true sentinel nodes in patients with FOM tumors. Many researchers believe that the close proximity of level I nodes to the primary tumor leads to "shine-through" radioactivity, thus masking signals from the relevant SLN [8, 9]. This is a considerable problem associated not only with anatomy but also the properties of the radiolabeled agent.

To overcome the disadvantages of radioactive agents, ICG fluorescence imaging has been applied for detection of SLN of head and neck cancer. SLN around the submandibular lymph nodes can be clearly identified by ICG fluorescence imaging [10, 11]. Additionally, the cost of ICG fluorescence imaging is minimal and does not result in exposure to irradiation as is the case in conventional procedures using technesium 99 m-labeled sulfur colloid.

5.3 ICG Fluorescence Imaging-Guided Surgery for Parapharyngeal Space Tumors

5.3.1 Introduction

In the narrow parapharyngeal space, it is exceedingly difficult to resect tumors without complications such as dysphagia and carotid artery rupture [12]. In order to minimize surgical complications and preserve organs, endoscopic or robotic surgery is often executed when performing head and neck surgery. While highly effective, a disadvantage of these procedures is that it is not possible for the surgeon to physically touch tumors or to directly observe diffusely invaded deep organs. As a result, we have proposed using ICG florescence method for navigation surgery and have demonstrated the advantageous and effectiveness of ICG fluorescent image-guided surgery for the safe resection of parapharyngeal space tumors [13].

5.3.2 Methods

0.5 mg/kg of ICG was injected via the cephalic vein. Observation of the fluorescent image was conducted with HEMS (Hyper Eye Medical System) at 10–30 min after injection. At first, the position of the tumor was marked over pharyngeal mucosa through the use of ICG fluorescence imaging with HEMS. We could confirm the submucosal tumor although obscured by fascia under HEMS imaging and then carried out resection.

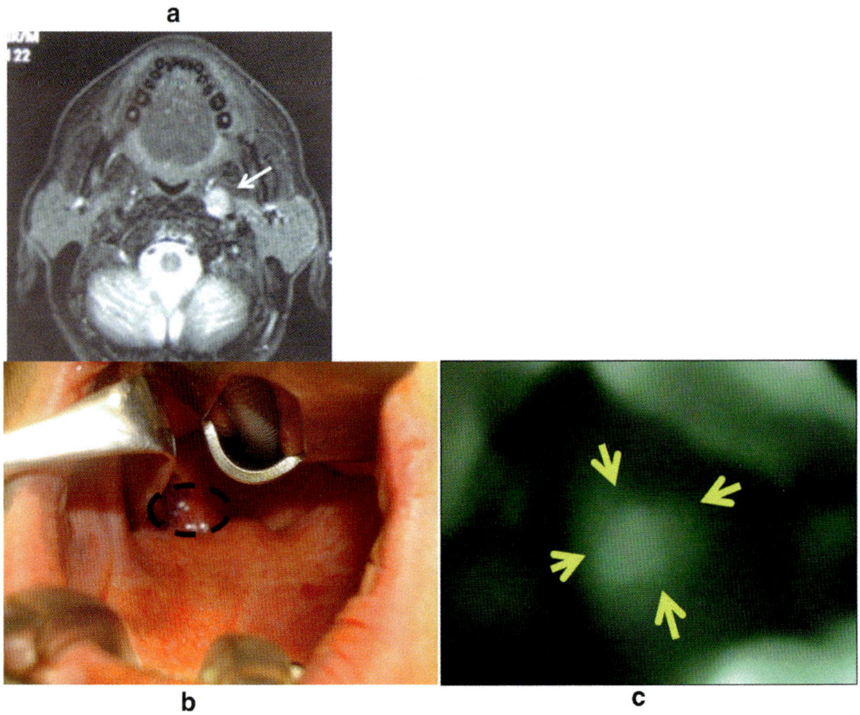

Fig. 5.1 Operative findings of metastatic parapharyngeal space from hypopharyngeal cancer
(**a**): Arrow represents a metastatic lymph node
(**b**): Dotted circle demonstrates the metastatic lymph node detected by ICG fluorescence Imaging over soft plate
(**c**): ICG fluorescence Imaging detects the metastatic lymph node (*arrows*)

5.3.3 Results

All tumors displayed bright fluorescence emissions which clearly contrasted with the surrounding normal structures. Even with the submucosal tumor covered with and obscured by fascia, we could observe the tumor clearly under HEMS imaging (Fig. 5.1). Tumors behind the carotid artery and lower cranial nerves also displayed bright fluorescence emissions and could therefore be clearly detected. Accordingly, we could remove the tumor safely and noninvasively which enabled successful preservation of pharyngeal functions.

5.3.4 Discussion

The handheld HEMS can significantly aid in the detection and visual confirmation of pharyngeal tumors located behind the oral cavity or nasal cavity by

ICG-enhanced imaging with vivid color. Of note is that it can be freely operated intraoperatively by surgeons. Because of the high sensitivity of ICG fluorescence imaging, ICG fluorescence imaging under HEMS can assist surgeons in the identification and resection of tumors which have invaded the parapharyngeal space behind the internal carotid artery, internal jugular vein, and lower cranial nerves.

We have demonstrated a successful method of distinguishing cancer from healthy tissue and the optimum surgical time with HEMS in animal models [14]. Application of endoscopic and robotic surgery for the parapharyngeal space lesions enables surgeons to perform minimally invasive surgery with superior results [15]. However, we need to be able to detect parapharyngeal tumors in deeper and invisible areas when palpation is not possible. This is required in order to resect tumors safely and can be aided through effective tumor detection carried out with ICG fluorescent imaging.

5.3.5 Conclusion

ICG fluorescence imaging is effective for the detection and resection of the parapharyngeal space tumors which enables greater preservation of functions.

5.4 Lymphatic Chemotherapy for Head and Neck Cancer

According to the sentinel theory, metastatic lymph nodes are directly connected with primary tumors via lymphatic canals. Lymphatic chemotherapy is defined as chemotherapy using lymphatic canals between metastatic lymph nodes and primary tumors. This therapy is viewed as an ultimate cancer treatment which is both highly effective and noninvasive.

(a) **Clinical N0 Cases (Occult Neck Metastasis)**

In the following, we consider a newly developed lymphatic chemotherapy procedure targeting the SLN using intra-arterial (I-A) chemotherapy for oral cancer in order to improve prognosis and to preserve organs while avoiding surgical complications [11, 16–18]. Our concept of lymphatic chemotherapy is shown in Fig. 5.2. Namely, the schema of lymphatic chemotherapy demonstrates an anticancer drug administered to the primary cancer which moves selectively to SLNs via lymphatic canals. As a result, the anticancer drug is accumulated in the SLNs and results in a higher anticancer drug concentration in the SLNs than non-SLNs. Because cis-diamminedichloroplatinum (CDDP) is the most promising drug for the treatment of head and neck cancers, we have adopted intra-arterial chemotherapy administered to the primary cancer so as to increase the CDDP concentration. To examine the potential advantages, we compared the CDDP concentration of SLNs with that of non-SLNs. The mean CDDP concentrations in the SLNs and

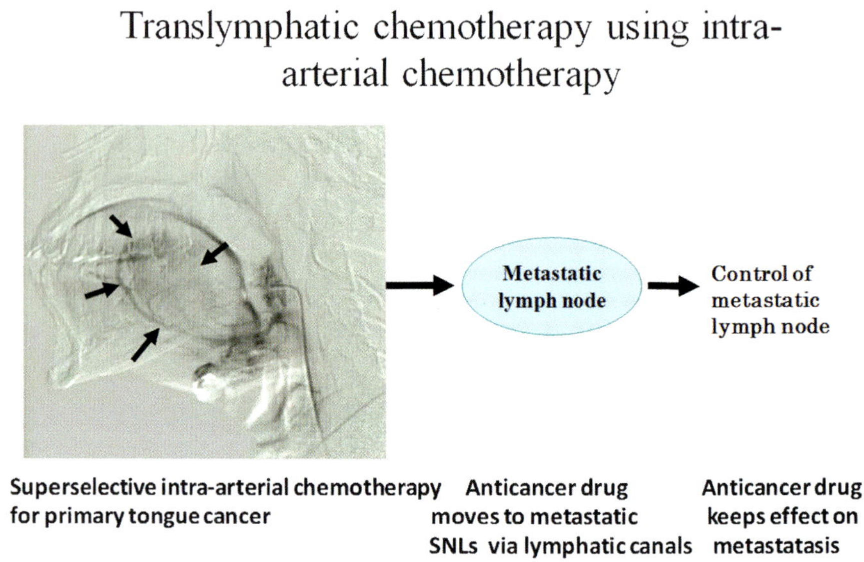

Fig. 5.2 Schema of lymphatic chemotherapy using intra-arterial chemotherapy

non-SLNs were 1.2 μg/g and 0.35 μg/g, respectively. Our ICG fluorescence procedure revealed that all metastatic lymph nodes, including SLNs, were without false-negative SLNs. However, of 7 metastatic lymph nodes, one was not identified by means of the conventional radiocolloid method [11]. Detection of SLNs was clearly demonstrated by ICG fluorescence imaging (Fig. 5.3). The mean number of SLNs was 5.6 (3–8). ICG fluorescence imaging showed a greater number of SLNs than seen when injecting radiocolloid intratumor (mean 3.4). SLNs detected by ICG fluorescence imaging included all of the SLNs detected by the conventional radioactive method.

(b) **Clinical Neck Metastasis Cases**

In the case of oral cancer with neck metastasis, modified radical neck dissection is often conducted to prevent cancer recurrence. However, this procedure can be the cause of severe postoperative complications. Instead of neck dissection and the associated surgical complications, minimally invasive lymphatic chemotherapy targeting neck metastasis based on the sentinel concept may contribute to the development of a revolutionary cancer treatment. This could potentially provide a superior method for the treatment of head and neck cancer which has been a key objective for researchers over many years. In our research, we consider I-A chemotherapy administered to primary oral cancers as not only organ preservation therapy but also a newly developed lymphatic chemotherapy targeting neck metastasis in order to improve prognosis.

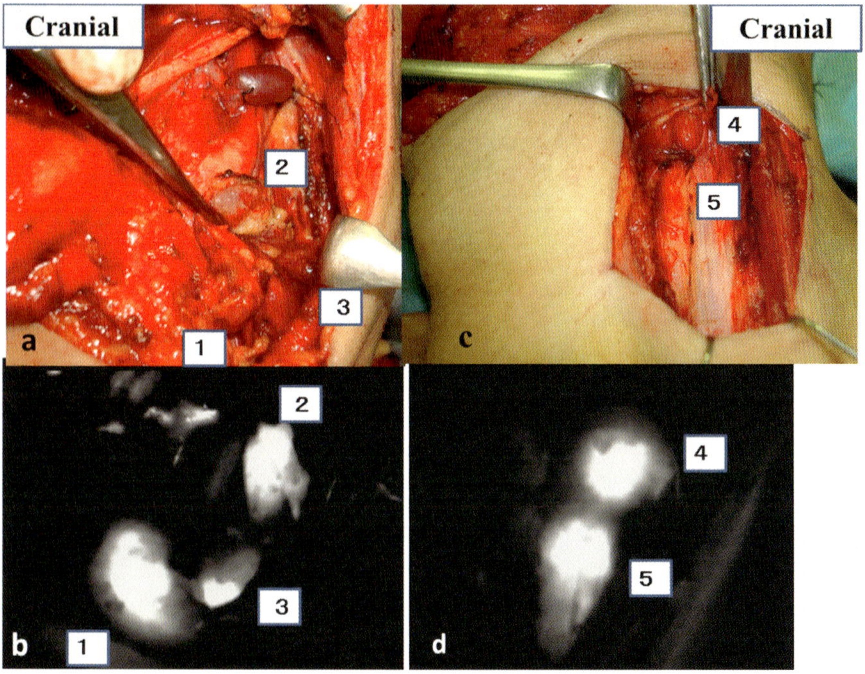

Fig. 5.3 Intraoperative navigation surgery using ICG fluorescence imaging
Upper figures (**a**, **c**) illustrate intraoperative navigation surgery by natural light; lower figures (**b**, **d**) illustrate intraoperative navigation surgery by ICG fluorescence imaging.
Number (1–5) means SLNs. (**a**) and (**b**) represent level II and III dissection. (**c**) and (**d**) represent level III and IV dissection

In our examination we evaluate the effect of lymphatic chemotherapy targeting neck metastases in patients with oral cancer (T3N2bM0) by measuring CDDP concentrations in metastatic lymph nodes and pathological effects [19].

5.4.1 Methods

Seven patients with tongue cancer (cT3N2bM0) were treated by intra-arterial chemotherapy as neoadjuvant chemotherapy. After a week of chemotherapy, patients underwent surgical treatment. Intra-arterial chemotherapy was administered at 75 mg/m^2 of CDDP two times weekly. At the beginning of surgery, 5 mg of ICG was administered to the lingual artery. SLNs were detected using ICG fluorescence imaging and a conventional radioactive method. The effect of lymphatic chemotherapy was evaluated based on the Ohboshi and Shimosato classification using the surgical specimens [20] and apoptosis using Trevigen's apoptosis detection kit.

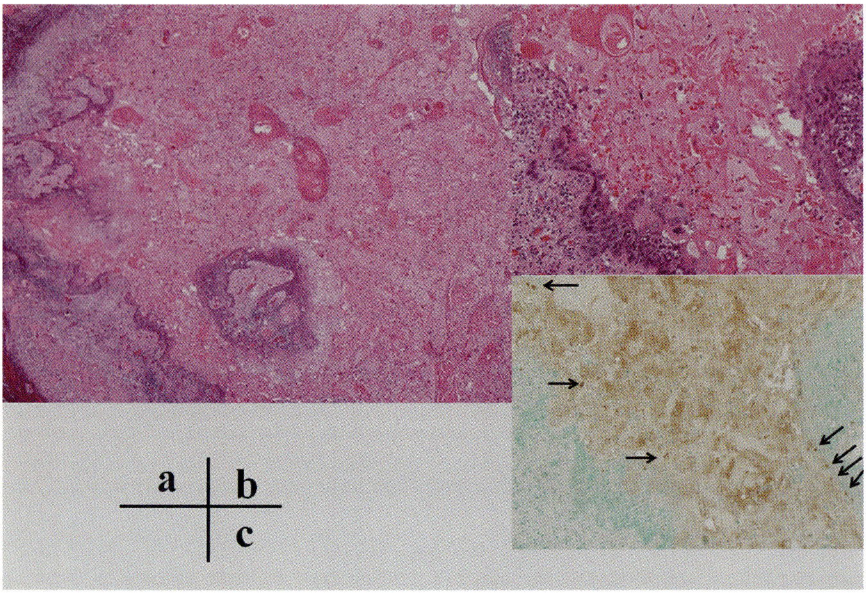

Fig. 5.4 Pathological findings of metastatic lymph nodes after chemotherapy
(**a**) Most of the metastatic cancer resulted in scar tissue; however, small cancer nests were residual (low-power magnification). (**b**) Cancer cells appeared to survive within small cancer nests (high-power magnification). (**c**) Many apoptotic bodies were detected within small cancer nests. *Arrows* indicate apoptotic cells

5.4.2 Results

The mean CDDP concentrations in the metastatic lymph nodes and non-SLNs were 2.35 μg/g and 1.08 μg/g, respectively ($p = 0.034$). Of 27 metastatic nodes, 24 (89 %) were identified by ICG fluorescence imaging; however, only 18 (67 %) were identified by the conventional method ($p = 0.043$). Of 22 measurable metastatic nodes, eight responded (partial response) and 14 did not respond (stable disease). Vast metastatic cancer was almost entirely diminished and resulted in scar tissue. Apoptosis was detected in all 27 metastatic lymph nodes and a pathological effect was achieved (Fig. 5.4).

5.4.3 Discussion

We have recently demonstrated that intra-arterial chemotherapy for the treatment of primary tongue cancers is also effective as a means of lymphatic chemotherapy as it aids in the control of the subclinical metastatic tumors in SLNs (11). All SLNs were detected by ICG fluorescence imaging infused via the lingual artery in cT3N0M0

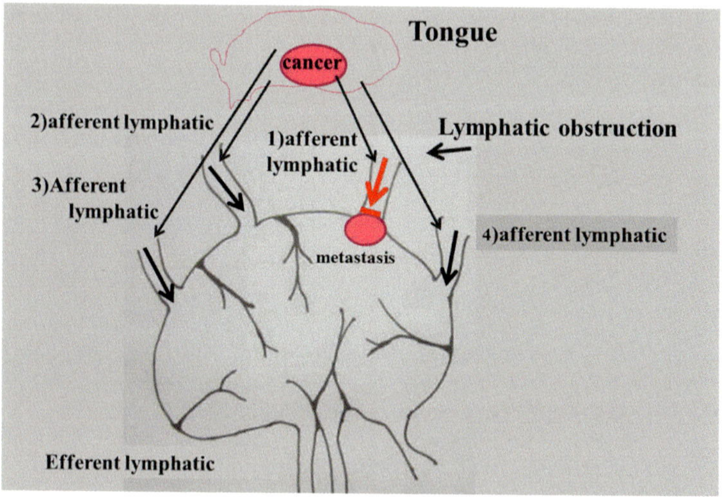

Fig. 5.5 Schema of increasing CDDP concentration of metastatic lymph nodes
Despite occlusion of afferent lymphatics from the tongue cancer, each lymph node has several afferent lymphatics, and ICG or CDDP could move to metastatic lymph nodes via several other afferent lymphatics in the case of intra-arterial infusion. (*1*) Occluded afferent lymphatics (*red arrow*). (*2–4*) Open afferent lymphatics (*black arrows*)

tongue cancer patients. However, of 27 metastatic lymph nodes, 24 (89 %) were detected by ICG fluorescence imaging infused via the lingual artery in seven cT3N2bM0 tongue cancer patients. The number of SLNs including metastatic lymph nodes resulting from I-A infusion was greater than that observed by means of a conventional injection into the tumor. Even in the case of micrometastatic SLNs, an afferent lymphatic canal was sometimes occluded by micrometastatic cancer based on sentinel navigation or CT lymphography [21]. In the current study, we also did not detect 9 (33 %) metastatic lymph nodes by conventional methods due to occlusion of afferent lymphatics from the tongue cancer (Fig. 5.5). However, the lymph nodes contained CDDP concentrations as high as 4.65 μg/g. This was because each lymph node has several afferent lymphatics and ICG or CDDP could move to metastatic lymph nodes via several other afferent lymphatics in the case of intra-arterial infusion. CDDP was released continuously from the primary tongue cancer via the lymphatic canal for a period of over more than 1 week. CDDP was selectively accumulated in metastatic lymph nodes and continued to affect metastatic lymph nodes over a long period.

Our intra-arterial chemotherapy is expected to contribute not only to primary organ preservation but also to positive prognosis by controlling the metastatic SLNs. Preservation of patients' quality of life in advanced cT3N2bM0 tongue cancer can be effectively achieved by intra-arterial chemotherapy and targeting metastatic lymph nodes with lymphatic chemotherapy.

As for ICG fluorescence imaging, metastatic SLNs were clearly detected even in close proximity to the primary tumor and "shine through" could be avoided. The ICG fluorescence imaging procedure demonstrated higher success rates for the detection of SLNs in patients with tumors located in the tongue than the radioactivity method.

5.4.4 Conclusion

CDDP concentrations in metastatic nodes were significantly higher than those in non-SLNs. This novel drug delivery system is feasible for lymphatic chemotherapy targeting metastatic nodes in patients with cT-3N2bM0 tongue cancer.

5.5 Significant Contribution to Superselective Intra-arterial Chemotherapy for Advanced Head and Neck Cancer

5.5.1 Introduction

For advanced paranasal sinus cancer, which is resistant to conventional systemic chemotherapy, superselective intra-arterial chemotherapy is believed to increase the concentration of anticancer drugs in the tumor [11, 22–24]. It is most important for I-A chemotherapy to obtain precise information about the blood supply to tumors. In 1998, we conducted CT angiography in order to accurately determine the blood supply to tumors in cases of head and neck cancer. This was the first time such a study had ever been conducted [25]. Our procedure can provide accurate and detailed information about the vascular supply to head and neck cancers [22, 26-29]. At the same time, it is difficult to confirm the drug distribution areas when the tumor is superficially invasive or the patient has undergone dental treatment involving metal fillings.

Recent advances in ICG fluorescence imaging have enabled visualization of the blood flow in tissues [11, 30, 31]. To date, the only report in which the ICG technique has been applied with intra-arterial chemotherapy was in a case involving oral cancer [32]. We have also utilized ICG fluorescence technique in combination with CT angiography in cases of advanced paranasal sinus cancer [33].

The purpose of this investigation was to assess the feasibility of the ICG fluorescence technique during intra-arterial chemotherapy for advanced paranasal sinus cancer.

Patients: Thirty-six patients with paranasal sinus cancer who were treated by intra-arterial chemotherapy were included in the study. Conventional CT angiography followed by 5 mg of ICG injection was performed to confirm the areas in which the drug had dispersed.

5.5.2 *Results*

Out of 36 cases, in 17 (47 %) the blood supply to the cancer was clearly detected by CT angiography (Fig. 5.6). By means of adding the infrared ICG evaluation, the blood supply to tumors could be easily confirmed in all cases without exposure to radiation. The information obtained from fluorescence imaging was advantageous when making decisions concerning the administration of chemo-agents for paranasal sinus cancers in cases involving dental metal fillings or skin invasion.

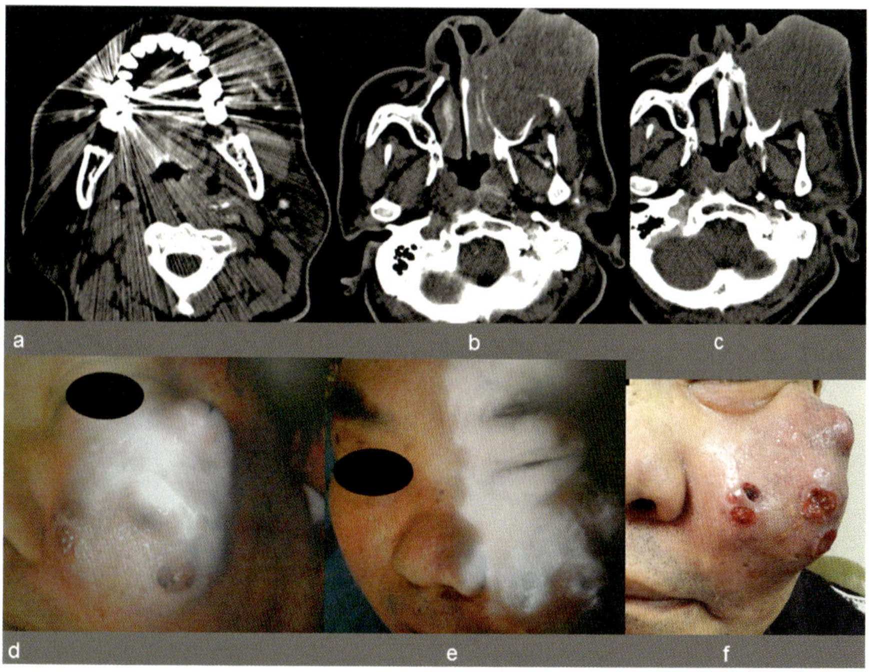

Fig. 5.6 CT angiography and ICG fluorescence imaging of maxillary cancer
(**a**) CT angiography obtained in the selected left side maxillary artery. It was difficult to confirm the vascular territory due to the presence of dental metals. (**b**) CT angiography obtained in the selected left side maxillary artery. It was difficult to confirm the vascular territory due to obstacle enhancement. (**c**) CT angiography obtained in the selected left side internal carotid artery. It was difficult to confirm the vascular territory due to obstacle enhancement. (**d**) ICG fluorescence imaging of the left maxillary artery. It was sufficiently clear to confirm the vascular territory. (**e**) ICG fluorescence imaging of the left internal carotid artery. Cancer involving the facial skin was clearly visible under fluorescent imaging of each vascular area. (**f**) Maxillary cancer invading the face before treatment

ICG fluorescence imaging combined with I-A chemotherapy compensated for the deficiencies of CT angiography for paranasal sinus cancer. ICG fluorescence provided greater clarity and more constructive information concerning the feeders to cancers (Fig. 5.6).

5.5.3 Discussion

Chemoradiotherapy for head and neck cancer plays an important role in organ preservation; nevertheless there are many cases, such as paranasal sinus cancer, for which conventional systemic chemotherapy does not work at all. For such chemo-resistant cancers including paranasal sinus cancer, superselective I-A chemotherapy is considered the most effective method by which to overcome these cancers due to increased concentrations of anticancer drugs in the cancer [11, 22–24]. To achieve effective therapeutic results for paranasal sinus cancer with I-A chemotherapy, precise evaluation of the tumor-feeding artery and drug distribution territories is required. CT angiography provides more precise identification of the blood supply to the tumor than digital subtraction angiography (DSA) [22, 25, 26, 32]. However, we are sometimes unable to confirm the tumor-feeding artery in paranasal sinus cancer patients with dental metal fillings or when the tumor has spread to oral cavities or superficially to the facial skin.

Recently the ICG fluorescence technique has been developed and applied to various fields [11, 30, 31]. We have reported that the ICG fluorescence technique can be a very useful method for treating oral cancers with I-A chemotherapy in patients with dental metal fillings [32]. We also reported our success in identifying the tumor-feeding arteries in paranasal sinus cancer by means of ICG fluorescence imaging. We found that the ICG fluorescence technique was a very useful method even in patients with dental metal fillings.

One of most problematic issues involving the application of I-A chemotherapy for advanced paranasal sinus cancers is that the tumors are often supplied by the internal carotid artery, and consequently, to prevent brain complications, I-A chemotherapies were previously not employed for such cases. However, tumors are often recurrences at the regions where CDDP is not administered by the internal carotid artery. These recurrent tumors in the skull base cannot be resected, and consequently, patient's prognosis is very poor. The development of ICG fluorescent image has enabled us to clearly detect tumor staining and evaluate the contribution to blood supplying for the tumor by the internal carotid artery. Minimal dose of CDDP via the internal carotid artery has enabled us to safely treat advanced paranasal sinus cancer, while improving patient prognosis and preserving organs.

5.6 Conclusion

ICG fluorescence imaging for intra-arterial chemotherapy reveals the blood supplies to paranasal sinus cancers more accurately than CT angiography, especially in cases of superficial spread or those involving dental metal. The application of ICG fluorescence together with CT angiography provides more accurate information about the feeding arteries to tumors and enables effective intra-arterial chemotherapy, while avoiding complications.

References

1. Morton DL, Wen DR, Wong JH et al (1992) Technical details of intraoperative lymphatic mapping for early stage melanoma. Arch Surg 127:392–399
2. Giuliano AE, Kirgan DM, Guenther JM et al (1994) Lymphatic mapping and sentinel Lymphadenectomy for breast cancer. Ann Surg 220:391–401
3. Morton DL, Thompson JF, Essner R et al (1999) Validation of the accuracy of intraoperative lymphatic mapping and sentinel lymphadenectomy for early-stage melanoma: a multicenter trial. Multicenter Selective Lymphadenectomy Trial Group. Ann Surg 230:453–463
4. Krag D, Weaver D, Ashikaga T et al (1998) The sentinel node in breast cancer – a multicenter validation study. N Engl J Med 339:941–946
5. Rinaldo A, Devaney KO, Ferlito A et al (2004) Immunohistochemical studies in the identification of lymph node micrometastases in patients with squamous cell carcinoma of the head and neck. ORL J Otorhinolaryngol Relat Spec 66:38–41
6. De Cicco C, Trifirò G, Calabrese L et al (2006) Lymphatic mapping to tailor selective lymphadenectomy in cN0 tongue carcinoma: beyond the sentinel node concept. Eur J Nucl Med Mol Imaging 33:900–905
7. Shah JP (1990) Patterns of cervical lymph node metastasis from squamous carcinomas of the upper aerodigestive tract. Am J Surg 160:405–409
8. Paleri V, Rees G, Arullendran P et al (2005) Sentinel node biopsy in squamous cell cancer of the oral cavity and oral pharynx: a diagnostic meta-analysis. Head Neck 27:739–747
9. Ross GL, Soutar DS, MacDonald DG et al (2004) Sentinel node biopsy in head and neck cancer: preliminary results of a multicenter trial. Ann Surg Oncol 11:690–696
10. Bredell MG (2010) Sentinel lymph node mapping by indocyanin green fluorescence imaging in oropharyngeal cancer – preliminary experience. Head Neck Oncol 2:31. doi:10.1186/1758-3284-2-31
11. Yokoyama J, Ito S, Ohba S et al (2011) A novel approach to translymphatic chemotherapy targeting sentinel lymph nodes of patients with oral cancer using intra-arterial chemotherapy-preliminary study. Head Neck Oncol 3:42
12. Carrau RL, Myers E, Johnson J (1990) Management of tumors arising in the parapharyngeal space. Laryngoscope 100:583–589
13. Yokoyama J, Ooba S, Fujimaki M et al (2014) Impact of indocyanine green fluorescent image-guided surgery for parapharyngeal space tumors. J Cranio-Maxillofacial Surg 42:835–838
14. Fujimaki M, Yokoyama J, Ohba S et al (2012) Dynamic imaging in determining the optimum surgical time for NIR fluorescent image-guided surgery. Head Neck Oncol 4:50
15. Desai SC, Sung CK, Genden EM (2008) Transoral robotic surgery using an image guidance system. Laryngoscope 118:2003e2005

16. Yokoyama J, Ohba S, Fujimaki M et al (2014) Impact of intra-arterial chemotherapy including internal carotid artery for advanced paranasal sinus cancers involving the skull base. Br J Cancer 1. doi: 10.1038/bjc.2014.501
17. Shiga K, Yokoyama J, Hashimoto S et al (2007) Combined therapy after superselective arterial cisplatin infusion to treat maxillary squamous cell carcinoma. Otolaryngol Head Neck Surg 136:1003–1009
18. Robbins KT (2000) The evolving role of combined modality therapy in head and neck cancer. Arch Otolaryngol Head Neck Surg 126:265–269
19. Yokoyama J, Ohba S, Ito S et al (2012) Impact of lymphatic chemotherapy targeting metastatic lymph nodes in patients with tongue cancer (T3, N2b, M0) using intra-arterial chemotherapy. Head Neck Oncol 4(2):64
20. Shimosato Y, Oboshi S, Baba K (1971) Histological evaluation of effects of radiotherapy and chemotherapy for carcinomas. Jpn J Clin Oncol 1:19–35
21. Matsuzuka T, Kano M, Ogawa H et al (2008) Sentinel node mapping for node positive oral cancer: potential to predict multiple metastasis. Laryngoscope 118(4):646–649
22. Kaketa S, Korogi Y, Miyaguni Y et al (2007) A cone-beam volume CT using a 3D angiography system with a flat panel detector of direct conversion type: usefulness for superselective intra-arterial chemotherapy for head and neck tumors. AJNR Am J Neuroradiol 28:1783–1788
23. Korogi Y, Hirai T, Nishimura R et al (1995) Superselective intraarterial infusion of cisplatin for squamous cell carcinoma of the mouth: preliminary clinical experience. AJR Am J Roentgenol 165:1269–1272
24. Bertino G, Benazzo M, Gatti P et al (2007) Curative and organ-preserving treatment with intra-arterial carboplatin induction followed by surgery and/or radiotherapy for advanced head and neck cancer: single-center five-year results. BMC Cancer 7:62
25. Yokoyama J (2002) Usefulness of CT-angiography for superselective intra-arterial chemotherapy for advanced head and neck cancers. Gan To Kagaku Ryoho 29:2302–2306
26. Miyayama S, Yamashiro M, Hattori Y et al (2002) Usefulness of C-arm CT during superselective infusion chemotherapy for advanced head and neck carcinoma. J Med Imaging Radiat Oncol 55:368–372
27. Hirai T, Korogi Y, Ono K et al (2001) Intra-arterial chemotherapy for locally advanced and/or recurrent hepatic tumors: evaluation of the feeding artery with an interventional CT system. Cardiovasc Intervent Radiol 24:176–179
28. Tomura N, Hashimoto M, Sashi R et al (1996) Superselective angio-CT of brain tumors. AJNR Am J Neuroradiol 17:1073–1080
29. Hirai T, Korogi Y, Ono K et al (2004) Preoperative embolization for meningeal tumors: evaluation of vascular supply with angio-CT. AJNR Am J Neuroradiol 25:74–76
30. Litvack ZN, Zada G, Laws ER Jr (2012) Indocyanine green fluorescence endoscopy for visual differentiation of pituitary tumor from surrounding structures. J Neurosurg 116:935–941
31. Shimada Y, Okumura T, Nagata T et al (2011) Usefulness of blood supply visualization by indocyanine green fluorescence during esophagectomy. Esophagus 8:259–266
32. Ohba S, Yokoyama J, Fujimaki M et al (2012) Significant improvement in superselective intra-arterial chemotherapy for oral cancer by using indocyanine green fluorescence. Oral Oncol 48:1101–1105
33. Yokoyama J, Ohba S, Fujimaki M et al (2012) Significant improvement in superselective intra-arterial chemotherapy for advanced paranasal sinus cancer by using Indocyanine green fluorescence. Eur Arch Otorhinolaryngol 271(10):2795–2801

Part IV
Cardiovascular Surgery

Chapter 6
Innovative SPY Intraoperative Imaging and Validation Technologies for Coronary Artery Bypass Graft Surgery

Masao Takahashi, Munetaka Masuda, Keisuke Miyajima, Toshihiro Ishikawa, Kazuyoshi Hatada, and Tsuyoshi Kobayashi

Abstract Off-pump Coronary Artery Bypass Graft (CABG) Surgery has rapidly increased in popularity, because of its less invasiveness and lower complication rates. However, graft patency rate highly depends on the operators' skill level due to technical difficulties associate with the technique.

The SPY® Intraoperative Imaging System ("SPY System") is an innovative device developed to assist surgeons in achieving 100 % graft patency. Introduced in 2002, the authors were the first site in the Asia-Pacific region to use the SPY system, as a noninvasive imaging device for intraoperative graft validation. After injection of Indocyanine Green (ICG) dye via a central venous line, real-time graft images can be obtained, without catheter insertion, X-rays, or iodine contrast media.

High contrast quality SPY images could be obtained in all 1921 distal anastomoses performed during 579 off-pump CABG cases. Twenty-four anastomoses (1.2 %) were revised intraoperatively, because of unfavorable SPY images. All revised grafts revealed patent in the post-CABG catheter angiography or 64-slice MDCT.

Using the SPY system, technical failures could be completely resolved before closing the chest incision. All heart team staff members can always monitor the surgeon's skill during surgery using the SPY system to assess graft patency much like assessing the interventionist's technique during PCI in the catheterization lab. We conclude that the use of SPY in the operating room eliminates the need for invasive post-CABG angiography except in the rare instance of symptomatic

---

M. Takahashi, M.D., Ph.D. (✉) • K. Miyajima
Department of Cardiovascular Surgery, Hiratsuka Kyosai Heart Center, 9-11 Oiwake, Hiratsuka, Kanagawa 254-8502, Japan
e-mail: airdonut@nifty.com

M. Masuda
Department of Surgery, Yokohama City University Hospital, Kanagawa, Japan

T. Ishikawa • K. Hatada
Department of Cardiovascular Surgery, Odawara Municipal Hospital, Kanagawa, Japan

T. Kobayashi
Clinical Engineering Section, Hiratsuka Kyosai Heart Center, Kanagawa, Japan

M. Kusano et al. (eds.), *ICG Fluorescence Imaging and Navigation Surgery*,
DOI 10.1007/978-4-431-55528-5_6

or eventful patients. The use of the SPY system for intraoperative graft validation during CABG may become the golden standard.

Keywords Off-pump CABG • Intraoperative graft assessment • Indocyanine green (ICG) • Intraoperative fluorescence imaging (IFI)

6.1 Introduction

A surgery, in general, is quite invasive however patients typically tolerate to some extent an incision made to his or her body. Nevertheless, the evolution of minimally invasive surgery has been one of the predomiant themes for surgeons in the twenty-first century. Ever since Dr. Ludwig Rehn [1] performed the first successful human heart surgery in 1896 in Frankfurt, it had been believed that cardiac surgery was the furthest from its application to the minimally invasive surgery. In 1996, however, minimally invasive direct coronary artery bypass (MIDCAB) was introduced in Japan, which opened the door to the minimally invasive cardiac surgery [2]. The MIDCAB procedure enabled cardiac surgeons to approach the epicardial coronary artery and perform an anastomosis on a beating-heart without using a cardiopulmonary bypass machine. MIDCAB acceptance became rapidly widespread in Japan because it was viewed as less invasive to the patient. In 1998, similarly, the safe approach to the coronary arteries located in the anterior and posterior regions of the heart through a median full sternotomy without the use of cardiopulmonary bypass pump was well established. This technique resulted in more than a 60 % of the adoption rate for off-pump coronary artery bypass grafting (OPCAB) throughout Japan [3] (Fig. 6.1).

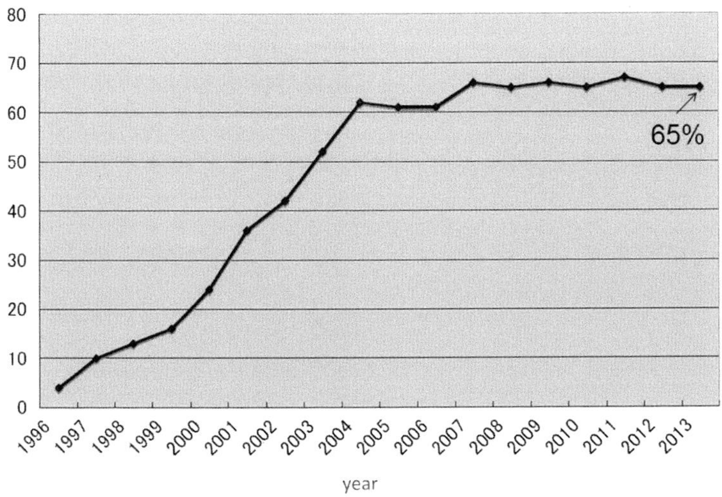

Fig. 6.1 Changes in OPCAB frequency rate of initial elective CABG in Japan

Since off-pump CABG is considered to be a more technically demanding surgery than traditional CABG, graft patency rate highly depends on the surgeon's skill level. The method for the graft assessment was either intraoperative angiography using portable digital subtraction angiography (DSA) or postoperative catheter angiography, both of which involve X-ray radiation exposure for the patient and staff members, potantial renal injury to patients due to the use of iodinated contrast media, and other complications due to the need for percutaneus catheter insertion. Furthermore, even if postoperative angiography were to comfirm graft occlusion, it would be impossible to immediately reopen the patient's chest to repair the technical graft failure. The SPY System (Novadaq Technologies Inc., Toronto, Canada) is the first commercially available fluorescence angiographic device which allows surgeons to assess the bypassed graft during the operation while the chest is still open without the concerns for radiation exposure or potentially harmful contrast agents. Intraoperative finding of technical errors using SPY system enables surgeons to revise the graft anastomosis during the operation.

6.2 About SPY System

The trend for the treatment of coronary artery diseases has been shifting from surgical CABG to percutaneous catheter intervention (PCI) with drug-eluting stents. The main reason for shifting to PCI may be its less invasiveness and immediate visual confirmation of the effectiveness of the treatment during its procedure through the use of X-ray angiography in the catheterization laboratory. As shown in Fig. 6.2, successful results can be confirmed quickly and easily during PCI; however, traditionally graft patency or

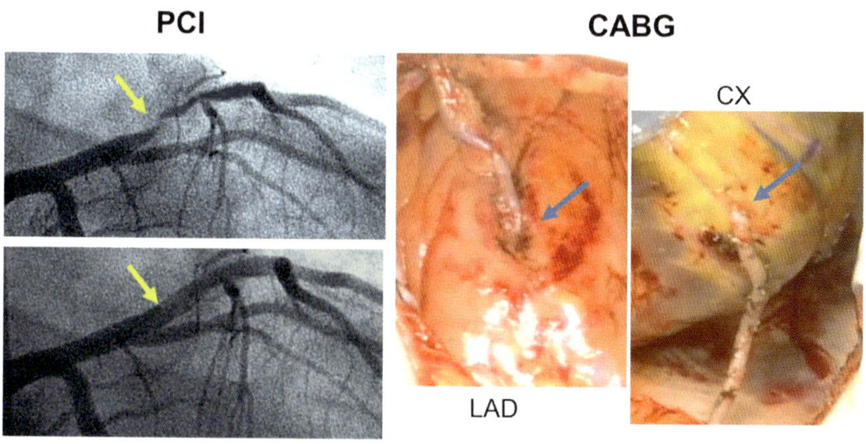

Fig. 6.2 Differences between PCI and CABG
Left: In PCI, blood flow and a successful result can be recognized at a glance using X-ray angiography.
Right: In CABG, using the human eye we can see there is no bleeding at the site of the graft anastomosis, but we cannot assess the quality of blood flow within the graft or graft patency

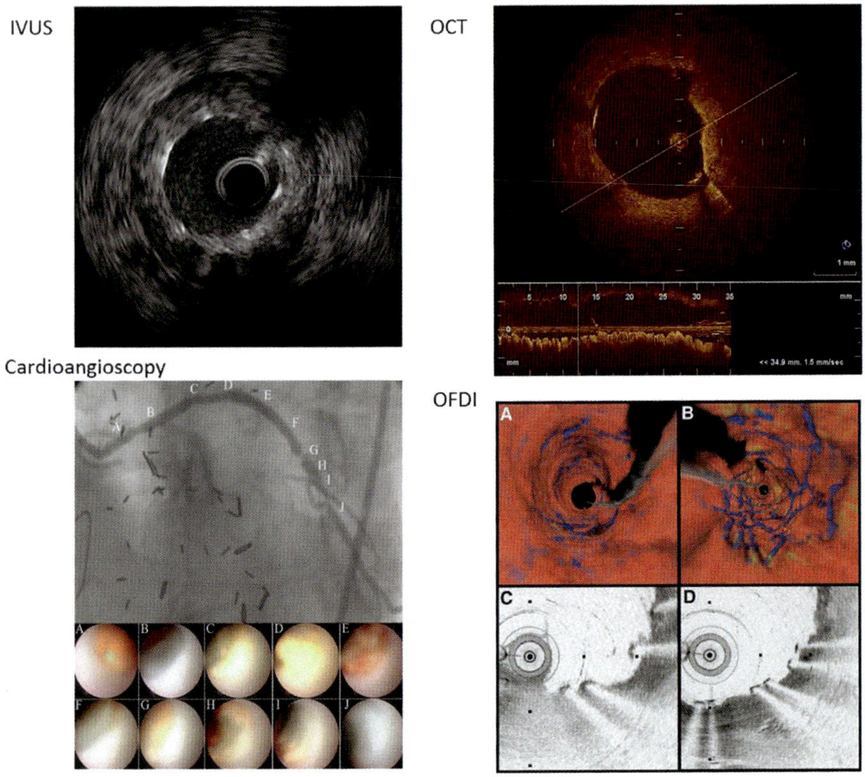

Fig. 6.3 Various imaging methods support procedure success in PCI

blood flow cannot be seen without significant difficulty during CABG surgery. Moreover, angiographic confirmation of the results of PCI can be seen by the human eye, but anastomotic quality and blood flow through a graft cannot be seen by the surgeon's eyes alone during CABG. In addition, there are other kinds of complementary technologies which can be used during PCI to evaluate the success of the procedure, such as intravascular ultrasound (IVUS), optimal coherence tomography (OCT), cardioangioscopy, and optical frequency domain imaging (OFDI) (Fig. 6.3).

In order to make CABG a standard treatment option for the coronary artery diseases, it has been believed that highly useful intraoperative graft assessment tools are essential to sustain higher rates of graft patency. With the exception of X-ray angiography which is extremely difficult to use during CABG, there had never been reliable easy to use tools to visualize blood flow in the native coronary arteries and bypass graft particularly under the beating-heart OPCAB circumstance. The SPY system (Fig. 6.4) is an innovative intraoperative graft patency assessment device that is ideal for use during both traditional CABG and OPCAB because of its ease of use and reliability. The SPY system was first introduced to the Asia Pacific region and to this author in 2002 [4, 5]. Since that time, the system has been further developed to improve the quality of the image, the ease of image capture, to provide objective analysis tools and to add other features that meet the needs of surgery.

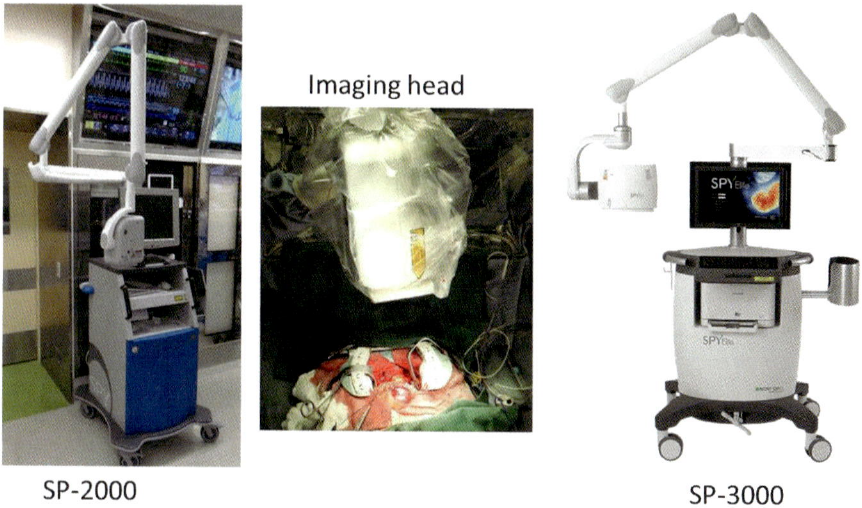

Fig. 6.4 SPY Intraoperative Imaging System
Left: First generation SPY system (SP-2000)
Center: In surgery, the imaging head is draped fixed 30 cm above the heart
Right: The latest generation SPY system (SP-3000)

The main characteristics of SPY system are:

1. It enables surgeons to visually assess blood flow in vessels and graft patency immediately after the anastomosis is created.
2. The real-time image of flow through the graft is equal or even superior to an X-ray angiogram.
3. It does not involve the need for catheter insertion, ionizing radiation exposure or potentially nephrotoxic contrast media.

How to capture SPY image:

1. After creating the anastomosis, the camera head is positioned approximately 30 cm above the area of the interest (Fig. 6.4 center).
2. 0.5 ~ 1.0 ml of 20 times diluted indocyanine green (ICG, 1.25 mg/ml) is injected through the central venous line followed by a 10 ml brisk bolus of saline (Fig. 6.5).
3. 10 ml of saline flush was administrated as a bolus injection following the ICG into the right atrium to ensure rapid circulation of the ICG. (Fig. 6.5).
4. High quality fluorescence image will then be shown up on the monitor in a few seconds.
5. ICG is excreted by the liver unchanged into the bile; hence, it does not have a negative affect on kidney function.

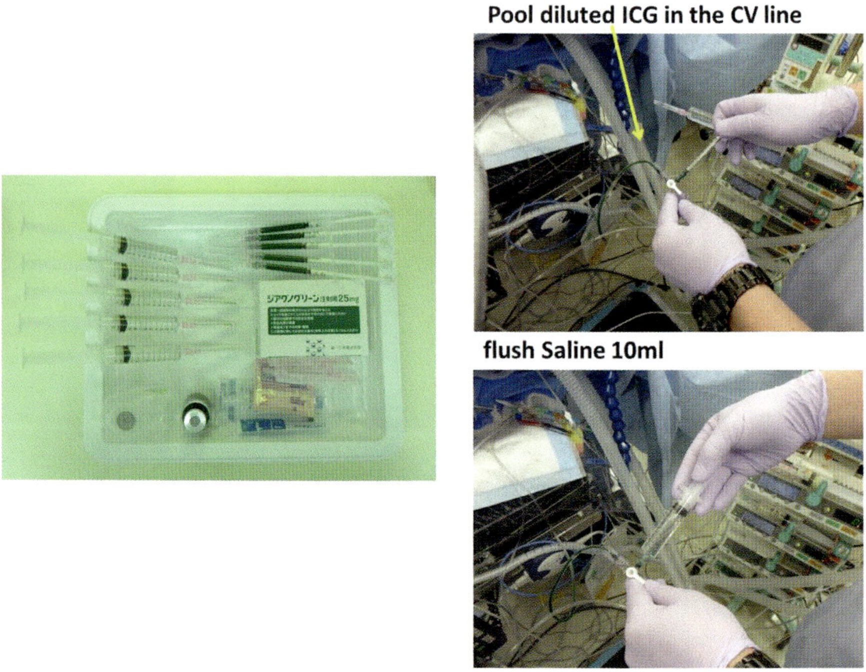

Fig. 6.5 How to inject the ICG imaging agent
Left: Prepare the required number of 0.5 ml or 1.0 ml of ICG diluted with 10 ml of aqueous solvent in 1.0 ml syringes and 10 ml of saline syringes for immediate bolus flush are prepared for SPY imaging
Right: Administer the diluted ICG in the central venous line, and flush it using 10 ml of saline

6. SPY imaging is used not only to assess the graft and coronary arteries, it is possible to detect and verify the course of coronary veins of less than 0.5mm diameter.
7. SPY imaging does not involve X-ray, but instead relies upon a laser (averaged output of 2.0 watt) to excite ICG which absorbs and emits light at 830nm which is then captured by the system's CCD camera and the video output is displayed on the monitor.

The adverse drug reaction rate of ICG has been known to be much lower than the conventional iohexol iodine contrast media (Table 6.1), and it has been reported to be safely usable.

Image sequences of this ICG fluorescence imaging (Fig. 6.6) are captured and saved in the computer of the SPY system in either AVI or MPEG format. The latest version of SPY system allows saving the sequences in compressed DICOM format, which enables the users to export the data of more than 20 patients into one CD-R.

Table 6.1 Adverse drug reaction (ADR) reporting rate comparison between iodine contrast media and ICG

	Contrast media (iohexol)	ICG
ADR reporting no./total no.	452/17,039	36/21,278
ADR %	2.65 %	0.17 %
Cardiovascular ADR %	0.33 %	0.023 %

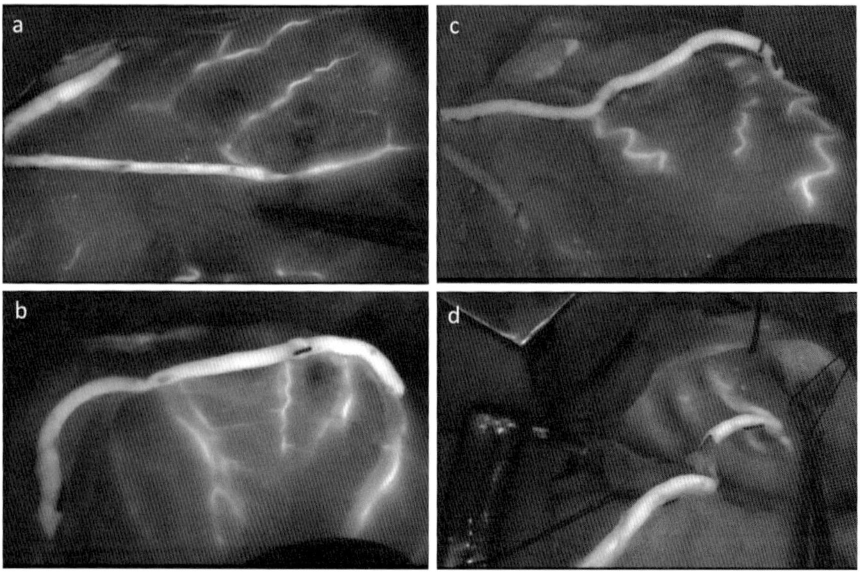

Fig. 6.6 Intraoperative SPY images
High quality graft images can be obtained wherever the distal anastomoses are performed in anterior, lateral, or inferior wall
(**a**) LITA-LAD, (b) SVG-HL-OM-PL, (**c**) RA-HL-OM, d GEA-4PD

6.3 Intraoperative SPY Images and Postoperative Angiography or MDCT

Several SPY system images utilizing the fluorescence properties of ICG were provided here (Figs. 6.7, 6.8, 6.9, and 6.10). The image quality of SPY system's fluorescence angiogram including the internal thoracic artery (ITA), the sequential graft of radial artery (RA), saphenous vein graft (SVG), and gastroepiploic artery (GEA) is excellent. The quality of the SPY image appears equivalent to the conventional X-ray angiogram [6–10]. The actual real time moving SPY image sequences available on the SPY system monitor at the time of surgery are of even higher quality that those that can be published in this textbook. The blood flow inside the patet graft is highly visible. The head camera of the SPY system can rotate freely so that the circumflex (CX) site and the distal site of the right coronary artery (RCA) can be also visible. As shown in Fig. 6.11, similar images can be revealed between intraoperative SPY image and postoperative MDCT scanning.

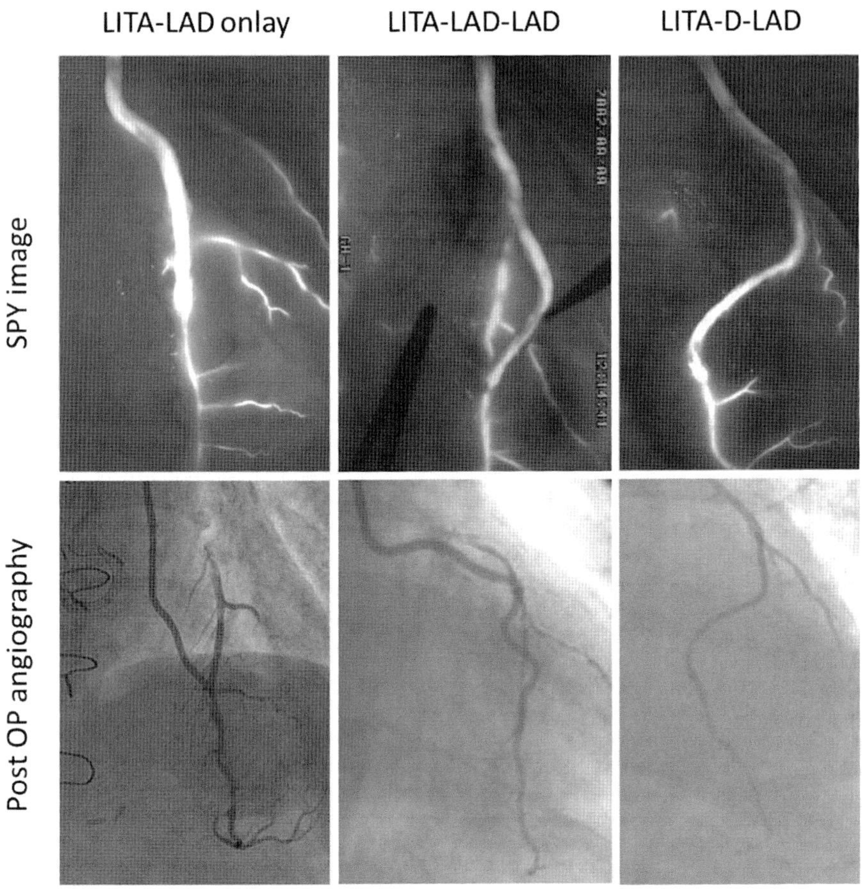

Fig. 6.7 SPY images and postoperative angiography of the left internal thoracic artery (LITA) graft
Almost same images could be seen in both SPY and angiography
Left: LITA-LAD on-lay patch graft
Middle: LTA-LAD-LAD sequential graft
Right: LITA-Diagonal-LAD sequential graft

6.4 Usefulness of the SPY System

Using the SPY system, we can revise a failed graft as soon as possible in the operation room while the chest is still open. Technical failures can be almost avoided through the use of the SPY system.

Figure 6.12 shows the tremendous effectiveness of the SPY system. Off-pump CABG with four anastomoses was performed in an 88-year-old female patient. Transit time flow measurement (TTFM) indicated an adequate flow (22 ml/min) on the sequential left ITA graft to the diagonal and on to the LAD. The SPY image, however, showed occlusion of the ITA graft between the diagonal and the LAD

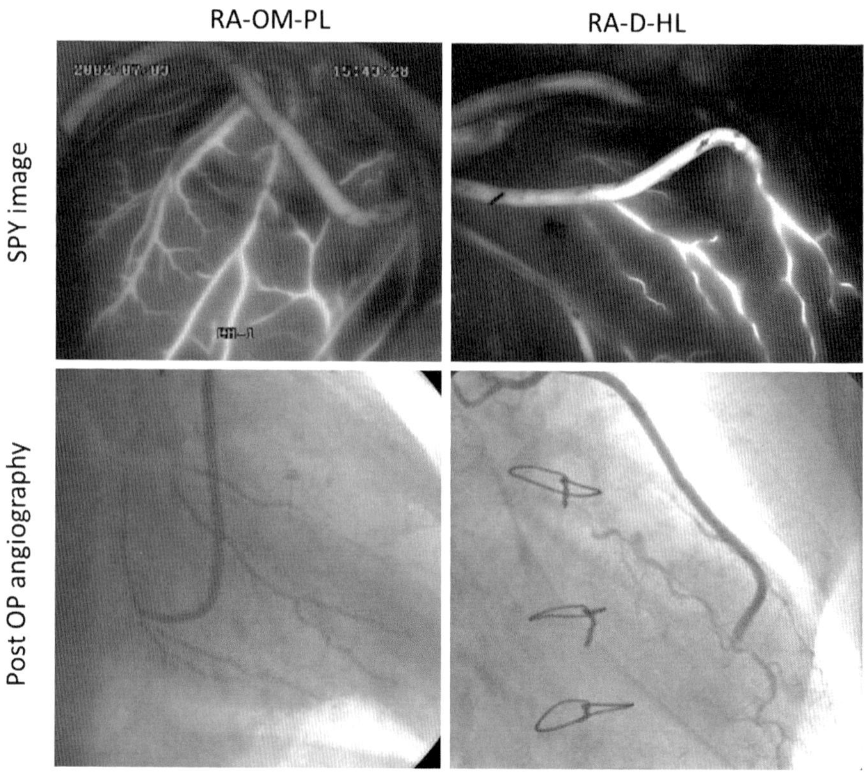

Fig. 6.8 SPY images and postoperative angiography of the radial artery (RA) graft
Left: RA-OM-PL sequential graft
Right: RA-Diagonal-HL sequential graft

(Fig. 6.12a). Following the revision of the anastomosis to the diagonal artery, excellent flow to the LAD could be observed (Fig. 6.12b). Detection of graft occlusion with the SPY system significantly affected the patient's prognosis. In fact, the patient lived to the age of 98 years old.

Effectiveness of the SPY system is also shown in Fig. 6.13. A 66-year-old male patient underwent emergency off-pump CABG with five distal anastomoses due to acute coronary syndrome. SVG graft was anastomosed from the aorta to the distal RCA sequentially. TTFM showed quite favorable diastolic flow waveform, but the SPY system image suggested that there was an occlusion of the SVG graft between 4PD and 4AV (Fig. 6.13 Left). After the revision of the 4AV anastomosis, the SPY system showed good fluorescence images of blood flow through the graft (Fig. 6.13 Right). The surgeon was able to close the chest with strong belief that there was no need for further revision of the anastomosis. The follow-up angiography at 1 year after surgery revealed good patency of the revised graft (Fig. 6.13 Lower).

In Fig. 6.14, LITA was anastomosed to the very thin chronic total occluded LAD less than 1 mm in a diameter. The SPY image could detect the toe-site occlusion of the LITA graft, although TTFM showed adequate flow (34ml/min). After revision,

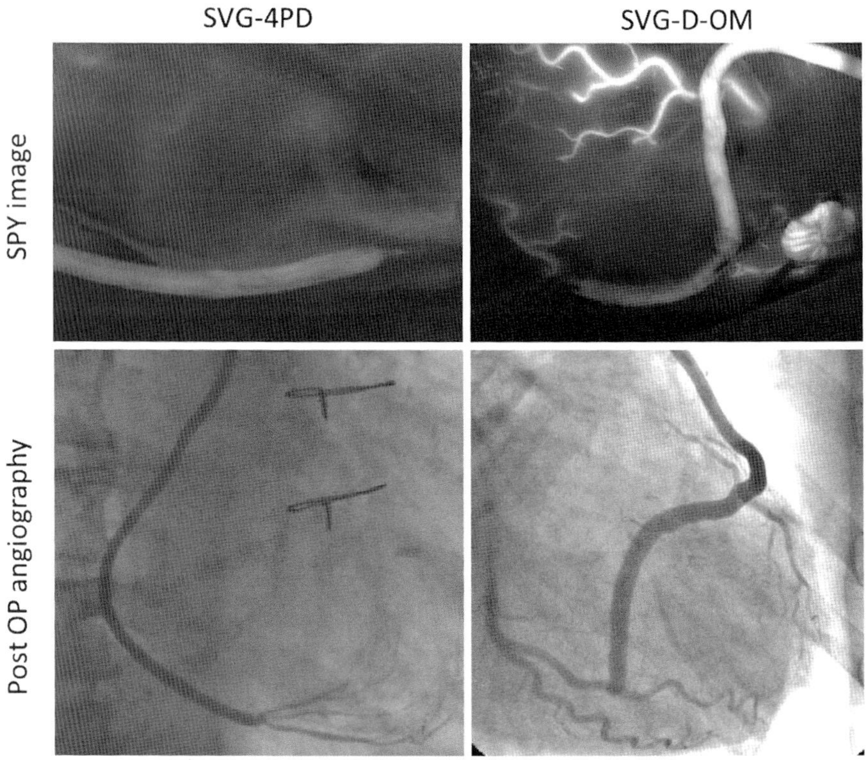

Fig. 6.9 SPY images and postoperative angiography of the saphenous vein graft (SVG)
Left: SVG-4PD
Right: SVG-Diagonal-OM sequential graft

the distal flow of the LITA to LAD was visible, and the TTFM increased up to 40 ml/min. Postoperative angiography showed a patent LITA to LAD graft.

A female patient who received steroids for a long period of time underwent LITA to LAD grafting via MIDCAB procedure. SPY detected retrograde dissection of the LITA graft as Fig. 6.15 Upper. Drastic change to the grafting operative plan was made and a radial artery graft from left axillary artery to the LAD was performed.

Thus, the clinical benefits of SPY system are summarized as follows:

1. The SPY system allows surgeons to intraoperatively identify bypass graft technical failure and to revise the anastomosis accordingly.
2. SPY allows surgeons to visualize the graft anastomoses to determine the need to perform graft revision.
3. It allows the surgeons to share visual information about intraoperative graft patency with the patients and his or her family just after the surgery.

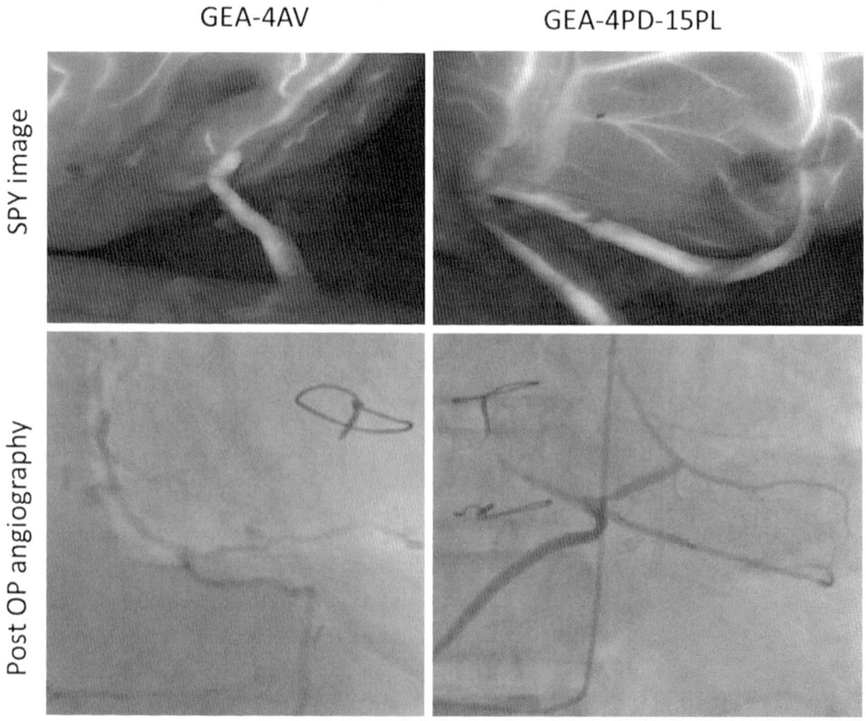

Fig. 6.10 SPY images and postoperative angiography of the gastroepiploic artery (GEA) graft
Left: GEA-4AV
Right: GEA-4PD-15PL sequential graft

6.5 Our Experiences Using SPY System

Since March 2002, off -pump CABG with SPY intraoperative graft validation was performed in 579 cases (Table 6.2). Total numbers of the distal anastomoses equaled 1921, and all anastomoses were evaluated using the SPY system.

In these series, 24 distal anastomoses could be revised intraoperatively, due to unfavorable SPY images (Table 6.3). That was 4.1 % of the total off-pump CABG cases and 1.2 % of the total numbers of distal anastomoses. Patency of revised grafts was confirmed in all cases by postoperative angiography or coronary CT scanning.

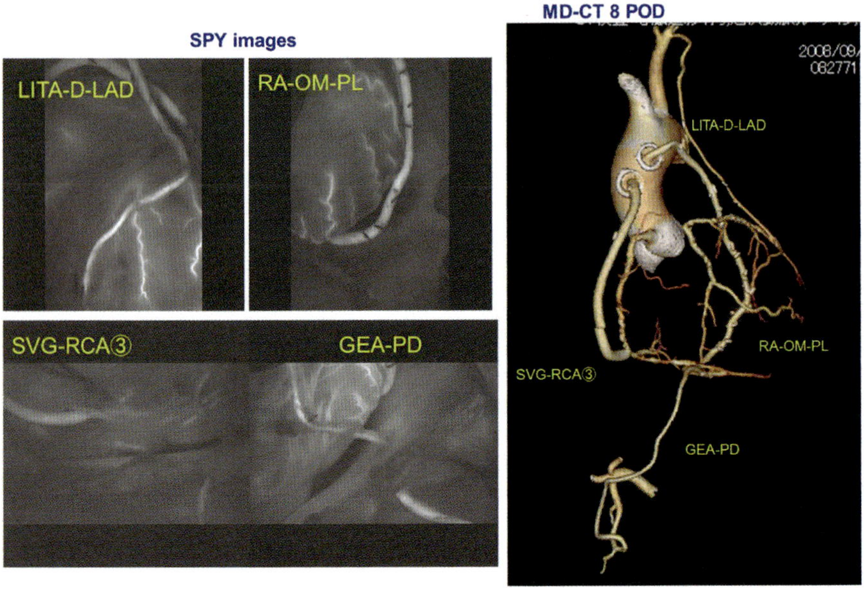

Fig. 6.11 SPY images and postoperative MDCT
Similar images could be seen in both SPY and MDCT

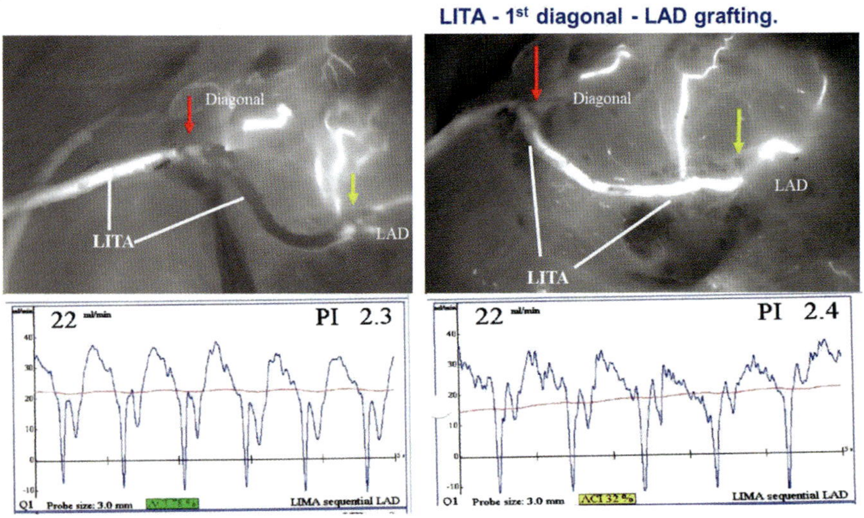

Fig. 6.12 Efficacy of the SPY system (LITA-diagonal sequential graft)
Left: SPY detected ITA graft occlusion between diagonal and LAD, although TTFM indicated an adequate flow
Right: After revision, excellent flow to the LAD could be observed

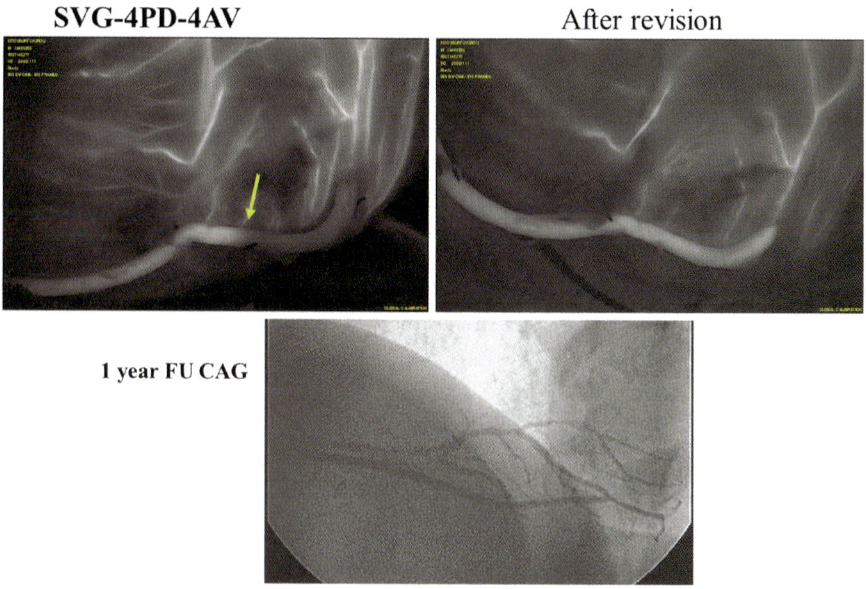

Fig. 6.13 Effectiveness of the SPY system (SVG-4PD-4AV sequential graft)
Left: SPY system detected occlusion of the SVG between 4PD and 4AV
Right: After revision, good blood flow could be obtained
Lower: Graft angiography 1 year after the surgery revealed good patency of the graft

6.6 The World's First Two Cases with Nine-Anastomosis Off-Pump CABG

In 2003, two cases received nine bypass grafting during off-pump CABG. They were the world's first two reported cases of maximum distal anastomoses in off-pump CABG. The first case was a 74-year-old male patient. Graft designs were LITA-Diag-LAD, RA-HL-OM-PL, RA-4PD-4PD-4AV, and RITA-RV branch. Intraoperative SPY angiography gave us confidence that all the grafts were patent. Ten years after surgery, all bypass grafts were still patent by coronary CT (Figs. 6.16, 6.17, and 6.18).

Another case was a 67-year-old male. Grafts were LITA-Diag1-Diag2-LAD, RA-HL-OM-CX, and RA-RV-4PD-15PL. Coronary CT 10 years after the surgery showed all of the grafts were patent (Figs. 6.19 and 6.20).

Using SPY system, we can completely avoid intraoperative technical failure. Consequently, long-term graft patency can be obtained like these cases.

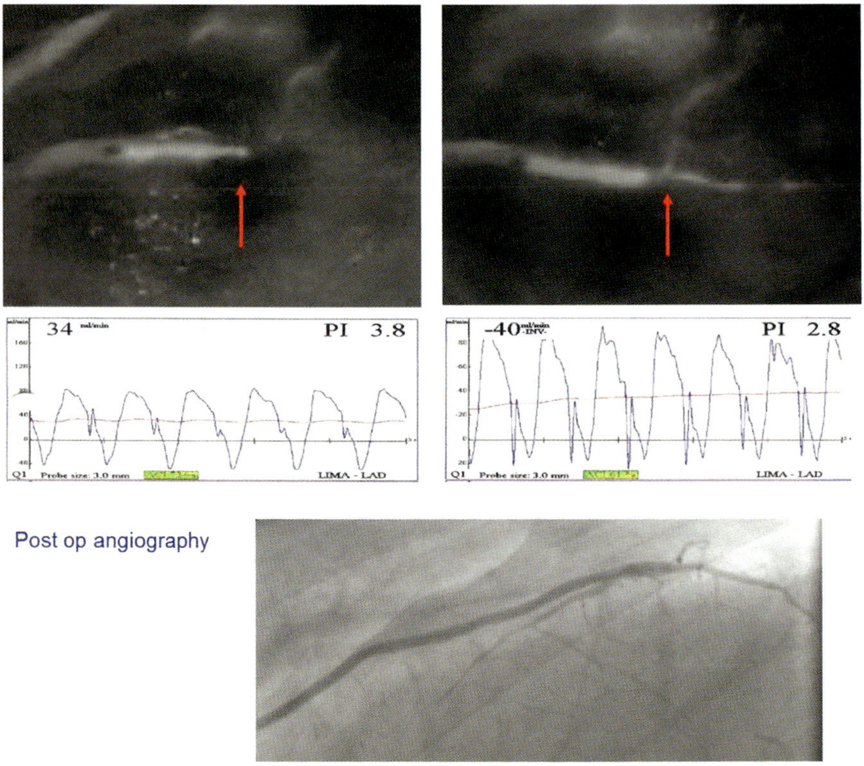

Fig. 6.14 Efficacy of the SPY system (LITA-LAD graft)
Left: SPY detected the toe-site occlusion of the LITA graft
Right: After revision, toe site can be visible, and TTFM flow increased
Lower: Postoperative angiography revealed excellent patency

6.7 Intraoperative Graft Assessment Tools Comparison

There have been several conventional methods for the intraoperative graft assessment such as:

1. Transit time flowmeter (TTFM)
2. Echo
3. IRIS (thermographic technology)
4. Portable DSA

However, there has been no graft assessment tool which is less invasive and fully visually assisted. Intraoperative graft assessment needs to be performed on each anastomosis during the peformance of every CABG operation, and in this way an echo, IRIS, and portable DSA are not really a convenient method. TTFM is a simple and convenient tool for the graft assessment, but it occasionally shows false

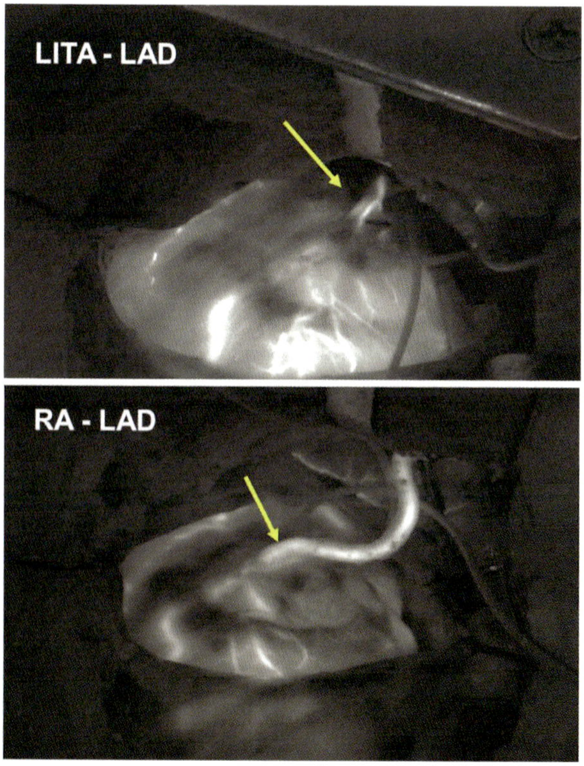

Fig. 6.15 Critical case of the MIDCAB
Upper: Retrograde dissection of the LITA anastomosis could be detected by the SPY image
Lower: After revision of the LAD anastomosis using the radial artery, an excellent image was obtained. The inflow of the radial artery was placed on the left axillary artery

Table 6.2 Case number using SPY system from March 2002 to December 2014

Off-pump CABG no.	579
MIDCAB/OPCAB	126/453
Age	69.2 +/− 9.5
Gender (f/m)	140/439
Total no. of distal anastomoses	1921
Mean distal anastomoses MIDCAB/OPCAB	1.5/3.8
Arrested CABG	6
Combined CABG with valve, aorta, LV	86

Table 6.3 Intraoperative graft revision due to unfavorable SPY image

Revision	/Cases	/Distal anastomosis
Total off pump	24/579, 4.1 %	24/1921, 1.2 %
MIDCAB	2/126, 1.6 %	2/184, 1.1 %
OPCAB	22/453, 4.9 %	22/1737, 1.3 %

positive. Therefore, the SPY system, which allows surgeons to identify any technical error related to the graft anastomosis and in which surgeons can visually confirm the patency of the graft. By reviewing a SPY movie sequence, makes it a unique and extremely efficient graft assessment tool (Table 6.4).

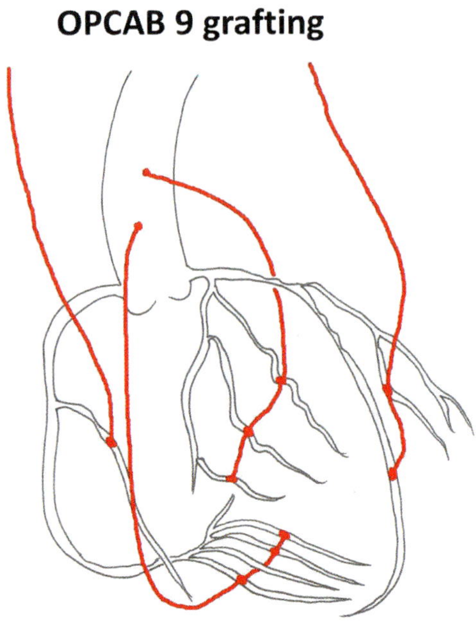

Fig. 6.16 Operative strategy of the OPCAB, nine grafting in a 74-year-old male patient

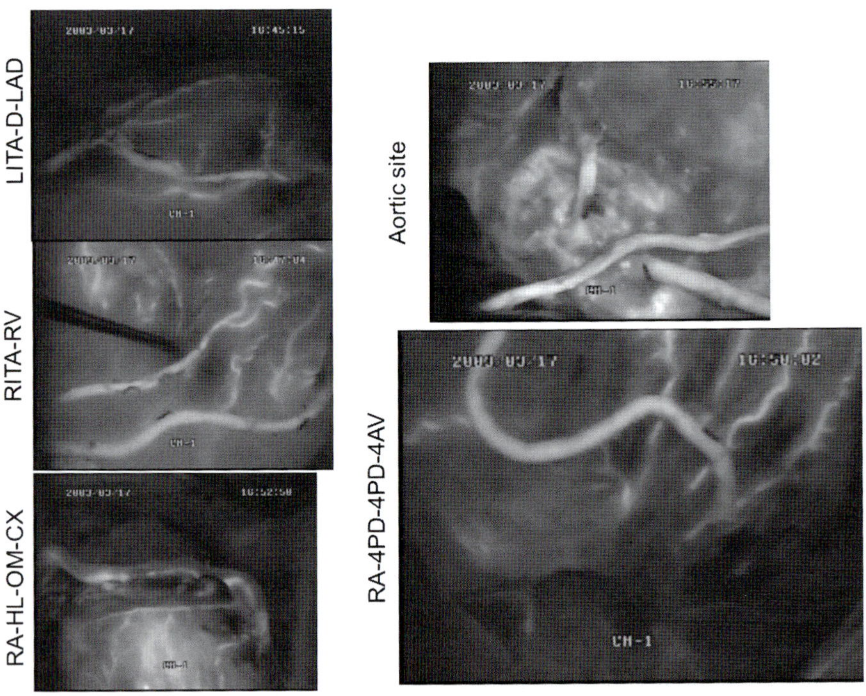

Fig. 6.17 SPY Intraoperative Imaging System could show all grafts patency
Especially, RA sequential graft to three distal right coronary arteries was shown excellent clear image

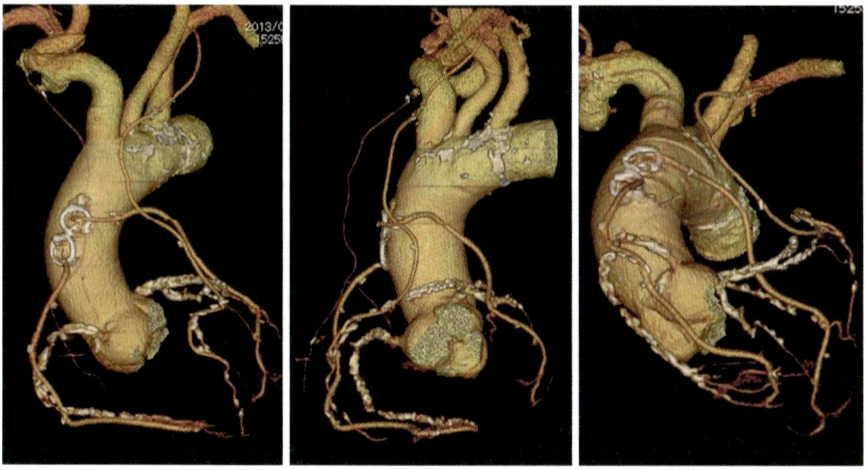

Fig. 6.18 Coronary CT scanning 10 years after surgery showed all patent grafts

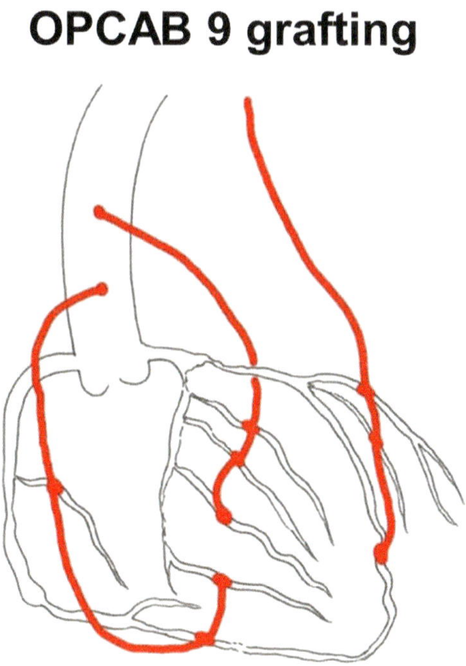

Fig. 6.19 Operative strategy of the OPCAB, nine grafting in a 67-year-old male patient

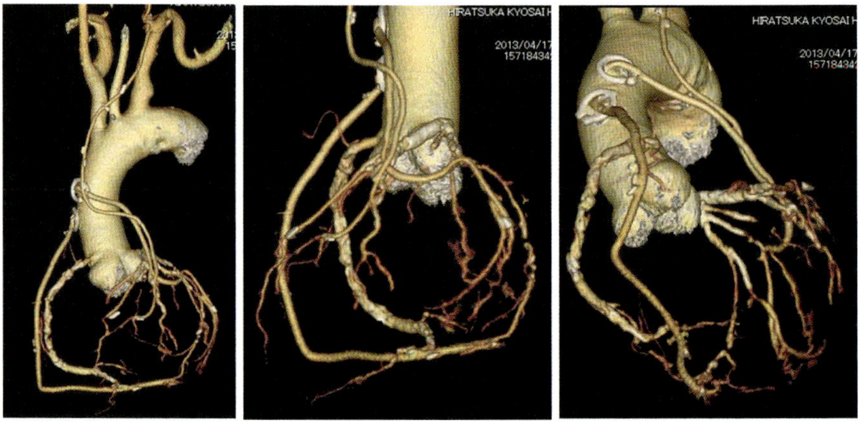

Fig. 6.20 Coronary CT scanning 10 years after surgery showed all patent grafts

Table 6.4 Comparison of intraoperative graft validation method

Method		Pros	Cons	Evaluation
TTFM	Quantification	Easy to use	Non-visually assisted	○
Echo	Visual assessment	Noninvasive	Not suitable for posterior wall	△
IRIS	Visual assessment	Noninvasive	Not clear Not suitable for posterior wall	△
Portable DSA	Visual assessment	Clear	Quite invasive	△
SPY system	Visual assessment	Noninvasive Clear	Needs graft skeletonization	◎

6.8 SPY System for Arrested Heart

Another examples highlighting the usefulness of the SPY system can be shown (Fig. 6.21) in arrested heart CABG surgery. In Fig. 6.21 left, diluted ICG with blood was injected directly from the proximal site of the saphenous vein graft. In Fig. 6.21 right, ICG was injected into the arterial filter of the cardiopulmonary bypass pump machine, and then LITA-LAD could be clearly shown.

6.9 DICOM Movie Network System

It is very essential to record and document any patients' intraoperative surgical data. The first generation of SPY system records its movie file of the fluorescence images with AVI file format, and the image can be exported only to CD-R. Each AVI file image has approximately 360 MB capacity, and it has not been convenient for the

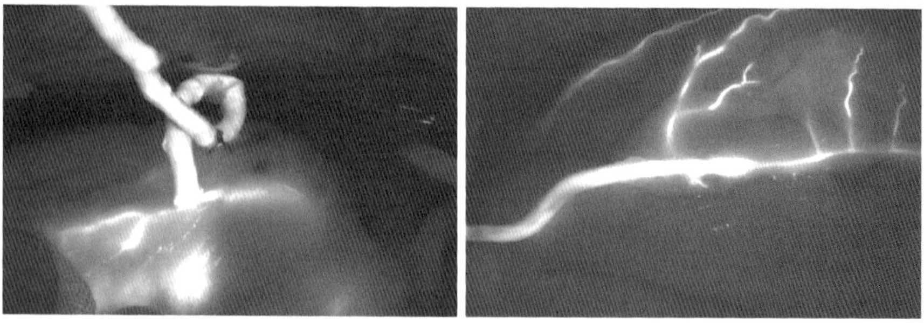

Fig. 6.21 SPY Intraoperative Imaging System for the arrested heart CABG surgery
Left: ICG diluted with blood was injected from the proximal saphenous vein graft
Right: ICG was injected into the arterial filter of the cardiopulmonary bypass machine

surgeons to show the intraoperative angiography images as a proof of the graft patency to the patients' family or referring physicians. The new operating SPY system software is now available with the excellent file compression with the file conversion from AVI to the compressed DICOM file format. As a result, moving image sequences can be now saved and exported into CD-R or other archiving programs.

We import SPY angiogram images through CD to our internal hospital network system and demonstrate its fluorescence images of each graft anastomosis to the patients' family immediately after the operation (Fig. 6.22). With the SPY system, surgeons can confirm the graft patency during the CABG procedure just as the interventional cardiologists can see the immediate result of PCI procedures. So, our explanation to the patients' family goes, thanks to this SPY system, "we have done XXX (number of anastomosis and) grafts and all of them were patent," while it used to be simply "we have done XXX (number of anastomosis) grafts." SPY system is a noninvasive, novel, and the most useful intraoperative graft assessment device.

6.10 Future Directions

The SPY system has been used to quantify perfusion improvements and image competitive flow. Because the intensity of fluorescence in a SPY image can be correlated with the volume of blood flow in an area, the SPY system and an investigational version of the SPY-Q analytical software, developed by Novadaq Technologies, Inc., can be used to compare epicardial blood flow before and after a bypass graft in a given segment of myocardium. To measure the perfusion improvement conferred by the bypass, the surgeon takes pre-bypass and post-bypass myocardial perfusion SPY images. Using the investigational analytical software (SPY-Q) in the SPY system, the surgeon compares the pre- and post-graft images using the criteria of fluorescence intensity (Fig. 6.23). In a series of 167 patients and

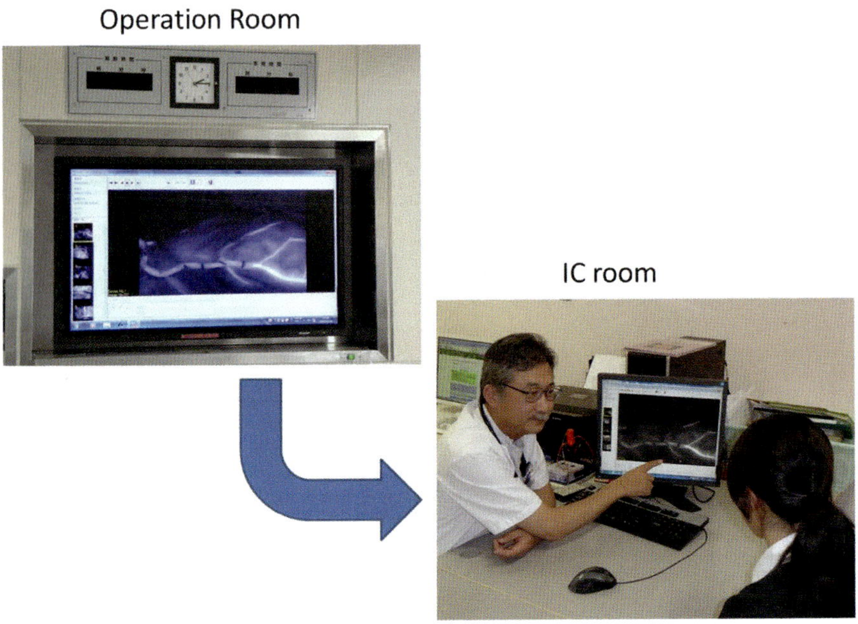

Fig. 6.22 SPY system and DICOM movie network system
DICOM movie file can be incorporated into the DICOM movie network system. We can show the SPY images to the patient's family, just after the surgery in the informed consent room

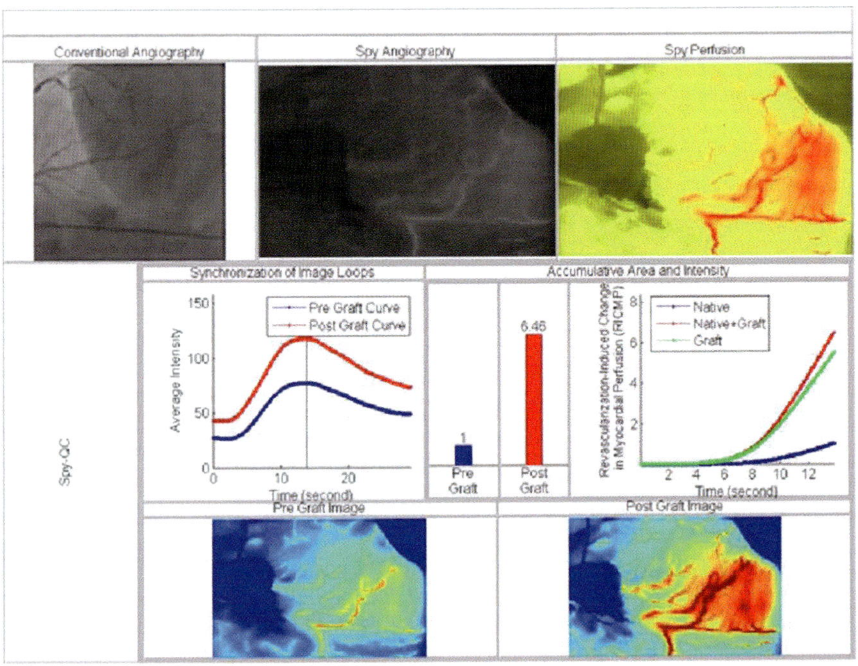

Fig. 6.23 SPY-Q analysis of LITA-LAD bypass graft demonstrating a significant improvement in post-graft tissue perfusion

359 grafts performed by T. Bruce Ferguson, Jr, MD, et al., all grafts were patent by SPY image, but 24 % of the arterial and 22 % of the saphenous vein grafts conferred no regional myocardial perfusion improvement. As more experience is gained with SPY and its analytic capabilities, surgeons may be better able to determine regional perfusion improvements offered by each graft, allowing surgeons to offer more or fewer grafts in each myocardial segment and provide the optimal revascularization procedure for each patient [11].

6.11 Conclusion

The SPY system produces real time images that can clearly show the quality of blood flow through native vessels and bypass grafts. SPY allow surgeons to assess graft patency and resolve technical graft failures before the chest is closed. The heart team staff members can also monitor the quality of the bypass grafts created during surgery in much the same way as the catheterization lab staff can assess the outcomes during PCI. We conclude that the need for invasive post-CABG X-ray angiography may be eliminated or needed only for a few symptomatic or eventful patients. The use of the SPY system for intraoperative graft validation during traditional CABG and OPCAB may become the golden standard.

References

1. Rehn L (1897) Ueber Penetrierende Herzwunden und Herznaht. Arch Klin Chir 55:315
2. Masuda M, Morita S, Tomita H et al (2002) Off-pump CABG attenuates myocardial enzyme leakage but not postoperative brain natriuretic peptide secretion. Ann Thorac Cardiovasc Surg 8:139–144
3. Japanese Associate for Coronary Artery Surgery (JACAS) Coronary Artery Surgery Results 2013, in Japan. Ann Thorac Cardiovasc Surg. 2014; 20(4):332–4. doi: 10.5761/atcs.sr.13-00001
4. Takahashi M, Ishikawa T, Higashidani K et al (2003) Off-pump coronary artery bypass grafting using DONUT and SPY. Kyobu Geka 56:611–618
5. Takahashi M, Ishikawa T, Higashidani K et al (2004) SPY™: an innovative intra-operative imaging system to evaluate graft patency during off pump coronary artery bypass grafting. Interact Cardiovasc Thorac Surg 3:479–483
6. Waseda K, Fitzgerald PJ, Takahashi M (2008) Intraoperative assessment of coronary grafts with fluorescent angiography. Heart 94:64
7. Waseda K, Ako J, Hasegawa T et al (2009) Intraoperative fluorescence imaging system for on-site assessment of off-pump coronary artery bypass graft. J AM Coll Imag 2:604–612
8. Honda Y, Fitzgerald PJ (2008) Frontiers in intravascular imaging technologies. Circulation 117(15):2024–2037
9. Rubens FD, Ruel M, Fremes SE (2002) A new and simplified method for coronary and graft imaging during CABG. Heart Surg Forum 5:141–144

10. Taggart DP, Choudhary B, Anastasiadis K et al (2003) Preliminary experience with a novel intraoperative fluorescence imaging technique to evaluate the patency of bypass grafts in total arterial revascularization. Ann Thorac Surg 75:870–873
11. Ferguson TB Jr, Chen C, Babb J et al (2013) Fractional flow reserve guided coronary artery bypass grafting: can intraoperative physiologic imaging guide intraoperative decision making? J Thorac Cardiovasc Surg 146:824–835

Chapter 7
Application of an Angiographic Blood Flow Evaluation Technique in Cardiovascular Surgery Using the Hyper Eye Medical System

Masaki Yamamoto, Kazumasa Orihashi, and Takayuki Sato

Abstract Anastomotic insufficiency of coronary artery bypass grafting (CABG) needs to be detected during surgery, to increase graft patency. The HyperEye Medical System (HEMS) provides a clear view of the blood flow and ischemic area with color visualization. The HEMS images are classified by smoothness of graft opacification into normal, delay, and occlusion during CABG. Though there are pitfalls of assessing graft, one is fluorescence permeability of indocyanine green (ICG), and the other is enhancement time lag by several parameters. Moreover, we described the concomitant use of HEMS and transit time flowmeter and showed the positive and negative predictive values were 100 and 97.6 %. Furthermore, this assessment technique was employed to revascularization surgery in arteriosclerosis obliterans. The other usage is to visualize ischemic region of the intestine in cases of acute or chronic ischemic colitis.

This chapter described the accuracy of HEMS angiography for cardiovascular surgeries.

Keywords Indocyanine green (ICG) • HyperEye Medical System (HEMS) • Coronary artery bypass grafting (CABG) • Arteriosclerosis obliterans (ASO) • Abdominal aortic aneurysm (AAA)

7.1 Introduction

Indocyanine green (ICG) exposed to near-infrared light at a wavelength of 760–780 nm generates fluorescence at a wavelength of 800–850 nm [1]. Although the fluorescence of ICG solution in plasma is weak, it increases after being

M. Yamamoto (✉) • K. Orihashi
Departments of Surgery II, Kochi Medical School, Kohasu, Oko-cho, Nankoku, Kochi 783-8505, Japan
e-mail: y-masaki@kochi-u.ac.jp

T. Sato
Cardiovascular Control, Kochi Medical School, Kohasu, Oko-cho, Nankoku, Kochi 783-8505, Japan

M. Kusano et al. (eds.), *ICG Fluorescence Imaging and Navigation Surgery*,
DOI 10.1007/978-4-431-55528-5_7

Table 7.1 Reported clinical studies on the indocyanine green imaging system in coronary artery bypass grafting

Investigators	Year	Patients	Graft no.	Sensitivity	Specificity
FD. Rubens	2002	20	–	–	–
O. Reuthebuch	2003	38	124	–	–
DP. Taggart	2003	84	213	–	–
L. Balacumaraswami	2004	200	533	–	–
M. Takahashi	2004	72	290	–	–
ND. Desai	2006	46	139	83.3	100
T. Handa	2009	39	116	100	100
T. Handa	2010	51	129	85.7	100

Reprinted from Surgery Today, 2011;41:1467–1474, Yamamoto M et al

combined with albumin and alpha1-lipoprotein. In 1960, Novotny first reported the use of ICG angiography and the effect of ICG fluorescence in ophthalmic fundoscopy [2]. Later, Rubens et al. reported the use of ICG angiography in coronary artery bypass grafting (CABG) in 2002 [3]. Since then, other ICG imaging devices have been developed and used for graft assessment of CABG, such as the SPY™ imaging system and photodynamic eye (PDE) imaging system [4–6]. Recently, Sato et al. developed the HyperEye Medical System (HEMS, model MNIRC-1000; Mizuho Ikakogyo, Co., Ltd., Tokyo, Japan) angiography ICG imaging system at Kochi Medical School [7]. Investigators have reported the reliability of ICG imaging system in clinical and experimental studies on CABG (Table 7.1) [3–5, 7–11].

Here we report our experience with bypass evaluation by HEMS angiography during CABG and peripheral arterial bypass grafting in cardiovascular surgery [8, 12, 13]. Furthermore, we introduce an appraisal method to evaluate intestinal blood flow for patients with acute intestinal ischemia [12].

7.2 Usefulness of HEMS Angiography in CABG

Off-pump coronary artery bypass grafting (OPCAB) was established as standard technique of CABG for treatment of angina patients, which has lowered the incidence of cerebral infarction and reduced operative mortality about 0.6 % [14]. On the other hand, OPCAB maintains heart rhythm for anastomosis during bypass of the coronary arteries. Moreover, the anastomotic site is displaced downward to the distal side of the coronary artery in OPCAB, compared to cardiac arrest in conventional CABG [15]. The difficulty of CABG is due to these two factors. As a result, a decrease in bypass patency in OPCAB and worsening of bypass anastomosis as an early operative result have been reported [15]. By evaluating bypass flow and the anastomotic state during surgery, surgeons are able to reanastomose the bypass intraoperatively. Such an approach was required by risk management and further clinical training of cardiovascular surgeons. Various types of flowmeters, echography systems, and X-ray coronary angiography (CAG) using a catheter have been used to evaluate bypass grafting during surgery. The transit time flowmeter (TTF) to evaluate the bypass graft by measuring the flow volume and flow pattern has been reported that noted the sensitivity and specificity of the device [16]. Even if there is a lot of flow volume of blood, it does not reflect the state of its anastomotic site. Although the anastomotic site can be visualized during CABG, manipulation of the catheter can be cumbersome during surgery, and X-ray imaging can be difficult to employ during surgery in a general hospital setting. The ICG angiography system using ICG fluorescence was developed to increase the precision of the bypass appraisal method by visualization of bypass flow in CAG to better describe the anastomosis. Although, several types of ICG imaging devices are commercially available, the HEMS angiography has two distinct advantages [7, 8, 13]. The first is visualization of blood flow, which is shown as ICG fluorescence of the bypass graft displayed on the monitor of the HEMS. Blood flow appears as fluorescent white in the bypass graft against a colored background of the surgical field on the monitor. As a second advantage, excitation light is generated from a light-emitting diode (LED), as opposed to a medical-grade laser; thus, the imaging time is unrestricted with the HEMS. An assessment method to describe and evaluate myocardial perfusion flow during CABG has also been reported [17]. Because an observation time of 30 s or more is required, this procedure by HEMS angiography is considered useful [7, 8, 13].

7.2.1 Setup and Imaging by HEMS Angiography for CABG

We recently developed the HEMS to resolve some problems with current ICG imaging devices [13]. The HEMS consists of an imaging unit, control unit, and monitor. The imaging unit consists of multiple LEDs around an ultrasensitive color charged-coupled device (CCD) imaging camera with non-Bayer color filter arrays (HyperEye Technology; SANYO Co., Ltd, Tokyo, Japan), which can detect near-infrared rays (380–1200 nm) and visible light at 30 frames/s at a time. The control unit consists of a computer and controller to record and adjust the focus and iris. The HEMS employs Diagnogreen (Daiichi Sankyo, Tokyo, Japan) as the ICG dye, which is prepared with 2.5 mg/mL dissolved in distilled water [8, 12]. The imaging head is draped by a sterile cover and placed 30–50 cm above the target (Fig. 7.1A). The LED illumination area is approximately 78.5 cm^2 on the surgical field. Conventionally, the standard dose of ICG solution is 5 mg per imaging sequence. The ICG solution is intravenously injected through a central or peripheral venous catheter and flushed with 10 mL of physiological saline (Fig. 7.1B). This allergy reaction has been reported to occur at an incidence of an approximately 1:40,000. The fluorescence of arterial blood flow is displayed on the monitor and recorded using a digital image-processing system with an audio video interweave or SmartDraw format.

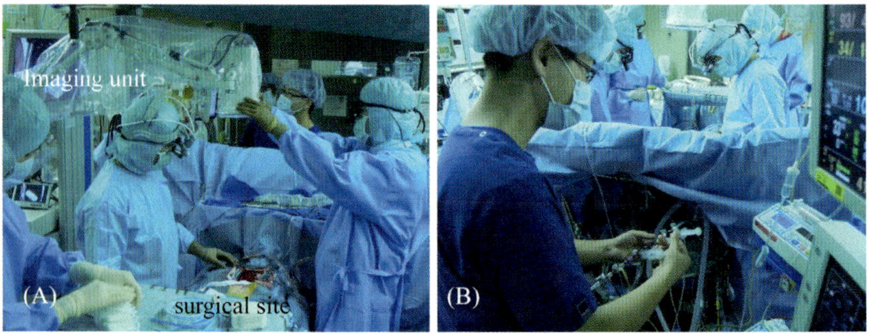

Fig. 7.1 HyperEye Medical System (HEMS). (**A**) The imaging head is draped by a sterile cover and placed 30–50 cm above the target. (**B**) ICG solution is injected through a central or peripheral venous catheter. *ICG* indocyanine green

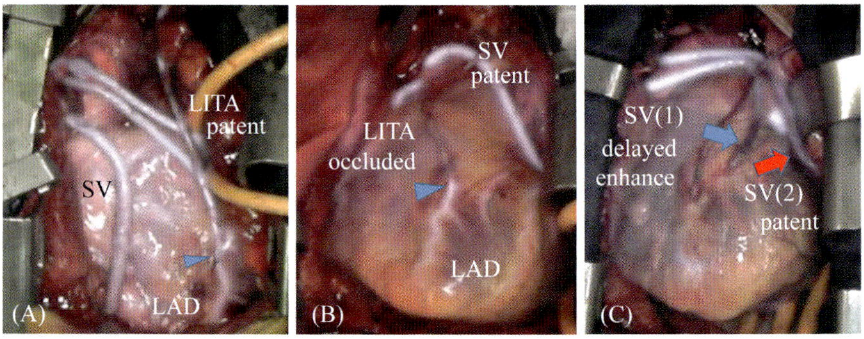

Fig. 7.2 The HEMS angiographic images are classified into three categories: (**A**) normal, smooth opacification of the graft and coronary artery; (**B**) occlusion, no enhancement of the graft; and (**C**) delay, delayed graft enhancement compared with other grafts. *Arrow head* shows anastomoses. *Arrow* showed the delayed enhanced bypass graft (*blue arrow*) and patent graft (*red arrow*)

7.2.2 Evaluation of Coronary Artery Bypass Patency by HEMS Angiography

The bypass graft of an anastomotic stenosis has a time lag from imaging of the graft to the distal side of the coronary artery. The HEMS angiographic images are classified into two categories, normal and abnormal opacification, with the latter subclassified into two categories, as follows [8]:

Normal: smooth opacification of the graft, coronary artery, and myocardium (Fig. 7.2A)
Abnormal: delayed or inadequate opacification of the graft
Occlusion: no enhancement of the graft (Fig. 7.2B)
Delay: delayed graft enhancement compared with other grafts (Fig. 7.2C)

Resolution of the HEMS angiograph showing arterial dissection of the bypass can distinguish a true lumen from a pseudo lumen. Although the flow competition from the coronary artery was classified as abnormal, it was considered an exception to these criteria because it was not a problem associated with anastomosis.

7.2.3 *Pitfalls of HEMS Angiography*

The setup and use of HEMS angiography are relatively simple, and the passage of blood flow can be observed with the monitoring screen; however, experience of HEMS is essential. Therefore, the surgeon should have knowledge of the properties of ICG and the features of each component of the ICG angiography apparatus. Several points to consider in the evaluation of HEMS angiography are discussed below.

7.2.3.1 Penetration Depth and Fluorescent Luminescence

There are differences between HEMS angiography and X-ray CAG because an X-ray passes through the human body to show an anastomotic site of the coronary artery, whereas ICG fluorescence is unable to pass through the thoracic wall; thus, its actual permeable depth is approximately 2–3 mm [13]. The accuracy of ICG angiography to estimate the degree of stricture of the lumen at an anastomotic site is limited. Moreover, ICG solution adheres to the vessel walls as it passes through the bypass grafts. Therefore, although the bypass and anastomotic site are imaged, only the vessel outline of the bypass graft can be observed. Figure 7.3 shows an image of three bypassed branches following OPCAB (left internal thoracic artery (LITA)/left anterior descending artery (LAD), radial artery/posterolateral branch, and greater saphenous vein (SV)/right posterior descending branch of a 69-year-old man with unstable angina) (Fig. 7.3A). The HEMS angiography showed no stenosis of anastomosis and bypass graft with smooth opacification (Fig. 7.3B). Though, X-ray CAG in the early postoperative stage showed that the distal end of the graft had a diffuse stricture and that blood flow was obstructed (Fig. 7.3C). In a review of HEMS angiography results, the rate of blood flow through the LITA was decreased in this case. However, although blood flowed through the entire graft, we were unable to identify the stricture by HEMS angiography. Therefore, we have developed a qualitative method to evaluate the time lag of flow passage [8, 13]. If ICG imaging of the bypass has delayed enhancement, it can be estimated with a delayed image called category "delay" (Fig. 7.2C). Fat deposits reflect ICG fluorescence; therefore, if the fat layer covers the arterial surface, it disrupts flow evaluation. Thus, although the ICG fluid adheres to the anastomotic surface, permeability is decreased. When the coronary artery, which is buried in the myocardium, and fat layer are thick, native coronary arterial blood flow cannot be visualized but is rather judged by influent and washout of ICG fluorescence passing through the grafts.

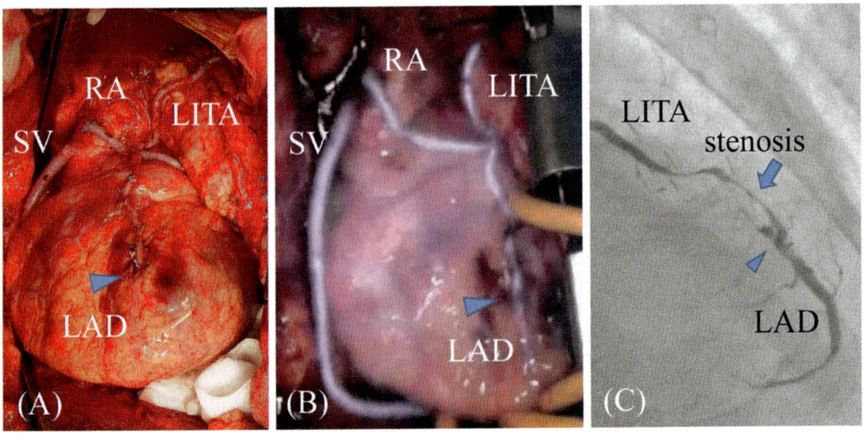

Fig. 7.3 Coronary arterial bypass grafting, left internal thoracic artery (LITA)/left anterior descending artery (LAD), radial artery/posterolateral branch, and greater saphenous vein (SV)/right posterior descending branch of a 69-year-old man with unstable angina. The LITA is indicated by anastomotic site with an *arrow head* (**A**). (**B**) HEMS showed the smooth opacification of the graft to coronary artery. (**C**) X-ray CAG in the early postoperative stage showed that the distal end of the graft had a diffuse stricture (*arrow*), although there was no anastomotic stenosis (*arrow head*)

Because the distal side of the LAD isn't often buried in the ventricular wall, the patency was evaluated by smoothness of flow from the ITA graft to LAD. On the other hand, it is often difficult to navigate the coronary artery downward. At the time of reoperation, the coronary artery is unobservable from the heart surface because of scar tissue on the coronary arteries. Although we examined the usefulness of angiography using the HEMS to navigate the target coronary artery during CABG, the ability to identify the coronary artery is decreased compared with that of echography of the cardiac surface because of its low ICG permeability. However, the coronary veins are thick with thin walls and run more superficially within the heart. Even when the coronary veins are covered with a scar layer, they can be visualized by HEMS angiography. In addition, the target coronary artery can be identified by contrasting the coronary vein described by the HEMS angiography with the coronary arteries identified by computed tomography and CAG before surgery. Furthermore, Shikayama reported that the penetration depth of the PDE imaging system is approximately 10 mm. The PDE system is maybe effective for observations at limited depths.

7.2.3.2 Time Lag of ICG Fluorescence

After intravenous injection of diluted ICG fluid from a central venous catheter, the right atrium, right ventricle, pulmonary artery, and lung gleam appeared white. Because the myocardium wall was thick, the left ventricle image appeared thin.

Then, the radial artery and saphenous vein, which were anastomosed to the ascending aorta, were imaged clearly. Finally, the internal thoracic arteries (ITAs) were identified in relation to the subclavian artery. After imaging of the bypass grafts, the image of the coronary artery appeared smooth, if there was no anastomotic stricture. Even if there was coronary stenosis, the native coronary blood flow reached the distal end earlier than the blood flow from the ITA graft, which is used as an in situ graft. For multiple aortocoronary bypass, which passes flow to the ascending aorta, a comparison of each bypass was useful [8]. However, ICG from the first images combines with proteins of the vessel wall and remains there, making evaluation difficult because of the increased ICG luminescence before passage of ICG blood flow. To achieve an accurate evaluation, it may be necessary to delete illumination from sources other than excitation by LEDs of the HEMS and to increase the contrast by changing the image from color to monochromatic.

7.2.3.3 Impact of Imaging Velocity and Fluorescent Luminescence

We sometimes experience a delay in HEMS angiography of grafts by administration of diluted ICG fluid because the concentration of ICG luminescence within a graft differs among individuals. We speculate that blood flow rate, diameter of the graft and native coronary artery, and myocardial runoff are factors that influence ICG luminescence of the bypass graft. In addition, ICG concentration, left ventricular volume, and stroke volume should be considered as general factors. Although qualitative evaluation during HEMS angiography is relatively simple, it requires a certain level of experience, and it also is necessary to consider the abovementioned factors.

7.2.4 General Assessment with Concomitant TTF

A TTF is often employed for graft assessment during CABG with HEMS angiography [7, 16]. The concurrent use of these modalities is possible during surgery; thus, we assessed them together [8]. Desai et al. reported a method to evaluate TTF, which included a 2-mm probe for the internal thoracic artery graft and a 3- or 4-mm probe for the other grafts [18]. The mean graft flow (MGF), pulsatile index (PI), and diastolic filling percentage (DF) were measured according to the criteria reported by previous reports [4, 7, 8, 18, 19]. The graft was classified as abnormal when at least one of these parameters was not within normal range ($MGF > 10$ mL/min, $PI < 5$, and $DF > 50$ %), as described in our previous reports. Moreover, in our previous report, we described the concomitant use of HEMS angiography and TTF. We also compared final imaging results of HEMS angiography and postoperative CAG and examined the final data from intraoperative HEMS angiography and TTF in all cases [8]. When the graft was judged as abnormal by either HEMS angiography or TTF, graft revision was performed. X-ray CAG showed that 130 of

133 normal grafts were patent, whereas nine of 11 abnormal grafts were occluded [8]. Therefore, the negative and positive predictive values were 97.7 % and 81.8 %, respectively, and the negative and positive predicting values were 100 % and 97.6 %, respectively. Conflicting results between the two assessment modalities were noted in 17 grafts. A total of eight cases were judged as normal by HEMS and abnormal by TTF; thus, we assessed the graft patency in all eight cases by X-ray CAG, which indicated a decrease in coronary arterial spasm and blood flow immediately after coronary anastomosis. Nine cases showed normal TTF data but abnormal HEMS angiographic findings, of which seven had occlusions. Although one graft showed graft dissection by HEMS angiography, it was not discovered during surgery. The other occlusions had unknown etiologies.

7.3 Application to Peripheral Artery Bypass Surgery

An increasing number of patients with critical limb ischemia caused by arteriosclerosis obliterans (ASO) require advanced revascularization of the perimalleolar arteries; however, this procedure carries the risk of limb amputation if the anastomosis is not successful [20]. If malperfusion in the distal region can be accurately assessed intraoperatively, revision of the anastomosis or placement of an additional graft can be performed. Unno et al. reported a series of nine ASO patients in which ICG angiography with monochromatic visualization was used to assess bypass grafts of the perimalleolar arteries [6]. We first reported the application of HEMS angiography for revascularization surgery in ASO patients [21]. Figure 7.4A is image of critical limb ischemia in a 70-year-old man who underwent end-to-side bypass of the posterior tibial artery with a saphenous vein graft. Angiographic imaging of peripheral artery bypass with the HEMS is possible using the same technique of graft evaluation by CABG, in which the graft image is obtained after ICG administration via a central venous catheter (Fig. 7.4A) [13, 21]. If a central venous catheter is not used, diluted ICG fluid can be intravenously injected into a peripheral vein of the upper limb and then flushed through with 20 mL of physiological saline solution. And, there are three points to consider with CABG. First, the concentration of ICG is more diluted because the imaging site is distal from the heart. Therefore, ICG fluid is further diluted and injected intravenously, although the ICG imaging luminescence is sufficient only to evaluate blood flow through the bypass grafts. Second, there are differences in graft types. For example, the SV is a good choice to image blood flow via ICG angiography. The blood flow in a vascular prosthesis, such as Dacron and polytetrafluoroethylene grafts, cannot be imaged in white because of poor penetration of fluorescence (Fig. 7.4C–F). Although the target artery is minimally dissected in peripheral vascular surgery, the anastomotic peripheral artery is peeled, and qualitative evaluation is performed by measurement of flow through the anastomotic site and bypass grafts. Third, stroke volume, blood

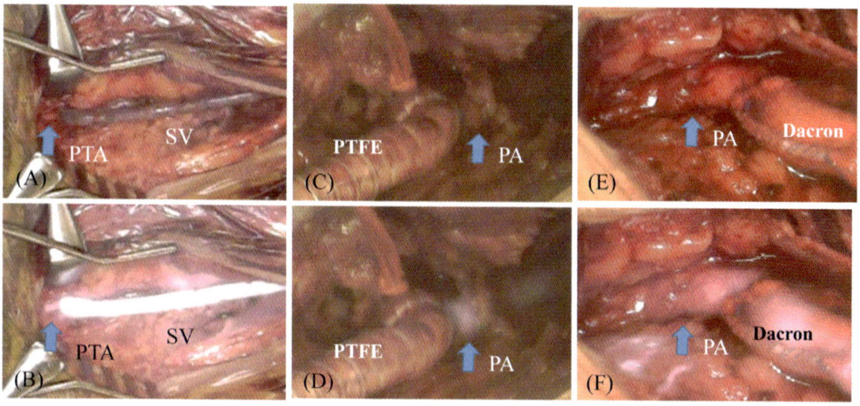

Fig. 7.4 HEMS assessment of graft in peripheral arterial surgery. Visual image and ICG angiogram in vein graft (**A**, **B**), PTFE graft (**C**, **D**), and Dacron graft (**E**, **F**). (**A**), (**C**), and (**E**) show pre-ICG imaging with HEMS. (**B**), (**D**), and (**F**) are color scale HEMS imaging. *Arrow* shows peripheral arteries. Opacification is poor in prosthesis grafts. *PTA* posterior tibial artery, *SV* saphenous vein, *PA* popliteal artery, *PTFE* polytetrafluoroethylene (Reprinted from © 2013 Masaki Yamamoto, Kazumasa Orihashi, Takayuki Sato Originally published in Artery Bypass, 2013; Chapter 5, 81–97 under CC BY 3.0 license. Available from: http://dx.doi.org/10.5772/55311)

pressure, and peripheral perfusion vary among patients; therefore, peripheral perfusion assessment should be carefully performed for each patient.

7.4 Evaluation of Blood Flow in Abdominal Organs

Abdominal aortic aneurysm (AAA) surgery has recently shifted to endovascular therapy following the development of some devices. However, aortic replacement is often required for a ruptured AAA, and patients with intestinal ischemia often require revascularization surgery of the abdominal organs. Intestinal ischemia is the most undesirable complication in AAA surgery [22]. Shock status in preoperative period is the most important predictor of ischemic colitis. The incidences of ischemic colitis after elective AAA surgery and ruptured AAA are reported to be 6 and 42 % [22]. Therefore, it is necessary to also maintain function of the intestine by performing suitable transection of necrotic intestine. We previously validated HEMS angiography to identify intestinal ischemia [13, 21]. Surgeons can monitor blood flow of the intestine by HEMS angiography. The ICG fluorescence can penetrate the mesentery to visualize flow through the mesenteric artery by HEMS angiography (Fig. 7.5). First, the mesenteric artery (arrow) was identified and the intestine wall enhanced. Although there was a time lag of ICG fluorescence enhancement in part of the ileum, the imaging effect was homogeneous

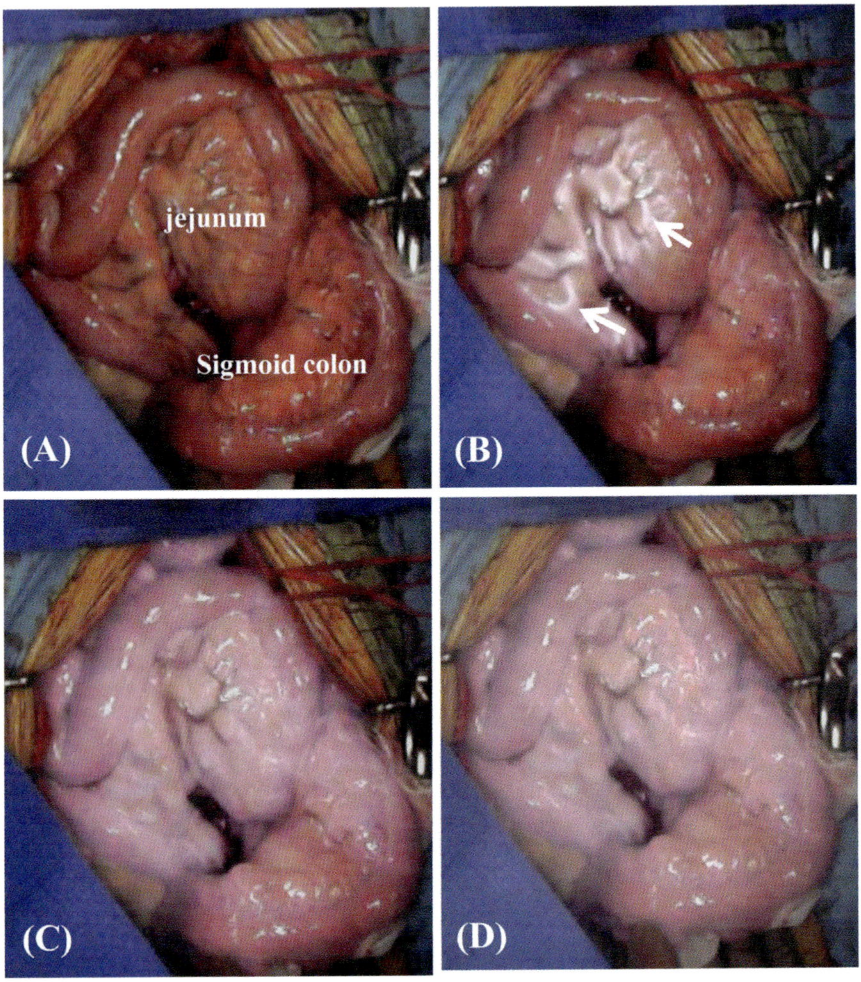

Fig. 7.5 Sequential HEMS images demonstrating mesenteric perfusion. (**A**) Pre-ICG imaging of ICG, (**B**) fluorescence in the mesenteric artery (*arrow*), (**C**, **D**) fluorescence in the intestinal wall with slightly in the sigmoid colon (Reprinted from Eur J Vasc Endovasc Surg, 2012; 43: 426–432, Yamamoto M et al.)

immediately afterward [21]. Furthermore, ischemic regions of the intestine can be identified by color imaging via HEMS angiography (Fig. 7.6). Although X-ray angiography can identify the exact site of the occlusion, it is difficult to detect the occluded regions of the entire intestine in the surgical field. Figure 7.6 is a HEMS angiographic image of the small intestine of a patient with acute intestinal ischemic syndrome because of "shaggy" aorta syndrome. In this case, HEMS angiography detected flow of ICG-stained blood to part of the small intestine and was useful to determine the extent of resection.

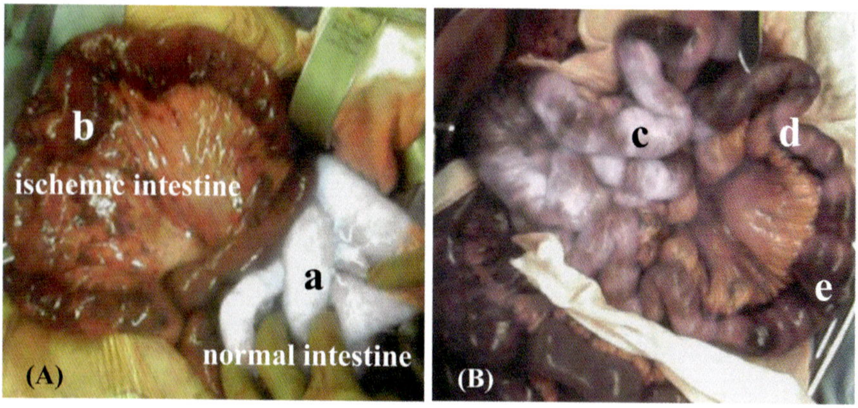

Fig. 7.6 HEMS imagings showing malperfused intestine in ruptured aneurysmal surgery. (**A**) No fluorescence in the ischemic intestine. Points (**A**) and (**B**) show the healthy and ischemic small intestine. (**B**) The spotty intestinal ischemia caused by nonobstructive mesenteric ischemia. Blood flow is maintained at point (**C**), is slightly diminished at point (**D**), and disappears at point (**E**) (Reprinted from Eur J Vasc Endovasc Surg, 2012; 43: 426–432, Yamamoto M et.al. and Surgery Today, 2011;41:1467–1474, Yamamoto M et al.)

7.5 Conclusion

Here we described the usefulness of an appraisal procedure of HEMS angiography during CABG. HEMS angiography is a useful technique to visualize bypass flow, although ICG fluorescence permeability varies among individuals.

In addition, we discussed our experience with HEMS angiography as well as differences between anastomosis inspection methods and measurement devices among hospitals. Moreover, peripheral artery surgery and assessment of blood flow to the abdominal organs were described.

References

1. Cherrick GR, Stein SW, Leevy CM et al (1960) Indocyanine green: observations on its physical properties, plasma decay, and hepatic extraction. J Clin Invest 39:592–600
2. Novotny HR, Alvis D (1960) A method of photographing fluorescence in circulating blood of the human eye. Technical documentary report SAM-TDR USAF School of Aerospace Medicine 60–82:1–4
3. Rubens FD, Ruel M, Fremes SE (2002) A new and simplified method for coronary and graft imaging during CABG. Heart Surg Forum 5(2):141–144
4. Desai ND, Miwa S, Kodama D et al (2006) A randomized comparison of intraoperative indocyanine green angiography and transit-time flow measurement to detect technical errors in coronary bypass grafts. J Thorac Cardiovasc Surg 132(3):585–594

5. Takahashi M, Ishikawa T, Higashidani K et al (2004) SPY: an innovative intra-operative imaging system to evaluate graft patency during off-pump coronary artery bypass grafting. Interact Cardiovasc Thorac Surg 3(3):479–483
6. Unno N, Suzuki M, Yamamoto N et al (2008) Indocyanine green fluorescence angiography for intraoperative assessment of blood flow: a feasibility study. Eur J Vasc Endovasc Surg 35 (2):205–207
7. Handa T, Katare RG, Sasaguri S et al (2009) Preliminary experience for the evaluation of the intraoperative graft patency with real color charge-coupled device camera system: an advanced device for simultaneous capturing of color and near-infrared images during coronary artery bypass graft. Interact Cardiovasc Thorac Surg 9(2):150–154
8. Yamamoto M, Orihashi K, Nishimori H et al (2014) Efficacy of intraoperative HyperEye Medical System angiography for coronary artery bypass grafting. Surg Today 45:996–972
9. Balacumaraswami L, Taggart DP (2004) Digital tools to facilitate intraoperative coronary artery bypass graft patency assessment. Semin Thorac Cardiovasc Surg 16(3):266–271
10. Reuthebuch O, Haussler A, Genoni M et al (2004) Novadaq SPY: intraoperative quality assessment in off-pump coronary artery bypass grafting. Chest 125(2):418–424
11. Taggart DP, Choudhary B, Anastasiadis K et al (2003) Preliminary experience with a novel intraoperative fluorescence imaging technique to evaluate the patency of bypass grafts in total arterial revascularization. Ann Thorac Surg 75(3):870–873
12. Yamamoto M, Orihashi K, Nishimori H et al (2012) Indocyanine green angiography for intra-operative assessment in vascular surgery. Eur J Vasc Endovasc Surg 43(4):426–432
13. Yamamoto M, Sasaguri S, Sato T (2011) Assessing intraoperative blood flow in cardiovascular surgery. Surg Today 41(11):1467–1474
14. Sakata R, Fujii Y, Kuwano H (2011) Thoracic and cardiovascular surgery in Japan during 2009: annual report by the Japanese Association for Thoracic Surgery. Gen Thorac Cardiovasc Surg 59(9):636–667
15. Shroyer AL, Grover FL, Hattler B et al (2009) On-pump versus off-pump coronary-artery bypass surgery. N Engl J Med 361(19):1827–1837
16. D'Ancona G, Karamanoukian HL, Ricci M et al (2000) Graft revision after transit time flow measurement in off-pump coronary artery bypass grafting. Eur J Cardiothorac Surg 17 (3):287–293
17. Detter C, Wipper S, Russ D et al (2007) Fluorescent cardiac imaging: a novel intraoperative method for quantitative assessment of myocardial perfusion during graded coronary artery stenosis. Circulation 116(9):1007–1014
18. Desai ND, Miwa S, Kodama D et al (2005) Improving the quality of coronary bypass surgery with intraoperative angiography: validation of a new technique. J Am Coll Cardiol 46 (8):1521–1525
19. Balacumaraswami L, Abu-Omar Y, Choudhary B et al (2005) A comparison of transit-time flowmetry and intraoperative fluorescence imaging for assessing coronary artery bypass graft patency. J Thorac Cardiovasc Surg 130(2):315–320
20. Conte MS (2010) Bypass versus Angioplasty in Severe Ischaemia of the Leg (BASIL) and the (hoped for) dawn of evidence-based treatment for advanced limb ischemia. J Vasc Surg 51 (5 Suppl):69S–75S
21. Funayama E, Minakawa H, Otani H et al (2012) Effectiveness of muscle coverage to manage osteomyelitis of very late onset in the irradiated chest wall. Surg Today 42(3):306–311
22. Champagne BJ, Darling RC 3rd, Daneshmand M et al (2004) Outcome of aggressive surveillance colonoscopy in ruptured abdominal aortic aneurysm. J Vasc Surg 39(4):792–796

Part V
Sentinel Node Navigation Surgery: Breast Cancer

Chapter 8
Principle and Development of ICG Method

Toshiyuki Kitai

Abstract Indocyanine green (ICG) fluorescence method is a modification of the dye method, in which the detection of sentinel node (SN) is facilitated by fluorescence navigation. Tissue penetration of near-infrared light is an important aspect of this method. Visualization of subcutaneous lymphatic vessels and lymph nodes during the dissection was useful to increase the accuracy of SN biopsy. However, pre-incisional localization of SN is sometimes difficult by ICG fluorescence method alone. Further improvement and investigation are necessary to be a possible replacement of radioactive colloid.

Keywords Sentinel node biopsy • ICG fluorescence imaging • Near-infrared light • Compression technique

8.1 Introduction

Numerous studies have been published during the last decade in which the optical imaging was applied for surgical navigation. There are several advantages in the intraoperative use of optical imaging: (1) real-time feedback is possible and (2) optical measurement provides unique biological information derived from the wavelength-dependent properties of the tracer. Among them, the usefulness of ICG fluorescence imaging has been demonstrated in the clinical settings. Especially, sentinel node biopsy is one of the platforms currently available.

Sentinel node biopsy (SNB) is an established procedure to access the lymph node status in early breast cancer to avoid unnecessary axillary dissection [1–3]. Radioisotope method is the worldwide standard. Dye method is also advantageous, because it is free from radiation exposure and does not require radioisotope facilities. Indocyanine green (ICG) fluorescence method is a modification of the dye method, in which the detection of sentinel nodes is facilitated by fluorescence navigation. Tissue penetration of near-infrared (NIR) light is an important aspect of this method. Under visible light, subcutaneous lymphatic vessels and the lymph

T. Kitai (✉)
Department of Surgery, Kishiwada City Hospital, 1001 Gakuhara-cho, Kishiwada, Osaka 596-8501, Japan
e-mail: kitait@kuhp.kyoto-u.ac.jp

M. Kusano et al. (eds.), *ICG Fluorescence Imaging and Navigation Surgery*,
DOI 10.1007/978-4-431-55528-5_8

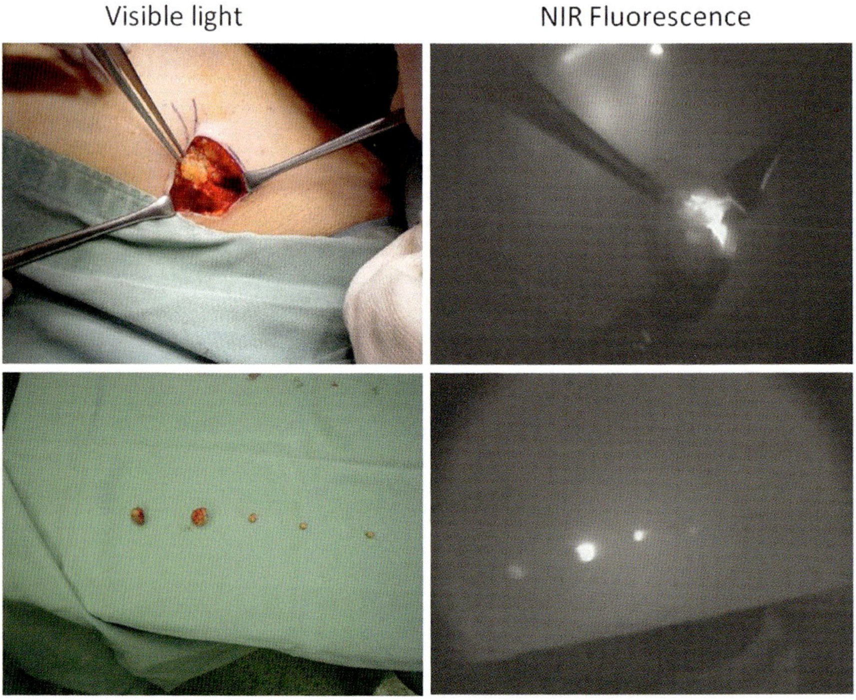

Fig. 8.1 Advantages of NIR fluorescence over visible light: Tissue penetration (*upper panel*): lymphatic vessels under the skin and lymph nodes in the fatty tissue can be detected by fluorescence. High sensitivity (*lower panel*): lymph nodes stained by ICG can be judged with high sensitivity

nodes in the fatty tissue are not visible to the naked eye, but fluorescence imaging makes these structures visible. High sensitivity is also beneficial. Even in cases where one can hardly tell which nodes are stained by the ICG color, fluorescence imaging clearly shows which nodes are sentinel nodes (Fig. 8.1). However, one of the main drawbacks is the difficulty in localization of the sentinel node before skin incision. The sentinel node is usually embedded in the axillary fatty tissue at a depth of 2 cm or more, and the fluorescence signal from the sentinel node is attenuated by light scattering in the tissue. In most cases, especially in the cases of fatty patients, the location of skin incision was decided with the help of radioisotope or by surgeon's experience. In this chapter, we describe the principle and the clinical development of the ICG fluorescence method for sentinel node biopsy in breast cancer.

8.2 Principle

8.2.1 Molecular Fluorescence of ICG

Molecular fluorescence of ICG consists of a two-step process, excitation and emission (Fig. 8.2). When light at 765 nm is emitted at ICG molecules, they move from ground state to excited state (excitation). When the molecules return to ground state, a part of the absorbed energy is radiated as fluorescent emission at 830 nm. The fluorescent emission is at a longer wavelength than the fluorescent excitation. Since the combination of these wavelengths is specific to the ICG molecule, highly sensitive measurement is possible by selecting proper wavelengths in the light source and the detector.

The general law of fluorescence spectroscopy is shown in the equation below [4]. The quantum efficiency shows that only 1.2 % of absorbed energy is emitted as fluorescence. The equation also indicates the nonlinear relationship between the fluorescence intensity and the ICG concentration, meaning that quantitative measurement is difficult. When the concentration of ICG is greater than 0.08 g/l, the fluorescence intensity becomes weaker (quenching effect). However, the quenching effect usually does not disturb the lymphatic detection in the clinical setting, since the administered ICG is adequately diluted by the lymphatic fluid.

$$F = \varphi P_0\{1 - \exp(-\varepsilon C b)\}$$

F: Intensity of fluorescent light
P_0: Intensity of excitation light

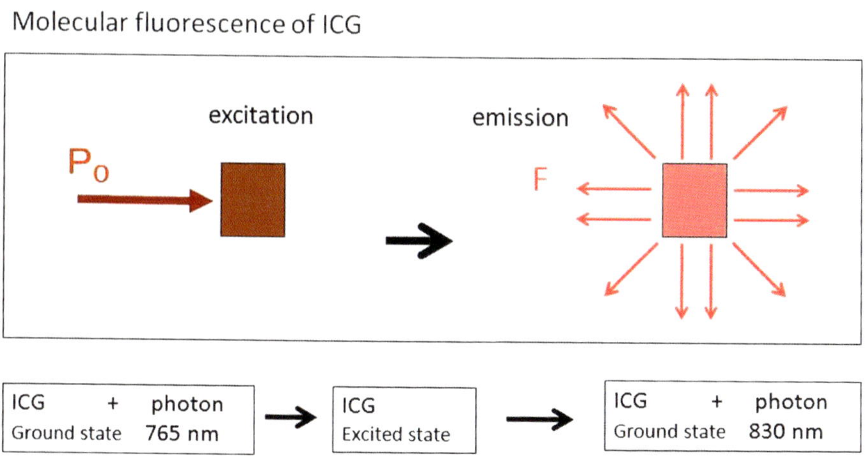

Fig. 8.2 Molecular fluorescence of indocyanine green (ICG): The wavelengths of fluorescent excitation and emission are specific to ICG. High signal-to-noise ratio can be obtained by fluorescence measurement. P_0 excitation light, F fluorescent light

φ: Quantum efficiency (ICG: 0.012)
exp: Natural log
ε: Absorption coefficient
C: ICG concentration
b: Cell size

8.2.2 Optical Properties of ICG in the Living Tissue

ICG has characteristic fluorescence spectra in the NIR wavelengths [5] (Fig. 8.3), ranging from 700 to 900 nm, which is called "an optical window." This is advantageous to clinical application, because the NIR light can penetrate deep into the tissue without being absorbed by hemoglobin or water. However, when applied to the living tissue, light scattering becomes an important issue [6] (Fig. 8.4). The fluorescent excitation and emission are attenuated by scattering when the light travels in the tissue. Fat droplets in the axilla are the main scatterers [7]. In the preliminary experiment, an ICG fluorescent signal at the depth of 1 cm in the breast phantom was detectable, but detection was difficult as the depth increases. The limit of detectable depth by fluorescence in the axilla is supposed to be 1–2 cm.

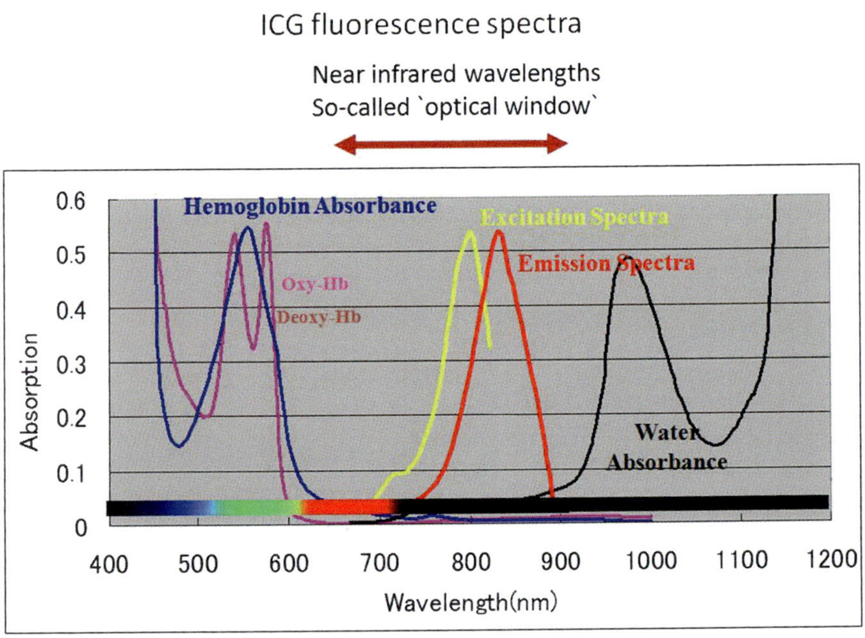

Fig. 8.3 Indocyanine green's fluorescence spectra in the near-infrared wavelengths: The wavelengths between 700 and 900 nm are called the "optical window," since the light at these wavelengths can penetrate deep into the tissue as escaped from the absorption by hemoglobin (Hb) and water

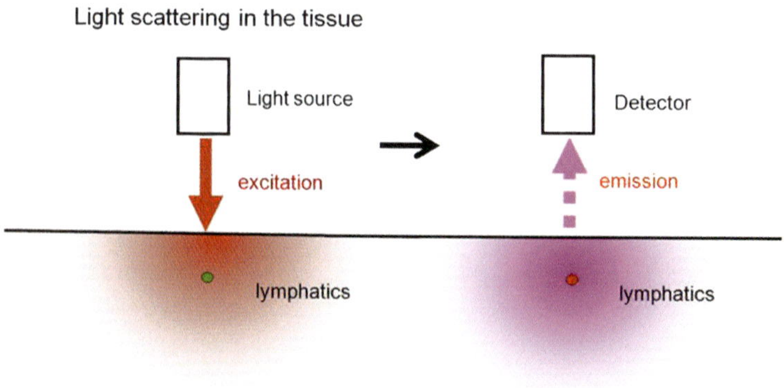

Fig. 8.4 Attenuation of fluorescence by scattering in living tissue: The fluorescent light is attenuated by scattering while traveling in the subcutaneous tissue. A main scatterer is subcutaneous fat droplets

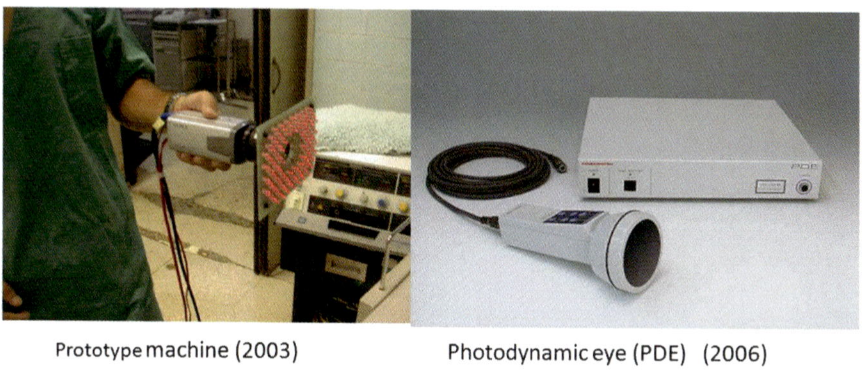

Fig. 8.5 Infrared fluorescence imaging system (Photodynamic eye, Hamamatsu Photonics, Japan): Prototype machine (*left*) and commercially available photodynamic eye (*right*)

8.3 Clinical Development for Sentinel Node Biopsy in Breast Cancer

8.3.1 Equipment

An infrared fluorescence imaging system (photodynamic eye, Hamamatsu Photonics, Japan), which consists of light-emitting diodes at 760 nm as a light source, and a charge-coupled device (CCD) camera with a cut filter below 820 nm as a detector were used to measure NIR fluorescence images [8] (Fig. 8.5).

8.3.2 Surgical Procedures

After induction of general anesthesia and sterilization of the operation site, 25 mg/5 ml indocyanine green (Diagnogreen 0.5 %; Daiichi Pharmaceutical, Tokyo, Japan) was injected in the subareolar breast tissue. Following a few seconds of massage, subcutaneous lymphatic drainage was then observed with fluorescent images (Fig. 8.6). Subcutaneous lymphatic streams could be detected over the skin usually within 1 or 2 min, and they disappeared before entering the axillary space. The subcutaneous lymphatic streams were marked again over the skin, and a 4-cm skin incision was made at the point where the lymphatic channels drained into the axilla. After skin incision, the subcutaneous lymphatics were more clearly observed. Green or fluorescent lymphatic channels were carefully dissected and traced until the first-drained lymph node was found in the axilla. The lymph node was then dissected with the surrounding fatty tissue. Usually, two or more lymph

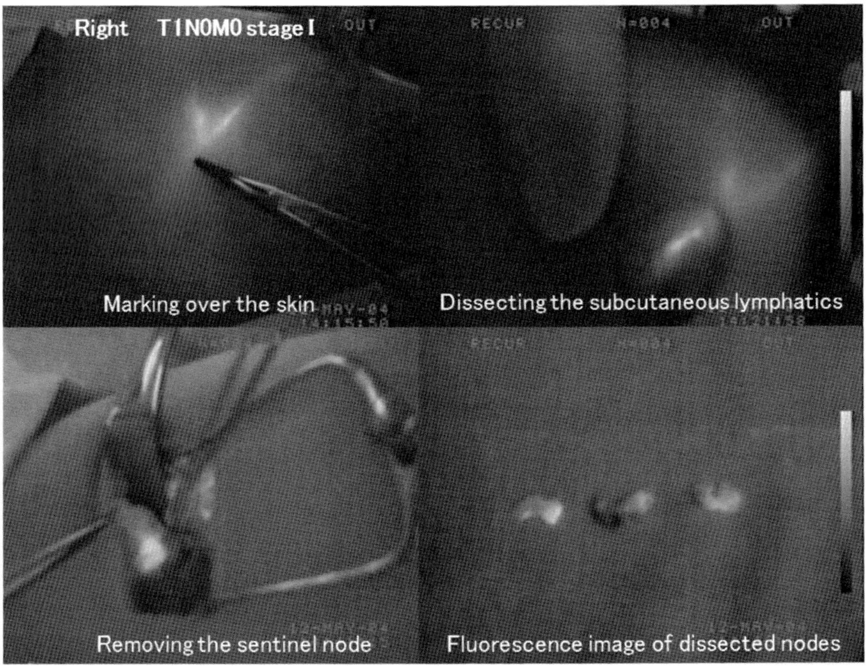

Fig. 8.6 (**a**) Subcutaneous lymphatic channels were detected by fluorescence. Two streams from the areola joined together before they drained into the axilla. The point to be incised was marked
(**b**) After skin incision, the subcutaneous lymphatics were more clearly visible by fluorescence
(**c**) The lymphatic channels and nodes that received ICG appeared as shining fluorescent streams and spots in the fluorescence image. The lymph node was dissected along with its surrounding fatty tissue
(**d**) Two of three dissected lymph nodes showed fluorescence signals inside the nodes (*right* and *left*). No fluorescence was seen inside the node but was observed in the surrounding fat with the other specimen (middle)

nodes embedded in the surrounding tissue were found. Fluorescence imaging was useful for the navigation of dissection. The lymphatic channels and nodes receiving ICG appeared as shining streams and spots with fluorescence in the fluorescence image. After removal, it was ensured that no fluorescent spot was left in the axilla. Lymph nodes in the dissected specimen were isolated from the surrounding fatty tissue, and we investigated whether each lymph node was fluorescent inside. All fluorescent lymph nodes were regarded as sentinel nodes.

8.3.3 Initial Results

Thirty-three patients with clinically node-negative breast cancer were examined from October 2003 to November 2004 at Osaka Red Cross Hospital [9]. Sentinel nodes were successfully identified in 31 of 33 cases (detection rate: 94 %), and the number of sentinel nodes was 2.7 on average (one to seven). Eleven patients had metastatic sentinel nodes. For one patient, the intraoperative pathological report was negative, but the permanent report was positive. Five out of 11 sentinel-positive patients were metastatic in the non-sentinel nodes. One patient was metastatic in the non-sentinel nodes among 20 sentinel-negative patients (negative predictive value, 95 %; false negative rate, 8.3 %).

Green lymphatic channels were visible in 24 of 33 patients. For eight patients in whom green lymphatic channels were not seen, further dissection was performed by fluorescent imaging. Green nodes were visible only in 13 patients, whereas fluorescence signals in the sentinel nodes were clearly observed in 30 patients.

8.4 Axillary Compression Technique

One of the main drawbacks of ICG fluorescence method was that the localization of the sentinel nodes could not be identified before skin incision. We introduced axillary compression technique to overcome this problem [10].

8.4.1 Principle and Procedures

The principle of the axillary compression technique is shown in Fig. 8.7. The fluorescence signal of a subcutaneous LV becomes invisible where it runs deeper in the axillary space (Fig. 8.7a). When the axillary skin is compressed against the chest wall with a transparent plastic device (Hamamatsu Photonics, Japan) (Fig. 8.8), a fluorescence signal appears at the bottom of the device because the LV or the LN comes near to the surface. As shown in Fig. 8.7b and c, the shape and intensity of the compression-inducible fluorescence signal depend on the

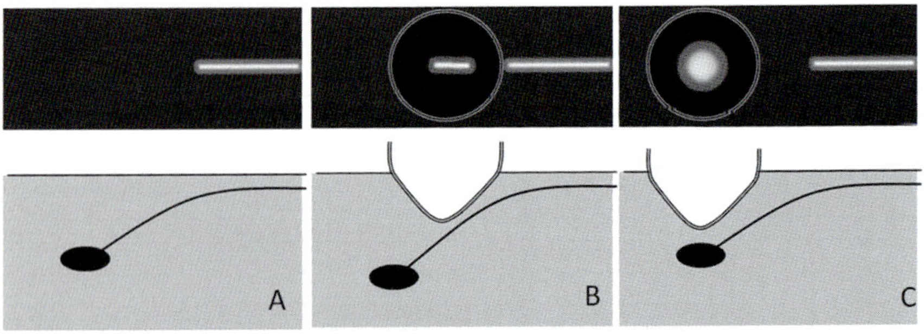

Fig. 8.7 Principle of axillary compression technique:
(**a**) Fluorescence signal of a subcutaneous lymphatic vessel becomes invisible where it runs deeper in the axillary space
(**b**) When the axillary skin is compressed against the chest wall with a transparent plastic device, a fluorescence signal appears at the bottom of the device. A linear-shaped and sharp signal represents a lymphatic vessel
(**c**) A round-shaped and intense signal represents a lymph node

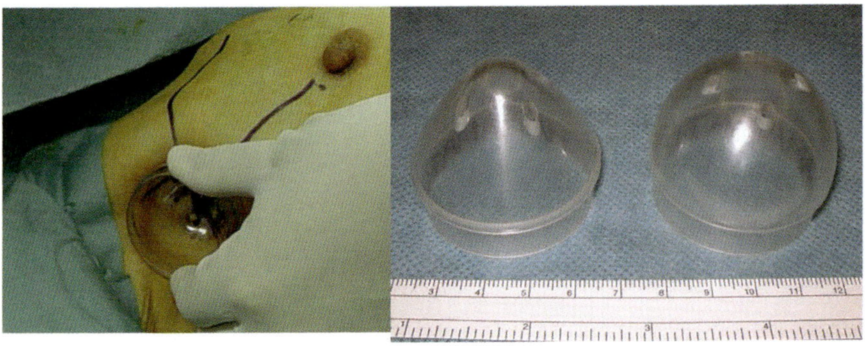

Fig. 8.8 (**a**) We used two types of compression devices, which were a hemispheric bowl with a diameter of 4 cm (*right*) and a cone-shaped device (*left*)
(**b**) The axillary skin was compressed against the chest wall by a plastic compression device

underlying structure. Typically, a linear-shaped and sharp signal represents a LV (B), and a round-shaped and intense signal represents a LN (C). Transcutaneous lymphatic mapping can be undertaken by tracing the compression-inducible fluorescence signal toward the axilla. The first pressure-inducible, round, and intense fluorescence signal is supposed to be the first SN. It usually takes several minutes after ICG injection until adequate amount of ICG is accumulated in the SNs. A skin incision is made at the estimated site, and the SN is directly approached without dissecting the LV. The dissecting procedure is as simple as severing the subcutaneous tissue and the axillary fascia toward the fluorescent signal. As the dissection plane becomes deep, the intensity of the fluorescence signal from the SN increases.

When the fluorescent nodes are extracted out of the wound, a subcutaneous LV draining to the nodes can be observed using a fluorescence image to ensure that the SNs are correctly excised. In most cases, when the first SL was pulled out of the wound with the surrounding fatty tissue, a few more fluorescent nodes were observed in the fat. We excised these nodes with the fatty tissue as a lymphatic basin. In order to clearly observe these SNs and draining LV without injury, it is important to widely open the axillary fascias and adequately pull them out of the wound by freeing the adjacent vessels and nerves. Electrical dissection was useful to minimize ICG contamination in the surgical field. In cases where only one node could be removed, the axillary space was observed again by fluorescence whether any fluorescent nodes were left after removal of the first node. The following procedures are the same as the original method.

8.4.2 Clinical Results

The axillary compression technique was used in 50 patients with clinically node-negative breast cancer who underwent SNB from January 2008 to August 2009. The mean age was 63.1 (41–93), and the body mass index (BMI) was 22.9 (17.6–36.4). Compression-inducible fluorescence signal in the axilla could be observed in all cases. Transcutaneous identification and direct approach to the SNs were successfully carried out in 47 cases. In the three other cases, where the SNs could not be directly approached, an axillary LV was first detected and then traced to the SNs following the original method. Finally, SNs were successfully removed in all cases. The average number of dissected nodes was 3.6 (1–8), and six cases were metastatic. It took 24.1 (10–47) minutes to remove the SNs after ICG injection. Transcutaneous detection and direct approach to the SN were also effective in twelve patients with BMI greater than 25. Three cases of unsuccessful results were nonobese and elderly patients.

Figure 8.9 shows a case of a 35-year-old female. Subcutaneous lymphatic drainage was observed, and the signal disappeared at the lateral edge of the pectoralis major muscle (A). Beyond the disappearing point, a linear-shaped fluorescence signal was seen by compression, representing a LV (B). Upon tracing toward the axilla, a round-shaped intense fluorescence signal was then observed and supposed to be the signal from the SN (C). A skin incision was made, and the subcutaneous tissue was dissected until a SN was exposed without tracing the LV (D, E). A LV draining to the SN was observed when the fluorescent node was extracted from the wound (F).

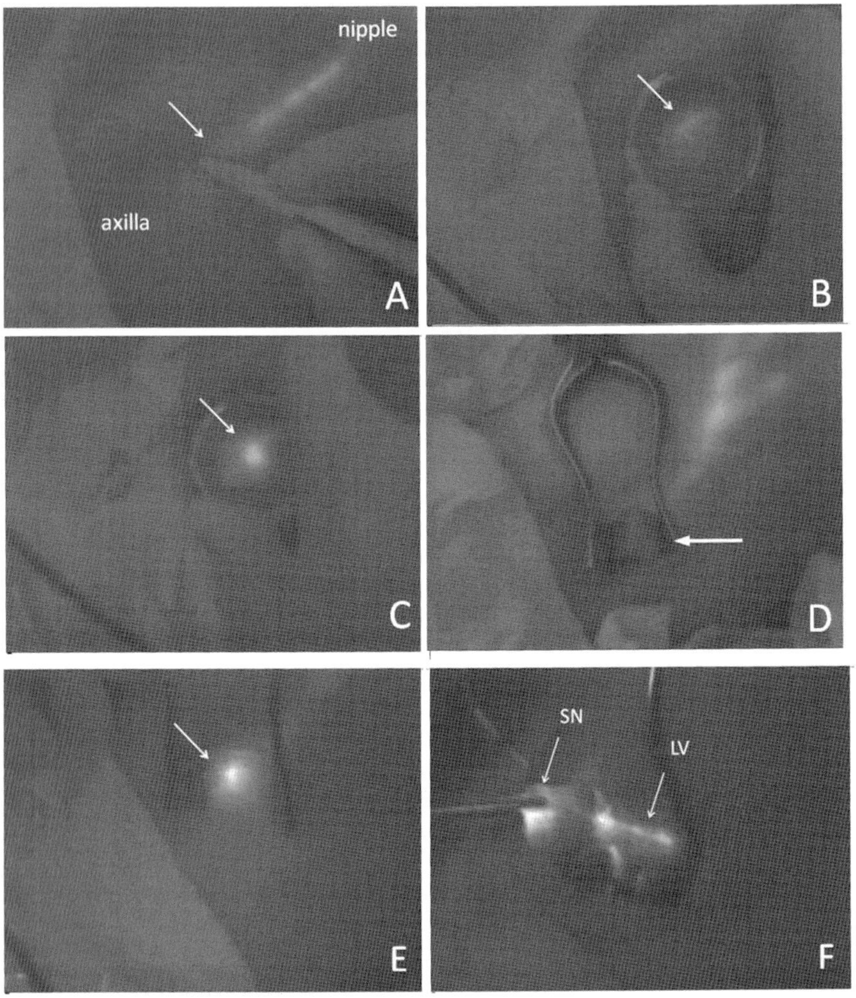

Fig. 8.9 Fluorescence images using the axillary compression technique:
(**a**) Subcutaneous lymphatic drainage was observed, and the signal disappeared beyond the lateral edge of the pectoralis major muscle (*arrow*)
(**b**) A linear-shaped fluorescence signal was seen by compression, representing a lymphatic vessel (*arrow*)
(**c**) A round-shaped intense fluorescence signal was observed, representing a sentinel node (*arrow*)
(**d**, **e**) After skin incision (**d**) and fascial dissection (**e**), the sentinel node showed more intense fluorescence signal (*arrows*)
(**f**) A lymphatic vessel (LV) draining to the sentinel node (SN) was observed

8.5 Conclusions

1. ICG fluorescence method was developed for the sentinel node biopsy in breast cancer.
2. Although the usefulness of the ICG fluorescence method has been demonstrated, it is not a replacement of the radioisotope method. Further improvement and investigation are necessary.

References

1. Veronesi U, Paganelli G, Viale G et al (2003) A randomized comparison of sentinel-node biopsy with routine axillary dissection in breast cancer. N Eng J Med 349:546–553
2. Krag DN, Anderson SJ, Julian TB et al (2010) Sentinel-lymph-node resection compared with conventional axillary-lymph-node dissection in clinically node-negative patients with breast cancer: overall survival findings from NSABP B-32 randomized phase 3 trial. Lancet Oncol 11:927–933
3. Giuliano AE, Jones RC, Brennan M et al (1997) Sentinel lymphadenectomy in breast cancer. J Clin Oncol 15:2345–2350
4. Wilson BC (1991) Optical properties of tissues. In: Encyclopedia of human biology, vol 5. Academic Press, St. Louis, pp 587–597
5. Benson RC, Kues HA (1978) Fluorescence properties of indocyanine green as related to angiography. Phys Med Biol 23:159–163
6. Sevick EM, Chance B, Leigh J et al (1991) Quantitation of time-and frequency-resolved optical spectra for the determination of tissue oxygenation. Anal Biochem 195:330–351
7. Beauvoit B, Chance B (1998) Time resolved spectroscopy of mitochondria, cells and tissues under normal and pathological condition. Moll Cell Biochem 184:445–455
8. Kitai T, Inomoto T, Shikayama T et al (2005) Fluorescence navigation with indocyanine green for detecting sentinel lymph nodes in breast cancer. Breast Cancer 12:211–215
9. Kitai T, Inomoto T, Miwa M et al (2005) Sentinel lymph node biopsy in breast cancer using fluorescence navigation by indocyanine green. Report of a validation study. Jpn J Breast Cancer 20:250–254 (Japanese)
10. Kitai T, Kawashima M (2011) Transcutaneous detection and direct approach to the sentinel node using axillary compression technique in ICG fluorescence-navigated sentinel node biopsy for breast cancer. Breast Cancer 19:343–348

Chapter 9
Practice of Fluorescence Navigation Surgery Using Indocyanine Green for Sentinel Lymph Node Biopsy in Breast Cancer

Kazuhiko Yamagami, Teruyuki Deai, Hajime Matumoto, and Takashi Hashimoto

Abstract The indocyanine green (ICG) navigation method enables a high detection rate and a low false-negative rate (FNR) in sentinel lymph node biopsy (SLNB). Unlike the blue dye-guided method (BD method), it emits a stronger fluorescence signal in the sentinel lymph node (SLN), contributing to its high detection rate and requiring less training. Unlike the radioisotope-guided (RI) method, it does not require radioactive colloids, expensive equipment, and legal permission. The ICG injection is diluted considering "quenching reaction," and this dilution shows that enough sensitivity for SLN detection is attainable even at lower-dose ICG. Compression of the chest wall and axilla using hemispherical transplant device enables the identification of fluorescent SLN locations prior to the skin incision. The reduced FNR observed with the ICG method is due to its high detection rate of involvement SLNs and its ability to aid examination of more than one or two SLNs at anatomical order. This paper describes the current clinical practice of the ICG fluorescence navigation method and its availability compared to conventional methods (BD or RI method).

Keywords Indocyanine green • ICG • Fluorescence • Sentinel lymph node • Breast cancer

---

K. Yamagami (✉) • T. Deai • H. Matumoto
Department of Breast Surgery, Shinko Hospital, 1-4-47 Wakinohama-cho, Chuo-ku, Kobe, Hyogo 651-0072, Japan
e-mail: kazu.yama.-0825@shinkohp.or.jp

T. Hashimoto
Department of Breast Surgery, Shinko Hospital, 1-4-47 Wakinohama-cho, Chuo-ku, Kobe, Hyogo 651-0072, Japan

Hashimoto Clinic, Hyogo, Japan

M. Kusano et al. (eds.), *ICG Fluorescence Imaging and Navigation Surgery*,
DOI 10.1007/978-4-431-55528-5_9

9.1 Sentinel Lymph Node Biopsy in Breast Cancer

Although axillary lymph node dissection (ALND) has long been a standard part of the local therapy of breast cancer, the rate of patients with axillary nodal metastases is not so high in daily clinical experience. The probability of axillary metastases increases with increasing tumor size. The TNM staging system is a cancer-staging notation system of the American Joint Committee on Cancer. The T category, which is the invasive components of the primary lesion, predicts the axillary nodal positivity (T1a:5 %, T1b: 16 %, T1c: 28 %, T2: 48 %) [1]. Therefore, considering the high rate of negative nodes, the uniform use of the ALND in all cases is irrational.

The sentinel lymph node (SLN) is defined as the first node that receives lymphatic drainage from the breast cancer cells, and hence, the most likely node to contain invading cancer cells. Sentinel lymph node biopsy (SLNB) in breast cancer is a promising surgical technique to assess the axillary nodal status, avoiding unnecessary ALND and leading to less morbidities, such as lymphedema, numbness, and pain. SLNB with nodal assessment in clinically node-negative patients is accepted as the standard technique by the American Society of Clinical Oncology (ASCO) guideline [2] and the National Comprehensive Cancer Network (NCCN) guideline.

9.2 Conventional Methods for SLN Detection

In general, three methods of SLN mapping are the current standards of care: the radioisotope method (RI method), the blue dye method (BD method), and a combination of both as the tracer. These conventional techniques have certain disadvantages.

The BD method alone does not require any special device and is therefore convenient. However, blue dye does not penetrate the dermis; therefore, it cannot provide the precise location of the SLNs prior to skin incision. Moreover, it is impossible to detect the small amount of dye in the SLNs with the naked eye. Additionally, the blue dye disperses easily, contributing to poor tissue contrast. The identification of deep SLNs is more difficult due to low penetration of blue color. All this results in lower detection rates of 73.8 % [3] and 83.1 % [4] compared to the RI method and combination method [4–6]. Additionally, two meta-analysis research studies reported higher false-negative rates (FNR) with the BD method alone compared to that of the RI method alone or the combination of both method [4, 7]. Visualization of the blue color is easily impaired because of dense fat, intraoperative bleeding, or rapid transition. For the reasons stated above, the breast surgeon needs a certain experience using dye method until a satisfactory identification rate.

Radioactive colloids are essential for stagnation of one or two nodes without spreading. Radionuclide scanning provides good accuracy allowing transcutaneous navigation from the skin to the more deeply located SLNs [8]. However, there are potential drawbacks associated with the use of radioactive colloids including the exposure of patients and health-care workers to a cumulative radiation dose and the use of expensive tracers and expensive equipment; therefore, radioactive colloids are not widely available [9]. Owing to the length of time it takes for the radioactive tracer to reach the SLN, all the necessary evaluation cannot be completed during the operation. In addition, radioactive signal from the injection site interferes with the detection of SLNs [10]. Moreover this method does not provide real-time visual guidance because it is guided by sound.

9.3 SLN Detection with the Indocyanine Green Fluorescence Navigation Method

Indocyanine green (ICG) as a tracer has been shown to be very safe and has low toxicity with iodine allergy (0.001 %) [11]. It does not require any special licensing, storage, or handling procedure. We proposed that ICG fluorescence navigation method (ICG method) has a great efficacy. It allows real-time transcutaneous and intraoperative visualization of lymphatic channels and superior recognition of SLN in early breast cancer patients [12, 13]. The ICG method has several characteristics that are advantageous for the SLNB procedure, including a higher detection rate for SLNs compared with that of the BD method alone, as outlined in Tables 9.1 [13] and Table 9.2 [11, 14–19]. The ability to observe subcutaneous lymphatic channels through the skin often helps to identify the optimal location for the skin incision. The high sensitivity and specificity of detection of the fluorescent nodes, without radiation exposure, is a clear advantage of this method. As a result, there is no need for any specialized training for detection of SLNs. The main weakness of ICG method is its poor tissue penetration (less than 2 cm) due to the excitation light and fluorescence of ICG. Unlike the RI method, it is generally necessary with the ICG method to separate subcutaneous tissue for identification of SLNs. The SLNs are usually located at a depth of 2 cm or more in the axilla. Observation of illuminated lymphatic channels and SLNs must be carried out with the shadowless light switched off, because of the interference from the near-infrared component of the shadowless light. However, the fluorescence image can be easily observed under the room light. Moreover, the higher number of SLNs captured due to the easy dispersal and high sensitivity of the fluorescence signal is considered a negative aspect of the treatment because of the possibility of the morbidity in the upper arm.

Table 9.1 Detection rate of sentinel lymph node using fluorescence and dye

Group	Characteristic	Patients, (%) ($n = 410$)	
A	(Flu+/Dye+)	381	(92.9 %)
B	(Flu+/Dye-)	18	(4.4 %)
C	(Flu-/Dye+)	0	(0 %)
D	(Flu-/Dye-)	11	(2.7 %)

Table 9.2 Comparison of detection rate (upper) and identified mean numbers (lower) in sentinel lymph nodes in clinical trials

Study	Year	ICG		BD		RI	
Tagaya et al. [14]	2008	100 %	(25/25)	92 %	(23/25)		
		5.5		2.3			
Abe et al. [15]	2011	100 %	(128/128)	66 %	(84/128)		
		3.1		1.0			
Hirano et al. [16]	2012	99 %	(107/108)	93 %	(100/108)		
		2.2		1.6			
Sugie et al. [17]	2013	99 %	(98/99)	78 %	(77/99)		
		3.4		2.4			
Hojo et al. [18]	2010	99 %	(140/141)	92.9 %	(105/113)	100 %	(28/28)
		3.8		1.9		2.0	
Wishart et al. [11]	2012	100 %	(104/104)	99 %	(103/104)	91 %	(95/104)
		–		–		–	
Jung et al. [19]	2014	100 %	(43/43)	91 %	(39/43)	100 %	(43/43)
		3.4		–		2.3	

9.3.1 Device Used

Fluorescence navigation of lymphatic channels and SLNs is achieved using a near-infrared fluorescence navigation device (Photodynamic Eye (PDE) camera or Photodynamic Eye-neo (PDE-neo) camera, Hamamatsu Photonics K.K., Hamamatsu, Japan).

9.3.2 Use of ICG as a Tracer

Figure 9.1 shows the strong illumination of diluted ICG. The dilution must be considered to be due to a "quenching reaction." All fluorophores exhibit fluorescence quenching if their concentration is too high, and near-infrared fluorophores are no exception [20]. That is, increasing the concentration actually decreases the fluorescence, so theoretically there would be no benefit to injecting a high concentration for SLN mapping [21]. It has been suggested that the degree of hypersensitivity symptoms resulting from diluted ICG is lower compared to a non-diluted dose; therefore the diluted ICG is also preferable from a safety perspective. In our

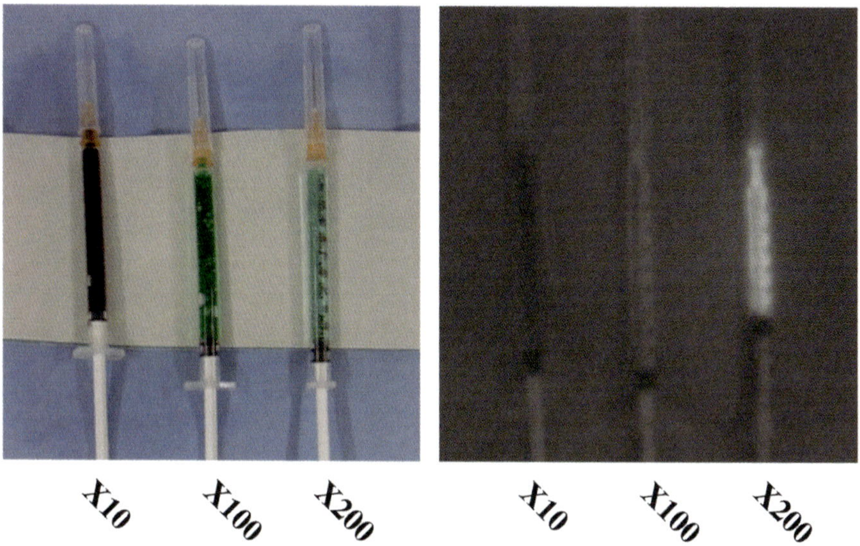

Fig. 9.1 Concentration-dependent quenching. The fluorescence intensity of changed in each sample (indocyanine green) when proportionally diluted with saline

previous study of 410 patients who received an intraoperative injection of ICG, none of these patients experienced any related adverse reactions or complications [13]. Careful attention to concentration and dilution is a factor that enables improved performance of the technology [22].

9.3.3 Tracer Preparation and Injection

ICG (25 mg/5 mL, Diagnogreen; Daiichi–Sankyo Co., Ltd., Tokyo, Japan) is diluted 100 times with saline considering "quenching reaction," resulting in ICG concentration of 0.05 mg/mL (0.064 mM). Then the mixture agents of 1.0 ml (0.05 mg) of diluted ICG and 1.0 ml of blue dye (indigo carmine (4 mg): Daiichi–Sankyo Co., Ltd., Tokyo, Japan) is injected subdermally into the areola. A thin injection needle (thinner than 27 gauge) is used for the purpose of taking pressure. If using ICG alone without using blue dye, 2.0 ml of diluted ICG has been found to be effective with this method.

9.3.4 Surgical Procedures

Within a couple of seconds after injection, the illuminated subcutaneous lymphatic channels and veins traveling toward the axilla can be visualized clearly. Gentle massage of the pomphus, which forms due to retention of the tracer, helps the lymphatic drainage. After a few minutes, only illuminated lymphatic channels remain visible (Fig. 9.2A); usually these lymphatic channels converge toward a single duct in the region of the axilla tail, and they can be traced to the axillary region where occasionally nodes can be seen percutaneously. These subcutaneous lymphatic channels are often invisible through the skin beyond the lateral edge of the greater pectoral muscle, where they extend deeper into the axillary space (Fig. 9.2A). To overcome the invisible SLNs from the skin, axillary compression technique was designed [23]. Use of a hemispherical transparent device (Hamamatsu Photonics K.K., Hamamatsu, Japan) enables the easy observation of deeper lymphatic structures. Figure 9.2B (left) depicts the principal of the technique and an actual observation. From the point where the illumination disappears, the chest wall is compressed by the hemispherical transplant device, allowing the observation of the liner fluorescence signals, which are lymphatic channels. Searching the illuminated lymphatic channels, the SLNs appear as round- or oval-shaped illuminated objects with intensity fluorescence signals as shown in Fig. 9.2B (middle). The site of the skin incision can be more precisely localized following this compression method. The major disadvantage of the ICG method compared to the RI method, the low penetration of the signal, is improved using this axillary compression technique. If transcutaneous identification of the SLNs is unsuccessful, the original method, in which a skin incision is made around 2 cm ahead from the vanishing point of fluorescence or at approximately 1–2 cm proximal to the hairline, is used. Once the axillary skin incision on the round- or oval-shaped illumination, following to the superficial connective tissue separation, has been performed. A vague, weak, and ill-defined fluorescence signal can be observed without a transparent device, affecting the fluorescence signal from the SLNs. As shown in Fig. 9.2C, in the combination of ICG and blue dye, a blue-stained structure is not clear, but a vague fluorescence is observed. When the tissue and fascia are dissected and separated toward the fluorescence signal, the intensity of the signal increases as the SLNs are approached. The illuminated fat tissues including SLNs are pulled from the surgical field, and the intensive fluorescence nodes are separated from any surrounding fatty tissue (Fig. 9.2D). The illuminated SLNs, with or without blue dye, are resected under the guidance of an ICG fluorescent image. A wide cut in the axillary fascia and the adequate pulling of the fluorescent fat tissue are effective in avoiding injury of the neighboring blood vessels and nerves. During dissection of the illuminated nodes, ICG sometimes can leak into the surgical field and produce nonspecific fluorescence staining, leading to difficulties in detection of other fluorescence nodes. As a solution, decreasing the excitation light leads to a line or disappearance of the nonspecific fluorescence staining. On the other hand, residual SLNs can remain as round- or oval-shaped illuminations even if the excitation light decreases. Finally, all dissected lymph nodes are investigated by the ICG camera (Fig. 9.2E).

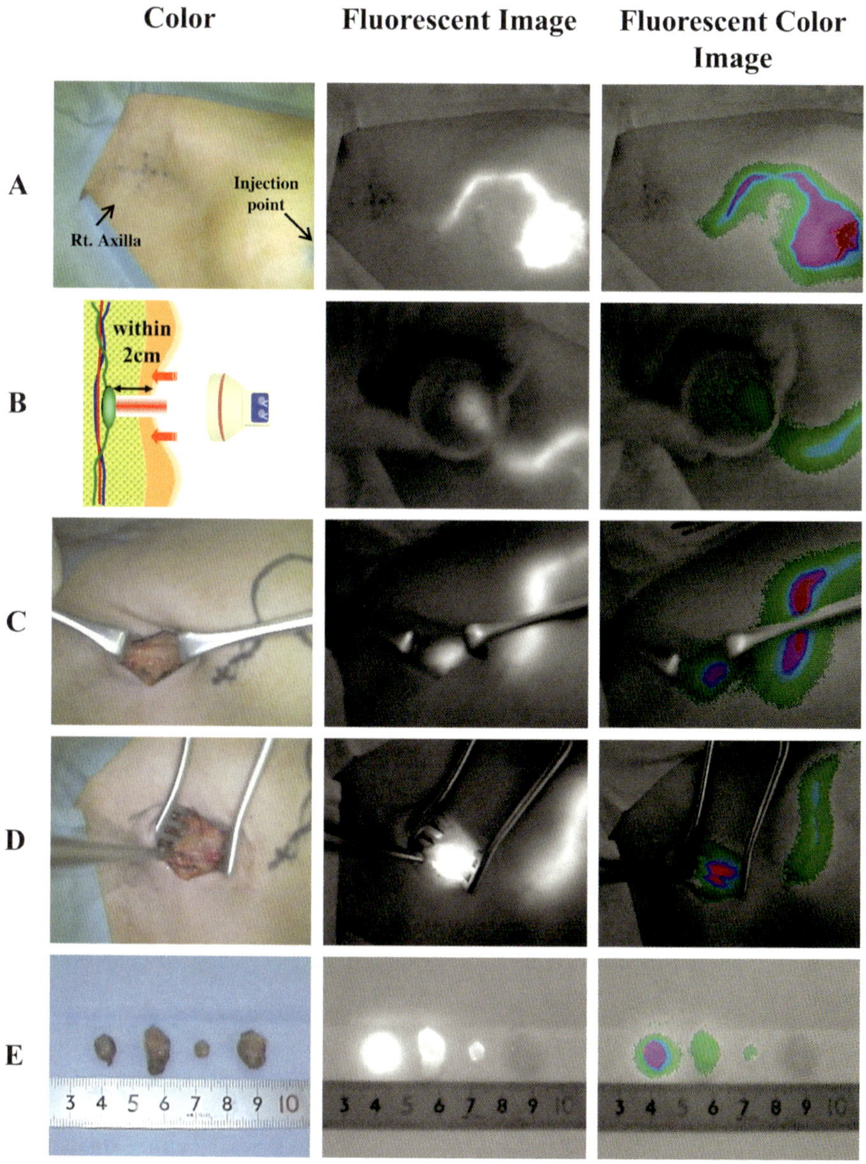

Fig. 9.2 Fluorescence-guided sentinel lymph node (SLN) mapping with a combination of indocyanine green (ICG) and blue dye by using a PDE-neo camera. Fluorescence-color imaging shows fluorescence intensity; red indicates strong intensity, while green indicates weak intensity. *Row A*: The fluorescent lymphatic channels were visualized percutaneously. The fluorescent line disappeared at the lateral edge of the greater pectoral muscle. *Row B*: A schema representing the principle of the axillary compression technique (*left panel*). Compression with a hemispherical transplant device enabled the detection of an intense, oval-shaped fluorescence signal depicting a SLN (*center* and *right panels*). *Row C*: After skin incision and superficial connective tissue separation, blue stained structures were not observed (*left panel*); however, a vague of fluorescence signal was visible (*center panel*). *Row D* Detection of the illuminated SLN (*center panel*). The red area in the fluorescent color image showed the accurate location of SLNs. *Row E*: Examination of

9.4 Comparison of SLNB Guided by the ICG Method Versus BD or RI Method

Table 9.1 shows the detection ratio of SLNs after applying the ICG and blue dye mixture method [13]. Although the detection rate (92.9 %) with the BD method (Group A and Group C) is relatively high compared with that of other reports (Table 9.2), 4.4 % of patients (Group B (Flu+/ Dye-)) could not be identified with blue dye alone. All SLNs stained with blue dye were identified by fluorescence (Group C (Flu-/ Dye+: 0 %)). Other reports also showed the higher detection rate of SLNs with the ICG method than the BD method (Table 9.2). In particular, the detection rate of SLNs with metastases was higher in the ICG method than in the BD method [11, 16, 18, 24], resulting in lower FNR in the ICG method [18]. The presence of tumor in the lymph nodes may interfere with their ability to take up the dye. Furthermore, one of other reasons for false-negative results may be a change in lymphatic flow due to a tumor cell embolism in the lymphatic systems. Unlike the BD method that needs large amounts of blue dye to visual recognition, very small amounts of ICG can illuminate the involvement of nodes that are occupied by tumor cells. Moreover, the weak signal of the BD method alone means it is sometimes necessary to search the blue stained lymphatic channels or SLNs in a large surgical field. Although it is difficult to express in data, all surgeons have experience to search for the weak blue-signal nodes with much stress resulting in considerable invasive searching operation. The ICG method requires less time than the BD method, which may prove the above indirectly [19, 24]. In the combination ICG and BD method, the fluorescence signal was particularly beneficial in difficult cases that were not readily identified using the dye method [18]. It is clear that the ICG fluorescence navigation method is superior to the dye method for the detection of SLNs.

How does the ICG method compare with the RI method in the detection of SLNs? The advantages in ICG method include no need of a radioactive facility, radiation exposure, and the high cost of a radioactive tracer. Visible ICG fluorescence guiding is effective without the need for extended tissue dissection [24] On the other hand, the fluorescent excitation and emission of ICG penetrates human tissue only to a depth of 2 cm, much less than radioactive tracers. In a study by Verbeek et al., axillary lymph nodes could be seen through the skin in only 31 % of cases (30/95) [22]. The axillary compression technique enabled transcutaneous detection (94 %: 47/50) and the mapping of a direct approach to the SLNs, independent of body mass index (mean 22.9 (17.6–36.4)) [23]. Other studies proved no difference in the detection rates between the ICG method and the RI method in keeping the high level (Table 9.2). A number of reports show that fluorescence

Fig. 9.2 (continued) all dissected lymph nodes. From *left* to *right*: Flu+/Dye+, Flu+/Dye-, Flu+/ Dye-, Flu-/Dye-. Using the ICG navigation method, the three nodes from the left were identified as SLNs

SLNs with macrometastases could not be identified by radioactivity [11, 22]. The ICG reagent is a 776-Da disulfonated small molecule and has an affinity-binding site on human serum albumin [25]. The hydrodynamic diameter of ICG tracer, which is defined as serum albumin (2–3 nm), and radioactive colloid (200–1000 nm) are vastly different and can have a major impact on performance [26]. Serum albumin-binding ICG has a potential access to the reduced lumen of afferent lymphatic and lymphatic channels occupied by tumor cell. ICG flows much faster and passes through the first SLN into secondary nodes due to the low molecular weight and the low hydrodynamic diameter. On the other hand, radioactive colloids require hours to travel but have excellent retention in the SLNs [22]. Table 9.2 shows the number of nodes removed using the ICG method is greater than those removed using the RI method. Evaluating additionally second or third SLN detection in the order of anatomical lymphatic flow reduces the FNR. In particular, fluorescent SLNs with macrometastases sometimes could not be detected by using conventional methods (blue dye and/or RI) [11, 22]. A small study ($n = 30$) showed the FNR for the ICG and RI method were 8 % and 23 %, respectively, including those with high rate of involvement nodes [27]. One of the criticisms made in the initial period of use with the ICG method is that the large number of sentinel nodes identified may lead to postoperative complications of the axilla and upper arm. Nonetheless, the surgeon can resect more than one or two SLNs, in the order of anatomical lymphatic flow without a random. Resection of more than one or two illuminated SLNs, which are not in a large field, does not appear to increase morbidity.

The American College of Surgeons Oncology Group (ACOSOG) Z0011 clinical trial was a randomized trial designed to compare overall survival and disease-free survival in SLN-positive patients with and without ALND [28]. If patients had limited SLN metastases, it was proposed that ALND was not useful [28]. Patients were ineligible for the Z-11 trial if they had three or more positive SLNs. Precisely, it is necessary to examine at least three SLNs to prove more than three metastases nodes. The ACOSOG Z1071 clinical trial determined the FNR for SLNB following chemotherapy in women initially presenting with biopsy-proven clinically node-positive patients [29]. SLNB using both blue dye and a radiolabeled colloid-mapping agent was encouraged. Although a high FNR (21.1 %, 19/90) was found in a two-SLN examination, examination of three or more SLNs reduced the FNR (9.1 %, 20/220). The ICG navigation method is effective in the identification of SLN involvement. Moreover examination of more than one or two SLNs, which are located in anatomical order, has the hidden potential of actually being a positive feature of the method instead of a negative.

Additionally, the radiocolloid tracers are produced as a bi-product of the nuclear industry, and a worldwide shortage of radioisotopes broke out in 2009. The decommissioning of deteriorated reactors means that there is a concern regarding unstable radioactive tracer supply. On the other hand, supply of ICG has not become a problem.

9.5 Summary

ICG fluorescence navigation for breast cancer patients does not require a radioisotope facility: it is safe, allows real-time and high-resolution imaging, provides a high detection rate and a low FNR, and does not require any specialized training. The axillary compression technique improved the transcutaneous detection of SLNs with ICG. Moreover, when more than one or two SLNs were identified in anatomical order compared with other methods, it provided a better outcome, including a reduction of the FNR. Considering the stable supply of ICG as a tracer, it will become a more and more promising method in the future.

References

1. Silverstein MJ, Skinner KA, Lomis TJ (2001) Predicting axially nodal positivity in 2282 patients with breast carcinoma. World J Surg 25:767–772. doi:10.1007/s00268001003x
2. Lyman GH, Giuliano AE, Somerfield MR et al (2005) American Society of Clinical Oncology. American Society of Clinical Oncology guideline recommendations for sentinel lymph node biopsy in early–stage breast cancer. J Clin Oncol 23:7703–7720
3. Motomura K, Inaji H, Komoike Y et al (1999) Sentinel node biopsy guided by indocyanine green dye in breast cancer patients. Jpn J Clin Oncol 29:604–607
4. Kim T, Giuliano AE, Lyman GH (2006) Lymphatic mapping and sentinel lymph node biopsy in early-stage breast carcinoma, a metaanalysis. Cancer 106:4–16
5. Noguchi M, Motomura K, Imoto S et al (2000) A multicenter validation study of sentinel lymph node biopsy by the Japanese Breast Cancer Society. Breast Cancer Res Treat 63:31–40
6. McMasters KM, Tuttle TM, Carlson DJ et al (2000) Sentinel lymph node biopsy for breast cancer: a suitable alternative to routine axillary dissection in multi-institutional practice when optimal technique is used. J Clin Oncol 18:2560–2566
7. Pesek S, Ashikaga T, Krag LE et al (2012) The false-negative rate of sentinel node biopsy in patients with breast cancer: a metaanalysis. World J Surg 36:2239–2251
8. Dauphine CE, Khalkhali I, Vargas MP et al (2006) Intraoperative injection of technetium-99m: sulfur colloid is effective in the detection of sentinel lymph nodes in breast cancer. Am J Surg 194:423–426
9. Stratmann SL, McCarty TM, Kuhn JA (1999) Radiation safety with breast sentinel node biopsy. Am J Surg 178:454–457
10. Cox CE, Pendas S, Cox JM et al (1998) Guidelines for sentinel node biopsy and lymphatic mapping of patients with breast cancer. Ann Surg 227:645–651
11. Wishart GC, Loh SR, Jones L et al (2012) A feasibility study (ICG-10) of indocyanine green (ICG) fluorescence mapping for sentinel lymph node detection in early breast cancer. Eur J Surg Oncol 38:651–656
12. Kitai T, Inamoto T, Miwa M et al (2005) Fluorescence navigation with indocyanine green for detecting sentinel lymph nodes in breast cancer. Breast Cancer 12:211–215
13. Yamagami K, Hashimoto T, Yamamoto M (2008) The efficacy of sentinel lymph node and lymphatic tracts detection using fluorescence navigation with indocyanine green in breast cancer. Analysis of 410 patients. J Clin Oncol 26 (Suppl 1): 39s
14. Tagaya N, Yamazaki R, Nakagawa A et al (2008) Intraoperative identification of sentinel lymph nodes by near-infrared fluorescence imaging in patients with breast cancer. Am J Surg 195:850–853

15. Abe H, Mori T, Umeda T et al (2011) Indocyanine green fluorescence imaging system for sentinel lymph node biopsy in early breast cancer patients. Surg Today 41:197–202
16. Hirano A, Kamimura M, Ogura K et al (2012) A comparison of indocyanine green fluorescence imaging plus blue dye and blue day alone for sentinel node navigation surgery in breast cancer patients. Ann Surg Oncol 19: 4112–4116. doi 10.1245/s1043401224780
17. Sugie T, Sawada T, Tagaya N et al (2013) Comparison of indocyanine green fluorescence and blue dye methods in detection of sentinel lymph nodes in early-stage breast cancer. Ann Surg Oncol 20:2213–2218. doi:10.1245/s1043401328909
18. Hojo T, Nagao T, Kikuyama M et al (2010) Evaluation of sentinel node biopsy by combined fluorescent and dye method and lymph flow for breast cancer. Breast 19:210–213
19. Jung SY, Kim SK, Kim SW et al (2014) Comparison of sentinel lymph node biopsy guided by the multimodel method of indocyanine green, fluorescence radioisotope, and blue dye versus the radioisotope method in breast cancer: a randomized controlled trial. Ann Surg Oncol 21:1254–1259. doi:10.1245/s1043401334370
20. Gioux S, Choi HS, Frangioni JV (2010) Image-guided surgery using invisible near-infrared light: fundamentals of clinical translation. Mol Imaging 9:237–255
21. Mieog JS, Troyan SL, Hutteman M et al (2011) Toward optimization of imaging system and lymphatic tracer for near-infrared fluorescent sentinel lymph node mapping in breast cancer. Ann Surg Oncol 18:2483–2491
22. Verbeek FPR, Troyan SL, Mieog JSD et al (2013) Near-infrared fluorescence sentinel lymph node mapping in breast cancer: a multicenter experience. Breast Cancer Res Treat 143:333–342. doi:10.1007/s1054901328029
23. Kitai T, Kawasima M (2012) Transcutaneous detection and direct approach to the sentinel node using axillary compression technique in ICG fluorescence-navigated sentinel node biopsy for breast cancer. Breast Cancer 19:343–348
24. Hirche C, Murawa D, Mohr Z et al (2010) ICG fluorescence-guided sentinel node biopsy for axillary nodal staging in breast cancer. Breast Cancer Res Treat 12:373–378
25. Moody ED, Viskari PJ, Coly CL (1999) Non-covalent labeling of human serum albumin with indocyanine green: a study by capillary electrophoresis with diode laser-induced fluorescence detection. J Chromatogr B Biomed Sci Appl 729:55–64
26. Ohnishi S, Lomnes SJ, Laurence RG et al (2005) Organic alternatives to quantum dots for intraoperative near-infrared fluorescence sentinel lymph node mapping. Mol Imaging 4:172–181
27. MurawaD HC, Dresel S et al (2009) Sentinel lymph node biopsy in breast cancer guided by indocyanine green fluorescence. Br J Surg 96:1289–1294
28. Giuliano AE, Hunt KK, Ballman KV et al (2011) Axillary dissection vs no axillary dissection in woman with invasive breast cancer and sentinel node metastasis: a randomized clinical trial. JAMA 305:569–575
29. Boughey JC, Suman VJ, Mittendorf EA et al (2013) Sentinel lymph node surgery after neoadjuvant chemotherapy in patients with node-positive breast cancer: the ACOSOG Z1071 (Alliance) clinical trial. JAMA 310:1455–1461. doi:10.1001/jama. 2013 278932

Chapter 10
A Perspective on Current Status and Future Directions of Sentinel Node Biopsy Using Fluorescence Imaging System in Breast Cancer

Tomoharu Sugie

Abstract Near-infrared (NIR) imaging using indocyanine green (ICG) fluorescence can localize sentinel lymph node (SLN) in context with lymphatic flows and leads to navigation surgery to identify SLN at high detection rate. Cumulative results of clinical trials demonstrate that this NIR fluorescence imaging could be good alternative to a standard SLN mapping using a radioactive tracer in breast cancer. Though there are some drawbacks for attenuation in the depth and larger number of SLN removed, NIR imaging using ICG achieves high SLN detection and has a potential to reduce false-negative study after neoadjuvant chemotherapy.

Keywords Near-infrared imaging • Sentinel lymph node biopsy • Indocyanine green • Breast cancer

10.1 Introduction

Sentinel lymph node (SLN) biopsy is now the standard of care for axillary staging in women with early breast cancer. Since Morton and colleagues [1] first applied SLN theory for melanoma in 1994, cumulative results demonstrated that completion of axillary lymph node dissection can be spared in early breast cancer without SLN involvement. Dual mapping using radioactive colloid and blue dye is currently the standard method for SLN mapping and can achieve a high detection rate and a low false-negative rate [2, 3]. However, these modalities have some drawbacks. Dye cannot be seen over the skin and often cause hypersensitivity. The RI method requires restricted facility and has to access to nuclear medicine. These logistical and legislative issues make SLN biopsy applicable in the high-volume center in urbanized countries.

T. Sugie (✉)
Department Surgery, Kansai Medical University, 2-3-1 Shinmachi, Hirakata, Osaka 573-1191, Japan
e-mail: sugiet@hirakata.kmu.ac.jp

M. Kusano et al. (eds.), *ICG Fluorescence Imaging and Navigation Surgery*,
DOI 10.1007/978-4-431-55528-5_10

There is an increasing evidence to support near-infrared (NIR) imaging using indocyanine green (ICG) applicable for SLN mapping in women with early breast cancer. ICG is an amphiphilic molecule and widely used in clinical practice for assessment of liver function and cardiac output. ICG binds to plasma proteins in the vascular compartment, and this protein-binding ICG obtains fluorescence brightness within a near-infrared optic window. NIR imaging using ICG utilizes these fluorescence spectra of ICG [4]. For the detection device, a photodynamic eye (PDE) is widely used in many clinical trial. PDE is composed of light-emitting diode (LED) producing light at a wavelength of 760 nm and a charged-couple device (CCD) camera which filters out a wavelength below 820 nm. This NIR fluorescence imaging system visualizes lymphatic channels over the skin and enables a real-time navigation surgery to harvest SLN [5].

This chapter presents a perspective on current status and discusses future directions of SLN biopsy using fluorescence imaging system in breast cancer.

10.2 A Perspective on Current Status of the ICG Fluorescence Imaging

10.2.1 Comparison Between ICG Fluorescence and Blue Dye

This novel ICG technique is currently adopted at the discretion of physicians in view of the following advantages: (1) no risk for exposure to irradiation, (2) applicable in a small-volume center because it does not require a mandatory licensing and a nuclear medicine department, (3) a real-time imaging of subcutaneous lymph flow that enables surgeon to the orderly and sequential dissection, and (4) requiring little skill.

When ICG is used in the daylight, the detection rate is no more than 73.8 % [6]. When ICG is used in PDE system, cumulative results in previous studies [7–13] demonstrated that the ICG fluorescence method is better than the blue dye method for SLN detection (Table 10.1). The recent meta-analysis confirmed that ICG fluorescence is significantly better for SLN detection (OR 18.37, 95 % CI 8.63–39.10) than the dye method [14]. Van der Vorst and colleagues [11] assessed the value of blue dye when used in combination with ICG and RI. Their study showed that an addition of blue dye does not provide any benefit to SLN biopsy, and they concluded that blue dye can be spared when ICG fluorescence is used in combination with radioactivity. Based on these results, blue dye can be spared when NIR imaging system is used.

Table 10.1 Surgical outcomes of SLN biopsy using blue dye and ICG

	N	SLN detection rate	
		Blue dye (%)	ICG (%)
Tagaya [7]	25	92	100
Abe [8]	128	65.4	100
Sugie [9]	99	78	100
Hojo [10]	113	93	100
Van der Vorst [11]	24	84	100
Shasfsma [12]	32	88	100
Wichart [13]	100	99	100

Table 10.2 Surgical outcome of SLN biopsy using RI and ICG

	N	SLN detection rate	
		RI (%)	ICG (%)
Hojo [10]	113	100	93.1
Van der Vorst [11]	24	95.8	95.8
Shasfsma [12]	32	100	100
Wishart [13]	100	91.3	100
Murawa [16]	20	85	100
Ballardinni [17]	134	99.2	100
Verbeek [18]	95	97.9	98.9
Samorani [19]	301	95.3	98.6

10.2.2 Comparison Between ICG Fluorescence and RI

Dual mapping involved with RI and blue dye is currently the standard technique for SLN localization. The detection rate for this technique was 96 % with low false-negative rate of 7.3 % [15]. Regardless of this clinical usefulness, the RI method has some drawbacks as mentioned above and cannot be uptaken in the small-volume center without involvement of nuclear medicine. As shown in Table 10.2, previous studies reported that ICG fluorescence was comparable or superior to RI for overall SLN detection [10–13, 16–19]. Two studies reported that SLN detection rate for ICG was 100 % compared with 88-89 % for RI and 78-88 % for blue dye [11, 12]. Wishart GC and colleagues [13] used tree tracer agents (ICG, RI, and blue dye) and compared SLN detection between these three techniques. In their study, the detection rates were 91.3 % for RI, 99 % for blue dye, and 100 % for ICG, and the combination of ICG and blue dye had the highest nodal sensitivity at 95.0 %. As blue dye does not have any impact for SLN detection when ICG is used simultaneously, the ICG fluorescence method has a potential to be an alternative to a dual technique with RI and blue dye. On the basis of these results, ICG fluorescence method alone is applicable as clinical practice if access to RI is not available.

10.2.3 Clinical Issue for the ICG Fluorescence Method

One drawback of the ICG fluorescence method is attenuation of fluorescence signal. As emitted fluorescence from ICG is scattered through fat droplets, detection of fluorescence signal deeper than 1 cm is difficult. As RI is superior to ICG fluorescence for tissue penetration, patients with high BMI is better subject for the RI method. Some previous studies reported that BMI was correlated with lower detection rate and longer time to identify SLN [8, 11]. In other studies, however, the detection rate for ICG fluorescence is independent of BMI and yields high detection rate regardless of high BMI [9, 19].

The second disadvantage was the larger number of SLN removed for the ICG fluorescence method. In previous studies, the mean number for SLN removed using ICG fluorescence ranged from 1.5 to 5.4 which was significantly higher than that using RI and/ or blue dye. ICG's small molecular size and spilt of ICG in the operation field might cause the larger number of fluorescence positive lymph nodes. To obtain an optimal concentration of ICG, Mieog JS and colleagues [20] examined the signal to background ratio (SBR) at the various concentration of human serum albumin-conjugated ICG (ICG: HSA), and they obtained the highest SBR at the concentration of 400–800 μM. The other study for melanoma also reported that a dose of 600 μM ICG: HAS was optimal to obtain high SBR [21]. A dose of 0.5 % (6.4 mM) which was widely used is approximately 10-fold higher than the optimal dose reported. Because the standard dose and concentration of ICG have not been determined yet, a larger study to address the optimal technique may be required.

10.3 Future Direction

SLN biopsy after neoadjuvant chemotherapy (NAC) is still controversial in terms of accuracy for axillary staging. The previous multicenter trial reported that the detection rate for SLN after NAC was 88.9 % for RI alone, 78.1 % for blue dye, and 87.6 % for the combination of RI and blue dye [22]. Three meta-analyses addressing accuracy for SLN biopsy after NAC reported that the RI and/or blue dye method provided a detection rate of 89.6–90.9 % and a false-negative rate of 8.4–12 % [23–25]. Updated ASCO clinical practice guideline reported that SLN may be offered after NAC [26]. The RI method after NAC, however, had a trend for a lower detection rate than before NAC. In the SENTIA trial [27], a false-negative rate for SLN mapping was 14.2 % for the patients who converted from clinically node-node positive to node-negative disease after NAC. This impairment of the SLN detection might be related with fibrosis and lymphatic obstruction by cytotoxic reagents.

For detection technique, additional use of blue dye tends to improve false-negative rate. This false-negative rate was associated with the number of SLN removed, and the accuracy for SLN biopsy was apparently improved when more than two nodes were removed. As the smaller size of ICG (<1 nm) can flow through narrowing lymphatic channels than the larger size of radio colloid (>50 nm), ICG potentially enables to reach the first SLN or the further tier more smoothly than RIafter NAC. A large-scale clinical trial is required to confirm the usefulness of theICG fluorescence method after NAC in the patients with clinically node-positive breast cancer.

References

1. Morton DL, Wen DR, Wong JH et al (1992) Technical details of intraoperative lymphatic mapping for early stage melanoma. Arch Surg 127:392–399
2. Krag DN, Anderson SJ, Julian TB et al (2007) Technical outcomes of sentinel-lymph-node resection and conventional axillary-lymph-node dissection in patients with clinically node-negative breast cancer: results from the NSABP B-32 randomized phase III trial. Lancet Oncol 8:881–888
3. Mansel RE, MacNeill F, Horgan K et al (2013) Results of a national training programmer in sentinel lymph node biopsy for breast cancer. Br J Surg 100:654–661
4. Benson RC, Kues HA (1978) Fluorescence properties of indocyanine green as related to angiography. Med Biol 23:159–163
5. Sugie T, Kassim KA, Takeuchi M et al (2010) A novel method for sentinel lymph node biopsy by indocyanine green fluorescence technique in breast cancer. Cancers 2:713–720
6. Motomura K, Inaji H, Komoike Y et al (1999) Sentinel node biopsy guided by indocyanine green dye in breast cancer patients. Jpn J Clin Oncol 29:604–607
7. Tagaya N, Yamazaki R, Nakagawa A et al (2008) Intraoperative identification of sentinel lymph node by near-infrared fluorescence imaging in patients with breast cancer. Am J Surg 195:850–853
8. Abe H, Mori T, Umeda T et al (2011) Indocyanine green fluorescence imaging system for sentinel lymph node biopsies in early breast cancer patients. Surg Today 41:197–202
9. Sugie T, Sawada T, Tagaya N et al (2013) Comparison of the indocyanine green fluorescence and blue dye methods in detection of sentinel lymph nodes in early-stage breast cancer. Ann Surg Oncol 20:2213–2218
10. Hojo T, Nagao T, Kikuyama M et al (2010) Evaluation of sentinel node biopsy by combined fluorescence and dye method and lymph flow for breast cancer. Breast 19:210–213
11. van der Vorst JR, Schaafsma BE, Verbeek FP et al (2012) Randomized comparison of near-infrared fluorescence imaging using indocyanine green and 99(m) technetium with or without patent blue for the sentinel lymph node procedure in breast cancer patients. Ann Surg Oncol 19:4104–4111
12. Schaafsma BE, Verbeek FP, Rietbergen DD et al (2013) Clinical trial of combined radio- and fluorescence-guided sentinel lymph node biopsy in breast cancer. Br J Surg 100:1037–1044
13. Wishart GC, Loh SW, Jones L, Benson JR (2012) A feasibility study (ICG-10) of indocyanine green (ICG) fluorescence map- ping for sentinel lymph node detection in early breast cancer. Eur J Surg Oncol 38:651–656
14. Ahmed M, Purushotham AD, Douek M (2014) Novel techniques for sentinel lymph node biopsy in breast cancer: a systematic review. Lancet Oncol 15:e351–e362
15. Kim T, Giuliano AE, Lyman GH (2006) Lymphatic mapping and sentinel lymph node biopsy in early-stage breast carcinoma. Cancer 106:4–16
16. Murawa D, Hirche C, Dresel S, Hünerbein M (2009) Sentinel lymph node biopsy in breast cancer guided by indocyanine green fluorescence. Br J Surg 96:1289–1294

17. Ballardini B, Santoro L, Sangalli C et al (2013) The indocyanine green method is equivalent to the ^{99}mTc-labeled radiotracer method for identifying the sentinel node in breast cancer: a concordance and validation study. Eur J Surg Oncol 39:1332–1336
18. Verbeek FP, Troyan SL, Mieog JS et al (2014) Near-infrared fluorescence sentinel lymph node mapping in breast cancer: a multicenter experience. Breast Cancer Res Treat 143:333–342
19. Samorani D, Fogacci T, Panzini I et al (2015) The use of indocyanine green to detect sentinel nodes in breast cancer: a prospective study. Eur J Surg Oncol 41:64–70
20. Mieog JS, Troyan SL, Hutteman M et al (2011) Toward optimization of imaging system and lym- phatic tracer for near-infrared fluorescent sentinel lymph node mapping in breast cancer. Ann Surg Oncol 18:2483–2491
21. Gilmore DM, Khullar OV, Gioux S et al (2013) Effective low-dose escalation of indocyanine green for near-infrared fluorescent sentinel lymph node mapping in patients with melanoma. Ann Surg Oncol 20:2357–2363
22. Mamounas EP, Brown A, Anderson S et al (2005) Sentinel node biopsy after neoadjuvant chemotherapy in breast cancer: results from National Surgical Adjuvant Breast and Bowel Project Protocol B-27. J Clin Oncol 23:2694–2702
23. Xing Y, Foy M, Cox DD et al (2006) Meta-analysis of sentinel lymph node biopsy after preoperative chemotherapy in patients with breast cancer. Br J Surg 93:539–546
24. Kelly AM, Dwamena B, Cronin P, Carios RC (2009) Breast cancer sentinel node identification and classification after neoadjuvant chemotherapy-systematic review and meta analysis. Acad Radiol 16:551–563
25. van Deurzen CH, Vriens BE, Tjan-Heijnen VC et al (2009) Accuracy of sentinel node biopsy after neoadjuvant chemotherapy in breast cancer patients: a systematic review. Eur J Cancer 45:3124–3130
26. Lyman GH, Temin S, Edge SB et al (2014) Practice. Sentinel lymph node biopsy for patients with early-stage breast cancer: American Society of Clinical Oncology clinical practice guideline update. J Clin Oncol 32:1365–1383
27. Kuehn T, Bauerfeind I, Fehm T et al (2014) Sentinel-lymph node biopsy in patients with breast cancer before and after neoadjuvant chemotherapy (SENTINA): a prospective, multicenter cohort study. Lancet Oncol 14:609–618

Chapter 11
Indocyanine Green Fluorescence Axillary Reverse Mapping for Sentinel Node Navigation Surgery in Breast Cancer

Takashi Sakurai

Abstract Introduction: We investigated whether indocyanine green (ICG) fluorescence axillary reverse mapping (ICG-ARM) is beneficial for evaluating the risk of lymphedema.

Patients and Methods: Between August 2009 and November 2013, 455 patients were enrolled in this study. Using a fluorescence camera, we checked the ICG accumulation of sentinel nodes and divided into corresponding group and non-corresponding group. Rate of concordance between ARM lymphatics and localization of SN was also investigated.

Results: Among the 455 axillary sites, 105 cases (23.1 %) were included in the corresponding group. Lymphedema developed in 6 of the 455 cases (1.3 %) in the overall population and in 6 of 105 cases (5.7 %) in the corresponding group, and no patient from the non-corresponding group developed lymphedema. In the upper side of the second intercostobrachial nerve (2ICBN), concordance rate of UE lymphatics and breast SN was 47/101 (46.5 %) and around the 2ICBN was 117/277 (42.2 %). On the other hand, only one patient observed UE lymphatics in the caudal side of 2ICBN.

Conclusion: ICG-ARM for sentinel node navigation surgery is useful for the selection of patients who are at risk for lymphedema.

Keywords Breast cancer • Axillary reverse mapping • Sentinel lymph node biopsy • Lymphedema • Fluorescence image

11.1 Introduction

In May 2014, the ASCO recommended against axillary dissection for macrometastases involving one or two sentinel lymph nodes (SNs); hence, axillary dissection for positive SNs has not been used during breast-conserving surgery.

T. Sakurai, M.D. (✉)
Division of Surgery, (JCHO), Saitama Medical Center, 4-7-9 Kitaurawa, Urawa-ku, Saitama 330-0074, Japan
e-mail: sakurai-ssih@umin.net

M. Kusano et al. (eds.), *ICG Fluorescence Imaging and Navigation Surgery*,
DOI 10.1007/978-4-431-55528-5_11

However, 0–13 % of patients undergoing only SNB were still at risk for postoperative upper extremity (UE) lymphedema. We investigated whether indocyanine green (ICG) fluorescence axillary reverse mapping (ICG-ARM) is beneficial for evaluating the risk of lymphedema.

11.1.1 History of Axillary Reverse Mapping

In the 1990s, SNB was developed for malignant melanoma surgery and breast axillary surgery. The technique of ARM is standard except when identifying UE lymphatics during breast axillary dissections.

Thompson and Nos first reported ARM results in 2007 [1, 2]. They used a dye method and discovered that there was a watershed at the axillary lymphatics that received drainage both from the breast and UE. Moreover, they concluded that lymph nodes draining from the UE had low risk for breast cancer metastasis.

In 2009, we reported a 46 % ARM lymphatic detection rate for 35 Japanese patients who underwent axillary dissection. Of all detected lymphatics, 94 % were in between the axillary vein and the second intercostobrachial nerve (2ICBN) [3]. This study highlighted that the detection rate for UE lymphatics and lymph nodes is low and that UE lymphatics sometimes flow near the 2ICBN. To solve these problems, we introduced the ICG fluorescence technique and started to evaluate the influence of lymphedema during SNB.

The usefulness of fluorescence imaging for detection of ARM nodes was first reported by Noguchi, who reported a 75 % identification rate for ARM nodes and/or lymphatics during SNB [4, 5].

11.2 Patients and Methods

11.2.1 Patients

Between August 2009 and November 2013, 455 patients who underwent surgery for Stage 0–IIB (Tis-T3, N0, and M0) primary breast cancer, without bilateral disease or primary chemotherapy, were enrolled in this study.

11.2.2 Methods

The procedure of ICG-ARM was as same as previously reported [6]. More than 2 h before SNB, 0.15 mL of ICG (25 mg of ICG plus 10 mL of 5 % glucose) was injected subcutaneously into the interdigital area of the affected side (Fig. 11.1). In

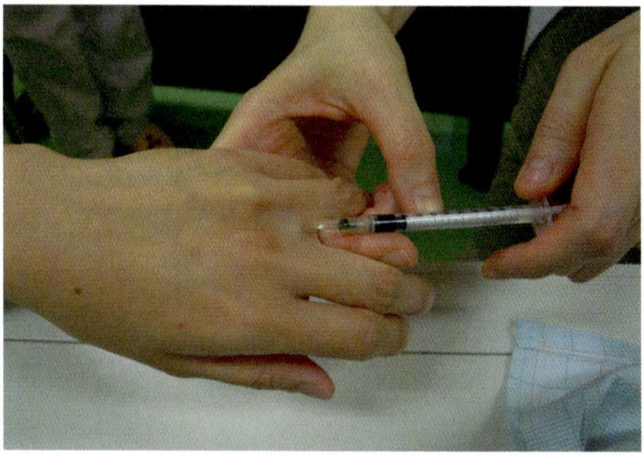

Fig. 11.1 Injection of 0.15 ml ICG at interdigital area subcutaneously

the operation room, we first detected the pattern of UE subcutaneous lymphatics using a fluorescence camera. Using the same detector, we checked the ICG accumulation of sentinel nodes. When a lymph node was clearly luminous, we considered this to be an SN draining both lymphatic routes from the breast and UE and counted this to the corresponding group; when the lymph node was not or only faintly luminous, we considered this to be draining a different lymphatic route and counted this to the non-corresponding group.

SNB procedures include preoperative lymphoscintigraphy and intraoperative radioisotope (RI) plus dye method (triple mapping method).

We assessed lymphedema in all patients at baseline and at 1, 6, and 12 months after surgery, and every 6 months thereafter. The measurement point was based on an international consensus on the best practice for the management of lymphedema [7]. Based on the average body size of a Japanese individual, we designated a 1–2 cm enlargement of the arm as mild edema and >2 cm enlargement as severe edema [8].

Rate of concordance between ARM lymphatics and localization of SN was also investigated. We divided the axillary region into three groups: (zone A) cranial side of the 2ICBN, (zone B) around the 2ICBN, and (zone C) caudal side or the 2ICBN.

11.3 Results

The baseline characteristics of 455 patients who underwent ICG-ARM were shown (Table 11.1). The median age, mean body mass index, mean number of removed lymph nodes, clinical stages, postoperative chemotherapy, and postoperative whole breast irradiation were not different between the two groups statistically.

Among the 455 axillary sites, 105 cases (23.1 %) were included in the corresponding group.

Table 11.1 A comparison of clinical features between the patients with (corresponding group) or without (non-corresponding group) lymphatics flowing into the breast sentinel node using ICG-ARM

	Corresponding group ($n=105$)	Non-corresponding group ($n=350$)	P-value
Age median (range)	58 (24–89)	56 (28–88)	NS
BMI mean (range)	22.2 (17.1–32.9)	22.3 (15.7–40.7)	NS
Number of removed nodes mean (range)	1.69 (1–6)	1.77 (1–6)	NS
Clinical stage (T stage)			
0 (Tis)	23	76	0.76
IA (T1)	52	191	
IIA (T2)	27	74	
IIB (T3)	3	9	
Chemotherapy			
No	98	311	0.18
Yes	7	39	
Breast irradiation			
No	19	56	0.61
Yes	86	294	

BMI body mass index, *NS* not significant

The difference in postoperative lymphedema rates between the corresponding group and non-corresponding group was reported in 2014 [6]. Now we updated the data of the total 455 cases, only 6 patients from the corresponding group and no patient from the non-corresponding group developed lymphedema (Table 11.2). Mild lymphedema was noted in 5 of 6 cases and only 1 case progressed to severe lymphedema.

In the non-corresponding group, we found 47 of 505 cases (9.3 %) with luminous non-SNs, which were dissected because of direct attachment to nonluminous SN.

In the zone A, concordance rate of UE lymphatics and breast SN was 47/101 (46.5 %) and in the zone B was 117/277 (42.2 %). On the other hand, only one patient observed UE lymphatics in the zone C, in this case, the lymphatic drainage around the third intercostobrachial nerve (Figure 11.2).

11.4 Discussion

As axillary dissection for positive SNs during breast-conserving surgery has been minimized, we must consider the risk of lymphedema during SNB procedures.

In this study, the rate of concordance between ARM lymphatics and SN (corresponding group) is almost same as that reported by Noguchi and Ikeda [5, 9]. It was thought that the high sensitivity of ICG-ARM technique contributed to this higher rate of concordance compared with other reports that used dye or RI

Table 11.2 Occurrence of lymphedema in the two groups

	Corresponding group ($n = 105$)	Non-corresponding group ($n = 350$)	P-value
Postoperative LE			
+	6	0	<0.0001
–	99	350	

LE lymphedema

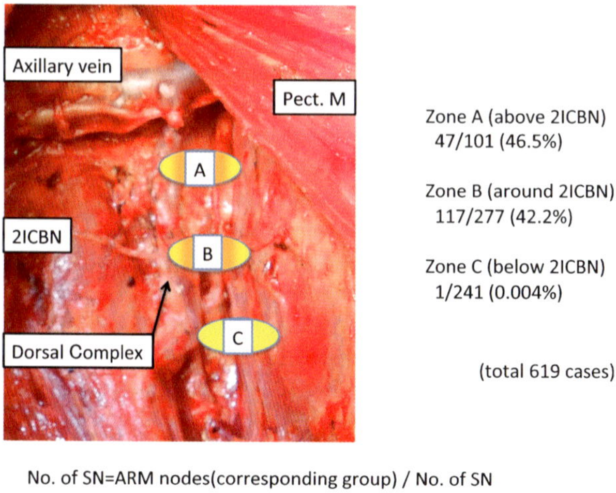

Fig. 11.2 Location of SN and ARM lymphatic concordance rate (No. of SN = ARM nodes (corresponding group)/No. of SN)

[10]. Initially, we used ICG-ARM combined with indigo carmine dye. Now we only use ICG-ARM because of the high ICG sensitivity rate (97.7 %).

Ikeda reported on the usefulness of ICG-ARM during axillary dissection on 76 patients. During a 24-month follow-up, 24 (32 %) patients developed lymphedema and 52 patients did not develop lymphedema. The positive node rate from UE lymphatics in the lymphedema group was 42 %; this is significantly greater than that of the no lymphedema group. He concluded that ICG-ARM could predict the incidence of postoperative lymphedema [11].

Lymphedema developed in 6 of the 455 cases (1.3 %) in the overall population and in 6 of 105 cases (5.7 %) in the corresponding group. All six cases that developed lymphedema belonged to the corresponding group. This shows the usefulness of ICG-ARM technique.

The low rate of lymphedema was the result of less SN pickup rates during less invasive surgery.

The 9.3 % rate of detecting luminous non-SNs indicates that dissection of lymph nodes other than the SNs was a risk for developing lymphedema.

Since the positional relationship between the 2ICBN and the SN cannot clearly delineate only two upper and lower positions, we used the 2ICBN as an important landmark to divide the location of the SN and ARM lymphatics into three groups: around, cranial, and caudal side of 2ICBN.

In the corresponding group, almost all SNs were located zone A or B. There were a few lymphatics found at zone C, signifying that if an SN was located in the caudal side of the 2ICBN, there will be no risk of developing lymphedema after operation.

The merit of ICG-ARM for sentinel node navigation surgery is the selection of patients who are at risk for lymphedema. It can be limited to approximately a quarter of patients who need to know the risk of LE. It can be effectively instructed by a medical human resources staff and can eliminate unnecessary care of the UE in non-corresponding group patients.

11.4.1 Prospects for the Future

At present, the proven merit of this procedure was limited to the identification of lymphedema risk group. In the near future, we must examine more limited risk groups in the corresponding group and develop more effective prophylactic therapy such as lymph-venous anastomosis [12].

References

1. Thompson M, Korourian S et al (2007) Axillary reverse mapping (ARM): a new concept to identify and enhance lymphatic preservation. Ann Surg Oncol 14:1890–1895
2. Nos C, Lesieur B et al (2007) Blue dye injection in the arm in order to conserve the lymphatic drainage of the arm in breast cancer patients requiring an axillary dissection. Ann Surg Oncol 14:2490–2496
3. Sakurai T, Sakoda T et al (2009) Axillary reverse mapping (ARM) may be useful in preventing lymphedema during axillary lymph node dissection for breast cancer patients. Jpn J Breast Cancer 24:737–740
4. Noguchi M, Yokoi M et al (2010) Axillary reverse mapping with indocyanine fluorescence imaging in patients with breast cancer. J Surg Oncol 101:217–221
5. Noguchi M (2010) Axillary reverse mapping for breast cancer. Breast Cancer Res Treat 119:529–535
6. Sakurai T, Endo M et al (2014) Axillary reverse mapping using fluorescence imaging is useful for identifying the risk group of postoperative lymphedema in breast cancer patients undergoing sentinel node biopsies. J Surg Oncol 109:612–615
7. MEP (2006) The lymphoedema framework: best practice for the management of lymphoedema. International consensus. London: Medical Education Partnership (MEP) Ltd
8. Kitamura K, Akazawa K (2010) Multi-center survey of breast cancer related arm lymphedema and future issues. J Jpn Coll Angiol 50:715–720
9. Ikeda K, Ogawa Y et al (2012) Evaluation of the metastatic status of lymph nodes identified using axillary reverse mapping in breast cancer patients. World J Surg Oncol 10:233–239

10. Connor C, McGinness M et al (2013) Axillary reverse mapping: a prospective study in women with clinically node negative and node positive breast cancer. Ann Surg Oncol 20:3303–3307
11. Ikeda K, Ogawa Y et al (2014) The influence of axillary reverse mapping related factors on lymphedema in breast cancer patients. Eur J Surg Oncol 40:818–823
12. Mitchell S, Klimberg VS et al (2014) Advanced locoregional therapies in breast. Ann Surg Oncol 21:3198–3203. doi:10.1245/s10434-014-3916-y, Epub 2014 Jul 30

Chapter 12
A New Concept for Axillary Treatment of Primary Breast Cancer Using Indocyanine Green Fluorescence Imaging

Masahiro Takada and Masakazu Toi

Abstract Sentinel lymph node (SLN) biopsy using fluorescence indocyanine green (fICG) method can visualize lymphatic vessels by real-time imaging and is technically straightforward. Identification and false-negative rates of SLN biopsy using fICG ranged from 93 to 100 % and 0 to 10 %, respectively, which were comparable to blue dye or radioisotope method. Four SLNs should be removed for the accurate staging of the axillary lymph node status. The fICG method seems to be advantageous for effective SLN dissection by the intraoperative visualization of a sentinel node bed. However, the number of SLNs removed can be adjusted by the risk of lymph node metastasis. SLN biopsy after preoperative systemic therapy (PST) in patients with clinical node positive is still challenging. There may be some advantage in fICG method for SLN detection after PST because the fICG method can identify an average of three SLNs. A prospective study to evaluate the accuracy of SLN identification using fICG after PST in node-positive patients is now warranted.

Keywords Sentinel lymph node biopsy • Fluorescence indocyanine green • Preoperative systemic therapy

12.1 Introduction

Sentinel lymph node (SLN) biopsy is now regarded as standard care for breast cancer patients with no clinical signs of metastasis in the axillary node. In fact, randomized trials have shown that patients with negative SLNs by SLN biopsy do not require further axillary lymph node dissection (ALND) [1, 2]. In a recent report, when limited SLN metastasis was detected by SLN biopsy in patients treated with

M. Takada
Department of Breast Surgery, Kyoto University Hospital, 54 Kawara-cho, Shogoin, Sakyo-ku, Kyoto 606-8507, Japan

M. Toi (✉)
Department of Breast Surgery, Graduate School of Medicine, Kyoto University, Kyoto, Japan
e-mail: toi@kuhp.kyoto-u.ac.jp

M. Kusano et al. (eds.), *ICG Fluorescence Imaging and Navigation Surgery*,
DOI 10.1007/978-4-431-55528-5_12

breast-conserving surgery and radiation therapy, the addition of ALND resulted in no survival benefit [3].

Current standard techniques for SLN detection are blue dye (dye), radioisotope (RI), and both (dual tracer). A meta-analysis including 63 trials from 1970 to 2003 comparing each method for SLN mapping and biopsy in early-stage breast carcinoma reported identification and false-negative rates of 83 % and 11 % for dye, 89 % and 9 % for RI, and 92 % and 7 % for dual tracer [4], respectively, suggesting additional benefits of the dual-tracer method. In the subsequent National Surgical Adjuvant Breast and Bowel Project (NSABP) B-32 trial comparing SLN resection plus ALND to SLN resection alone (in which dual-tracer imaging was a recommended method), the identification rate was 97.2 % and the false-negative rate 9.8 % [5].

In the fluorescence indocyanine green (fICG) method, subcutaneous lymphatic flow is observed using a near-infrared light camera after subareolar injection of ICG [6]. Real-time images of lymphatic flow into the axilla are then obtained. After skin incision, subcutaneous lymphatics are clearly observed by both real-time fluorescent imaging and macroscopic lymphatic mapping. The fICG method involves no radiation exposure and no scheduling of injection before surgery. Furthermore, it is technically straightforward.

In light of these advantages, we review the accuracy of fICG imaging and describe a new concept for axillary surgery using fICG.

12.2 Sentinel Node Identification by the fICG Method

Identification and false-negative rates from recent clinical trials of SLN biopsy using the fICG method are summarized in Table 12.1. Identification rates ranged from 93 to 100 %, which is within the range reported in dye, RI, and dual-tracer studies. However, only two randomized controlled trials actually compared the identification rates of the fICG method to the dye or RI methods. In the trial conducted by van der Vorst et al., patients were randomly assigned to undergo SLN biopsy involving fICG and RI with or without dye. They reported no additional benefit of dye for SLN identification [7]. Similarly, Jung et al. compared the identification rate for SLN biopsy using a mixture of fICG, RI, and dye with that obtained using RI alone and found identification rates of 100 % in both arms [8]. In contrast, we conducted a multicenter prospective study of SLN identification using both fICG and dye methods in 99 patients and found a substantially higher identification rate using the fICG method (99 % vs. 78 %, $p < 0.001$) [9]. Moreover, although a recent meta-analysis found no statistically significant difference in identification rate between the fICG and RI methods, the identification rate tended to be higher using fICG [10]. Five out of 16 studies reported the false-negative rate of the fICG method, which ranged from 0 to 10 %. The number of SLNs removed varied from 1.5 to 5.4 per patient.

Age and body mass index (BMI) can affect the accuracy of SLN biopsy. A retrospective study of 1356 patients showed that the odds of successful SLN biopsy

Table 12.1 Clinical studies of SLN biopsy using fICG method

First author	Study type	Patients (*N*)	SLN technique	Identification rate (%)	False-negative rate (%)	SLNs (N)	References
Kitai	Cohort	18	fICG	94	NA	2.8	[6]
Tagaya	Cohort	25	fICG	100	0	5.4	Am J Surg, 2008.
			Dye	92	25	2.3	
Murawa	Cohort	30	fICG	97	10	1.75	Br J Surg, 2009.
		20	RI	85	23	1.35	
Abe	Cohort	128	fICG	100	0	3.1	Surg Today, 2011.
			Dye	65.4	42	1	
Hojo	Cohort	113	fICG	100	NA	3	Breast, 2010.
			Dye	92.9	NA	1.9	
		29	fICG	93.1	NA	3	
			RI	100	NA	2	
Hirche	Cohort	43	fICG	97.7	NA	2	Breast Cancer Res Treat, 2010.
Aoyama	Cohort	312	fICG	100	NA	3.41	World J Surg Oncol, 2011.
Tagaya	Cohort	50	fICG + dye	100	NA	3.7	World J Surg, 2011.
Wishart	Cohort	100	fICG	100	0	1.93	Eur J Surg Oncol, 2012.
			RI	91.3	0	1.5	
			Dye	99	0	1.84	
Polom	Cohort	28	fICG + RI	96	NA	2	Eur J Surg Oncol, 2012.
		21	fICG:HAS + RI	100	NA	2	

(continued)

Table 12.1 (continued)

First author	Study type	Patients (*N*)	SLN technique	Identification rate (%)	False-negative rate (%)	SLNs (N)	References
Hirche	Cohort	47	fICG	97.9	5.3	2	J Surg Oncol, 2012.
Van der Vorst	RCT	12	fICG	100	NA	1.6	[7]
			RI	100	NA		
			Dye	84	NA		
		12	fICG	100	NA	1.5	
			RI	100	NA		
Schaafsma	Cohort	32	fICG	100	NA	1.5	Br J Surg, 2013.
			RI	100	NA		
			Dye	88	NA		
Sugie	Cohort	99	fICG	99	NA	3.4	[9]
			Dye	78	NA	2.4	
Jung	RCT	43	fICG + dye + RI	100	NA	3.4	[8]
		43	RI	100	NA	2.3	
Sugie	Cohort	821	fICG	97.4	NA	2.3	In press
			RI	97	NA	1.7	

Abbreviations: *fICG* fluorescent indocyanine green, *dye* blue dye, *RI* radioisotope, *SLN* sentinel lymph node, *RCT* randomized controlled trial, *NA* not available decreased with age and higher BMI [11]. In the validation phase of the ALMANAC study using the dual-tracer method, an inverse relationship between BMI and success rate of SLN biopsy was also reported [12]. On the other hand, the identification rate of SLN using the fICG method was independent of age and BMI [9].

Most clinical trials of the fICG method are cohort studies, and no randomized trial has directly compared the efficacy of the fICG method to that of the dual-tracer technique for SLN identification. According to recent studies and our own experience, the capability of the fICG method for SLN identification appears equal to that of the RI method; however, limited data is available on the adverse effects of fICG imaging, such as arm edema. Therefore, to clarify the clinical usefulness of the fICG method, further prospective studies with long-term follow-up are required.

12.3 Axillary Staging by the fICG Method

SLN biopsy involves examination of the axillary lymph node because it receives direct lymphatic flow from the mammary gland. In reality, however, tumor cells do not always pass from the primary tumor into a single lymph node followed by sequential passage to second and third echelon nodes. Rather, lymphatics from primary tumors initially drain into a group of three to five lymph nodes [13]. Using the fICG method, fluorescent images of lymphatic flow through multiple nodes in cutaneous and subcutaneous tissue are acquired almost in real time. Multiple lymphatic routes into axilla were identified in 47 % of patients by the fICG method [14]. Thus, intraoperative visualization of a sentinel node bed is advantageous for effective sentinel lymph node dissection, and this is possible using fICG.

At the MD Anderson Cancer Center, the relationship between the order of the SLN and metastatic status was examined in detail among 777 patients with positive SLNs. In 579 patients (74.5 %), the first SLN removed contained metastatic disease. However, tumor cells skipped the first SLN in 198 patients. In 16 patients (2.1 %), the metastasis was detected only after 4 or more SLNs were removed [15]. In our study, skip metastasis to the second or third SLN was detected in 6 of 28 patients, while no patients had skip metastasis in the fourth SLN. Therefore, four SLNs should be removed for the accurate staging of the axillary lymph node status.

It was suggested that ICG travels to deeper echelon nodes than dye or RI. We reported an average of 3.4 SLNs identified using the fICG method, which is significantly higher than when using the dye method [9]. In the same study, all positive SLNs were detected by fICG. When the first SLN was the only metastatic lymph node, no residual metastasis was detected in non-SLNs. However, 50 % of patients with positive second or higher-echelon SLNs had non-SLN metastasis [9]. Thus, four-node dissection of SLNs using fICG may be useful for risk stratification of non-SLN metastasis in patients with positive SLNs.

There is a trade-off between the number of SLNs removed and the invasiveness of the SLN biopsy procedure, so the number removed should be adjusted according to the risk of SLN metastasis. In patients with a low risk of lymph node metastasis, we can minimize the number removed. Alternatively, four-node SLN dissection

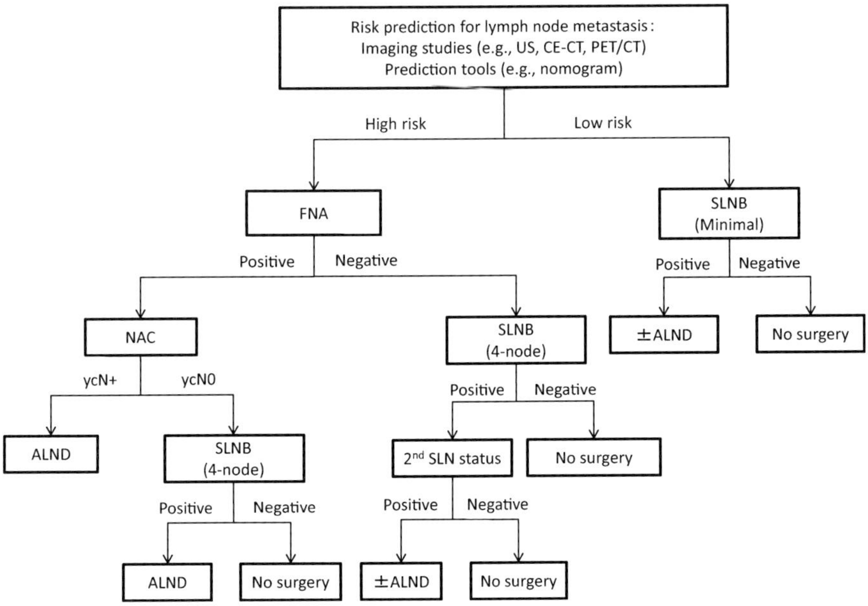

Fig. 12.1 Axillary management algorithm including sentinel lymph node biopsy using fluorescence indocyanine green method. Abbreviations: *FNA* fine needle aspiration, *SLNB* sentinel lymph node biopsy, *ALND* axillary lymph node dissection, *NAC* neoadjuvant chemotherapy

should be considered for patients at a higher risk of lymph node metastasis and also possibly following preoperative systemic therapy (Fig. 12.1).

12.4 SLN Biopsy After Preoperative Systemic Therapy

Preoperative systemic chemotherapy (PST) increases the rate of breast conservation by downstaging the breast tumor [16]. It was reported that about 40 % of patients with axillary lymph node metastasis at diagnosis were node-negative after conventional PST [17]. The node-negative conversion rates could be even higher following more potent combination therapy such anti-HER-2 therapy and dose-dense chemotherapies if, as presumed, node-negative conversion rate correlates with pathological complete response (pCR) rate. In general, at the time of post-PST, ALND is frequently considered for patients who were clinically node positive before PST. A meta-analysis of retrospective and prospective cohort studies (1993–2003) evaluating SLN biopsy after PST for clinically node-positive breast cancer reported an identification rate of 89 % and false-negative rate around 14 % [18].

The American College of Surgeons Oncology Group (ACOSOG) Z1071 trial evaluated the accuracy of SLN biopsy after PST in patients with clinically node-positive breast cancer. Here, dual tracer was the recommended method for SLN biopsy. The identification rate was 92.7 % and false-negative rate was 12.6 %, higher than the predefined threshold of 10 % [17]. In the exploratory analysis, however, the false-negative rate was reduced to 9.1 % in patients with three or more SLNs removed.

In the SENTINA trial, the accuracy of SLN biopsy after PST in node-positive patients was also evaluated, but the dual-tracer method was used in only 28 % of the participants. In this case, the identification rate was markedly lower at 80.1 % and false-negative rate higher at 14.2 % [19]. In patients with three or more SLNs examined, however, the false-negative rate was below 10 %.

A recent exploratory study using fICG reported that the lymphatic pathway changed after preoperative chemotherapy in 42.8 % of the examined cases. Nonetheless, the location of sentinel nodes was not changed substantially. Thus, if the location of the sentinel node bed is identified and marked before PST, sentinel node dissection after PST may be more accurate [20].

In summary, SLN could not be examined in 10–20 % of node-positive patients after PST in these trials, and such patients did not benefit from axillary node downstaging by PST. When only one or two SLNs were removed, estimated false-negative rate was unacceptable and ALND was unavoidable. In the NSABP B-32 trial using the dual-tracer method, a median of two SLNs was removed [5]. Therefore, few node-positive patients may benefit from SLN biopsy after PST using dual-tracer imaging.

Alternatively, using the fICG method, SLNs were systemically excised and a median of 3 SLNs was examined. In the exploratory analysis of Sugie et al., the identification rate of metastatic SLNs after PST was 100 % using fICG and 91 % using RI. A prospective study to evaluate the accuracy of SLN identification using fICG after PST in node-positive patients is now warranted.

12.5 Conclusions

SLN biopsy using fICG is at least as accurate as the RI or dye method, but is technically easier and does not require special management like the RI method. The fICG method can become an alternative to RI or dye method in the presence of standard systemic treatment. Four-node SLN dissection using fICG may contribute to optimal axillary management, especially in patients who undergo preoperative systemic therapy.

References

1. Krag DN, Anderson SJ, Julian TB, Brown AM, Harlow SP, Costantino JP et al (2010) Sentinel-lymph-node resection compared with conventional axillary-lymph-node dissection

in clinically node-negative patients with breast cancer: overall survival findings from the NSABP B-32 randomised phase 3 trial. Lancet Oncol 11(10):927–933
2. Veronesi U, Paganelli G, Viale G, Luini A, Zurrida S, Galimberti V et al (2003) A randomized comparison of sentinel-node biopsy with routine axillary dissection in breast cancer. N Engl J Med 349(6):546–553
3. Giuliano AE, Hunt KK, Ballman KV, Beitsch PD, Whitworth PW, Blumencranz PW et al (2011) Axillary dissection vs no axillary dissection in women with invasive breast cancer and sentinel node metastasis: a randomized clinical trial. JAMA 305(6):569–575
4. Kim T, Giuliano AE, Lyman GH (2006) Lymphatic mapping and sentinel lymph node biopsy in early-stage breast carcinoma: a metaanalysis. Cancer 106(1):4–16
5. Krag DN, Anderson SJ, Julian TB, Brown AM, Harlow SP, Ashikaga T et al (2007) Technical outcomes of sentinel-lymph-node resection and conventional axillary-lymph-node dissection in patients with clinically node-negative breast cancer: results from the NSABP B-32 randomised phase III trial. Lancet Oncol 8(10):881–888
6. Kitai T, Inomoto T, Miwa M, Shikayama T (2005) Fluorescence navigation with indocyanine green for detecting sentinel lymph nodes in breast cancer. Breast Cancer (Tokyo, Japan) 12 (3):211–5
7. van der Vorst JR, Schaafsma BE, Verbeek FP, Hutteman M, Mieog JS, Lowik CW et al (2012) Randomized comparison of near-infrared fluorescence imaging using indocyanine green and 99(m) technetium with or without patent blue for the sentinel lymph node procedure in breast cancer patients. Ann Surg Oncol 19(13):4104–4111
8. Jung SY, Kim SK, Kim SW, Kwon Y, Lee ES, Kang HS et al (2014) Comparison of sentinel lymph node biopsy guided by the multimodal method of indocyanine green fluorescence, radioisotope, and blue dye versus the radioisotope method in breast cancer: a randomized controlled trial. Ann Surg Oncol 21(4):1254–1259
9. Sugie T, Sawada T, Tagaya N, Kinoshita T, Yamagami K, Suwa H et al (2013) Comparison of the indocyanine green fluorescence and blue dye methods in detection of sentinel lymph nodes in early-stage breast cancer. Ann Surg Oncol 20(7):2213–2218
10. Ahmed M, Purushotham AD, Douek M (2014) Novel techniques for sentinel lymph node biopsy in breast cancer: a systematic review. Lancet Oncol 15(8):e351–e362
11. Cox CE, Dupont E, Whitehead GF, Ebert MD, Nguyen K, Peltz ES et al (2002) Age and body mass index may increase the chance of failure in sentinel lymph node biopsy for women with breast cancer. Breast J 8(2):88–91
12. Goyal A, Newcombe RG, Chhabra A, Mansel RE, Group AT (2006) Factors affecting failed localisation and false-negative rates of sentinel node biopsy in breast cancer--results of the ALMANAC validation phase. Breast Cancer Res Treat 99(2):203–208
13. Benson JR, della Rovere GQ, Axilla Management Consensus G (2007) Management of the axilla in women with breast cancer. Lancet Oncol 8(4):331–348
14. Takeuchi M, Sugie T, Abdelazeem K, Kato H, Shinkura N, Takada M et al (2012) Lymphatic mapping with fluorescence navigation using indocyanine green and axillary surgery in patients with primary breast cancer. Breast J 18(6):535–541
15. Yi M, Meric-Bernstam F, Ross MI, Akins JS, Hwang RF, Lucci A et al (2008) How many sentinel lymph nodes are enough during sentinel lymph node dissection for breast cancer? Cancer 113(1):30–37
16. Mauri D, Pavlidis N, Ioannidis JP (2005) Neoadjuvant versus adjuvant systemic treatment in breast cancer: a meta-analysis. J Natl Cancer Inst 97(3):188–194
17. Boughey JC, Suman VJ, Mittendorf EA, Ahrendt GM, Wilke LG, Taback B et al (2013) Sentinel lymph node surgery after neoadjuvant chemotherapy in patients with node-positive breast cancer: the ACOSOG Z1071 (Alliance) clinical trial. JAMA 310(14):1455–1461
18. Fu JF, Chen HL, Yang J, Yi CH, Zheng S (2014) Feasibility and accuracy of sentinel lymph node biopsy in clinically node-positive breast cancer after neoadjuvant chemotherapy: a meta-analysis. PLoS One 9(9), e105316

19. Kuehn T, Bauerfeind I, Fehm T, Fleige B, Hausschild M, Helms G et al (2013) Sentinel-lymph-node biopsy in patients with breast cancer before and after neoadjuvant chemotherapy (SENTINA): a prospective, multicentre cohort study. Lancet Oncol 14(7):609–618
20. Tsuyuki S, Yamaguchi A, Kawata Y, Kawaguchi K (2015) Assessing the effects of neoadjuvant chemotherapy on lymphatic pathways to sentinel lymph nodes in cases of breast cancer: usefulness of the indocyanine green-fluorescence method. Breast 24(3):298–301

Part VI
Sentinel Node Navigation Surgery and Other Applications for Gastrointestial Tract Cancers: Stomach Cancer

Chapter 13
Function-Preserving Curative Gastrectomy Guided by ICG Fluorescence Imaging for Early Gastric Cancer

Shinichi Kinami

Abstract Recently, the SNNS study provided proof of the sentinel node (SN) concept in gastric cancer. The result highlights the credibility of the clinical application of SN biopsy for indicating function-preserving curative surgery in early gastric cancer. In the SNNS study, combination mapping with technetium-99 m tin colloid and isosulfan blue was used and has been adopted as a temporary standard. Nevertheless, blue dye deteriorates quickly, and radioactive colloids exhibit a shine-through effect during gamma probe detection of hot nodes in the surgical field. These limitations increase the difficulty in performing laparoscopic SN biopsy. In contrast, ICG seemed to be a promising tracer candidate for laparoscopic SN biopsy. ICG fluorescence imaging was developed after the recent invention of Photodynamic Eye. The advantages of ICG fluorescence imaging are as follows: obvious visualization, easier detection of bright nodes and lymphatic canals than with the naked eye, very high sensitivity to detect minute concentrations of ICG, and signal stability. ICG fluorescence imaging for SN biopsy might be feasible in both open and laparoscopic surgery for early gastric cancer; therefore, laparoscopic function-preserving curative gastrectomy would be a good alternative to the commonly used D1+ gastrectomy for patients with node-negative gastric cancer.

Keywords Gastric cancer • Sentinel lymph node biopsy • Indocyanine green • Fluorescence imaging

13.1 The Need for Function-Preserving Gastrectomy

Early gastric cancer is a curable cancer for the following reasons: rare distant metastasis, low rate of nodal metastasis, and high curability with nodal dissection even in metastatic cases. Some cases diagnosed as node negative based on

S. Kinami (✉)
Department of Surgical Oncology, Kanazawa Medical University, 1-1 Daigaku, Uchinada-machi, Kahoku-gun, Ishikawa 920-0293, Japan
e-mail: kinami@kanazawa-med.ac.jp

M. Kusano et al. (eds.), *ICG Fluorescence Imaging and Navigation Surgery*,
DOI 10.1007/978-4-431-55528-5_13

clinicopathological findings are treated by endoscopic submucosal dissection [1]. Therefore, the standard curative procedure for early gastric cancers falling outside the indication parameters for endoscopic resection is gastrectomy with lymph node dissection. A nodal dissection extent of D1+ is recommended by the Gastric Cancer Treatment Guidelines [2].

The standard lymph node dissection technique results in wide-area resection of the stomach because it eliminates some of the main arteries feeding this region. Patients undergoing standard gastrectomy with lymph node dissection experience postgastrectomy symptoms [3]. These symptoms often pose lifelong problems for patients. Thus, lymph node dissection should be avoided to preserve the stomach, alleviate the aforementioned symptoms, and improve postoperative quality of life. At present, sentinel lymph node (SN) biopsy is the most reliable method for identification of node-negative cases and recommendation of oncologically safe, function-preserving gastrectomy.

13.2 SN Concept in Early Gastric Cancer

An SN is defined as a node that directly receives lymphatic drainage from a primary tumor [4]. SN biopsy has two main roles in the treatment of various cancers: ultrastaging and determining if lymph node dissection is needed. In malignant melanoma and colorectal cancer management, SN biopsy is primarily used for ultrastaging [4, 5]. On the other hand, SN biopsy is mainly used to determine if lymph node dissection should be performed in breast cancer surgery [6].

Gastric cancer is one of the cancers that are well investigated by many researchers whether the SN concept is valid. Over the past few decades, the application of SN mapping in gastric cancer, which has relatively complicated lymphatic flow, has been controversial [7]. However, recent prospective studies have successfully demonstrated the utility of SN biopsies in gastric cancer [8–12]. Two large-scale, nationwide, multicenter prospective studies were conducted to establish the usefulness of SN biopsy in gastric cancer: the JCOG0302 [13] study and the SNNS study [14]. Unfortunately, the JCOG0302 trial was terminated because of the high proportion of false-negative results obtained from intraoperative histological examinations. On the other hand, the SNNS study provided proof of the SN concept in gastric cancer. In this study, the sensitivity and specificity of SN biopsy were 93 % and 99 %, respectively. The major difference between these two multicenter trials was study design. The JCOG0302 trial was designed to evaluate the usefulness of intraoperative SN biopsy for guiding local resection in early gastric cancer and not specifically to verify the SN concept. Therefore, the results of this study were influenced not only by the SN concept but also by intraoperative SN detection techniques and the intraoperative diagnosis of nodal metastasis. This trial demonstrated that a learning curve exists in conducting SN biopsies and that intraoperative histological examination using a single plane is not suitable for clinical application. On the other hand, the sole purpose of the SNNS study was to scientifically verify the SN concept in gastric cancer. Therefore, learning curve issues and the intraoperative diagnostic ability of SN biopsy for nodal metastasis did not influence the results of this study. The hospitals that participated in the study were highly skilled in SN biopsy, with over 30 procedures performed at each institution. Metastasis was diagnosed using permanent sections, and the sensitivity of intraoperative frozen section diagnosis was 79 %. Based on these findings, the SN node concept seems to be scientifically valid, even in patients with small-sized early gastric cancers.

13.3 Clinical Application of SN Navigation Surgery

The results of the SNNS study highlight the credibility of the clinical application of SN biopsy for indicating function-preserving curative surgery without lymph node dissection in early gastric cancer. However, the decision to exclude lymph node dissection should be carefully considered, because standard lymph node dissection has been shown to improve prognoses in patients with gastric cancer [15]. Furthermore, in contrast to breast cancer, reoperation for additional nodal dissection is rarely performed for gastric cancers.

These issues could be resolved by lymphatic basin dissection. The lymphatic basin is defined as the lymphatic zone divided by the stream of the dyed lymphatic canals in dye mapping; the proximal border is the fatty tissue attached to the stomach wall, and the distal border is the front of the blue node furthest from the stomach. The lymphatic basins are thought to be the primary lymphatic drainage areas in each patient, and patients with gastric cancer often have two or three basins. All sentinel nodes exist within the lymphatic basin. Lymphatic basin dissection is a selective lymphadenectomy to dissect lymphatic basins *en bloc*, containing lymph nodes and lymphatic vessels stained with dye [16, 17]. Lymphatic basin dissection is considered a standard SN biopsy technique for gastric cancer, unlike for other cancers. SNs are retrieved after lymphatic basin dissection and subjected to intraoperative pathological analysis. Lymphatic basin dissection is superior to the ordinary pickup method in not only minimizing the rate of missed SNs, but also in terms of oncological safety as it complements intraoperative pathological diagnosis by serving as a backup dissection [17–19]. Kinami et al. reported that there were no recurrent cases, including two false-negative cases, in 190 patients diagnosed as node negative by SN biopsy intraoperatively and treated by function-preserving gastrectomy with lymphatic basin dissection.

From these findings, the most optimal and oncologically safe surgery indicated by SN biopsy would appear to be small-area gastrectomy with lymphatic basin dissection.

13.4 Technical Difficulty of Combination Mapping for Laparoscopic Gastrectomy

SN biopsy is a complex multistep surgical technique. This technique requires limited indication, the selection of an adequate tracer, a proper tracer injection method, the objective detection of tracer uptake by the nodes, a reliable biopsy technique for the nodes that have taken up the tracer, and the precise intraoperative detection (micrometastasis level) of nodal metastasis. Many studies have provided recommendations regarding the suitable indication and tracer injection method for SN biopsy in gastric cancer. In a meta-analysis of SN biopsy for gastric cancer by Wang et al. [20], early T stage, combined tracers, the submucosal injection method, conventional open surgery, and immunohistochemistry were found to be associated with a higher SN identification rate and sensitivity. In the SNNS study, an indication of clinically early stage cancers less than 4 cm in diameter, the dual-tracer method, and endoscopic submucosal injection were adopted. Based on the findings of these studies, the indication of SN biopsy for gastric cancer should be limited to clinical T1 cancers less than 4 cm in diameter, and endoscopic submucosal injection into four points surrounding the tumor should be adopted as the tracer injection method. As mentioned in the previous chapter, lymphatic basin dissection is thought to be the appropriate SN biopsy technique. In contrast to these solvable issues, the precise intraoperative detection of nodal metastasis is a serious problem. Therefore, the molecular diagnosis of metastasis must be investigated.

In comparison with these technical issues, the selection of an appropriate tracer and the objective detection of tracer uptake by the nodes are important issues in the treatment of gastric cancer. In the SNNS study, combination mapping with technetium-99 m tin colloid and isosulfan blue was used and has been adopted as a temporary standard. Combination mapping is thought to be superior to single-tracer mapping because of its synergistic effect [21]. However, blue dye deteriorates quickly, and radioactive colloids exhibit a shine-through effect during gamma probe detection of hot nodes in the surgical field. These limitations increase the difficulty in performing laparoscopic SN biopsy by impairing lymphatic basin visualization and hot node detection. Thus, this type of combination mapping has limited clinical use in laparoscopic surgery, which is the most commonly used approach for early gastric cancers in Japan.

13.5 Feasibility of ICG Fluorescence Mapping for Early Gastric Cancer

ICG is a promising tracer candidate for laparoscopic gastrectomy. ICG is a widely used diagnostic reagent that is clinically approved for use in the assessment of hepatic function and cardiac output. ICG was formerly used as a dye tracer for gastric cancer [9, 11]. However, ICG is generally thought to be less visible than blue dye because of its weaker contrast against the background adipose tissue. On the other hand, ICG absorbs light in the near-infrared range, with maximum absorption at a wavelength of 800 nm. ICG also emits maximal fluorescence at a wavelength of 840 nm when it binds to plasma proteins. Nimura et al. developed an infrared ray electronic endoscopy system for ICG detection and invented a new SN biopsy technique known as the infrared ray method. This electro-optic system can detect minute concentrations of ICG with high sensitivity and is considered to be suitable for performing SN biopsy in laparoscopic gastrectomy [22, 23]. The other method is ICG fluorescence imaging. This technique was developed after the recent invention of the camera system known as the Photodynamic Eye (PDE; Hamamatsu Photonics Co. Ltd., Hamamatsu, Shizuoka, Japan). The PDE has been widely used in various cancer surgeries in the past several years [24–35]. Kusano et al. demonstrated the high sensitivity of this ICG fluorescence imaging system for SN mapping in gastric cancer [36].

The advantages of ICG fluorescence imaging are as follows: lower cost, lower equipment costs than that for radioactive tracers, does not require radioactivity, lower frequency of allergic reactions than that with blue dye, ability to detect bright nodes under thick adipose tissue [36], obvious visualization, easier detection of bright nodes and lymphatic canals than with the naked eye or infrared ray imaging [29], very high sensitivity to detect minute concentrations of ICG [34, 37], and signal stability [29, 34, 37]. Signal stability is a unique characteristic of ICG fluorescence imaging. After injection into the submucosa, ICG binds to plasma lipoproteins and is trapped in the peripheral sinus and lymphatic labyrinth of the SN. The stability of ICG fluorescence imaging allowed us to successfully use preoperative injections for SN detection. Tajima et al. found signal stability to be the most important advantage of ICG fluorescence imaging over dye- and radioisotope-guided methods [37].

We performed feasibility tests of ICG fluorescence imaging for SN biopsy for early gastric cancer. From October 2009, patients with histologically confirmed clinical type 0 (superficial type) adenocarcinoma of the stomach, single primary lesions less than 5 cm in diameter, no history of chemotherapy, and no distant metastasis (cM0) or obvious nodal metastasis (cN0) and those who did not satisfy the criteria for endoscopic submucosal dissection were enrolled in the study. All patients provided written informed consent. The PDE or PDE neo (a newer version of the PDE with similar sensor sensitivity) was used to detect ICG fluorescence. The day before surgery, ICG solution was endoscopically injected into four quadrants of the submucosal layer of the primary lesion using an endoscopic puncture needle. To determine the adequate ICG concentration for SN biopsy, 0.5 mL × 4 injection points of 2.5 mg/mL, 125 μg/mL, 50 μg/mL, and 5 μg/mL ICG were preliminarily assessed in one or two cases. After identifying the adequate concentration, ICG injection volumes of 0.5 mL × 4 points and 0.2 mL × 4 points were evaluated. Bright nodes were defined as obvious fluorescent nodes. The bright nodes were thought to contain SNs. The number and direction of the lymphatic basins were observed and recorded intraoperatively by the surgeon. The patients underwent standard gastrectomy with lymph node dissection up to D1+ or D2

Table 13.1 Patient characteristics

Patient characteristics	
Age (years)	68 (47–82)
Male/female	26/16
Tumor location	
Upper/middle/lower	5/23/14
Less/ant/post/gre	24/5/3/10
Pathological depth of invasion	
T1a(M)/T1b(SM)/T2(MP)/T3(SS)	16/17/8/1
Tumor size after gastrectomy (mm)	27 (10–65)
Surgical approach	
Open/laparoscopic	15/27

M mucosal, *MP* proper muscle, *SM* submucosal, *SS* subserosal

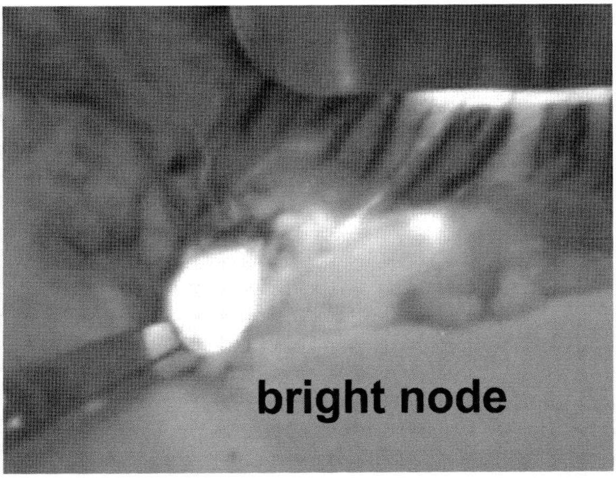

Fig. 13.1 Bright node detected by ICG fluorescence imaging with the Photodynamic Eye. An intraoperative image obtained after distal partial gastrectomy with standard lymph node dissection up to D2 is shown. The tumor is seen at the greater curvature of the middle third of the stomach. Fluorescence is noted in the lymphatics and lymph nodes. In this case, the lymphatic basin is in the right gastroepiploic artery area, and bright nodes are No. 4d

according to the Gastric Cancer Treatment Guidelines. Postoperatively, the only one well-trained surgeon (S.K.) managed all resected specimens, harvested the dissected nodes, and mapped them. The regional lymph nodes of the stomach were classified into numbered stations according to the Japanese Classification of Gastric Carcinoma.

Forty-two patients were enrolled. Patient characteristics are shown in Table 13.1. A laparoscopic approach was performed in 64 % of patients. No serious allergic reactions were observed after tracer injection. Bright nodes and lymphatic basins were detected in all cases (Fig. 13.1), and the detection rate of ICG fluorescence imaging was therefore 100 %. Bright node detection was performed postoperatively in the initial 16 patients. The other 26 patients underwent intraoperative bright node biopsy and intraoperative frozen section diagnosis. In this series, seven patients had lymph node metastasis, and all patients were diagnosed using bright node biopsy.

Table 13.2 Bright node biopsy results

	Status of all dissected nodes	
Bright node biopsy	Metastasis	No metastasis
Metastasis	7	0
No metastasis	0	35

Table 13.3 Relationship between the number of bright nodes and ICG concentration

Concentration	Volume	No. of cases	No. of bright nodes (median)
×2 (2.5 mg/mL)	0.5 mL × 4	1	17
×40 (125 μg/mL)	0.5 mL × 4	2	8 (8, 8)
×100 (50 μg/mL)	0.5 mL × 4	4	5 (4–7)
×1000 (5 μg/mL)	0.5 mL × 4	1	3
×100 (50 μg/mL)	0.5 mL × 4	15	6 (3–11)
×100 (50 μg/mL)	0.2 mL × 4	19	6 (2–7)

The sensitivity, specificity, and accuracy of ICG fluorescence SN mapping were all 100 % (Table 13.2). Of these seven metastatic patients, four were diagnosed postoperatively using permanent pathological sections, and three were diagnosed intraoperatively using frozen sections.

13.6 Unsolvable Issues of ICG Fluorescence Mapping

Our results suggested that ICG fluorescence imaging for SN biopsy might be feasible in both open and laparoscopic surgery for early gastric cancers. On the other hand, some disadvantages of ICG fluorescence imaging were also obvious in our analysis, the subjectivity of SN evaluation and potential secondary node contamination because of the high sensitivity of the PDE system.

In the preliminary phase of our study, we attempted intraoperative mapping. However, intraoperative mapping was difficult because of pollution of the surgical field by ICG leakage from the edge of the dissected lymphatic basin (data not shown). A reduction in ICG dose is essential when performing SN biopsy for gastric cancer, as this region has a rich lymphatic flow. We thought that the PDE was sensitive enough to detect minute ICG concentrations. We next changed the timing of injection from intraoperative to preoperative (the day before surgery). A marked reduction in the pollution of the surgical field was achieved with this modification. The adequate concentration of ICG was determined in the initial eight cases, which were all node negative. Table 13.3 shows the relationship between the number of bright nodes and ICG concentration. At an ICG concentration of 5 μg/mL (×1000), bright lymphatics and bright nodes were detected despite the weak fluorescence. Therefore, the adequate concentration of ICG was determined to be 50 μg/mL (×100). Next, we determined the adequate injection volume. Fifteen and 19 sequential patients were injected with 0.5 mL × 4 points and 0.2 mL × 4 points of

50 μg/mL ICG, respectively. The visualization of bright nodes and bright lymphatics was similar between the two groups. The median number of bright nodes was not significantly different between the two groups. Therefore, the adequate injection volume of ICG solution was determined to be 0.5 mL × 4 points because of its technical reliability.

The numbers of bright nodes depended on the concentration of the ICG solution injected. Therefore, the bright nodes detected by the PDE seemed to contain a few secondary nodes. Secondary node contamination is a significant drawback of ICG fluorescence imaging resulting from its high sensitivity, because true SNs are difficult to distinguish from secondary nodes. In the radioisotope method, the threshold for distinguishing true SNs from secondary nodes is determined by measuring the radioactive count of hot nodes. This is because the SNs receive much greater lymphatic flow and take up more radioactive colloid than secondary nodes. We hypothesize that ICG-lipoprotein complexes might behave in the same manner as radioactive colloids and, therefore, the threshold level for true SN detection could be determined by measuring ICG fluorescence intensity. Further investigation is needed to validate our hypothesis and to overcome this limitation of ICG fluorescence imaging.

13.7 The Future of Laparoscopic Gastric Surgery

At present, laparoscopic gastrectomy merely replicates standard gastrectomy. It is difficult to perform function-preserving curative gastrectomy using the laparoscopic approach. However, if ICG fluorescence mapping for early gastric cancer becomes feasible, laparoscopic function-preserving curative gastrectomy would be a good alternative to the commonly used D1+ gastrectomy for patients with node-negative gastric cancer. Schematic diagrams of function-preserving gastrectomy with lymphatic basin dissection are shown in Fig. 13.2.

Our results were obtained using the PDE, so a small incision at the upper abdomen was needed to assess the direction of the lymphatic basins. However, several ICG fluorescence imaging systems have been developed and are available,

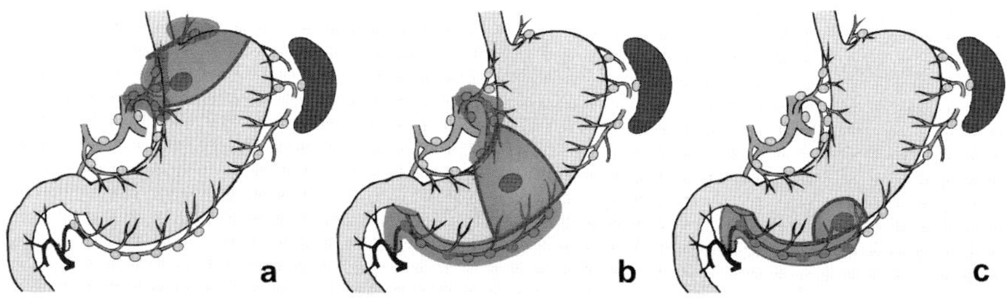

Fig. 13.2 Schematic diagrams of function-preserving gastrectomy with lymphatic basin dissection. (**a**) Limited proximal gastrectomy, (**b**) segmental gastrectomy, (**c**) local resection

including the IMAGE 1 HD system by Karl Storz, the IRI system by Olympus, the ICG fluorescent laparoscope by Shinko-Optical, and the PINPOINT system by Novadaq. The use of these systems would allow avoidance of the upper abdomen incision and promote widespread proliferation of ICG fluorescence imaging and function-preserving curative gastrectomy. Nevertheless, the proper concentration of ICG should be reexamined if these detection devices are to be used.

A limitation of ICG fluorescence imaging is the subjectivity of SN evaluation and potential secondary node contamination. Nevertheless, the elimination of secondary node contamination will be possible by using new agents. New fluorescence agents with both fluorescence and colloid particle characteristics have been developed [38–42]. These agents detect only fluorescent SNs and not secondary nodes and could potentially be useful in laparoscopic SN biopsy in cases of gastric cancer. Furthermore, they may be used alone as a standard tracer instead of in combination with other SN mapping tracers.

References

1. Gotoda T, Yamamoto H, Soetikno RM et al (1999) Endoscopic submucosal dissection of early gastric cancer. J Gastroenterol 41:929–942
2. Japanese Gastric Cancer Association (2011) Japanese gastric cancer treatment guidelines 2010 (ver. 3). Gastric Cancer 14:113–123
3. Eagon JC, Miedema BW, Kelly KA (1992) Postgastrectomy syndromes. Surg Clin N Am 72:445–465
4. Morton DL, Wen DR, Wong JH, Economou JS et al (1992) Technical details of intraoperative lymphatic mapping for early stage melanoma. Arch Surg 127:392–399
5. Sirop S, Kanaan M, Korant A et al (2011) Detection and prognostic impact of micrometastasis in colorectal cancer. J Surg Oncol 103:534–537
6. Giuliano AE, Haigh PI, Brennan MB et al (2000) Prospective observational study of sentinel lymphadenectomy without further axillary dissection in patients with sentinel node-negative breast cancer. J Clin Oncol 18:2553–2559
7. Maruyama K, Sasako M, Kinoshita T et al (1999) Can sentinel node biopsy indicate rational extent of lymphadenectomy in gastric cancer surgery? Fundamental and new information on lymph-node dissection. Langenbecks Arch Surg 384:149–157
8. Miwa K (2000) Sentinel node concept and its application for cancer surgery. Nihon Geka Gakkai Zasshi 101:307–310
9. Hiratsuka M, Miyashiro I, Ishikawa O et al (2001) Application of sentinel node biopsy to gastric cancer surgery. Surgery 129:335–340
10. Carlini M, Carboni F, Petric M et al (2002) Sentinel node in gastric cancer surgery. J Exp Clin Cancer Res 21:469–473
11. Ichikura T, Morita D, Uchida T et al (2002) Sentinel node concept in gastric carcinoma. World J Surg 26:318–322
12. Kitagawa Y, Fujii H, Mukai M et al (2002) Radio-guided sentinel node detection for gastric cancer. Br J Surg 89:604–608
13. Miyashiro I, Hiratsuka M, Sasako M et al (2014) High false-negative proportion of intraoperative histological examination as a serious problem for clinical application of sentinel node biopsy for early gastric cancer: final results of the Japan Clinical Oncology Group multicenter trial JCOG0302. Gastric Cancer 17:316–323

14. Kitagawa Y, Takeuchi H, Takagi Y et al (2013) Sentinel node mapping for gastric cancer: a prospective multicenter trial in Japan. J Clin Oncol 31:3704–3710
15. Songun I, Putter H, Kranenbarg EM et al (2010) Surgical treatment of gastric cancer: 15-year follow-up results of the randomised nationwide Dutch D1D2 trial. Lancet Oncol 11:439–449
16. Miwa K, Kinami S, Taniguchi K et al (2003) Mapping sentinel nodes in patients with early-stage gastric carcinoma. Br J Surg 90:178–182
17. Kinami S, Fujimura T, Ojima E et al (2008) PTD classification: proposal for a new classification of gastric cancer location based on physiological lymphatic flow. Int J Clin Oncol 13:320–329
18. Kelder W, Nimura H, Takahashi N et al (2010) Sentinel node mapping with indocyanine green (ICG) and infrared ray detection in early gastric cancer: an accurate method that enables a limited lymphadenectomy. Eur J Surg Oncol 36:552–558
19. Lee YJ, Ha WS, Park ST et al (2008) Which biopsy method is more suitable between a basin dissection and pick-up biopsy for sentinel nodes in laparoscopic sentinel-node navigation surgery (LSNNS) for gastric cancer? J Laparoendosc Adv Surg Tech A 18:357–363
20. Wang Z, Dong ZY, Chen JQ et al (2012) Diagnostic value of sentinel lymph node biopsy in gastric cancer: a meta-analysis. Ann Surg Oncol 19:1541–1550
21. Hayashi H, Ochiai T, Mori M et al (2003) Sentinel lymph node mapping for gastric cancer using a dual procedure with dye- and gamma probe-guided techniques. J Am Coll Surg 196:68–74
22. Nimura H, Narimiya N, Mitsumori N et al (2004) Infrared ray electronic endoscopy combined with indocyanine green injection for detection of sentinel nodes of patients with gastric cancer. Br J Surg 91:575–579
23. Tajima Y, Murakami M, Yamazaki K et al (2010) Sentinel node mapping guided by indocyanine green fluorescence imaging during laparoscopic surgery in gastric cancer. Ann Surg Oncol 17:1787–1793
24. Aoyama K, Kamio T, Ohchi T et al (2011) Sentinel lymph node biopsy for breast cancer patients using fluorescence navigation with indocyanine green. World J Surg Oncol 9:157
25. Crane LM, Themelis G, Arts HJ et al (2011) Intraoperative near-infrared fluorescence imaging for sentinel lymph node detection in vulvar cancer: first clinical results. Gynecol Oncol 120:291–295
26. Fujisawa Y, Nakamura Y, Kawachi Y et al (2012) Indocyanine green fluorescence-navigated sentinel node biopsy showed higher sensitivity than the radioisotope or blue dye method, which may help to reduce false-negative cases in skin cancer. J Surg Oncol 106:41–45
27. Gilmore DM, Khullar OV, Gioux S et al (2013) Effective low-dose escalation of indocyanine green for near-infrared fluorescent sentinel lymph node mapping in melanoma. Ann Surg Oncol 20:2357–2363
28. Imai K, Minamiya Y, Saito H et al (2013) Detection of pleural lymph flow using indocyanine green fluorescence imaging in non-small cell lung cancer surgery: a preliminary study. Surg Today 43:249–254
29. Miyashiro I, Miyoshi N, Hiratsuka M et al (2008) Detection of sentinel node in gastric cancer surgery by indocyanine green fluorescence imaging: comparison with infrared imaging. Ann Surg Oncol 15:1640–1643
30. Rossi EC, Ivanova A, Boggess JF (2012) Robotically assisted fluorescence-guided lymph node mapping with ICG for gynecologic malignancies: a feasibility study. Gynecol Oncol 124:78–82
31. Schaafsma BE, van der Vorst JR, Gaarenstroom KN et al (2012) Randomized comparison of near-infrared fluorescence lymphatic tracers for sentinel lymph node mapping of cervical cancer. Gynecol Oncol 127:126–130
32. Tagaya N, Aoyagi H, Nakagawa A et al (2011) A novel approach for sentinel lymph node identification using fluorescence imaging and image overlay navigation surgery in patients with breast cancer. World J Surg 35:154–158

33. van der Vorst JR, Hutteman M, Gaarenstroom KN et al (2011) Optimization of near-infrared fluorescent sentinel lymph node mapping in cervical cancer patients. Int J Gynecol Cancer 21:1472–1478
34. Yoshida M, Kubota K, Kuroda J et al (2012) Indocyanine green injection for detecting sentinel nodes using color fluorescence camera in the laparoscopy-assisted gastrectomy. J Gastroenterol Hepatol 27(Suppl 3):29–33
35. Kubota K, Yoshida M, Kuroda J (2013) Application of the HyperEye Medical System for esophageal cancer surgery: a preliminary report. Surg Today 43:215–220
36. Kusano M, Tajima Y, Yamazaki K et al (2008) Sentinel node mapping guided by indocyanine green fluorescence imaging: a new method for sentinel node navigation surgery in gastrointestinal cancer. Dig Surg 25:103–108
37. Tajima Y, Yamazaki K, Masuda Y et al (2009) Sentinel node mapping guided by indocyanine green fluorescence imaging in gastric cancer. Ann Surg 249:58–62
38. Brouwer OR, Buckle T, Vermeeren L et al (2012) Comparing the hybrid fluorescent-radioactive tracer indocyanine green-99mTc-nanocolloid with 99mTc-nanocolloid for sentinel node identification: a validation study using lymphoscintigraphy and SPECT/CT. J Nucl Med 53:1034–1040
39. Frontado LM, Brouwer OR, van den Berg NS et al (2013) Added value of the hybrid tracer indocyanine green-99mTc-nanocolloid for sentinel node biopsy in a series of patients with different lymphatic drainage patterns. Rev Esp Med Nucl Imagen Mol 32:227–233
40. Heuveling DA, Visser GW, de Groot M et al (2012) Nanocolloidal albumin-IRDye 800CW: a near-infrared fluorescent tracer with optimal retention in the sentinel lymph node. Eur J Nucl Med Mol Imaging 39:1161–1168
41. Kong SH, Noh YW, Suh YS et al (2015) Evaluation of the novel near-infrared fluorescence tracers pullulan polymer nanogel and indocyanine green/γ-glutamic acid complex for sentinel lymph node navigation surgery in large animal models. Gastric Cancer 18:55–64
42. Toyota T, Fujito H, Suganami A et al (2014) Near-infrared-fluorescence imaging of lymph nodes by using liposomally formulated indocyanine green derivatives. Bioorg Med Chem 22:721–727

Part VII
Sentinel Node Navigation Surgery and Other Applications for Gastrointestial Tract Cancers: Stomach and Colon Cancer

Chapter 14
Fluorescent Navigation Surgery for Gastrointestinal Tract Cancers: Detection of Sentinel Nodes, Tumor Tattooing, and Harvesting of Lymph Nodes

Mitsuo Kusano, Hiromi Ono, Yasushi Danjo, Futoshi Kawamata, Yusuke Tajima, Seiji Ohtsubo, Shingo Shimada, and Kaname Koyanagi

Abstract The applications of indocyanine green (ICG) fluorescence imaging (IFI) for fluorescent-guided surgery have been expanding. Here we assessed the use of IFI in gastrointestinal tract surgeries. We first evaluated the feasibility of sentinel lymph node (SLN) mapping guided by IFI in gastrointestinal cancers. Twenty-two gastric cancer patients and 26 colorectal cancer patients who had undergone standard surgical resection were enrolled. The SLN detection rate in our preliminary study was 90.9 % and the mean number of SLNs was 3.6 in the gastric cancer patients, and the corresponding values in the colorectal cancer patients were 88.5 % and 2.6. Among the gastric cancer patients, the accuracy was 88.9 % and the false-negative rate was 33.3 %. Secondly, we assessed the efficacy of a new method for tattooing the tumor location using IFI instead of India ink. We succeeded in the ICG marking of early-stage stomach cancer and colon cancer, and our results may lead to the establishment of a new marking procedure instead of the conventional India

M. Kusano (✉)
Department of Surgery, Seiwa Memorial Hospital, 1-5-1-1, Kotoni, Nishi-ku, Sapporo, Hokkaido 063-0811, Japan
e-mail: kusanomitsuo@me.com

H. Ono
Department of Medicine, Seiwa Memorial Hospital, 1-1, 1-Jo, 5-Chome, Kotoni, Nishi-ku, Sapporo, Hokkaido 063-0811, Japan

Y. Danjo • F. Kawamata • S. Ohtsubo
Department of Surgery, Seiwa Memorial Hospital, 1-1, 1-Jo, 5-Chome, Kotoni, Nishi-ku, Sapporo, Hokkaido 063-0811, Japan

Y. Tajima
Department of Oral and Maxillofacial Surgery, Kanto Rosai Hospital, Kanagawa, Japan

S. Shimada
Department of Gastroenterological Surgery I, Hokkaido University, Graduate School of Medicine, Sapporo, Hokkaido, Japan

K. Koyanagi
Department of Surgery, KKR Hospital, Hokkaido, Japan

M. Kusano et al. (eds.), *ICG Fluorescence Imaging and Navigation Surgery*,
DOI 10.1007/978-4-431-55528-5_14

ink and clipping methods. Lastly, we evaluated whether an IFI method of harvesting lymph nodes (LNs) from resected specimens could improve the accuracy of LN staging. ICG fluorescence-labeled LNs were found even though the ICG solution was injected ex vivo. The IFI method thus improved the LN harvest from resected specimens. This method will provide precise evaluations of the pathological status of LNs.

Keywords Sentinel node navigation surgery • Tumor tattooing • Fluorescent endoscope • Lymph node harvest

14.1 Introduction

Sentinel lymph nodes (SLNs) drain directly from primary lesions and the initial sites of metastasis (Fig. 14.1). When there is no metastasis in the SLNs, the dissection area of lymph nodes can be minimized. SLN navigation surgery (SLNNS) for malignancies has been used in breast cancers [1] and melanomas [2]. The feasibility of SLNs for gastrointestinal (GI) malignancies, gastric cancer, and colon cancers has not yet been established. Various dye-guided [3] and radioisotopic radio-guided methods [4] have been used to detect SLNs, but each method has some technical and cost-benefit disadvantages. Here, we evaluated the usefulness of indocyanine green (ICG) fluorescence imaging (IFI) for the detection of SLNs in GI tract malignancies (Fig. 14.2a).

The correct marking of the tumor lesion is essential for the laparoscopic or other minimally invasive surgery for GI tract cancers. Tattooing by India ink and a

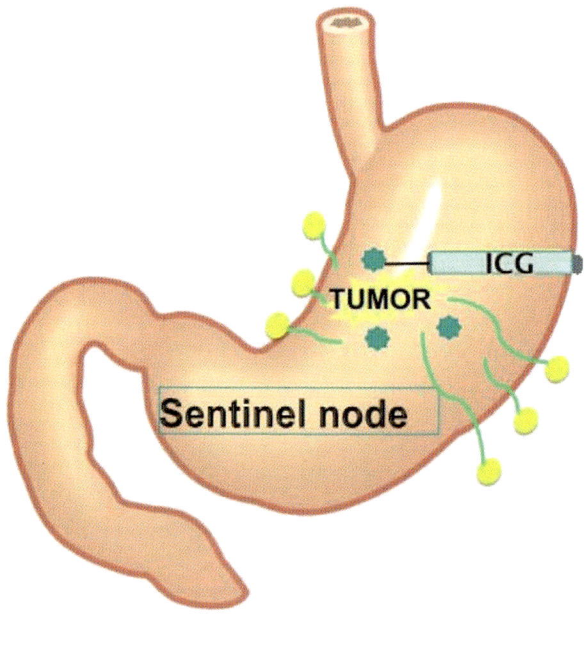

Fig. 14.1 The identification of SLNs. ICG can be injected around a tumor by endoscopy prior to surgery or by the direct injection of ICG during the surgery

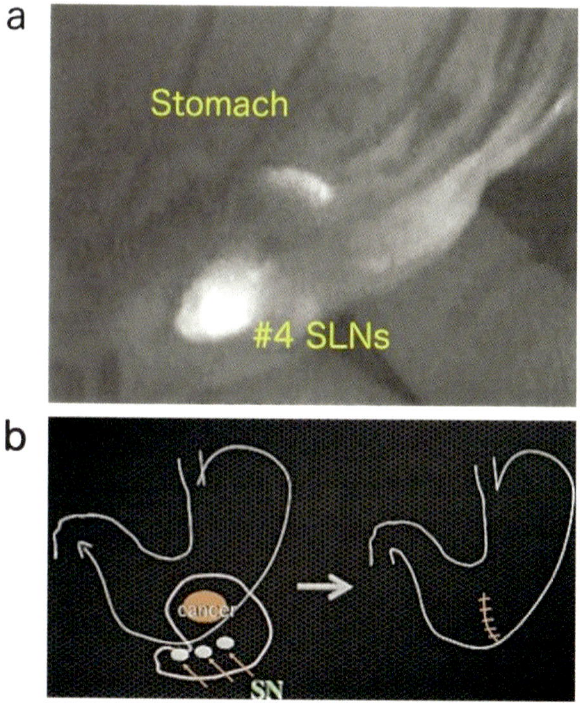

Fig. 14.2 (a) Intraoperative detection of SLNs. (b) When no micrometastasis is detected in SLNs, is the partial resection of stomach acceptable?

clipping procedure have been widely employed, but they present risks of dirty staining or the leakage of India ink into the abdominal cavity [5] and the dropout of clips. We developed a novel endoscopic device [6], and here we evaluated the ICG fluorescence marking method as a new way to tattoo a GI tumor.

Several studies [7–9] have reported a significant correlation between the number of lymph node (LN) metastases and the number of retrieved LNs, and the number of metastatic LNs is the main prognostic factor in patients with gastric cancers. It is thus mandatory to harvest LNs from resected specimens very precisely for the accurate determination of the clinical stage in gastric cancer.

In this study, we tested the efficacy of the IFI method for the retrieval of LNs from resected GI cancer specimens.

14.2 Materials and Methods

14.2.1 The Detection of SLNs

Fluorescence images were obtained after an injection of ICG using a charge-coupled device fluorescent endoscope with a cut filter as the detector and light-emitting xenon at 840 nm as the light source. There are two ICG injection approaches. In one approach, ICG is injected into the subserosa around the tumor. In the present study, 0.3 mL of ICG solution was injected at three points around the tumor prior to the patients' surgeries. In the second approach, the ICG is injected intraoperatively.

The patient series in our preliminary study consisted of 22 patients with gastric cancer and 26 patients with colorectal cancer, all of whom had undergone a standard surgical resection [10]. In the open laparotomy cases, we observed the SLNs using a fluorescence imaging device (photodynamic emission [PDE] camera) after the laparotomy. In the laparoscopy-assisted gastrectomy cases, a fluorescent endoscope was used.

14.2.2 Tattooing the Tumor Region Using ICG Fluorescence

ICG injections were given to the patients undergoing preoperative gastrectomy or colectomy for early-stage stomach and colon cancers or adenomas. After the laparotomy, the stomach or colon was first observed with the naked eye, and then the PDE camera or fluorescent endoscope was used.

14.2.3 ICG Fluorescence-Assisted Ex Vivo Lymph Node Harvest in Gastric Cancer

Three timings for the ICG injection have been explored: preoperative, intraoperative, and postoperative injection. Here we focused on the ex vivo injection of ICG in 20 patients with proven gastric cancer. After resection, 0.3 mL of ICG solution was injected into four or five points of the submucosal areas. LNs were then harvested by the conventional procedure. We reexamined whether there were any LNs left behind, using the PDE camera. Lastly, we evaluated IF-labeled LNs in paraffin-embedded specimens from the patients.

14.3 Results

14.3.1 The Detection of SLNs

We observed that during the surgeries, soon after the laparotomy, the tumors were easily recognized and lymphatic channels draining from the tumor to the SLNs were clearly visible by fluorescence and the SLNs' bighting fluorescence (Fig. 14.2a). Even the SLNs that were not fluorescent green in color could be easily and clearly visualized by the IFI imaging. The SLN detection rate in our preliminary study was 90.9 % and the mean number of SLNs was 3.6 in the gastric cancer patients, and the corresponding values in the colorectal cancer patients were 88.5 % and 2.6.

14.3.2 The Tattooing of the Tumor Region by ICG Fluorescence

After the laparotomy, we observed the tattooing areas by using the PDE camera or fluorescent endoscope (Figs. 14.3 and 14.4). In our preliminary study we combined the injection of ICG and India ink and the clipping method in an attempt to identify the marking spots without fail. However, when we injected India ink prior to the ICG injection, we could not detect the tattooing points due to the ink's obstruction of the ICG pathway to the LNs.

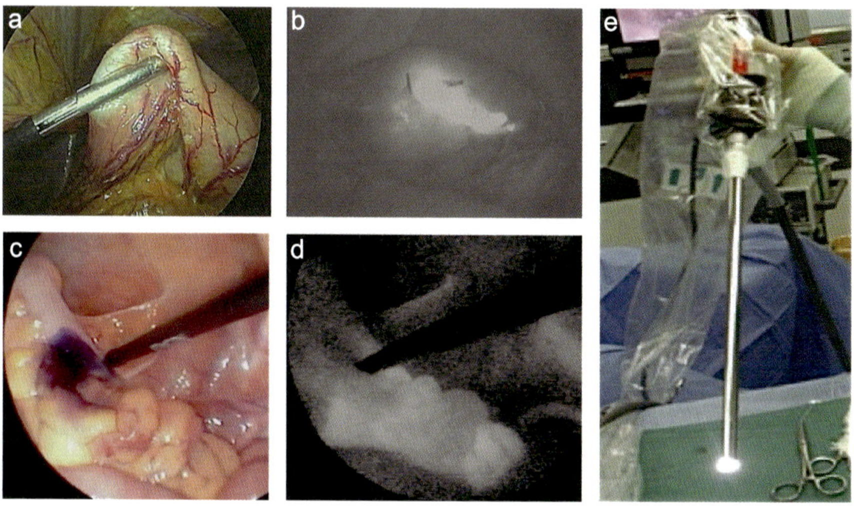

Fig. 14.3 Tattooing the tumor region by ICG fluorescence in the early gastric cancer. The stomach was mobilized laparoscopically and exteriorized through a minilaparotomy incision (**a**). The fluorescence-marked tumor localization was clearly visualized (**b**). (**c–e**) Fluorescent laparoscopic findings during a colon surgery. The fluorescent area around the tumor (**a**) was clearly visualized by fluorescent endoscopy (**e**). After marking using pyoktanin dye (**d**), a segmental colectomy was performed

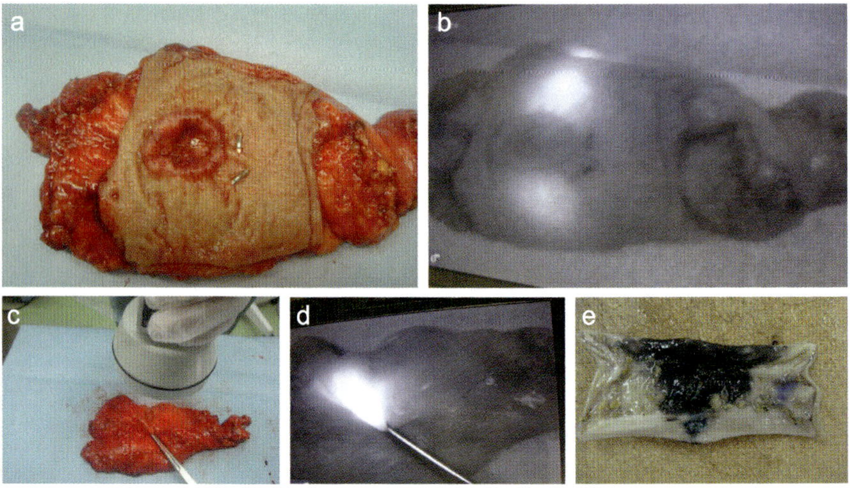

Fig. 14.4 Rectum cancer with tattooing by ICG. (**a**, **b**) The marking spot cannot be seen by the naked eye, but fluorescent spots were clearly observed at the upper and lower sides of the tumor by the PDE camera (see Fig. 14.4b). (**c**) The observation of fluorescent-tattoo spot by PDE camera. (**d**) The marking spot cannot be seen by the naked eye (Fig. 14.4c), but fluorescent spots were clearly detected (serous side, Fig. 14.4d). (**e**) Resected specimen tattooed by India ink (the case shown in Fig. 14.4e)

14.3.3 ICG Fluorescence-Assisted Ex Vivo Lymph Node Harvest in Gastric Cancer

Soon after the gastrectomies, we injected ICG at several points in submucosal areas around the tumors in resected specimen. A few minutes later, the lymphatic ducts and lymph nodes that generated fluorescence were detectable by the PDE camera (Fig. 14.5d–f). LNs were found by IFI even after the conventional harvesting of LNs.

Of the 20 gastric cancer patients in our patient series, eight patients had early-stage cancer and 12 had advanced-stage cancer. The mean number of residual LNs in the early cancers was 3.1, and that in advanced cancers was 6.2. Residual lymph nodes were detected in 19 of the 20 gastric cancer cases. Pathology-based upstaging was done for one patient. In that case, at primary harvest, we found 19 lymph nodes, and two were metastatic. At the patient's secondary harvest, 19 more lymph nodes were detected and three were metastatic. The pathological stage of this patient was thus upstaged form stage 2B to 3A.

This result prompted us to conduct a further study of the relationship between fluorescence and lymph nodes, using paraffin-embedded specimens (Fig. 14.6).

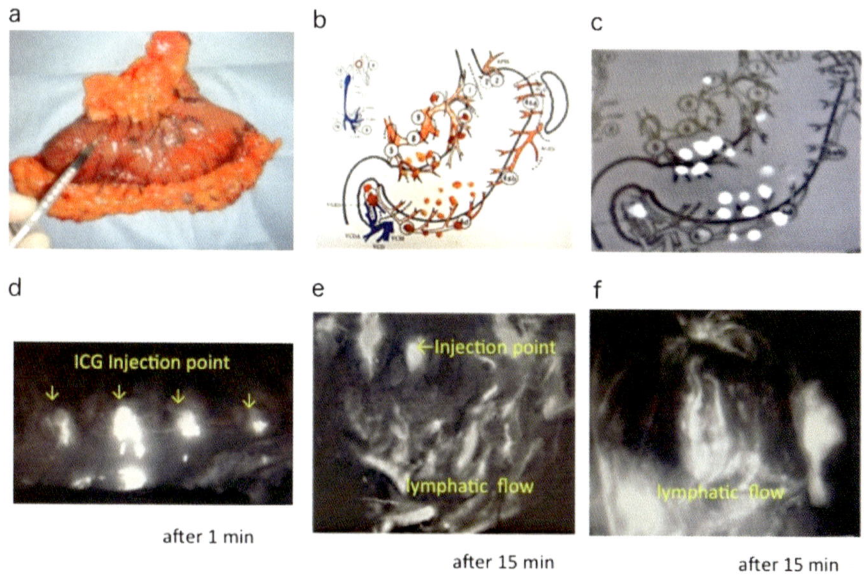

Fig. 14.5 ICG fluorescence-assisted ex vivo lymph node harvest in GI tract cancers. (**a–c**) Ex vivo ICG injection (gastric cancer). ICG was injected directly into the subserosa. A conventional LN harvest (**b**) and additional LN harvest (**c**) were then performed. (**d–f**) Ex vivo ICG injection (colon cancer). After the injection of ICG, the lymphatic flows appeared gradually. One min (**d**) and 15 min (**e**, **f**) after the injection

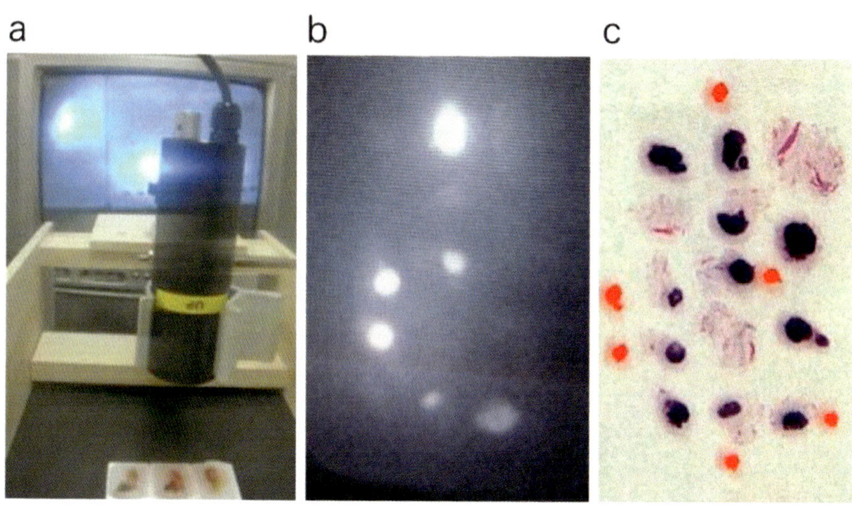

Fig. 14.6 Observation of paraffin-embedded LNs. (**a**) Observation of the fluorescence of LNs by the prototype PDE system. (**b**, **c**) Observation of fluorescent LNs (**b**) and LNs with hematoxylin and eosin stain. *Red spots*: LNs with metastasis

14.4 Discussion

We confirmed the efficacy of navigation surgery using the ICG fluorescent imaging, but several questions remain unanswered. Sentinel navigation surgery in breast cancer and malignant melanoma has been recognized as an established method, but there is no evidence regarding sentinel navigation surgery in stomach [11, 12] or colon cancer [10]. However, Takeuchi et al. [13] reported promising data from both a meta-analysis and a prospective multicenter trial of SLN mapping for early-stage gastric cancer. In their report, the SLN detection rates and the accuracy of the determination of lymph node status were acceptable for the establishment of the concept of SLNNS in gastric cancer. In the study [13], a dual-tracer method that uses blue dyes [3] and radioactive colloids [4] was used, but the authors emphasized that new technologies such as ICG infrared or fluorescence imaging might be a promising approach for the SLN mapping procedures in gastric cancer.

The concept of sentinel navigation surgery not only in early gastric cancers but also in early colon cancer may be beneficial for patients by preventing various complications related to unnecessary prophylactic regional LN dissection in patients with cancer-negative SLNs. When sentinel navigation surgery in gastric cancer is established, the partial resection of the stomach also becomes possible as a minimally invasive surgery for cancers of the gastrointestinal tract (Fig. 14.2b).

Regarding the tracer used to detect the SLNs, three tracers have been used: dye, RI, and ICG. Each tracer has its respective disadvantages. The disadvantages of the dye method are a low recognition rate and a short leveling time. The high cost and the exposure problem of radioactivity are disadvantages of RI tracers. The use of the ICG fluorescence method has officially been approved in Japan in SLNNS of breast cancer and malignant melanoma, and it thus appears that ICG can be an acceptable tracer for the detection of SLNs in gastric and colon cancer.

In the present examination of 110 cases, we found that the ICG tattooing method was very useful for the marking of the early gastric and colonic cancers, especially when using a laparoscopic approach (Fig. 14.3). Our clinical experience of successful ICG marking of early-stage stomach and colon cancers may lead to the establishment of new marking procedures that could be used as alternatives to the conventional India ink and clipping methods.

The injection of India ink has been used frequently for marking tumors, but there are some disadvantages of India ink [5]. One is that the marking portion is stained black (Fig. 14.4e), and the leakage of India ink into the abdominal cavity is an additional disadvantage. In the clipping method, the clips are likely to fall off. The ICG fluorescence method does not have these disadvantages. In addition, the fluorescence images obtained by this method are maintained even 10 days following ICG injection, and thus additional endoscopic approaches are not needed for the tattooing of tumors. Moreover, in colon cancer case it is easy to confirm the excision site when the ICG tattooing area is observed with the PDE camera after the colon is exteriorized.

We recommend this reliable tattooing procedure because it provides a more secure approach and a clean marking area. We also want to emphasize the development of the fluorescence endoscope [14] (Fig. 14.3e). The use of laparoscopic surgery in stomach and colon surgery has spread widely. When we want to perform minimally invasive ICG fluorescent navigation surgery, the fluorescence endoscope is an essential tool [14] in the SLNNS as described above. The ICG fluorescence endoscope enables a promising approach for the detection of SLNs and for marking early-stage tumors [15, 16]. The endoscope was developed first in Japan, and the tattooing method of colorectal cancer using the fluorescence endoscope has been reported [17]. The endoscope is now being tested in Europe. The new ICG fluorescence endoscope is also a potential approach for laparoscopic image-guided cholecystectomies [6].

In the present investigation we evaluated LN mapping by ICG fluorescence imaging using an ex vivo injection of ICG into resected specimens. We found that this imaging enabled the precise evaluation of harvested LNs (including SLNs) after surgery. The imaging makes it possible to conduct a more accurate retrieval of LNs, especially those that are very small in size.

Lastly, we discuss the harvest of LNs from resected specimens in cases in which metastatic LNs are defined as a prognostic factor [8]. According to the TNM [18] and Japanese staging systems for gastric cancer [19], N-staging is defined as follows: N0, no regional lymph node metastasis; N1, metastasis in 1–2 regional lymph nodes; N2, metastasis in 3–6 regional lymph nodes; N3, metastasis in >7 regional lymph nodes; N3a, 7–15; and N3b, >16. The Japanese lymph node staging system is the same as the TNM classification. It is necessary to evaluate the exact numbers of lymph nodes and metastatic lymph nodes that are correlated with the prognosis of stomach and colon cancer patients.

Our present findings demonstrated that ICG fluorescence-labeled LNs were detectable even though the ICG solution was injected ex vivo, which greatly improved the accuracy of the LN harvest from resected specimens. This improvement will enable more precise evaluations of the pathological status of LNs. Thus, ICG fluorescence imaging is a highly effective method for LN harvest for the determination of more accurate staging not only in stomach cancer but also in colon cancer. To our surprise, the lymphatic flows in the resected specimens remained even 30 min after the resection. The dynamics of lymph flows should be evaluated pathophysiologically in resected specimens with the use of ICG fluorescence imaging.

References

1. Veronesi U, Paganelli G, Viale G et al (2006) Sentinel-lymph-node biopsy as a staging procedure in breast cancer: update of a randomised controlled study. Lancet Oncol 7 (12):983–990
2. Morton DL, Wen DR, Wong JH, Economou JS, Cagle LA, Storm FK, Foshag LJ, Cochran A (1992) Technical details of intraoperative lymphatic mapping for early stage melanoma. Arch Surg 127(4):392–399

3. Fattahi AS, Tavassoli A, Rohbakhshfar O et al (2014) Can methylene blue dye be used as an alternative to patent blue dye to find the sentinel lymph node in breast cancer surgery? J Res Med Sci 19(10):918–922
4. Ahmed M, Purushotham AD, Horgan K et al (2015) Meta-analysis of superficial versus deep injection of radioactive tracer and blue dye for lymphatic mapping and detection of sentinel lymph nodes in breast cancer. Br J Surg 102(3):169–181
5. Singh S1, Arif A, Fox C, Basnyat P (2006) Complication after pre-operative India ink tattooing in a colonic lesion. Dig Surg 23(5–6):303
6. Kusano M, Yasuda D, Watanabe M et al (2008) Novel fluorescence endoscope for minimally invasive surgery SAGES (Society of American Gastrointestinal Endoscopic Surgeons) 2008. Emergency technology poster session proceedings, vol 2, p 304
7. Saito H, Fukumoto Y, Osaki T, Fukuda K et al (2007) Prognostic significance of level and number of lymph node metastases in patients with gastric cancer. Ann Surg Oncol 14:1688–1693
8. Karpeh MS, Leon L, Klimstra D, Brennan MF (2000) Lymph node staging in gastric cancer: is location more important than Number? An analysis of 1,038 patients. Ann Surg 232:362–371
9. Espin F, Bianchi A, Llorca S et al (2012) Metastatic lymph node ratio versus number of metastatic lymph nodes as a prognostic factor in gastric cancer. Eur J Surg Oncol 38:497–502
10. Kusano M, Tajima Y, Yamazaki K et al (2008) Sentinel node mapping guided by indocyanine green fluorescence imaging: a new method for sentinel node navigation surgery in gastrointestinal cancer. Dig Surg 25(2):103–108
11. Tajima Y, Yamazaki K, Masuda Y et al (2009) Sentinel node mapping guided by indocyanine green fluorescence imaging in gastric cancer. Ann Surg 249:58–62
12. Kitagawa Y, Takeuchi H, Takagi Y et al (2013) Sentinel node mapping for gastric cancer: a prospective multicenter trial in Japan. J Clin Oncol 31:3704–3710
13. Takeuchi H1, Kitagawa Y (2015) Sentinel lymph node biopsy in gastric cancer. Cancer J 21 (1):21–24
14. Nimura H, Narimiya N, Mitsumori N et al (2004) Infrared ray electronic endoscopy combined with indocyanine green injection for detection of sentinel nodes of patients with gastric cancer. Br J Surg 91:575–579
15. Tajima Y, Murakami M, Yamazaki K et al (2010) Sentinel node mapping guided by indocyanine green. Ann Surg Oncol 17(7):1787–1793
16. Cahill RA, Anderson M, Wang LM et al (2012) Near-infrared (NIR) laparoscopy for intraoperative lymphatic road-mapping and sentinel node identification during definitive surgical resection of early-stage colorectal neoplasia. Surg Endosc 26(1):197–204
17. Miyoshi N, Ohue M, Noura S et al (2009) Surgical usefulness of indocyanine green as an alternative to India ink for endoscopic marking. Surg Endosc 23(2):347–351
18. Sobin LHGM, Wittekind C (2009) TNM classification of malignant tumors, 7th edn. Wiley-Blackwell, Oxford
19. Japanese Gastric Cancer A (2011) Japanese classification of gastric carcinoma, 3rd English Edition. Gastric Cancer 14:101–112

Part VIII
Sentinel Node Navigation Surgery and Other Applications for Gastrointestial Tract Cancers: Colon Cancer

Chapter 15
Sentinel Node Navigation Surgery for Rectal Cancer: Indications for Lateral Node Dissection

Shingo Noura, Masayuki Ohue, and Norikatsu Miyoshi

Abstract *Background*: Lateral node dissection (LND) for lower rectal cancer is beneficial in a limited number of patients. If sentinel node navigation surgery could be applied in cases of lower rectal cancer, unnecessary LND procedures could be avoided. The aim of this study was to confirm the efficacy of sentinel node (SN) surgery for lateral lymph node (LLN) involvement of lower rectal cancer.

Methods: We investigated the existence of a lateral pelvic region SN in 53 lower rectal cancer patients. Indocyanine green (ICG) was injected into the submucosa along the dentate line, and the lateral pelvic region was observed using a near-infrared camera system (PDE, photodynamic eye). Bilateral LND was performed in cases in which the lateral SN demonstrated metastasis, whereas mesorectal excision only was performed in cases in which the lateral SN had no metastasis.

Results: Using PDE, the LNs that received ICG appeared as shining fluorescent spots on the fluorescence images. The lateral SNs were successfully identified in 49 (92.5 %) of the 53 patients; the mean number of lateral SNs per patient was 2.0 (range, 1–4). Of the 49 patients in whom lateral SNs were identified, four (8.2 %) had LLN metastases.

Conclusions: We were able to correctly identify patients with LLN metastases using PDE. It is difficult to predict LLN metastasis based on the findings of preoperative images or traditional criteria. Therefore, obtaining an intraoperative diagnosis is essential for selecting patients exhibiting LLN metastases.

Keywords Sentinel node navigation surgery • Rectal cancer • Lateral node dissection • ICG • Near-infrared camera system

---

S. Noura • M. Ohue (✉) • N. Miyoshi
Department of Surgery, Osaka Medical Center for Cancer and Cardiovascular Diseases, 1-3-3 Nakamichi, Higashinari-ku, Osaka 537-8511, Japan
e-mail: ohue-ma@mc.pref.osaka.jp

M. Kusano et al. (eds.), *ICG Fluorescence Imaging and Navigation Surgery*,
DOI 10.1007/978-4-431-55528-5_15

15.1 Introduction

In 1895, Gerota described the lateral and upward lymphatic flow in the rectum, as visualized using the dye injection method [1]. However, abdominopelvic lymph node (LN) dissection has failed to provide any significant benefits in patient survival [2, 3]. Therefore, in the West, extended surgery for rectal cancer has generally been abandoned. In Japan, Senba et al. reported the results of an anatomic study of the lymphatics of the rectum in which dye was injected into fetal cadavers and concluded that the lateral lymphatic vessels are distributed around the internal iliac arteries and inside the obturator space [4]. It is generally understood that some lymphatic vessels, mostly those originating from the lower rectum, easily penetrate the extramesenteric lymphatic vessels via the lateral ligament and ascend along the internal iliac arteries. Lateral node dissection (LND) is performed to treat middle or lower rectal cancer and has been shown to be associated with a lower rate of local recurrence than conventional surgery [5–7]. LND is indicated when the lower border of the tumor is located distal to the peritoneal reflection and has invaded beyond the muscularis propria [8]. However, the lateral lymph node (LLN) metastasis rate in patients treated with LND according to these criteria is only 20.1 % [9]. In the JCOG0212 trial, Fujita et al. reported that mesorectal excision (ME) with LND requires a significantly longer operative time (median, 360 min vs. 254 min) and results in significantly greater blood loss (median, 576 ml vs. 337 ml) than ME alone. Therefore, the routine adoption of LND in patients with advanced lower rectal cancer remains controversial.

The sentinel node (SN) is defined as the first node in the regional lymphatic basin that drains the primary tumor and is detected with a radioisotope and/or dye. A SN biopsy (SNB) is the standard procedure for determining the axillary stage in patients with breast cancer with clinically negative LNs [10, 11]. Recently, the SNB technique has been applied to cancers of the gastrointestinal tract [12–15], and numerous studies, including these reports, have used radioactive colloid tracers (e.g., 99mTc sulfur colloid) or visible blue dye (e.g., isosulfan blue) [16]. Furthermore, a promising new technique that uses SNB guided by indocyanine green (ICG) fluorescence imaging has recently been reported for the treatment of gastric cancer [17, 18]. If sentinel node navigation surgery (SNNS) could be successfully applied in cases of advanced lower rectal cancer, unnecessary LND procedures could be omitted, and the use of personalized lymphadenectomy may be possible.

The aim of this study was therefore to confirm the efficacy of lateral pelvic SN surgery for lower rectal cancer.

15.2 Patients and Methods

15.2.1 Patients

A total of 53 rectal cancer patients in whom the lower border of the tumor was located distal to the peritoneal reflection and invaded beyond the muscularis propria on preoperative images were investigated. No subjects exhibited extramesorectal lymph node enlargement (i.e., lymph nodes with a short-axis diameter of less than 10 mm on CT or MRI were not regarded as indicating lymph node enlargement) and had received either chemotherapy or irradiation preoperatively. This study was approved by the Human Ethics Review Committee of Osaka Medical Center for Cancer and Cardiovascular Diseases, and signed informed consent was obtained from each patient.

15.2.2 Detection of the SN with ICG Using the Near-Infrared Camera System

ICG fluorescence imaging was carried out using the near-infrared camera system (photodynamic eye (PDE), Hamamatsu Photonics, Hamamatsu, Japan) (Fig. 15.1a). The light source was a light-emitting diode that emitted light at a wavelength of 760 nm, and the detector was a charge-coupled device camera with a filter used to filter out light with a wavelength of 820 nm. The fluorescence signals were sent to a digital video processor to be displayed on a TV monitor in real time (Fig. 15.1b). The camera unit of the device was covered with a sterilized transmissive cover (Fig. 15.1c) and held directly by the surgeon, placed approximately 20 cm ahead of the pelvic side wall (Fig. 15.1d).

Before performing laparotomy, a fine needle (26 gauge) was inserted into the submucosal layer via the anus, and ICG dye (Diagnogreen, Daiichi Sankyo Co., Ltd., Tokyo, Japan) was gently injected at four sites along the dentate line circumferentially. The total amount of injected dye was 1 ml (5 mg, 0.5 % ICG) in each patient. After the rectal cancer was resected, the lateral vesical and obturator spaces were opened via the extraperitoneal approach between the lateral aspect of the internal iliac vessels and the pelvic wall. The adipose tissue surrounding the common-internal iliac arteries and obturator space was observed with PDE, which allowed for the identification of SN in the lateral pelvic region.

15.2.3 Division of the Lateral Pelvic Region

According to the Japanese Classification of Colorectal Carcinoma [19], the lateral pelvic region can be classified into three divisions: (1) the common iliac region along the common iliac artery, (2) the internal iliac region along the internal iliac artery, and (3) the obturator region along the obturator nerve, artery, and vein (Fig. 15.2).

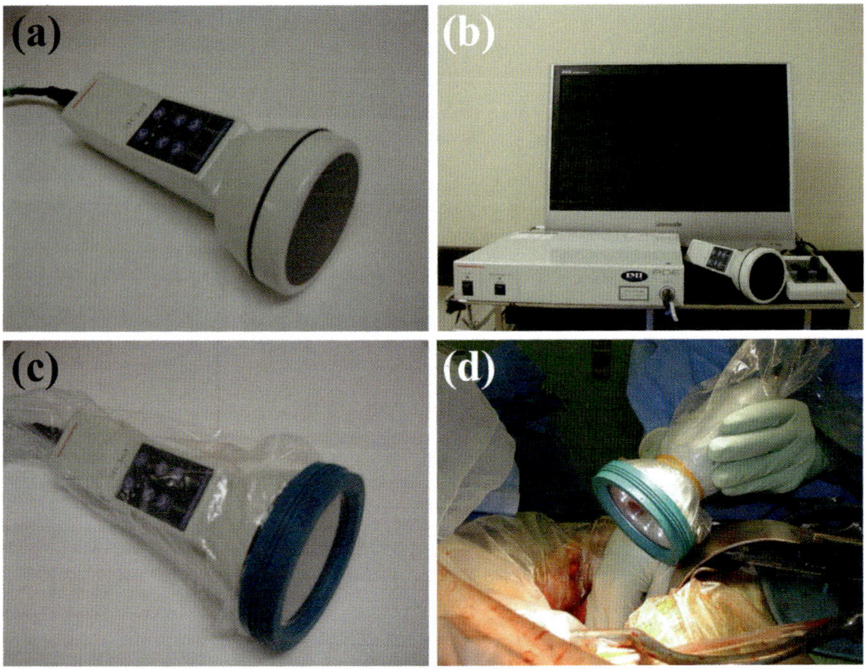

Fig. 15.1 (**a**) Near-infrared camera system (PDE, photodynamic eye). (**b**) PDE system. (**c**) The camera unit was covered with a sterilized transmissive cover. (**d**) The camera was handled directly by the surgeon

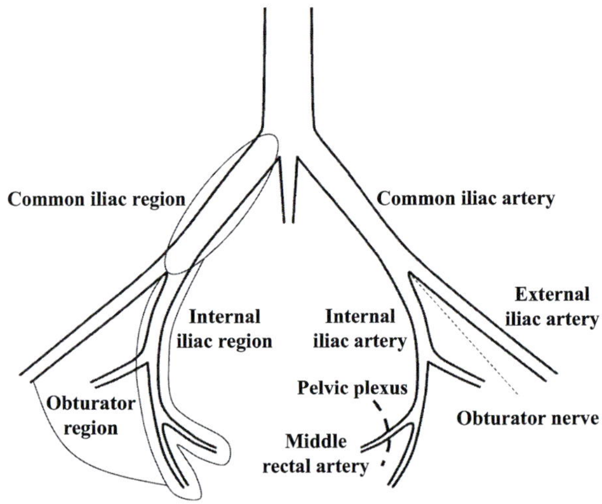

Fig. 15.2 Diagram showing the division of the lateral pelvic region

15.2.4 *Statistical Analysis*

The statistical analyses were performed using the StatView version 5.0 software package (Abacus Concepts, Berkeley, CA). The data are presented as the mean ± standard deviation and were analyzed using the χ^2 test for discrete variables. If the sample size was small, Fisher's exact test was used. A P value of <0.05 denoted the presence of a statistically significant difference.

15.3 Results

15.3.1 *Patient Characteristics*

The patients included 36 males (67.9 %) and 17 females (32.1 %), with an average age of 59.8 ± 11.5 (range, 32–83) years. The anal edge of all tumors at the lower level was located either at or below the peritoneal reflection. The distance from the dentate line to the lower border of the tumor was 2.9 ± 2.1 (range, −2.0 to 6.0) cm, and the tumor size was 4.6 ± 1.7 (range, 1.2–11.0) cm. Most tumors were moderately differentiated adenocarcinomas (N = 38), followed by well-differentiated adenocarcinomas ($N = 13$) and poorly differentiated adenocarcinomas ($N = 2$) (Table 15.1).

15.3.2 *Feasibility*

No adverse events related to the ICG injections were noted. As previously described [20], the optimal concentration of ICG was 0.5 %, and a total of 1 ml (5 mg) of ICG solution was injected. PDE clearly visualized the LNs and lymphatic vessels that received ICG; however, the PDE-positive LNs were not detected with the naked eye. The LNs and lymphatic vessels not seen under ordinary white light were visualized on PDE in the surrounding adipose tissue around the common-internal iliac arteries and obturator space (Fig. 15.2). The preparation of the device, injection of the ICG solution, and observation of the fluorescence images took less than 30 min.

15.3.3 *Detection of Lateral SNs*

The LNs and lymphatic vessels that received ICG appeared as shining fluorescent spots and streams on the fluorescence images of PDE. The lateral SNs were successfully identified in 49 (92.5 %) of the 53 patients; the total number of lateral

Table 15.1 Clinicopathological findings of the 53 patients with rectal cancer

Age (years)	59.8 ± 11.5 (32–83)
Gender	
Male	36 (67.9 %)
Female	17 (32.1 %)
Distance from dentate line (cm)	2.9 ± 2.1 (−2.0–6.0)
Tumor size (cm)	4.6 ± 1.7 (1.2–11.0)
Histological grade	
Well	13 (24.5 %)
Mod	38 (71.7 %)
Por	2 (3.8 %)
Primary tumor	
pT1	3 (5.7 %)
pT2	13 (24.5 %)
pT3/T4	37 (69.8 %)
Regional lymph nodes	
pN0	25 (47.2 %)
pN1	17 (32.1 %)
pN2	11 (20.8 %)
pTNM stage	
I	10 (18.9 %)
II	15 (28.3 %)
III	22 (41.5 %)
IV	6 (11.3 %)
Lymphatic invasion	
No	20 (37.8 %)
Yes	33 (62.3 %)
Venous invasion	
No	14 (26.4 %)
Yes	39 (73.6 %)

Well well-differentiated adenocarcinoma, *Mod* moderately differentiated adenocarcinoma, *Por* poorly differentiaterd adenocarcinoma

SNs was 94, and the number of lateral SNs per patient was 1.9 ± 0.8 (range, 1–4). Of the 94 SNs, 51 (54.3 %) were detected in the internal iliac region, 40 (42.5 %) were detected in the obturator region, two (2.1 %) were detected in the external iliac region, and one (0.1 %) was detected in the common iliac region. The parameters age, sex, distance from the dentate line, tumor size, histological grade, depth of the primary tumor, upward LN status, pTNM stage, lymphatic invasion, and venous invasion did not affect the successful identification of the lateral SNs (Fig. 15.3, Table 15.2).

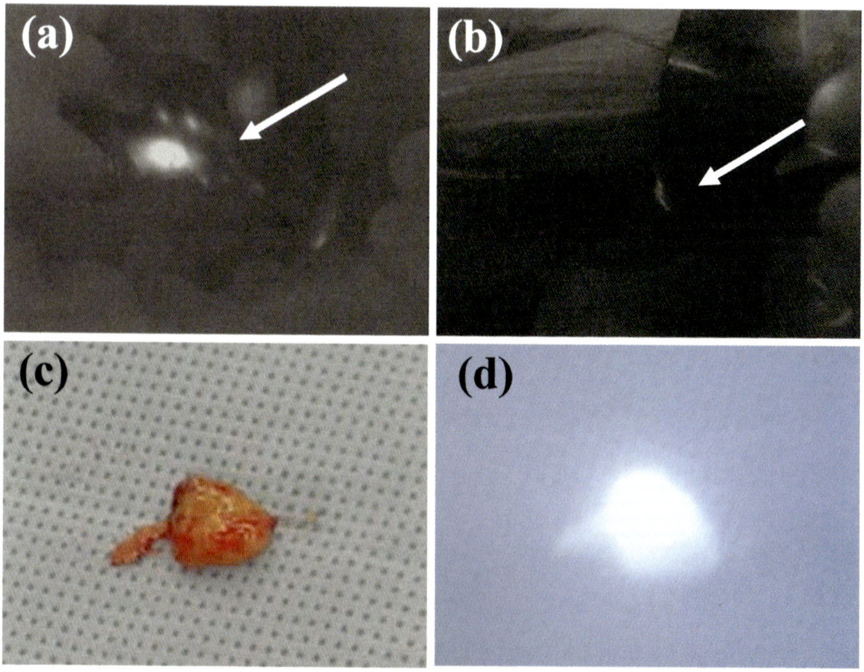

Fig. 15.3 Detection of SNs around the left internal iliac artery. (**a**) On PDE, the LNs that received ICG appeared as shining fluorescent spots (*arrow*). (**b**) On PDE, the lymphatic vessels that received ICG appeared as shining fluorescent streams (*arrow*). (**c**) The SNs that received ICG were not stained green in the naked eye examination. (**d**) The same SNs that received ICG appeared as shining fluorescent spots on PDE

15.3.4 Correlations Between the Tumor-Positive Lymph Nodes and Dissected Lymph Nodes

Lateral SNs were detected in 49 of the 53 patients. Figure 15.4 shows the therapeutic courses of these 49 patients. Patients in whom we detected lateral SNs on PDE were diagnosed with or without metastasis in the lateral SNs based on the results of HE staining. LND was performed in nine of the 49 patients with lateral SNs, four (8.2 %) of whom showed metastasis in the lateral SNs on HE staining. Although the remaining five patients demonstrated no metastasis in the lateral SNs on HE staining, LND was performed prophylactically in these cases.

Of the nine patients who received ME with LND, four had tumor-positive lateral SNs. In two of these four patients, tumor-positive LNs were detected in the dissected lateral non-SNs. In contrast, in the five patients with tumor-negative lateral SNs, all of the dissected lateral non-SNs were negative. Therefore, the negative predictive value in the patients with tumor-negative lateral SNs was 100 %.

Table 15.2 Clinicopathological features and rate of success in identifying lateral SNs

Clinicopathological features	No. of cases examined ($N=53$)	No. of SNs detected in cases ($N=49$)	Success rate (%)	*P* value
Age				
<60 years old	30	28	93.3	>0.9999
≥60 years old	23	21	91.3	
Gender				
Male	33	31	93.9	0.6274
Female	20	18	90.0	
Distance from the dentate line				
<3.0 cm	22	20	90.9	0.1241
≥3.0 cm	31	29	89.0	
Tumor size				
<4.5 cm	24	22	91.6	>0.9999
≥4.5 cm	29	27	93.1	
Histological grade				
Well/Mod	51	47	92.2	>0.9999
Por	2	2	100	
Depth of the primary tumor				
pT1	3	3	100	0.8772
pT2	13	12	92.3	
pT3/T4	37	34	91.9	
Upward LN status				
negative	28	26	92.9	>0.9999
positive	25	23	92.0	
pTNM stage				
I	10	9	90	0.7766
II	15	14	93.3	
III	22	21	95.5	
IV	6	5	100	
Lymphatic invasion				
No	20	19	95.0	>0.9999
Yes	33	30	90.9	
Venous invasion				
No	14	13	92.9	>0.9999
Yes	39	36	92.3	

Well well-differentiated adenocarcinoma, *Mod* moderately differentiated adenocarcinoma, *Por* poorly differentiated adenocarcinoma, *LN* lymph node, *SN* sentinel node

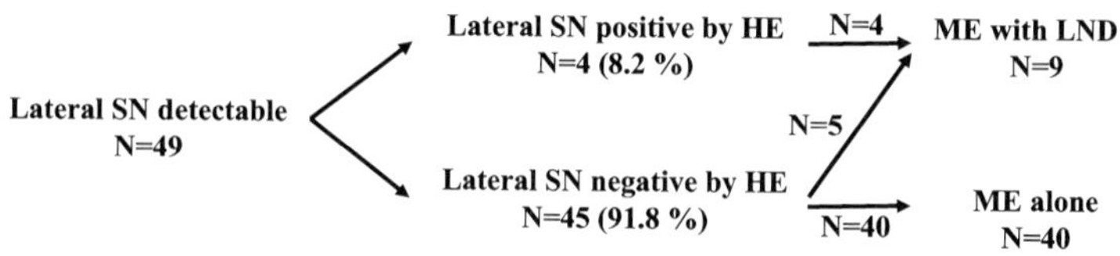

Fig. 15.4 Number of LND procedures and status of SN and non-SN cases based on hematoxylin and eosin (HE) staining

15.4 Discussion

One of the most common sites of recurrence after curative resection for rectal cancer is the pelvis, and local control is a major goal of surgical treatment. Several trials comparing the efficacy of LND with preoperative chemoradiotherapy (CRT) found no differences in the rates of either locoregional recurrence or survival. In contrast, the operative time, amount of blood loss and frequency of urinary dysfunction, and male sexual disorders were observed to be increased in the LND group versus the ME-alone group [6, 21–25]. In a multi-institutional study conducted in Japan, LLN metastasis was found to have a positive association with overall survival in a multivariate analysis, and the prognosis of these patients was similar to that of the subjects with N2b disease and better than that of the subjects with stage IV disease. The authors concluded that LLN involvement can be regarded as a regional condition that may benefit from LND [26]. In addition, Kim et al. reported LLN metastasis to be a major cause of locoregional recurrence in patients with rectal cancer treated with preoperative CRT and curative resection [27]. In the context of clinically suspected LLN disease, dissection should be attempted to remove these nodes, if technically feasible [28]. For this reason, there is currently no consensus regarding the implementation of LND based on the lack of high-level evidence. If lateral SNs to which the fluid first spreads from the primary tumor of lower rectal cancer could be detected accurately, it would be possible to omit unnecessary LND procedures.

The SN is defined as the first node in the regional lymphatic basin that drains the primary tumor, and either radionuclide tracer or vital dye is used to detect these nodes. Although ICG was initially developed as a drug to assess the liver and circulatory function, it also is used for lymphography, angiography, and SN detection due to its diagnostic value and ready availability [12, 29–33]. Moreover, the ICG method is convenient and safe compared with the radioisotope method [17]. Avoiding the use of radioisotopes is also beneficial, especially in institutes where the use of radioisotopes is limited. The clinical applicability of SNNS has been investigated extensively in cases of gastrointestinal tract cancer [12–15], and the usefulness of dye-guided SN detection in patients with colon cancer has previously been reported [34], showing the high efficacy (70–99 %) of assessment of SNs. However, there are few reports regarding lateral SNs in cases of rectal cancer. Recently, Kawahara et al. reported conducting initial lateral pelvic LN assessments for lower rectal cancer using infrared ray electronic endoscopy (IREE) with ICG [35]. However, the rate of detection of SN in that study was not high (43 %, six of 14). Detection via absorption spectroscopy is more sensitive than that based on color perception, and some surgeons have reported that IREE with ICG injection is useful for identifying SNs [36, 37]. In contrast, Ishikawa et al., using the IREE system, reported the case of an obese patient with a falsely negative SN detected with laparoscopic SN navigation, although infrared rays are capable of penetrating fatty tissues up to a depth of 3 mm [37]. Kitai et al. noted, in their preliminary report of ICG fluorescence imaging in the setting of breast cancer surgery, that the sensitivity of fluorescence spectroscopy is much greater than that of absorption spectroscopy. In addition, they reported detecting fluorescence from an ICG solution embedded 1 cm deep in the material with optical properties compatible to that of human tissue in a preliminary study using a phantom [38]. Similarly, Miyashiro et al. recently reported that the sensitivity of ICG fluorescence imaging appears to be much greater than that of infrared ray imaging [17]. In fact, the rate of detection of lateral SNs on PDE in the present study was 2.2 times greater (92.5 % vs. 43 %) than that reported by Kawahara [35]. In our previous study, the lateral SNs for lower rectal cancer tumors were investigated using ICG with an examination with the naked eye. However, lateral SNs were identified in only seven (28 %) of 25 patients [39]. Because the previous detection rate was so low, it was hard to apply this method in clinical practice. In the current study, PDE was successfully used to detect the lateral SNs for lower rectal cancer, thus improving the detection rate. The rate of success in detecting the lateral SNs by means of ICG using PDE was 92.5 %, which was 3.3 times greater than that obtained in examinations with the naked eye based on our previous data. Due to the high sensitivity of PDE, both tumor-negative and tumor-positive SNs can be clearly detected using PDE.

The JCOG0212 trial [40] is a randomized controlled non-inferiority trial evaluating the efficacy of ME alone against ME with LND in patients with clinical stage II/III lower rectal cancer without lateral pelvic LN enlargement. In that study, 7 % patients in the ME with LND group without lateral pelvic LN enlargement on preoperative images had lateral pelvic LN metastasis. These results show that, even in patients without clinically evident lateral pelvic LN metastasis, such metastasis is sometimes present pathologically. In the current study, the incidence of tumor-positive lateral SNs was 8.2 % (four of 49), which is approximately the same as that observed in the JCOG0212 trial. There is a limitation in predicting LLN metastasis on preoperative imaging. Akiyoshi et al. reported that the incidence of LLN metastases is 20 % among all patients undergoing preoperative CRT [41]. This rate of LLN metastasis is similar to the findings of previous reports in which patients received surgery alone [9, 26].

Based on these observations, when performing LND according to the traditional guidelines [8], approximately 80 % of patients are negative for lateral pelvic LN [9]. In addition, when LND is conducted in patients with negative lateral pelvic LN findings on preoperative images, 7 % of these patients are found to have lateral pelvic LN metastasis [40]. Furthermore, among patients who receive preoperative

CRT, the incidence of lateral pelvic LN metastasis is 20 % [41]. Judging from these reports, LLN metastasis cannot be cured with CRT alone. In order to reduce the rate of lateral recurrence, LND is a necessary operative procedure in patients with LLN metastases.

Although further studies with larger sample populations are needed to validate the oncologic outcomes, the dye-guided method using the ICG fluorescent imaging system is considered to be a potentially safe and convenient tool. In the current study, the negative predictive value was 100 %, and we were able to correctly identify patients with LLN metastasis using PDE.

References

1. Gerota D (1895) Die Lymphgefaesse des Rectums und des Anus. Arch Anat Physiol Anat Abt:240–256
2. Blair JB, Holyoke EA, Best RR (1950) A note on the lymphatics of the middle and lower rectum and anus. Anat Rec 108(4):635–644
3. Stearns MW Jr, Deddish MR (1959) Five-year results of abdominopelvic lymph node dissection for carcinoma of the rectum. Dis Colon Rectum 2(2):169–172
4. Senba Y (1927) An anatomical study of lympatic system of the rectum [in Japanese]. J Hukuoka Med Col 20:1213–1268
5. Suzuki K, Muto T, Sawada T (1995) Prevention of local recurrence by extended lymphadenectomy for rectal cancer. Surg Today 25(9):795–801
6. Moriya Y, Sugihara K, Akasu T, Fujita S (1995) Patterns of recurrence after nerve-sparing surgery for rectal adenocarcinoma with special reference to loco-regional recurrence. Dis Colon Rectum 38(11):1162–1168
7. Mori T, Takahashi K, Yasuno M (1998) Radical resection with autonomic nerve preservation and lymph node dissection techniques in lower rectal cancer surgery and its results: the impact of lateral lymph node dissection. Langenbecks Arch Surg 383(6):409–415
8. Sugihara K, Kobayashi H, Kato T, Mori T, Mochizuki H, Kameoka S, Shirouzu K, Muto T (2006) Indication and benefit of pelvic sidewall dissection for rectal cancer. Dis Colon Rectum 49(11):1663–1672. doi:10.1007/s10350-006-0714-z
9. Watanabe T, Itabashi M, Shimada Y, Tanaka S, Ito Y, Ajioka Y, Hamaguchi T, Hyodo I, Igarashi M, Ishida H, Ishiguro M, Kanemitsu Y, Kokudo N, Muro K, Ochiai A, Oguchi M, Ohkura Y, Saito Y, Sakai Y, Ueno H, Yoshino T, Fujimori T, Koinuma N, Morita T, Nishimura G, Sakata Y, Takahashi K, Takiuchi H, Tsuruta O, Yamaguchi T, Yoshida M, Yamaguchi N, Kotake K, Sugihara K (2012) Japanese Society for Cancer of the Colon and Rectum (JSCCR) guidelines 2010 for the treatment of colorectal cancer. Int J Clin Oncol 17 (1):1–29. doi:10.1007/s10147-011-0315-2
10. Giuliano AE, Kirgan DM, Guenther JM, Morton DL (1994) Lymphatic mapping and sentinel lymphadenectomy for breast cancer. Ann Surg 220(3):391–398; discussion 398–401
11. Veronesi U, Paganelli G, Galimberti V, Viale G, Zurrida S, Bedoni M, Costa A, de Cicco C, Geraghty JG, Luini A, Sacchini V, Veronesi P (1997) Sentinel-node biopsy to avoid axillary dissection in breast cancer with clinically negative lymph-nodes. Lancet 349 (9069):1864–1867, doi:S0140673697010040 [pii]
12. Hiratsuka M, Miyashiro I, Ishikawa O, Furukawa H, Motomura K, Ohigashi H, Kameyama M, Sasaki Y, Kabuto T, Ishiguro S, Imaoka S, Koyama H (2001) Application of sentinel node biopsy to gastric cancer surgery. Surgery 129(3):335–340. doi:10.1067/msy.2001.111699, S0039-6060(01) 02450-3 [pii]

13. Saha S, Wiese D, Badin J, Beutler T, Nora D, Ganatra BK, Desai D, Kaushal S, Nagaraju M, Arora M, Singh T (2000) Technical details of sentinel lymph node mapping in colorectal cancer and its impact on staging. Ann Surg Oncol 7(2):120–124
14. Joosten JJ, Strobbe LJ, Wauters CA, Pruszczynski M, Wobbes T, Ruers TJ (1999) Intraoperative lymphatic mapping and the sentinel node concept in colorectal carcinoma. Br J Surg 86(4):482–486. doi:10.1046/j.1365-2168.1999.01051.x
15. Kitagawa Y, Fujii H, Kumai K, Kubota T, Otani Y, Saikawa Y, Yoshida M, Kubo A, Kitajima M (2005) Recent advances in sentinel node navigation for gastric cancer: a paradigm shift of surgical management. J Surg Oncol 90(3):147–151. doi:10.1002/jso.20220; discussion 151–142
16. Saha S, Dan AG, Bilchik AJ, Kitagawa Y, Schochet E, Choudhri S, Saha LT, Wiese D, Morton D, Kitajima M (2004) Historical review of lymphatic mapping in gastrointestinal malignancies. Ann Surg Oncol 11(3 Suppl):245S–249S
17. Miyashiro I, Miyoshi N, Hiratsuka M, Kishi K, Yamada T, Ohue M, Ohigashi H, Yano M, Ishikawa O, Imaoka S (2008) Detection of sentinel node in gastric cancer surgery by indocyanine green fluorescence imaging: comparison with infrared imaging. Ann Surg Oncol 15(6):1640–1643. doi:10.1245/s10434-008-9872-7
18. Tajima Y, Yamazaki K, Masuda Y, Kato M, Yasuda D, Aoki T, Kato T, Murakami M, Miwa M, Kusano M (2009) Sentinel node mapping guided by indocyanine green fluorescence imaging in gastric cancer. Ann Surg 249(1):58–62. doi:10.1097/SLA.0b013e3181927267, 00000658-200901000-00010 [pii]
19. Japanese Society for Cancer of the Colon and Rectum. (2009). Japanese classification of colorectal carcinoma (Second English edn.). Kanehara, Tokyo
20. Noura S, Ohue M, Seki Y, Tanaka K, Motoori M, Kishi K, Miyashiro I, Ohigashi H, Yano M, Ishikawa O, Miyamoto Y (2010) Feasibility of a lateral region sentinel node biopsy of lower rectal cancer guided by indocyanine green using a near-infrared camera system. Ann Surg Oncol 17(1):144–151. doi:10.1245/s10434-009-0711-2
21. Pilipshen SJ, Heilweil M, Quan SH, Sternberg SS, Enker WE (1984) Patterns of pelvic recurrence following definitive resections of rectal cancer. Cancer 53(6):1354–1362
22. Nagawa H, Muto T, Sunouchi K, Higuchi Y, Tsurita G, Watanabe T, Sawada T (2001) Randomized, controlled trial of lateral node dissection vs. nerve-preserving resection in patients with rectal cancer after preoperative radiotherapy. Dis Colon Rectum 44 (9):1274–1280
23. Watanabe T, Tsurita G, Muto T, Sawada T, Sunouchi K, Higuchi Y, Komuro Y, Kanazawa T, Iijima T, Miyaki M, Nagawa H (2002) Extended lymphadenectomy and preoperative radiotherapy for lower rectal cancers. Surgery 132(1):27–33, doi:S0039606002000387 [pii]
24. Kobayashi H, Mochizuki H, Sugihara K, Morita T, Kotake K, Teramoto T, Kameoka S, Saito Y, Takahashi K, Hase K, Oya M, Maeda K, Hirai T, Kameyama M, Shirouzu K, Muto T (2007) Characteristics of recurrence and surveillance tools after curative resection for colorectal cancer: a multicenter study. Surgery 141(1):67–75. doi:10.1016/j.surg.2006.07.020, S0039-6060(06)00456-9 [pii]
25. Georgiou P, Tan E, Gouvas N, Antoniou A, Brown G, Nicholls RJ, Tekkis P (2009) Extended lymphadenectomy versus conventional surgery for rectal cancer: a meta-analysis. Lancet Oncol 10(11):1053–1062. doi:10.1016/S1470-2045(09)70224-4, S1470-2045(09)70224-4 [pii]
26. Akiyoshi T, Watanabe T, Miyata S, Kotake K, Muto T, Sugihara K (2012) Results of a Japanese nationwide multi-institutional study on lateral pelvic lymph node metastasis in low rectal cancer: is it regional or distant disease? Ann Surg 255(6):1129–1134. doi:10.1097/SLA.0b013e3182565d9d
27. Kim TH, Jeong SY, Choi DH, Kim DY, Jung KH, Moon SH, Chang HJ, Lim SB, Choi HS, Park JG (2008) Lateral lymph node metastasis is a major cause of locoregional recurrence in rectal cancer treated with preoperative chemoradiotherapy and curative resection. Ann Surg Oncol 15(3):729–737. doi:10.1245/s10434-007-9696-x

28. Nelson H, Petrelli N, Carlin A, Couture J, Fleshman J, Guillem J, Miedema B, Ota D, Sargent D (2001) Guidelines 2000 for colon and rectal cancer surgery. J Natl Cancer Inst 93 (8):583–596
29. Caesar J, Shaldon S, Chiandussi L, Guevara L, Sherlock S (1961) The use of indocyanine green in the measurement of hepatic blood flow and as a test of hepatic function. Clin Sci 21:43–57
30. Cherrick GR, Stein SW, Leevy CM, Davidson CS (1960) Indocyanine green: observations on its physical properties, plasma decay, and hepatic extraction. J Clin Invest 39:592–600
31. Unno N, Inuzuka K, Suzuki M, Yamamoto N, Sagara D, Nishiyama M, Konno H (2007) Preliminary experience with a novel fluorescence lymphography using indocyanine green in patients with secondary lymphedema. J Vasc Surg 45(5):1016–1021. doi:10.1016/j.jvs.2007.01.023, S0741-5214(07)00037-7 [pii]
32. Unno N, Suzuki M, Yamamoto N, Inuzuka K, Sagara D, Nishiyama M, Tanaka H, Konno H (2008) Indocyanine green fluorescence angiography for intraoperative assessment of blood flow: a feasibility study. Eur J Vasc Endovasc Surg 35(2):205–207. doi:10.1016/j.ejvs.2007.09.001, S1078-5884(07)00585-0 [pii]
33. Motomura K, Inaji H, Komoike Y, Kasugai T, Noguchi S, Koyama H (1999) Sentinel node biopsy guided by indocyanine green dye in breast cancer patients. Jpn J Clin Oncol 29 (12):604–607
34. Saha S, Nora D, Wong JH, Weise D (2000) Sentinel lymph node mapping in colorectal cancer–a review. Surg Clin North Am 80(6):1811–1819
35. Kawahara H, Nimura H, Watanabe K, Kobayashi T, Kashiwagi H, Yanaga K (2007) Where does the first lateral pelvic lymph node receive drainage from? Dig Surg 24(6):413–417. doi:10.1159/000108323, 000108323 [pii]
36. Nimura H, Narimiya N, Mitsumori N, Yamazaki Y, Yanaga K, Urashima M (2004) Infrared ray electronic endoscopy combined with indocyanine green injection for detection of sentinel nodes of patients with gastric cancer. Br J Surg 91(5):575–579. doi:10.1002/bjs.4470
37. Ishikawa K, Yasuda K, Shiromizu A, Etoh T, Shiraishi N, Kitano S (2007) Laparoscopic sentinel node navigation achieved by infrared ray electronic endoscopy system in patients with gastric cancer. Surg Endosc 21(7):1131–1134. doi:10.1007/s00464-006-9062-2
38. Kitai T, Inomoto T, Miwa M, Shikayama T (2005) Fluorescence navigation with indocyanine green for detecting sentinel lymph nodes in breast cancer. Breast Cancer 12(3):211–215
39. Noura S, Ohue M, Seki Y, Yamamoto T, Idota A, Fujii J, Yamasaki T, Nakajima H, Murata K, Kameyama M, Yamada T, Miyashiro I, Ohigashi H, Yano M, Ishikawa O, Imaoka S (2008) Evaluation of the lateral sentinel node by indocyanine green for rectal cancer based on micrometastasis determined by reverse transcriptase-polymerase chain reaction. Oncol Rep 20(4):745–750
40. Fujita S, Akasu T, Mizusawa J, Saito N, Kinugasa Y, Kanemitsu Y, Ohue M, Fujii S, Shiozawa M, Yamaguchi T, Moriya Y (2012) Postoperative morbidity and mortality after mesorectal excision with and without lateral lymph node dissection for clinical stage II or stage III lower rectal cancer (JCOG0212): results from a multicentre, randomised controlled, non-inferiority trial. Lancet Oncol 13(6):616–621. doi:10.1016/S1470-2045(12)70158-4, S1470-2045(12)70158-4 [pii]
41. Akiyoshi T, Ueno M, Matsueda K, Konishi T, Fujimoto Y, Nagayama S, Fukunaga Y, Unno T, Kano A, Kuroyanagi H, Oya M, Yamaguchi T, Watanabe T, Muto T (2014) Selective lateral pelvic lymph node dissection in patients with advanced low rectal cancer treated with preoperative chemoradiotherapy based on pretreatment imaging. Ann Surg Oncol 21 (1):189–196. doi:10.1245/s10434-013-3216-y

Part IX
Sentinel Node Navigation Surgery: Skin Cancer

Chapter 16
Indocyanine Green Fluorescence-Navigated Sentinel Node Navigation Surgery (SNNS) for Cutaneous Malignant Melanoma and Extramammary Paget's Disease

Taiki Isei

Abstract Sentinel node navigation surgery (SNNS) has been developed as a beneficial procedure to detect clinically-negative early regional lymphatic metastases in various types of skin cancers. Recently, a novel method was developed using a near-infrared imaging system to visualize indocyanine green (ICG)-induced fluorescence and to detect sentinel lymph nodes (SLN) in breast cancer. Herein, we describe the critical techniques of this new method in the patients with cutaneous melanoma and nonmelanoma skin cancers.

For sentinel node biopsy, intra-operative observation of ICG-induced fluorescence image is easily performed by infrared camera system. Cutaneous lymphatic tracts to SNs become visible shortly after intracutaneous ICG injection. This method is more ideal for detecting SLNs because of the higher intensity, contrast, and penetrability of ICG compared with conventional vital dyes and can be suitable for SNNS in melanoma and nonmelanoma skin cancers.

Keywords Sentinel node • Sentinel node navigation surgery • Melanoma • Paget disease • Extramammary • Indocyanine green • ICG • Infrared

16.1 Introduction

Since Morton et al. [1] proposed the concept of sentinel lymph nodes (SLN) concept in cutaneous malignant melanoma, pre-operative lymphatic mapping and lymphadenectomy of SLNs (sentinel lymph node biopsy, SLNB) has been developed and has been proven to be a minimally invasive procedure that provides important prognostic information; thus, allowing the detection of early nodal metastases of thin to intermediate-thickness melanoma [2]. This method is now

T. Isei, M.D., Ph.D. (✉)
Division of Dermatology, Osaka National Hospital, 2-1-14 Hoenzaka, Chuo-ku, Osaka 540-0006, Japan
e-mail: iseit@onh.go.jp

M. Kusano et al. (eds.), *ICG Fluorescence Imaging and Navigation Surgery*,
DOI 10.1007/978-4-431-55528-5_16

applied widely to a variety of nonmelanoma skin cancers, i.e., Merkel cell carcinoma (MCC) [3] and extramammary Paget's disease (EMPD) [4]. As such, using this concept to limit the extent of surgical tissue dissection, sentinel node navigation surgery (SNNS) is now also applied to the treatment of several internal malignancies. SNNS involves preoperative imaging with radioisotope (RI) lymph scintigraphy to detect the SLNs, and intra-operative detection of the SLN. The RI tracer-guided method using gamma probe detection is the most accurate intra-operative procedure, but this requires special facilities and equipment, which can be expensive. Although the conventional vital dye method for intra-operative SLN detection is simple and inexpensive, it requires somewhat intensive training to obtain a suitable detection rate. These have a common limitation, as they cannot visualize the lymph vessels and lymph nodes from the skin surface during SNNS.

Recently, the novel method (ICG-NIR method) using a near-infrared (NIR) imaging system to visualize indocyanine green (ICG)-induced fluorescence (Fig. 16.1) was developed to detect SLN in breast cancer [5]. This system uses

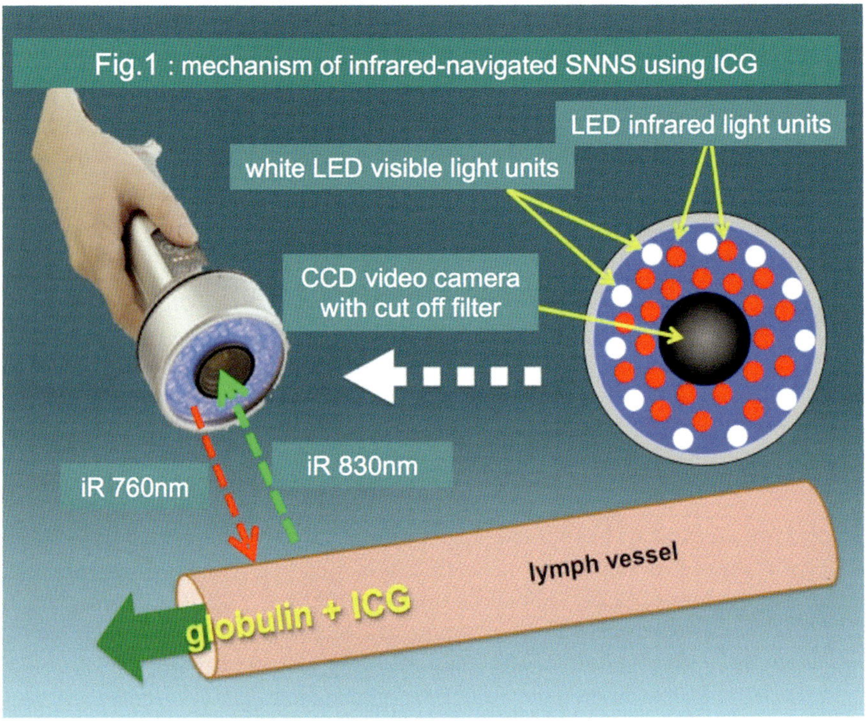

Fig. 16.1 The mechanism for detecting ICG-induced fluorescence by NIR camera system
Once binding with plasma protein, ICG can emit fluorescence of maximum wavelength around 845 nm when it is excited by near-infrared light wavelength of 750–810 nm. This fluorescence of ICG can be detected at least 10 mm beneath the skin surface by infrared camera unit. This camera system has a NIR camera, which has a cutoff filter wavelength below 830 nm, in the center to capture the fluorescence from lymphatic tracts, surrounded by many light-emitting diode (LED) units of wavelength 760 nm to excite protein-binding ICG

the properties of ICG that absorbs wavelength mainly between 600 and 900 nm and emits fluorescence between 750 and 950 nm. This method has also been applied to the treatment of several types of skin cancers, and has been reported to be useful for the accurate detection of SLNs in both cutaneous melanomas as well as non-melanoma skin cancers, e.g., squamous cell carcinoma (SCC), MCC, and EMPD. Herein, we review the essential techniques of this new method in the patients with cutaneous melanoma and nonmelanoma skin cancers on the extremities and trunks.

16.2 Objectives

SLNB using ICG-NIR method can be applied for melanoma as well as for various types of nonmelanoma skin cancers tend to lead to lymphatic metastases, e.g., MCC, EMPD, SCC, and porocarcinoma; although the efficacy of SLNB for nonmelanoma skin cancers has not been well proven. For SLNB, patients who exhibited clinically- or radiographically- obvious metastasis of the regional lymph nodes or other organs must be excluded. However, in patients with tumors in the midline of the trunk, who are diagnosed as having hemilateral regional lymph node metastases, clinical stage can be evaluated using the contralateral SLNs.

16.3 Methods

16.3.1 Administration of ICG

As a tracer, 25 mg of ICG was diluted into 5 ml of sterile distilled water. The concentration of ICG was reduced based upon the distance between the injection sites and the SLNs. Up to 1.0 ml of this solution was injected intracutaneously into several locations around the tumor. The desirable points for tracer administration in skin cancers, other than some cases of EMPD, are in the vicinity of the tumor or the scar following excisional biopsy (Fig. 16.2a). For EMPD, the sites for tracer administration should be carefully determined according to the size and surface configuration of the plaque. For flattened small lesions (less than 5 cm in maximum diameter), the tracer should be injected nearby. For large plaques (over 5 cm in maximum diameter), the tracer can be injected in the proximity of the most elevated or eroded lesions, which suggest histopathologic intradermal cancer invasion, within or besides the plaque (Fig. 16.3a and c). In order to reduce the pain of intracutaneous injection, local anesthetic tape may be pasted at the estimated injection sites one hour prior to administration. During intradermal injections of ICG, oozing ICG should be absorbed or wiped off immediately to avoid unnecessary illumination of the skin surface and operative field. Surgical gloves that

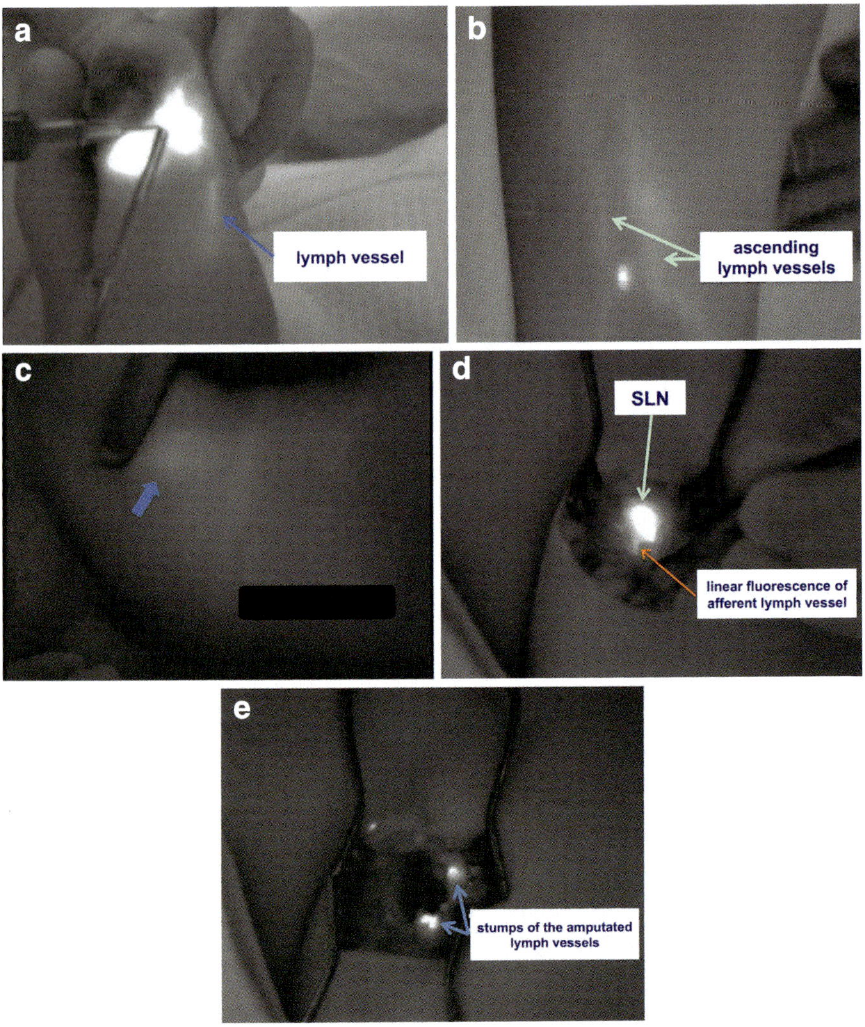

Fig. 16.2 (**a**) Linear fluorescence of lymph tract appeared shortly after intradermal injection of ICG. (**b**) Fluorescence of ascending lymph vessels observed on the lower leg (*light-green arrows*). (**c**) Within 10 min, fluorescence from inguinal node (*blue arrow*) becomes visible from the surface. (**d**) After incision, round fluorescence of SLN and linear fluorescence of afferent lymph vessels (*red arrow*) become visible. (**e**) Stumps of the amputated lymph vessels can be observed after SLN dissection

become contaminated with ICG should be changed for the same reason. Another type of vital dye, i.e. 0.4 % (w/v) indigo carmine or 2 % isosulfan blue could be administered several minutes prior to ICG injection in order to support the blue staining of the lymphatic tracts.

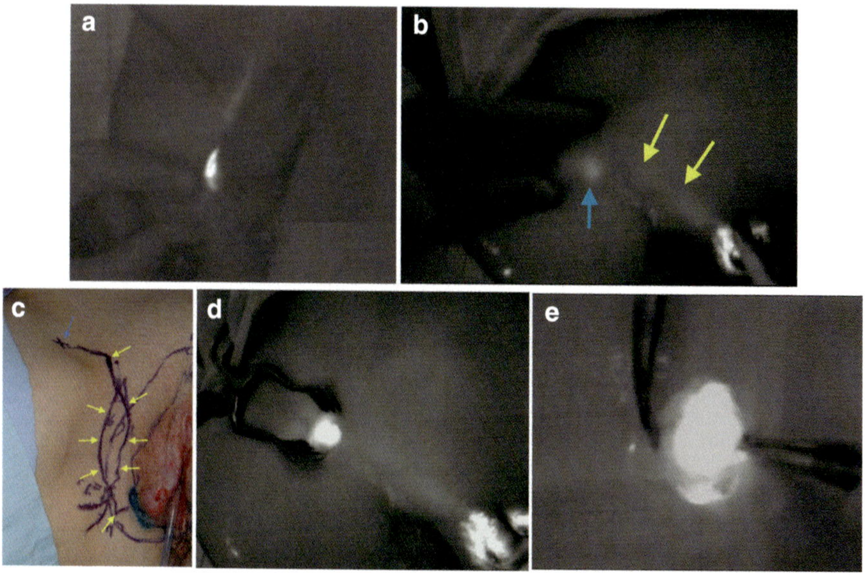

Fig. 16.3 (**a**) Linear fluorescence of lymph tract appeared during intradermal injection of ICG. (**b**) Fluorescence of ascending lymph vessels (*yellow arrows*) and fluorescence from inguinal node (*blue arrow*) become visible within several minutes after ICG administration. (**c**) Clinical feature of detected lymph tracts (*yellow arrows*) to SLN (*blue arrow*). (**d**) After incision, round fluorescence of SLN becomes visible. (**e**) Resected SLN still generates fluorescence

16.3.2 Observation of the Lymph Tracts (Fig. 16.1)

Immediately after injection of the ICG, fluorescence of the lymphatic channels to the SLNs can be observed from the skin surface (Figs. 16.2b–c and 16.3b–c) using the infrared camera system [PDE (Photodynamic Eye) or PDE-neo, Hamamatsu Photonics K.K., Hamamatsu, Japan] under normal room light. Only the operating lamps needed to be switched off for the ICG-INR guided observation. The required time for detecting fluorescence of SLNs is within 5 min for inguinal nodes. For the trunk, head, neck, and upper limbs, a rather longer detecting time tends to be necessary. Diffuse fluorescence of the skin overlying the regional lymph nodes (Fig. 16.4), which reflects the dermal backflow and pooling of tracer caused by lymphatic obstruction, sometimes suggests the existence of regional node metastasis. In the axillary region, observation of the fluorescence from the SLNs is more difficult than the inguinal area because of the deeper location of the SLNs covered by thicker fat tissues. In such cases, the overlying skin and subcutaneous tissue should be pressed in order to reduce the distance from the skin surface to the SLNs.

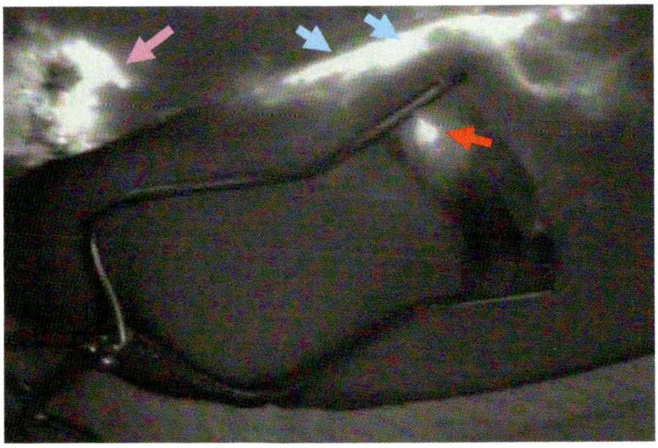

Fig. 16.4 Dermal backflow observed at left inguinal region of EMPD patient. SLN could not be observed from the surface because it was masked by the brighter fluorescent pooling of the skin (*blue arrows*), which is called "dermal backflow." SLN (*red arrow*) could be visible only after skin incision was made. *Pink arrow* shows the ICG-injected genital site

16.3.3 Surgical Resection of SLNs

Detected SLNs should be removed surgically (Fig. 16.3d) for histological examination. After making the incision, the linear fluorescence of the afferent lymph vessels to SLNs is observed (Fig. 16.2d). To avoid diffuse illumination that can interfere with observation of the lymphatic flow and the SLNs, surgery for lymph node detection must be performed carefully. The detected lymph vessels (Fig. 16.2d) must be carefully ligated or cauterized to avoid the leakage of the ICG that led to the disseminated fluorescence at the biopsy basin and disturbed the further detections of other SLNs. This series of lymph node dissections should be completed as quickly as possible within about 30 minutes to avoid the spread of the fluorescence to second-tier lymph nodes. After completion of the dissection of the SLNs, residual lymph nodes must be examined by gamma-prove and the NIR camera system. At this time, punctate illumination, which suggests the stumps of amputated lymph vessels, should be detected and ligated in order to avoid lymphorrhea. This procedure for detecting disrupted lymph tracts is also useful for the operation of lymph node dissection in order to reduce the occurrence of both postoperative leakage from lymph tracts and seroma formation (Fig. 16.2e). The resected SLN, which still generates fluorescence under NIR camera observation (Fig. 16.3e), can be used for RI counting with the gamma-probe to determine whether or not it is SLN.

16.3.4 Histopathologic Evaluation of SLNs

In order to detect metastatic cancer cells, surgically resected SLNs are evaluated histopathologically and immunohistopathologically. Immunohistopathological evaluation is useful not only for the differential diagnosis among cancers but also for detecting metastasized cancer cells in SNs. The resected lymph nodes are fixed with formalin, embedded in paraffin, and stained with hematoxylin-eosin and /or monoclonal antibodies for histological and immunohistochemical examinations. In nonmelanoma skin cancers in which dermal invasion is suspected, immediate histological diagnosis of the resected SLNs should be considered using frozen sections from the largest dimension of the specimen obtained during surgery.

For the immunohistopathologic evaluation of melanoma, NSE and several melanoma-specific monoclonal antibodies (e.g., HMB-45, MART-1) must be used. When evaluating metastasis of epithelial malignancies, monoclonal antibodies to pan-cytokeratin can be helpful. CEA, cytokeratin 7 (CK7), and GCDFP-15 antibodies are beneficial for detecting faint metastatic cells of EMPD. In order to detect MCC, cytokeratin 2 (CK20) and neuron-specific enolase (NSE) are beneficial. Both antibodies are stained in conjunction in the rare case of a CK20-negative MCC. Chromogranin A and synaptophysin, which suggest neuroendocrine differentiation, are useful for more precise evaluation of MMC.

16.4 Discussion

Sentinel lymph node biopsy (SLNB) was developed as a minimally invasive procedure to detect clinically-negative regional lymphatic metastases. The evaluation of SLNs is based on the hypothesis that efferent lymphatic flow from solid tumors is not random but rather follows a pattern in which there is spread to an initial node. This concept was first introduced for penile carcinoma by Cabanas in 1977 [6], but has been recently been developed or patients with cutaneous melanoma. The procedure for detecting SLNs, which consists of pre-operative and intra-operative detection of SLNs and surgical resection of the detected SLNs, is called sentinel node navigation surgery (SNNS). The techniques of SNNS have been developed for SLNB in cutaneous melanoma and are now widely used for SNB in skin cancers as well as for SNNS in various organs.

For the intraoperative detection of SLN, the combination of RI detection by gamma probe and visible observation using conventional vital dyes is now widely regarded as the standard procedure for SNNS. Although the RI-tracer guided method using gamma probe detection is the easiest and most accurate intra-operative SNB procedure, this method has some limitations in that it cannot be used to visualize lymph tracts and that it requires expensive facilities. In addition, the so-called "shine through" effects, which make detection of active SLN in the vicinity of the injection site more difficult, occasionally occurs due to the sensitive nature of the gamma probe. By contrast, the conventional vital dye method, which makes lymph tracts visible by blue staining, is a more simple and low-cost approach for intra-operative detection. Nevertheless, this method requires somewhat intensive training to obtain a reliable detection rate.

ICG-NIR using NIR-imaging after intracutaneous ICG injection has been developed to detect SLN in breast cancer [5]. Because of its higher intensity, contrast, and penetrability, ICG can provide more accurate visible images of the lymph tracts compared with conventional vital dyes. Without using RI, it does not result in any "shine through" effect similar to the RI method. Therefore, the ICG-INR method is recognized as an ideal lymphatic tracing procedure for skin cancers [7]. By contrast, these advantages can lead to limitations. For example, the good penetrability makes the surgical procedure a bit more difficult, as SLN must be dissected more quickly in order to avoid quick spreading of the ICG-induced fluorescence to second-tier nodes. During lymphadenectomy, detected lymph vessels should be firmly ligated or cauterized to avoid dissemination of fluorescence due to leakage of the ICG.

For skin cancers, ICG-INR method has been mainly applied in cutaneous melanoma [[8], [9]], and it has subsequently been used in other skin malignancies. The SLN detection rates for cutaneous melanoma before skin incision by the ICG-NIR method were reported to vary from 100 % in the groin region draining from the trunk to 15.8 % in the axillary region from the upper limb [10]. The factors that influenced the failure of ICG to identify positive SLNs were suspected to be the axillary node field and a high body mass index (BMI). In addition, misdiagnosis of sentinel node metastasis could occur due to obstruction of the lymph tracts and the pooling of tracers, which appear as dermal back flow.

Although the efficacy of SNB in EMPD has not been determined, it may be safe and feasible may play an important role in the management of extramammary Paget's disease with clinically-negative lymph node metastasis [11]. EMPD appears as a cutaneous adenocarcinoma that presents with eczema-like erythematous and/or depigmented lesions in the groin, genitalia, perineum, or perianal area. In spite of the poor prognosis for patients with lymph node metastasis, management of EMPD without clinical evidence of the involved nodes is a matter of ongoing discussion [12], and the efficacy of SNB has not been well elucidated.

Normally, cancer resection surgery is not indicated for EMPD patients with bilateral regional lymph node metastases, as Japanese guidelines for the treatment of malignant skin tumors do not recommend surgical treatment for EMPD with clinically evident bilateral inguinal lymph node metastases because of the poor prognosis. In contrast, a recent retrospective study of Japanese EMPD patients [13] revealed that SLB and subsequent lymph node dissection could improve the survival of invasive EMPD patients with early-stage lymphatic spread; thus, the authors proposed that SLB should be considered for invasive EMPD without clinically-obvious lymphadenopathy. This suggests the possibility of SLB and subsequent lymph node dissection for the clinically-negative bilateral inguinal lymph node basin in EMPD.

Although the protocols of SLB for nonmelanoma skin cancers has been established based upon investigations for cutaneous melanoma, it remains to be established for EMPD. EMPD sometimes develops into large plaque-containing elevated tumors and/or eroded areas, which suggest the dermal invasion of cancer cells. Such diversity of appearances makes it difficult to determine the adequate points for tracer injection. As the ICG-INR method can be recognized as a unique variation of conventional vital dye method, the procedure of SNB by ICG-NIR for nonmelanoma solid skin cancers is virtually the same as that for cutaneous melanoma. By contrast, the protocols for NIR detection of EMPD have not been well established since the first feasibility report of this method for EMPD [14].

As this newly developed ICG-NIR method has both advantages and disadvantages over conventional methods, its use in combination with other SNNS methods will allow the improvement of the SLB outcome. Usage of this method for various types of lymphatic surgeries, i.e., lymphadenectomy and lymph node dissection, will also be beneficial in reducing the after-effects such as lymphorrhea and seroma. Further development of SNNS with ICG-NIR in the field of skin surgery is anticipated.

References

1. Morton DL, Wen DR, Wong JH et al (1992) Technical details of intra-operative lymphatic mapping for early stage melanoma. Arch Surg 127:392–399
2. Morton DL, Thompson JF, Cochran AJ et al (2014) Final trial report of sentinel-node biopsy versus nodal observation in melanoma. N Engl J Med 370:599–609
3. Messina JL, Reintgen DS, Cruse CW et al (1997) Selective lymphadenectomy in patients with Merkel cell (cutaneous neuroendocrine) carcinoma. Surg Oncol 4:389–395
4. Nakamura Y, Fujisawa Y, Ishikawa M et al (2012) Usefulness of sentinel lymph node biopsy for extramammary Paget disease. Br J Dermatol 167:954–956
5. Kitai T, Inomoto T, Miwa M, Shikayama T (2005) Fluorescence navigation with indocyanine green for detecting sentinel lymph nodes in breast cancer. Breast Cancer 12:211–215
6. Cabanas RM (1977) An approach for the treatment of penile carcinoma. Cancer 39:456–466
7. Fujisawa Y, Nakamura Y, Kawachi Y et al (2012) Indocyanine green fluorescence-navigated sentinel node biopsy showed higher sensitivity than the radioisotope or blue dye method, which may help to reduce false-negative cases in skin cancer. J Surg Oncol 106:41–45
8. Namikawa K, Yamazaki N (2011) Sentinel lymph node biopsy guided by indocyanine green fluorescence for cutaneous melanoma. Eur J Dermatol 21:184–190
9. Fujiwara M, Mizukami T, Suzuki A et al (2009) Sentinel lymph node detection in skin cancer patients using real-time fluorescence navigation with indocyanine green: preliminary experience. J Plast Reconstr Aesthet Surg 62:e373–378. (e-pub)
10. Namikawa K1, Tsutsumida A, Tanaka R et al (2014) Limitation of indocyanine green fluorescence in identifying sentinel lymph node prior to skin incision in cutaneous melanoma. Int J Clin Oncol 19:198–203
11. Hatta N, Morita R, Yamada M, Takehara K et al (2004) Sentinel lymph node biopsy in patients with extramammary Paget's disease. Dermatol Surg 30:1329–1334
12. Pierie JP, Choudry U, Muzikansky A, Finkelstein DM et al (2003) Prognosis and management of extramammary Paget's disease and the association with secondary malignancies. J Am Coll Surg 196:45–50
13. Fujisawa Y, Yoshino K, Kiyohara Y et al (2015) The role of sentinel lymph node biopsy in the management of invasive extramammary Paget's disease: multi-center, retrospective study of 151 patients. J Dermatol Sci, 2015 Apr 18. [Epub]
14. Isei T, Okamoto H (2008) Fluorescence navigation with indocyanine green for sentinel lymph node biopsy in acral melanoma and genital extramammary Paget's carcinoma. Ann Surg Oncol 15:233

Chapter 17
Regional Lymph Node Dissection Assisted by Indocyanine Green Fluorescence Lymphography and Angiography for Stage III Melanoma

Hiroshi Furukawa, Toshiyuki Hayashi, and Yuhei Yamamoto

Abstract Lymph node dissection is a standard treatment for Stage III melanoma. Indocyanine green fluorescence lymphography and angiography may help to perform en-bloc dissection, to decide the levels to be excised, and to prevent postoperative wound dehiscence especially in groin dissection.

Keywords Lymph node dissection • Stage III melanoma • Indocyanine green fluorescence lymphography • Indocyanine green fluorescence angiography • En-bloc dissection • Levels in regional nodal basin • Postoperative wound dehiscence

17.1 Introduction

Lymph node dissection is a standard treatment for Stage III melanoma; however, surgeon should consider the following: (1) application of en-bloc excision to high-risk cases, (2) the proximal boundary in regional nodal basin, and (3) how to prevent postoperative skin flap complications. In this chapter, we proposed regional lymph node dissection assisted by indocyanine green (ICG) fluorescence lymphography and angiography to resolve those three problems.

H. Furukawa, M.D., Ph.D. (✉) • T. Hayashi, M.D., Ph.D. • Y. Yamamoto, M.D., Ph.D.
Department of Plastic and Reconstructive Surgery, Graduate School of Medicine, Hokkaido University, Kita-15, Nishi-7, Kita-ku, Sapporo, Hokkaido 060-8638, Japan
e-mail: hfuru@med.hokudai.ac.jp

M. Kusano et al. (eds.), *ICG Fluorescence Imaging and Navigation Surgery*,
DOI 10.1007/978-4-431-55528-5_17

17.2 En-bloc Lymph Node Dissection

If the primary melanoma is located in the thigh or upper arm, and nodal basin is including clinical metastasis, it has high risk of regional recurrence, and subcutaneous lymph vessels between the primary site and basin, possible sites for in-transit metastases that may develop later, should be excised (Fig. 17.1). The excised areas

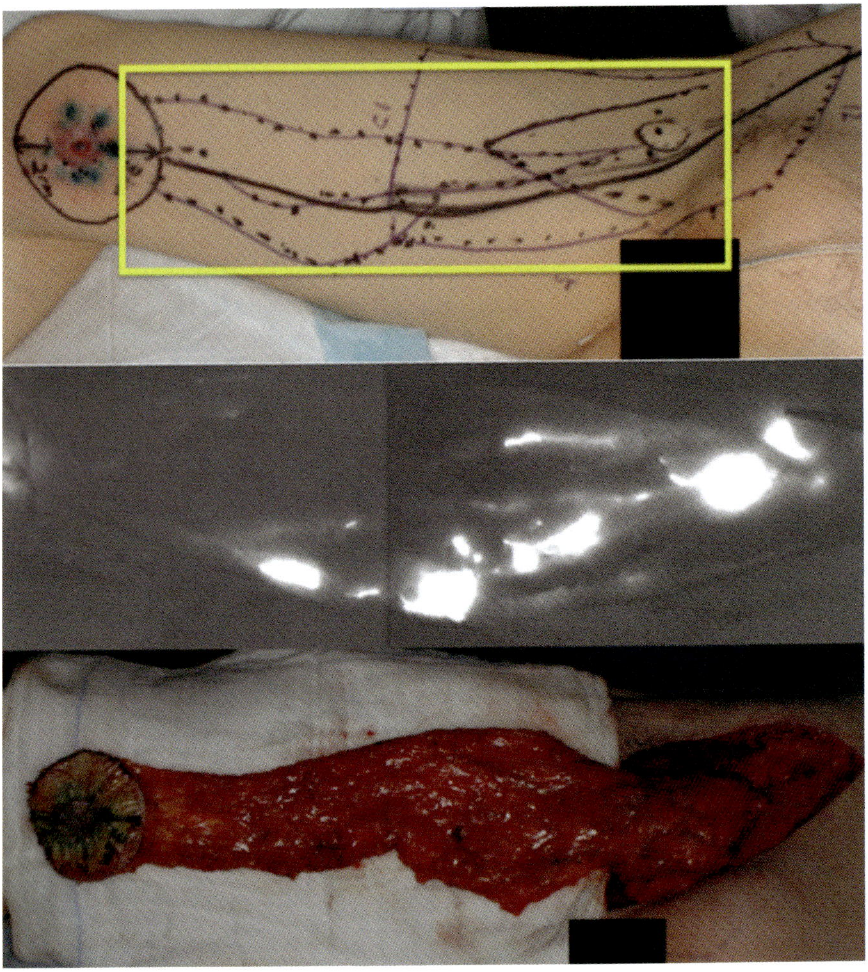

Fig. 17.1 *Above*: The design for en-bloc excision in Stage III melanoma case. The primary site is distal thigh. Clinical metastatic node was involved in regional groin nodal basin. Before en-bloc excision, the lymph vessels running through subcutaneous tissue were detected by ICG fluorescence lymphography and marked by black pen. *Middle*: A view of lymph vessels through PDE (Photodynamic Eye®, PDE; Hamamatsu Photonics, Hamamatsu, Japan) after elevation of skin flap. *Below*: Intraoperative view of en-bloc excision of lymph vessels and primary lesion (Figure 17.1 were previously published in leaflet for PDE and reprinted in this chapter with permission of Hamamatsu Photonics, Hamamatsu, Japan)

of lymph vessels (and skin) are decided using real-time fluorescence navigation with ICG [1, 2].

Before en-bloc excision, the ICG was injected evenly around a tumor lesion at a distance of 5 mm from the primary tumor margin. The ICG is dissolved at a concentration of 2.5 mg/mL in aqueous solution. 0.1 mL was injected at each of the four sites and the total dosage was 0.4 mL (ICG 1 mg). Lymph vessels, running from primary lesion into nodal basin, are detected by a near-infrared camera system (Photodynamic Eye®, PDE; Hamamatsu Photonics, Hamamatsu, Japan).

17.3 Decision of the Levels of Dissection of Regional Lymph Basin

For planning lymph node dissection, detection of lymph flow entering into lymph basin is important for decision of the excised levels in lymph basin. The axilla basin consists of three levels divided by edges of pectoralis minor muscle. In the case that primary lesion is located in upper extremity, lymph flow from primary lesion is usually entering level I of axilla, and dissection area includes levels I and II. If primary lesion is located near the shoulder, the additional lymph flow may run over pectoralis major muscle into level III (Fig. 17.2). The information of lymphography may help to decide whether the level III should be excised or not.

17.4 Blood Flow Evaluation of Skin Flap in Groin Dissection

The incidence of postoperative wound dehiscence following inguinal lymph node dissection (ILND) is higher than lymph node dissections in other anatomic regions (Fig. 17.3a) [3]. In the prospective study of melanoma patients undergoing ILND, 53 % had some degree of wound dehiscence (wound dehiscence was defined as poor wound healing with a measured defect of at least 1 cm.) [3].

To resolve postoperative wound dehiscence, we introduced intervention with ICG fluorescence angiography into ILND for blood flow evaluation of skin flap. During ILND, the area of ischemic skin around groin wound just after dissection was detected based on ICG fluorescence angiography. One mL of ICG (a concentration of 2.5 mg/mL in aqueous solution) was injected intravenously. Three minutes after injection, areas of non-fluorescence were marked using the pen (Fig. 17.3b, c). The edge of skin flaps with non-fluorescence was trimmed off while preserving the other part of skin flap with fluorescence. Our intraoperative intervention based on ICG fluorescence angiography was effective for preventing postoperative wound dehiscence after ILND (Fig. 17.3d), and the outcome was reported recently in our article [4].

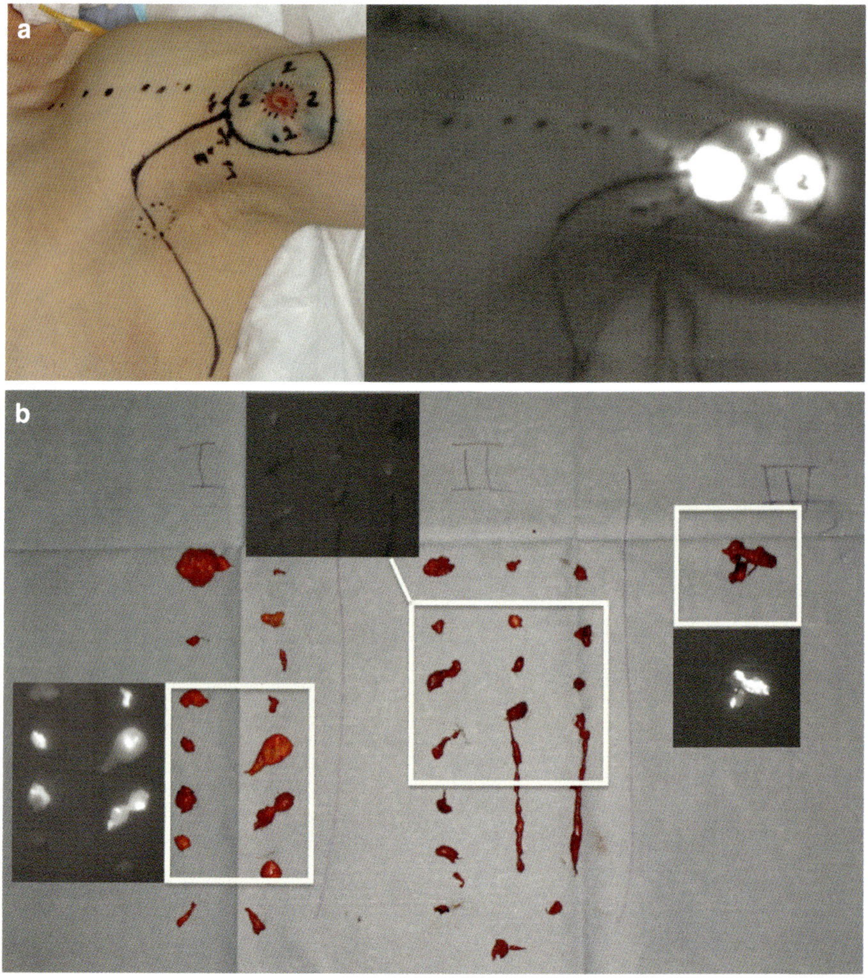

Fig. 17.2 (**a**) *Left*: The design for axilla dissection in Stage III melanoma. Primary lesion located in proximal arm. Clinical metastatic node was involved in the axilla basin. Before dissection, ICG was injected intradermally around the primary site. *Right*: Same view as left photo through PDE. The lymph vessels running on pectoralis major muscle were detected and marked by black pen. (**b**) After dissection of levels I, II, and III, the lymph nodes were enucleated from dissected tissue at back table and divided into three levels. Small flames are view through PDE. Lymph nodes of levels I and III had fluorescence and level II did not. This confirmed the two lymph flows entering the axilla basin from primary tumor, one is into level I and the other is directly into level III (Figure 17.2 were previously published in leaflet for PDE and reprinted in this chapter with permission of Hamamatsu Photonics, Hamamatsu, Japan)

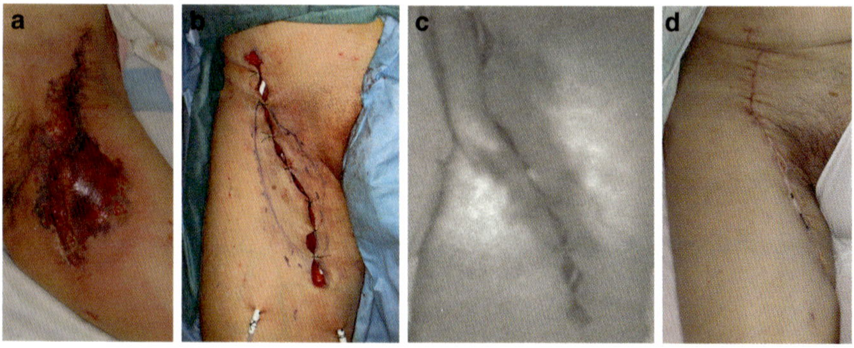

Fig. 17.3 (**a**) Figure shows typical postoperative complication in groin dissection. Skin necrosis and wound breakdown required debridement and skin graft. (**b**) Intraoperative view of other case of groin dissection is presented. After dissection, both the lateral and medial flaps were roughly closed using several silk stitches. Ischemic edge of skin flap was marked using a purple pen, depending on fluorescence angiography. (**c**) Same view as Fig. 17.3b through PDE is presented. Three minutes after ICG venous injection, the fluorescence sequentially shows the illumination of the blood flow as the dye passes through the microcirculation. The edges of the flaps lack any fluorescence, and they were trimmed off at the line marked with a *purple pen*. (**d**) There was no necrosis or breakdown measuring more than 1 cm width of the remnant skin flap postoperatively at 3 weeks after groin dissection (Figure 17.3 was in press in Reference 4 and reprinted in this chapter with permission of the publisher)

References

1. Hayashi T, Furukawa H, Oyama A, Funayama E, Saito A, Yamao T, Yamamoto Y (2012) Sentinel lymph node biopsy using real-time fluorescence navigation with indocyanine green in cutaneous head and neck/lip mucosa melanomas. Head Neck 34:758–761
2. Furukawa H, Hayashi T, Oyama A, Takasawa A, Yamamoto Y (2012) Tailored excision of in-transit metastatic melanoma based on Indocyanine green fluorescence lymphography. Eur J Plast Surg 35:329–332
3. Chang SB, Askew RL, Xing Y, Weaver S, Gershenwald JE, Lee JE, Royal R, Lucci A, Ross MI, Cormier JN (2010) Prospective assessment of postoperative complications and associated costs following inguinal lymph node dissection (ILND) in melanoma patients. Ann Surg Oncol 17:2764–2772
4. Furukawa H, Hayashi T, Oyama A, Funayama E, Murao N, Yamao T, Yamamoto Y (2015) Effectiveness of intraoperative indocyanine-green fluorescence angiography during inguinal lymph node dissection for skin cancer to prevent postoperative wound dehiscence. Surg Today 45:973–978

Part X
Assessment of Blood Supply to Tissue & Reconstructed Organ with Application of Plastic Surgery

Chapter 18
Blood Supply Visualization for Reconstruction During Esophagectomy

Yutaka Shimada, Tomoyuki Okumura, Makoto Moriyama, Takuya Nagata, Koshi Matsui, Ryusuke Osada, and Kazuhiro Tsukada

Abstract An adequate blood supply to reconstructed organs is important for safe esophagogastric anastomosis during esophagectomy. We previously reported that the vascular network could be visualized in the gastric wall, colonic grafts, and free jejunal grafts by indocyanine green (ICG) fluorescence. ICG fluorescence could be used to select patients who do not need additional vessel anastomosis. However, anastomotic leakage was not reduced; its rate was 7.5 % (3/40). In the present study, we accumulated further patients and reviewed recent research regarding ICG fluorescence. Although the number of patients examined was increased from 40 to 70, further reductions in the rate of anastomotic leakage were not achieved. The rate of anastomotic leakage was 7.1 % (5/70). Thus, we reconfirmed that microcirculation detected by ICG fluorescence did not necessarily provide an adequate blood supply for viable anastomosis. Although blood supply as well as other conditions in patients may affect viable anastomosis, combination analyses such as ICG and laser Doppler flowmetry may improve the outcome of anastomotic leakage.

Keywords ICG fluorescence • Anastomotic leakage • Vessel anastomosis • Esophagectomy • Esophageal reconstruction

---

Y. Shimada, M.D., Ph.D., F.A.C.S. (✉)
Department of Surgery and Surgical Science, Graduate School of Medicine & Pharmaceutical Sciences for Research, University of Toyama, Toyama, Japan

Department of Nanobio Drug Discovery, Graduate School of Pharmaceutical Sciences, Kyoto University, 46-29 Yoshida-Shimoadachi-cho, Sakyo-ku, Kyoto 606-8501, Japan
e-mail: yshimada@pharm.kyoto-u.ac.jp

T. Okumura, M.D., Ph.D. • M. Moriyama, M.D., Ph.D. • T. Nagata, M.D., Ph.D. • K. Matsui, M.D., Ph.D. • K. Tsukada, M.D., Ph.D.
Department of Surgery and Surgical Science, Graduate School of Medicine & Pharmaceutical Sciences for Research, University of Toyama, Toyama, Japan

R. Osada, M.D., Ph.D.
Department of Orthopedics, Graduate School of Medicine & Pharmaceutical Sciences for Research, University of Toyama, Toyama, Japan

M. Kusano et al. (eds.), *ICG Fluorescence Imaging and Navigation Surgery*,
DOI 10.1007/978-4-431-55528-5_18

18.1 Introduction

18.1.1 Background

Reconstruction of the gastrointestinal tract still represents a major issue in patients with gastrointestinal malignancies. Anastomotic leakage is one of the main causes of death in esophageal cancer surgery [1], at a rate of between 0 and 35 % [2]. The most recent Japanese National Clinical Database (NCD) registry revealed that the rate of anastomotic leakage was 13.3 % (711/5354) in 2011 [3]. Among several causes of anastomotic leakage, ensuring an adequate blood supply is the most important point for safely performing anastomosis after esophagectomy.

18.1.2 Laser Doppler Flowmetry

Although laser Doppler flowmetry (LDF) has been used to assess the blood supply to reconstructed organs, sufficiently reliable measurements have not yet been obtained [4, 5]. We also investigated whether the LDF system improved the outcome of anastomotic leakage (Fig. 18.1a–d). Blood supply to the antrum of the gastric tube was reduced by 30 % at the top of the gastric tube; however, we could not establish the usefulness of the LDF system in esophagectomy because leakage was not observed in over 100 consecutively performed esophagectomies.

18.1.3 Intraoperative Fluorescent Imaging

Recent advances have led to the development of intraoperative fluorescent imaging (IFI) using the SPY™ system, which allows the patency of a coronary artery bypass graft to be evaluated intraoperatively based on the detection of indocyanine green (ICG) fluorescence [6, 7]. We began using ICG fluorescence in July 2008 to visualize the blood supply to reconstructed organs during esophagectomy and found that it was very useful [8]. We have since accumulated more patients who underwent esophagectomy and esophageal reconstruction. In the present study, we reevaluated the efficacy of ICG fluorescence and reviewed a recent clinical evaluation of the ICG method in the field of esophagectomy.

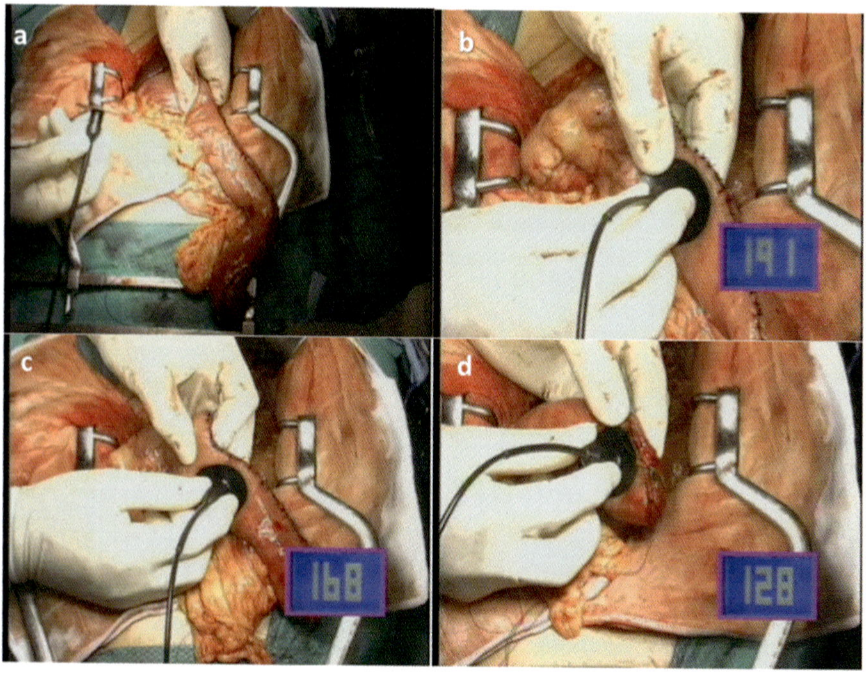

Fig. 18.1 Measurement of blood supply in the gastric tube by LDF. Whole gastric tube (**a**). Antrum of the gastric tube (**b**). *Middle* portion of the gastric tube (**c**). *Top* of the gastric tube (**d**). The *right lower* corner of each figure indicates the relative measurement data of LDF

18.2 Methods

18.2.1 Patient Characteristics

Sixty-two patients underwent esophagectomy for thoracic esophageal cancer, three were treated for cervical esophageal cancer, and five had double cancer in the thoracic and cervical regions (Table 18.1). There were 56 men and 14 women with an average age of 67 years (range, 44–86 years). Twenty-one patients received preoperative chemotherapy, two received preoperative chemoradiotherapy, and two had received radiotherapy several years before surgery. Three patients who had undergone jejunal graft reconstruction and two patients who had undergone esophageal bypass were evaluated at this time. Two patients who underwent partial resection for gastric tube cancer in the reconstructed gastric tube were also evaluated (Table 18.2).

Table 18.1 Characteristics of patients who underwent esophagectomy

	Number
Age	67 (44–86)
Sex	
Male	56
Female	14
Tumor location[a]	
PhMt	3
CeMt	2
Ce	3
Ut	3
Mt	34
LtAe	25
TNM stage[b]	
1	18
2a	11
2b	8
3	30
4	3
Preoperative treatment	
Chemotherapy	21
Chemoradiotherapy	2
Radiotherapy	2
None	45

Table 18.2 Characteristics of patients who underwent reconstructive surgery or resection for gastric tube cancer

	Number
Age	66 (45–79)
Sex	
Male	6
Female	1
Procedure	
Bypass	2
Free jejunal graft	3
Partial resection of the gastric tube	2
Preoperative treatment	
Chemotherapy	1
Chemoradiotherapy	2
Radiotherapy	0
None	4

[a]*Ph* pharynx, *Ce* cervical esophagus, *Ut* upper thoracic esophagus, *Mt* middle thoracic esophagus, *Lt* lower thoracic esophagus, *Ae* abdominal esophagus
[b]UICC TNM 6th edition

18.2.2 Operative Procedures

After esophagectomy, we made a gastric tube or colonic graft and pulled it up via the retrosternal, posterior mediastinal, or subcutaneous route depending on the patient. We routinely used the retrosternal route. A gastric tube was commonly fashioned with a width of 4 cm. Anastomosis was performed in the cervical region by hand sewing or using a circular stapler (25-mm EEA) [9]. We used a subcutaneous route for esophageal bypass. When a free jejunal graft was used, we first made a hand-sewn pharyngo-jejuno anastomosis, followed by microvascular anastomosis, and then jejuno-esophago anastomosis.

18.2.3 Modified Procedure

After preparing the gastric tube, the end of the short gastric vein was cut and we assessed the status of bleeding. Additional venous drainage was considered if bleeding was not continuous or very weak. We performed ICG fluorescence of the gastric tube in order to determine whether additional drainage was likely to be effective. If ICG fluorescence revealed a strong microvascular network, we concluded that the gastric tube did not need additional venous drainage or arterial anastomosis. If ICG fluorescence first appeared or became stronger after cutting the short gastric vein, we concluded that additional venous drainage would be effective. If ICG fluorescence did not appear after cutting the short gastric vein, additional arterial anastomosis was performed. If additional drainage or anastomosis was needed, anastomosis was performed between the short gastric vein or artery and the external cervical or superficial cervical vein [8].

18.2.4 ICG Imaging

Before and after pulling up the reconstructed organ, 2.5 mg of ICG dye (Diagnogreen; Dai-Ichi Pharm, Tokyo, Japan) was injected as a bolus. ICG fluorescence imaging was then performed using a near-infrared camera system (Photodynamic Eye; Hamamatsu Photonics K.K., Hamamatsu, Japan) and images were recorded. Briefly, images were obtained with a charge-coupled device (CCD) camera using a light-emitting diode with a wavelength of 760 nm as the light source and a filter to eliminate light with wavelengths below 820 nm before detection [10]. Images were sent to a digital video processor and displayed on a monitor. [8]. In the case of gastric tube cancer, ICG fluorescence was performed before and after partial resection of the gastric tube.

18.3 Results

18.3.1 Operative Procedures

Twenty-six patients underwent thoracoscopic-assisted right thoracotomy in the left lateral position, one underwent left thoracotomy because of a right aortic arch, 41 underwent esophagectomy in the prone position, and two underwent cervical esophagectomy in the supine position. Regarding the method used to reconstruct the esophagus, a gastric tube was employed in 57 patients, gastric tube plus free jejunal graft in two patients, free jejunal graft in two patients, and colonic graft in nine patients. Reconstruction was performed via the posterior mediastinal route in two patients, by the subcutaneous route in 15 patients, and the retrosternal route in 51 patients (Table 18.3).

18.3.2 Intraoperative Fluorescent Imaging

Fluorescence in the gastric tube wall was easily detected in all patients 1 min after the ICG injection. Both arteries and veins were effectively visualized (Fig. 18.2a, b). Furthermore, microvessels in the reconstructed esophagus could be clearly visualized approximately 2 min after the ICG injection (Fig. 18.3a, b). Anastomosis was added between the short gastric vein and vessels in the necks of seven patients based on the results of ICG fluorescence. We could also effectively visualize blood flow in free jejunal grafts and colonic grafts [8].

18.3.3 Patient Outcomes

No severe complications were observed in this series; however, three minor and two major anastomotic leakages occurred. The subcutaneous route was used for reconstruction in four out of five patients with anastomotic leakage. Additional vascular anastomosis was performed in three out of these five patients. The details of these patients were summarized in Table 18.4. Anastomotic leakage was not detected in patients who underwent bypass, reconstruction, and partial resection of the gastric tube.

Table 18.3 Operative procedures performed on patients

	Number
Method of esophagectomy	
VATS (right thoracotomy)	26
VATS (left thoracotomy)	1
Prone position esophagectomy	41
Cervical esophagectomy	2
Reconstruction organ	
Gastric tube	57
Gastric tube plus free jejunal graft	2
Free jejunal graft	2
Colonic graft	9
Reconstruction route	
Retrosternal route	51
Subcutaneous route	15
Posterior mediastinal route	2
Cervical anastomosis	2
Vessel anastomosis	
Supercharge	6
Venous drainage	7

VATS Video-assisted thoracoscopic surgery

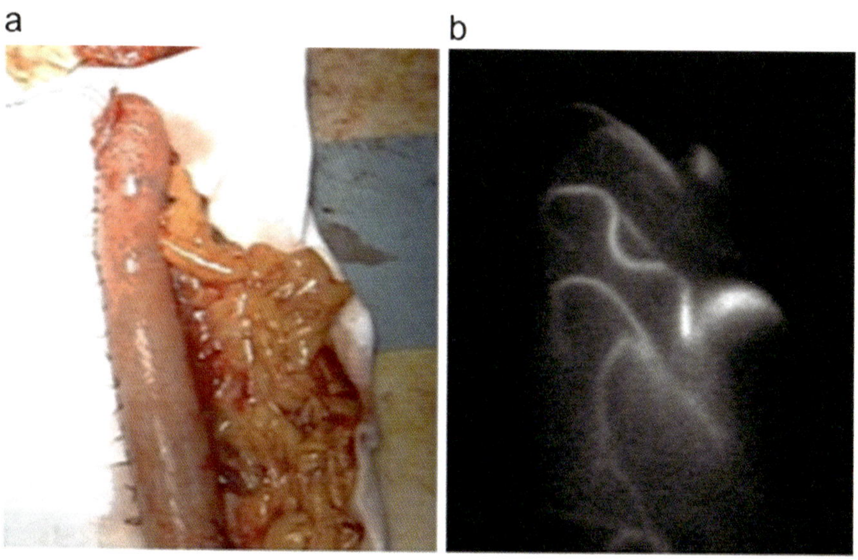

Fig. 18.2 ICG fluorescence image of a gastric tube before anastomosis. Blood flow in the arteries and veins was clearly visualized. (**a**) The gastric tube. (**b**) ICG fluorescence image. (From Shimada Y et al. [8] Esophagus 8:259–266)

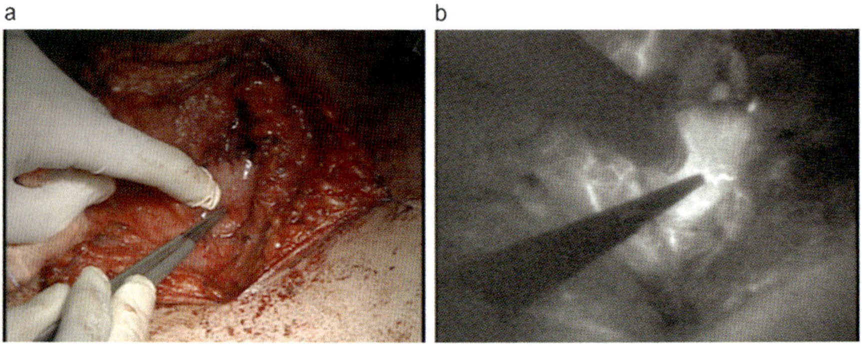

Fig. 18.3 ICG fluorescence image of a gastric tube after anastomosis. Image obtained under normal light (**a**). Blood vessels and microcirculation in the gastric tube (**b**). The forceps indicates a small blood vessel in the gastric wall (From Shimada Y et al. [8] Esophagus 8:259–266)

18.4 Discussion

18.4.1 Intraoperative Visualization of Blood Supply

Previous studies have employed LDF to assess the blood supply to reconstructed organs [4, 5]. However, there are currently no numerical criteria regarding safety margins in the LDF method. Thermography could also not evaluate the blood supply to the gastric tube. Recent advances have led to the development of IFI using the SPY^{TM} system, which has allowed the patency of a coronary artery bypass graft to be evaluated intraoperatively based on the detection of ICG fluorescence [6, 7]. However, this has not yet been extensively examined in the microcirculation in gastrointestinal organs [11–13].

18.4.2 Rate of Anastomotic Leakage

We previously reported that ICG fluorescence could detect organ blood flow before reconstruction and assist in evaluating appropriate anastomotic sites [8]. Although the average anastomotic leakage rate between 1994 and 2008 was 4.8 % (20/416), we reported an increase to 7.5 % (3/40) [8]. The reason why the rate of anastomotic leakage increased may be attributed to differences in patient backgrounds. In the present study, the total rate of anastomotic leakage decreased to 7.1 % (5/70), which was not significant. Thus, the microvessels detected by ICG fluorescence did not always provide an adequate blood supply for viable anastomosis.

Table 18.4 Characteristics of patients in whom anastomotic leakage was detected

Patient number	Age/gender	Stage	Tumor location[a]	Substitute organ[b]	Pulling-up route[c]	Preoperative treatment[d]	Coexisting diseases	Vessel anastomosis
1	70/M	T3N1M0 stage 3	Lt	G	S	–	Colon cancer	+
2	71/M	T2N0M0 stage 2a	Mt	G	S	–	Right aortic arch	–
3	67/M	T4N1M0 stage 3	Mt	G	S	DCF	–	–
4	74/M	T1aN0M0 stage 1	Ut	C	S	–	–	+
5	69/M	T3N0M0 stage 2a	Ae	G	R	FP	–	+

[a]*Ut* upper thoracic esophagus, *Mt* middle thoracic esophagus, *Lt* lower thoracic esophagus, *Ae* abdominal esophagus
[b]*G* gastric tube, *C* colonic graft
[c]*R* retrosternal, *S* subcutaneous
[d]*FP* 5-FU plus cisplatin, *DCF* FP plus docetaxel

18.4.3 Evaluation of Microvascular Anastomosis

Regarding additional microvascular anastomosis, a significant increase in tissue blood flow was observed after additional venous anastomosis (mean, 19 %) and also after combined arterial and venous anastomosis (mean, 43 %) [14]. Additional anastomosis between the short gastric vessels and vessels in the neck resulted in reductions in the rate of anastomotic leakage [15]. We achieved good outcomes in a previous series; therefore, ICG fluorescence may provide useful information to the surgeon regarding whether patients require additional microvascular anastomosis. However, anastomotic leakage was detected in three patients who underwent microvascular anastomosis. Thus, the recovery of blood circulation to the gastric tube was not sufficient for viable anastomosis in these three patients.

18.4.4 Literature Review

After publishing our findings, several studies described ICG fluorescence in the field of blood supply visualization during esophagectomy. Murawa D et al. reported that although ICG fluorescence imaging of the gastric tube allowed for intraoperative modifications, patient comorbidities and general health may also increase the risk of anastomosis leakage [16]. Ishiguro T et al. described a case of gastric tube necrosis and suggested that ICG angiography was useful for evaluating perfusion in a reconstructed gastric tube [17]. Furthermore, the blood route to the reconstructed stomach was analyzed by ICG fluorescence imaging and the splenic hiatal vessels were identified as the major blood supply for anastomosis in most patients [18]. Kumagai Y et al. measured the time from the initial enhancement of the root of the right gastroepiploic artery until that of the most cranial branch of the left gastroepiploic artery and tip of the gastric tube. They found that the gastric tube was divisible into three zones according to the dominant arteries present in the greater curvature using ICG fluorescence. They suggested that preserving the whole vessel arcade of the greater curvature was essential for achieving good blood perfusion in the gastric tube [19].

18.4.5 Evaluation of ICG Fluorescence

These findings and our results indicate that ICG fluorescence can evaluate real-time blood circulation to the gastric tube; however, the ICG method is limited because it cannot quantify blood flow to the gastric tube. In order to improve the efficacy of this evaluation, the combination of ICG fluorescence with the LDF method was found to be effective for preventing anastomotic leakage and stricture [20].

ICG fluorescence is also useful for evaluating blood supply in the case of gastric tube cancer and esophagogastric bypass [21, 22]. In our series, two patients with gastric tube cancer and two with esophagogastric bypass achieved good results.

18.4.6 Benefits of ICG Fluorescence

Imaging with the photodynamic eye had the following benefits. ICG fluorescence is a simple and easy procedure. ICG is almost completely washed out within 20 min of being injected; therefore, ICG fluorescence can be assessed several times during surgery. We can detect microcirculation in a target organ as well as adjacent organs. Patients who do not need additional vessel anastomosis can be selected using ICG fluorescence [8].

18.5 Conclusions

Imaging with ICG fluorescence can be used to evaluate the blood supply to reconstructed organs and select patients who do not need additional vessel anastomosis. However, the microcirculation detected by ICG fluorescence does not necessarily provide an adequate blood flow to maintain viable anastomosis.

References

1. Alanezi K, Urschel JD (2004) Mortality secondary to esophageal anastomotic leak. Ann Thorac Cardiovasc Surg 10:71–75
2. Blencowe NS, Strong S, McNair AG et al (2012) Reporting of short-term clinical outcomes after esophagectomy: a systematic review. Ann Surg 255:658–666
3. Takeuchi H1, Miyata H, Gotoh M et al (2014) A risk model for esophagectomy using data of 5354 patients included in a Japanese nationwide web-based database. Ann Surg 260:259–266
4. Miyazaki T, Kuwano H, Kato H et al (2002) Predictive value of blood flow in the gastric tube in anastomotic insufficiency after thoracic esophagectomy. World J Surg 26:1319–1323
5. Ikeda Y, Niimi M, Kan S et al (2001) Clinical significance of tissue blood flow during esophagectomy by laser doppler flowmetry. J Thorac Cardiovasc Surg 122:1101–1106
6. Taggart DP, Choudhary B, Anastasiadis K et al (2003) Preliminary experience with a novel intraoperative fluorescence imaging technique to evaluate the patency of bypass grafts in total arterial revascularization. Ann Thorac Surg 75:870–873
7. Balacumaraswami L, Abu-Omar Y, Choudhary B et al (2005) A comparison of transit-time flowmetry and intraoperative fluorescence imaging for assessing coronary artery bypass graft patency. J Thorac Cardiovasc Surg 130:315–320
8. Shimada Y, Okumura T, Nagata T et al (2011) Usefulness of blood supply visualization by indocyanine green fluorescence for reconstruction during esophagectomy. Esophagus 8:259–266

9. Imamura M, Ohishi K, Mizutani N et al (1987) Retrosternal esophagectomy with EEA stapler after subtotal resection of the esophagus: Application and results. Dig Surg 4:101–105
10. Kusano M, Tajima Y, Yamazaki K et al (2008) Sentinel node mapping guided by indocyanine green fluorescence imaging: a new method for sentinel node navigation surgery in gastrointestinal cancer. Dig Surg 25:103–108
11. Okamoto K, Muguruma N, Kimura T et al (2005) A novel diagnostic method for evaluation of vascular lesions in the digestive tract using infrared fluorescence endoscopy. Endoscopy 37:52–57
12. Nobuhisa T, Sato S (2009) Application of indocyanine green fluorescence method to esophagus cancer surgery. Geka 71:939–942 (in Japanese)
13. Ebihara Y, Okushiba S, Miyasaka D et al (2010) Technical device for reconstruction after thoracic esophagectomy. Geka Chiryo 102:156–160 (in Japanese)
14. Murakami M, Sugiyama A, Ikegami T et al (1999) Additional microvascular anastomosis in reconstruction after total esophagectomy for cervical esophageal carcinoma. Am J Surg 178:263–266
15. Murakami M, Sugiyama A, Ikegami T et al (2000) Revascularization using the short gastric vessels of the gastric tube after subtotal esophagectomy for intrathoracic esophageal carcinoma. J Am Coll Surg 190:71–77
16. Murawa D, Hunerbein M, Spychała A et al (2012) Indocyanine green angiography for evaluation of gastric conduit perfusion during esophagectomy–first experience. Acta Chir Belg 112:275–280
17. Ishiguro T, Kumagai Y, Ono T et al (2012) Usefulness of indocyanine green angiography for evaluation of blood supply in a reconstructed gastric tube during Esophagectomy. Int Surg 97:340–344
18. Rino Y, Yukawa N, Sato T et al (2014) Visualization of blood supply route to the reconstructed stomach by indocyanine green fluorescence imaging during esophagectomy. BMC Med Imaging 14:18. doi: 10.1186/1471-2342-14-18
19. Kumagai Y, Ishiguro T, Haga N et al (2014) Hemodynamics of the reconstructed gastric tube during esophagectomy: assessment of outcomes with indocyanine green fluorescence. World J Surg 38:138–143
20. Uchikado Y, Okumura H, Omoto I et al (2014) The blood flow evaluation of gastric tube by ICG fluorescence method and Laser doppler method in esophagectomy for esophageal cancer. Dis Esophagus 27(Suppl):164A
21. Saito T, Yano M, Motoori M et al (2012) Subtotal gastrectomy for gastric tube cancer after esophagectomy: A safe procedure preserving the proximal part of gastric tube based on intraoperative ICG blood flow evaluation. J Surg Oncol 106:107–110
22. Ariyoshi Y, Fujiwara H, Shiozaki A et al (2013) Minimally invasive surgery for cancer arising in a reconstructed gastric tube after esophagectomy based on evaluation of blood and lymphatic flow by indocyanine green fluorescence imaging. Gan To Kagaku Ryoho 40:2170–2172 (In Japanese)

Chapter 19
Evaluation of Viability of Reconstruction Organs During Esophageal Reconstruction

Daisuke Saikawa and Shunichi Okushiba

Abstract A considerable percentage of morbidity and mortality after esophagectomy for esophageal cancer is due to leakage of esophageal reconstruction, which is mainly caused by ischemia of reconstruction organ such as the stomach, free intestine, and pedunculated intestine. Therefore, we use a light-emitting diode (LED) excitation indocyanine green (ICG) fluorescence video navigation system to visually evaluate the reconstruction organ after esophagectomy, and we attempt anastomosis at a site that shows the best perfusion and for which the best possible elevation can be achieved.

The greatest advantage of using an LED-excitation ICG-fluorescence video navigation system during esophageal reconstruction is that it becomes possible to observe, in real time, the circulatory conditions in the reconstruction organ via luminescence of the incoming blood, and it is very useful for the evaluation of the risk of anastomotic leakage.

We urgently need to establish both a useful intraoperative strategy for patients who are at high risk of anastomotic leakages and a means of perioperative monitoring.

Keywords Esophagectomy • Esophageal reconstruction • Indocyanine green (ICG) fluorescence imaging

19.1 Background

Esophageal reconstruction after radical surgery for thoracic esophageal cancer remains one of the most challenging gastrointestinal reconstructions, despite advances in medical techniques. In addition, the development of potent, multidisciplinary neoadjuvant therapies for esophageal cancer may have further increased the difficulty of esophageal reconstruction. Although various reconstruction organs (stomach, free intestine, pedunculated intestine) are used during esophageal

D. Saikawa (✉) • S. Okushiba
Department of Surgery, KKR Sapporo Medical Center Tonan Hospital, N1, W6, Chuo-ku, Sapporo, Hokkaido 060-0001, Japan
e-mail: d.saikawa@tonan.gr.jp

M. Kusano et al. (eds.), *ICG Fluorescence Imaging and Navigation Surgery*,
DOI 10.1007/978-4-431-55528-5_19

reconstruction, the most common reconstruction involves use of the stomach. This is because the stomach provides superior perfusion and anastomotic tension, and there are few complications associated with esophagogastric anastomosis.

The stomach cannot be used as a reconstruction organ in patients who have undergone gastrectomy or who have another primary cancer, such as gastric cancer, so pedunculated jejunum or pedunculated colon is used for esophageal reconstruction in these cases. However, there are a number of patients in whom perfusion of the distal part of a pedunculated intestine fails, and we believe that vascular anastomosis is an important additional measure in these cases. The incidences of reconstruction organ necrosis and anastomotic leakage have decreased with the development of automatic anastomotic devices and supplementary vascular anastomosis, but at present anastomotic leakage still occurs in 10–20 % of esophagectomy patients. During esophageal reconstruction with pedunculated intestine and/or stomach, perfusion decreases as the distance from the intraperitoneal vascular pedicle increases; therefore, it is vital to select an anastomotic site that facilitates both perfusion at the anastomotic site and low tension. For this reason, we use a light-emitting diode (LED) excitation indocyanine green (ICG) fluorescence video navigation system to visually evaluate the reconstruction organ after esophagectomy, and we attempt anastomosis at a site that shows the best perfusion and for which the best possible elevation can be achieved.

19.2 The LED-Excitation ICG-Fluorescence Video Navigation System

The molecular weight of ICG is 774.96 g/mol, and 95–97 % is bound to plasma proteins in vivo. It is excreted by the liver almost exclusively.

LED excitation of ICG that is administered in vivo results in fluorescence at 840 nm, and the molecule enters a ground state. This ICG fluorescence in biological tissues can be observed in real time by means of the Photodynamic Eye (PDE, Hamamatsu Photonics, KK), an infrared camera system. There are few self-fluorescent materials that have the same excitation maximum and emission maximum as that provided by this system, which characteristically produces good contrast, even in biological tissues.

19.2.1 Application of the LED-Excitation ICG-Fluorescence Video Navigation System

Steps involve in application of the LED-excitation ICG-fluorescence video navigation system are as follows:

1. ICG (2.5 mg) is administered intravenously before a 5-mL physiological saline flush.
2. ICG fluorescence is observed at the roots of the arteries supplying the reconstruction organ, and, while it is fluorescent, the arterial perfusion is tracked as it passes distally to the destination of the arterial flow, and the extent of arterial perfusion is identified.
3. After the arterial phase, the extent of contrast enhancement in the wall of the reconstruction organ is identified. The timing and strength of contrast enhancement are both observed in the organ wall.
4. The presence of arterial ICG in the veins is confirmed. Frequently, there is no contrast enhancement of the veins in distal regions of the reconstruction organ.

19.3 Surgical Procedure

Since 2008, we have treated esophageal cancer by means of thoracoscopic esophagectomy with the patient in a prone position and under bilateral lung ventilation. We intubate the patient with a standard single-lumen tracheal tube and establish bilateral ventilation to create artificial CO_2 pneumothorax at 6–8 mmHg, promoting lung collapse [1].

The patient is placed in the prone position; airtight ports are placed in the third, fifth, seventh, and ninth intercostal spaces on the right, and, after esophagectomy, the patient is placed in the supine position with legs spread apart. Lymph node dissection and gastric mobilization are performed laparoscopically. We then elevate the entire stomach and the esophagus extracorporeally via the umbilical incision.

We create a small-diameter gastric tube by removal of a portion of the stomach along the greater curvature, as illustrated in Fig. 19.1a. The greater omentum is separated at the point of attachment to the transverse colon, and as much of the vascular network within the omentum as possible is preserved. In addition, where possible, the gastrosplenic ligament is separated at the point of attachment to the spleen, and we make a point of preserving the delicate vascular network. After we finish creating the stomach tube, we use the ICG-fluorescence video navigation system to evaluate the perfusion of the gastric tube, and we attempt anastomosis at a site where there is good contrast in both the arterial phase and mural contrast phase. We use a retromediastinal reconstruction route and perform cervical esophagogastric anastomosis with a linear stapler.

If we do not use the stomach for reconstruction, we use pedunculated jejunum or pedunculated ileocolic bowel and perform antethoracic reconstruction. In this case, we use the ICG-fluorescence video navigation system to evaluate perfusion of the elevated intestine, and, thereafter, we perform microscopic vascular anastomosis of the internal thoracic vessels and the relevant neck vessels, as required.

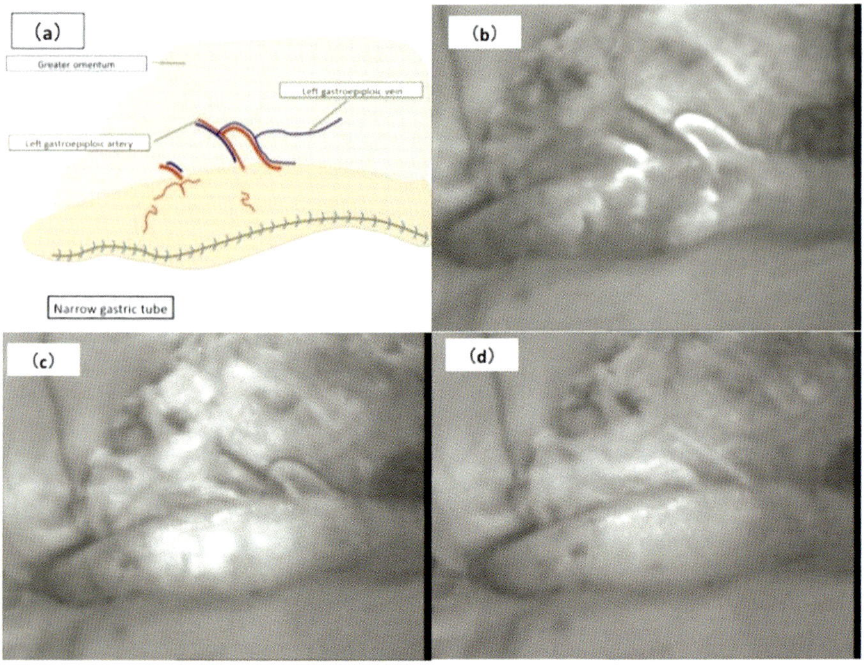

Fig. 19.1 Intraoperative ICG contrast enhancement of the greater curvature gastric tube. (**a**) Schematic diagram of the small-diameter gastric tube. (**b**) Arterial phase. Rapid contrast enhancement of a part of the left gastroepiploic artery and short gastric artery is seen. (**c**) Mural contrast phase. Extensive contrast enhancement of the gastric tube wall and greater omentum is seen. There is no contrast in the distal portion of the gastric tube. (**d**) Venous phase. Contrast has reached the left gastroepiploic vein

19.4 ICG-Based Assessment of Perfusion of the Small-Diameter Gastric Tube

Five to ten seconds after intravenous administration of ICG, Tcontrast is produced, first in the gastroepiploic artery arcade and then in the root of the right gastroepiploic artery (arterial phase: Fig. 19.1b). Several seconds after administration of the ICG, the small-diameter gastric tube wall is contrast enhanced (mural contrast phase: Fig. 19.1c), and, at approximately 10 s after administration of the ICG, venous outflow of the agent is observed (venous phase: Fig. 19.1d).

Table 19.1 Quality of blood flow in the left gastroepiploic artery and corresponding anastomotic patency status

	Blood flow in the left gastroepiploic artery		
	Delayed or poor	Rapid	Total
Leak	4	3	7
No Leak	6	35	41
Total	10	38	48

Number of cases is shown. Quality of blood flow was determined by intraoperative ICG contrast enhancement

19.4.1 *Assessment of Gastric Tube Perfusion: Results in 48 Patients*

We reviewed the results of gastric tube perfusion assessment obtained by means of the LED-excitation ICG-fluorescence video navigation system in 48 patients for whom a small-diameter gastric tube was created when thoracoscopic esophagectomy is performed. The surgeries were performed at our hospital, starting in 2010. Good contrast enhancement of the right gastroepiploic artery and the small-diameter gastric tube wall in the same region was achieved in 47 of the 48 patients. In 38 of the 48 patients, blood flow from the right gastroepiploic artery root rapidly reached the left gastroepiploic artery. In the remaining ten patients, there was a delay of ≥3 s or poor contrast enhancement.

Rapid contrast enhancement was seen in the region of the short gastric artery in six patients, but poor contrast enhancement accounted for more than half of the patients.

A ≥ grade 3 (Clavien-Dindo classification) anastomotic leakage developed in 7 of the 48 patients (14.5 %). A significant difference occurred in the development of anastomotic leakages between patients in whom contrast enhancement of the left gastroepiploic artery was delayed or insufficient and those in whom this contrast enhancement was rapid, with anastomotic leakages being more common in the former group ($p = 0.027$, OR = 7.8) (Table 19.1).

19.5 ICG-Based Assessment of Intestinal Perfusion Associated with Vascular Anastomosis

Results of vascular evaluation after anastomosis of the ileocolic vessels and the internal thoracic vessels during pedunculated ileocolic reconstruction are shown in Fig. 19.2a, b. The ICG contrast image in Fig. 19.2a shows obstruction of the vascular anastomosis by a thrombus. Weak enhancement revealed poor flow from the middle colic artery to the internal thoracic vein via the venous anastomosis site. After the arterial anastomosis was recreated, there was a rapid spread of contrast agent through the graft site from the anastomosed artery, the intestinal wall

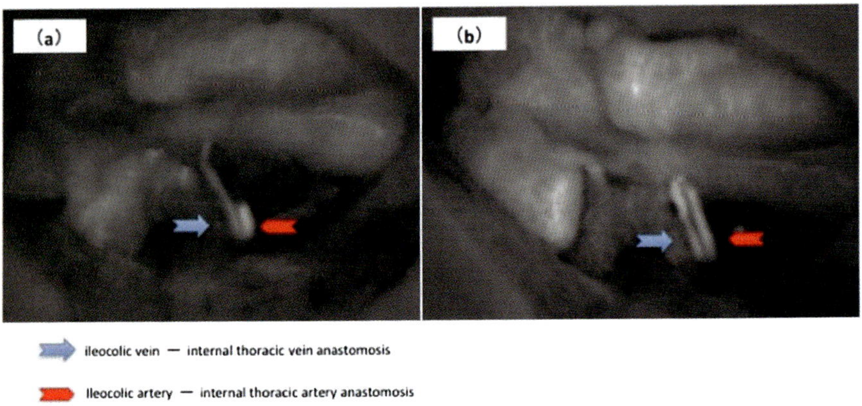

Fig. 19.2 ICG-based intraoperative evaluation of perfusion after vascular anastomosis. (**a**) Stasis observed in an ileocolic artery-internal thoracic artery anastomosis (*red arrow*). (**b**) Findings after repeat arterial anastomosis. Strong enhancement of the entire reconstructed intestine is seen

appeared bright, and rapid drainage via the venous anastomosis was confirmed (Fig. 19.2b).

19.6 Discussion

The esophageal reconstruction distance is extremely long, and it necessitates the reconstruction of blood supply routes; therefore, anastomotic leakage occurs at a high rate, and this type of gastrointestinal reconstruction remains one of the most difficult. When anastomotic leakages occur, the start of oral intake is substantially delayed, and this has a major impact on the patient's quality of life. In addition, potentially fatal complications such as mediastinitis and empyema can develop.

Historically, the causes of anastomotic leakage have been excessive tension at the anastomotic site and impaired perfusion, and, thus, various devices and techniques have adopted to resolve and even avoid these problems. The greatest advantage of using an LED-excitation ICG-fluorescence video navigation system during esophageal reconstruction is that it becomes possible to observe, in real time, the circulatory conditions in the reconstruction organ via luminescence of the incoming blood. Other methods used to date are incapable of depicting organ status and vascular pulsation, or they are indirect, e.g., Doppler ultrasound.

ICG rarely causes an allergic reaction, and there are no major adverse drug reactions. Its application is minimally invasive, and, because it is rapidly excreted from the liver, it can be used during surgery as many times as needed.

Jorg et al. confirmed perfusion of the stomach tube by means of ICG-fluorescence intraoperative angiography and reported an anastomotic leakage rate of 2 % when anastomosis was performed at sites where there was good perfusion. By comparison, the anastomotic leakage rate when anastomosis was performed at sites with poor perfusion was 45 % [2]. During our investigation, we documented anastomotic leakages in 4 of 7 patients (57 %) with poor contrast enhancement of the left gastroepiploic artery. Meanwhile, we documented anastomotic leakages in 3 of 38 patients (7.9 %) in whom the left gastroepiploic artery showed rapid and good contrast enhancement, indicating that anastomotic leakages were significantly more common in the poor enhancement group.

Intraoperatively, ICG fluorescence is useful for the identification of patients who should undergo additional vascular anastomosis even when imaging is performed on a small-diameter gastric tube, but there is at least one report indicating that ICG-fluorescence imaging does not reduce the incidence of anastomotic leakage [3]. This is because reconstruction for esophagectomy occurs over a very long distance, and anastomosis cannot always be limited to sites showing good perfusion during ICG-fluorescence imaging.

We may encounter patients in whom the use of ICG for intraoperative observation of gastric tube perfusion indicates that additional vascular anastomosis would be ideal, but, depending on the case, it may be necessary to consider a two-stage reconstruction with modifications to the reconstruction route, or to consider risk management, which would involve perioperative monitoring in patients who are at high risk for anastomotic leakages and minimizing the injury after anastomotic leakages have occurred.

Meanwhile, if vascular anastomosis is performed at the time of pedunculated intestine or free intestine reconstruction, observations that are performed using the LED-excitation ICG-fluorescence video navigation system are very useful because the system is capable of accurately confirming the success or failure of vascular anastomosis as well as recovery of reconstruction organ perfusion in real time.

19.7 Conclusion

LED-excitation ICG-fluorescence video navigation is simple and noninvasive, and it has the advantage of providing for intraoperative, real-time evaluation of perfusion of the reconstruction organ, and we believe it is very useful for the evaluation of the risk of anastomotic leakage. Going forward, we urgently need to establish both a useful intraoperative strategy for patients who are at high risk of anastomotic leakages and a means of perioperative monitoring.

References

1. Saikawa D, Okushiba S, Kawada M et al (2014) Efficacy and safety of artificial pneumothorax under two-lung ventilation in thoracoscopic esophagectomy for esophageal cancer in the prone position. Gen Thorac Cardiovasc Surg 62:163–170

2. Jorg Z, Steven RD, Evan TA et al (2014) Intraoperative assessment of perfusion of the gastric graft and correlation with anastomotic leaks after esophagectomy. Ann Surg 00:1–5
3. Shimada Y, Okumura T, Nagata T et al (2011) Usefulness of blood supply visualization by indocyanine green fluorescence for reconstruction during esophagectomy. Esophagus 8:359–366

Chapter 20
ICG Fluorescence Navigation Surgery in Breast Reconstruction with TRAM Flaps

Meisei Takeishi

Abstract Free TRAM flaps (transverse rectus abdominis myocutaneous flaps), including DIEP flaps (deep inferior epigastric perforator flaps), are among the most useful flaps in breast reconstruction. Vascular territory varies among individuals. We sometimes encounter partial fat necrosis of the TRAM flap after a breast reconstruction. Partial fat necrosis is a minor complication, but it can influence the contour of the reconstructed breast in some cases. When partial fat necrosis occurs, it develops in the hypo-vascularity region of the TRAM flap's fat layer. It is very difficult for us to determine the presence and exact location of regions of hypo-vascularity in TRAM flaps intraoperatively.

Intraoperative ICG fluorescence angiography is the best method of identifying the viable vascular territory of TRAM flaps.

Keywords ICG fluorescence angiography • Breast reconstruction • TRAM flap • Fat necrosis

20.1 Methods

A skin incision is made around the TRAM flap. The flap is elevated from the abdominal fascia and the deep epigastric vessels which feeding the skin & fat layer flap are dissected. Two milliliters of ICG (2.5 mg/ml) are injected transvenous systemically, before the vascular pedicle of the flap is cut. Ten milliliters of saline solution is injected, continually. Room lights and operating lights are then turned off. The flap is enhanced and the enhanced area is observed with a PDE camera. The PDE camera should be positioned directly above the flap so the whole flap is in the frame.

M. Takeishi, M.D., Ph.D. (✉)
Breast Reconstruction Institute, 2-25-11-904 Chiyoda, Naka-ku, Nagoya, Aichi 460-0012, Japan
e-mail: meisei.takeishi@gmail.com

M. Kusano et al. (eds.), *ICG Fluorescence Imaging and Navigation Surgery*,
DOI 10.1007/978-4-431-55528-5_20

20.2 Observation

The enhancement starts from the individual perforators. Several lines can be observed going horizontally or radially from each perforator (Fig. 20.1). In some cases, a few lines extend to the contralateral side beyond the center line.

The TRAM flap is enhanced from Zone I diffusely, when the movement of the line stops (Fig. 20.2: Zone Classification of a TRAM Flap). On the ipsilateral side of the vascular pedicle, the diffuse enhancement extends toward the Zone III, and in most of the cases, the whole of the Zone III is enhanced. On the contralateral side of the vascular pedicle, the diffuse enhancement extends beyond the center line, and the enhancement stops between Zone II and the lateral edge of Zone IV (Fig. 20.3).

Diffuse enhancement starts and stretches between the linear enhancement. And then, the diffuse enhancement stagnates in 1–2 s (Fig. 20.4).

The enhanced area starts to spread laterally again, after the movement of the enhanced region stops or move very slowly in a few minutes. But the movement of the enhanced region after the stagnation is slower than it was before the stagnation. This extension moves slower than the former extension. The enhanced region spreads slowly toward the lateral edge of the TRAM flap and the whole region is eventually enhanced in most flaps. But, in some cases, the spread of the enhancement stops between Zones II and IV of the flap (Figs. 20.5 and 20.6).

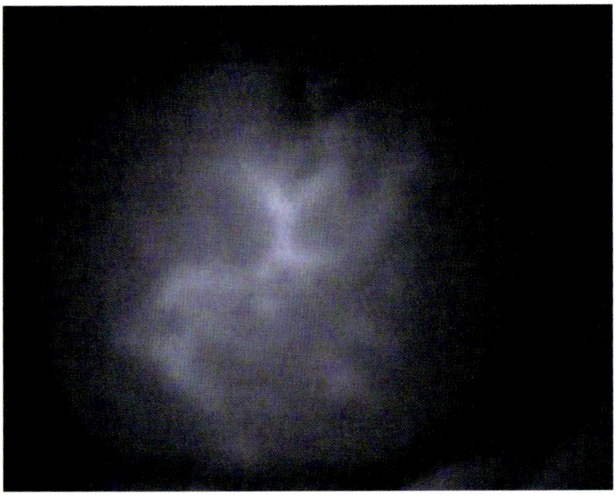

Fig. 20.1 Some linear enhancement from each of the perforators is observed in the TRAM flap

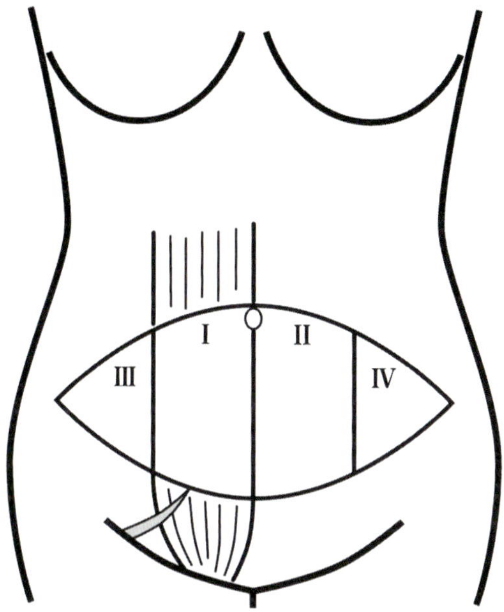

Fig. 20.2 Zone classification of the TRAM flap

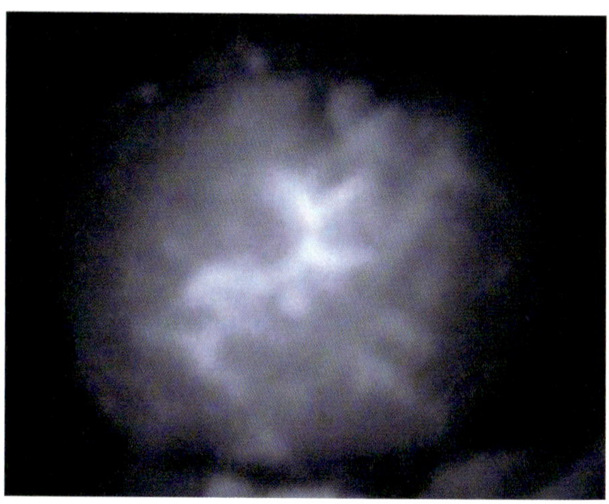

Fig. 20.3 The TRAM flap is enhanced diffusely

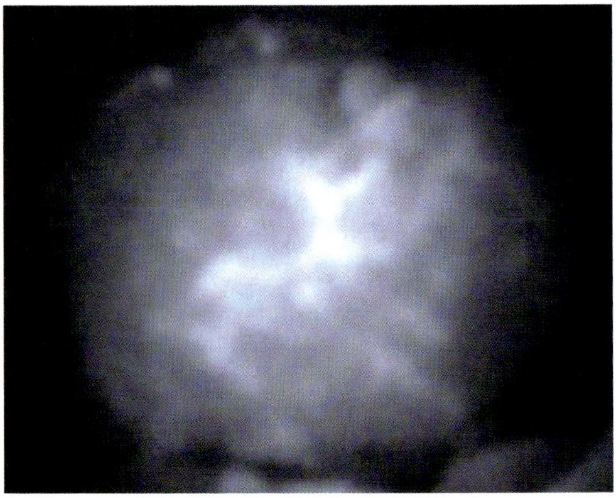

Fig. 20.4 The enhancement stagnates. Three seconds after Fig. 20.3, enhanced region is almost the same as Fig. 20.3

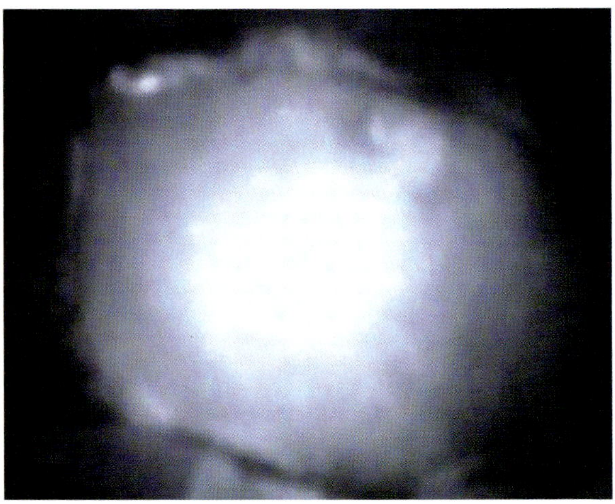

Fig. 20.5 Thirty seconds after Fig. 20.4, enhanced region extends and almost all of the region of the TRAM flap is enhanced

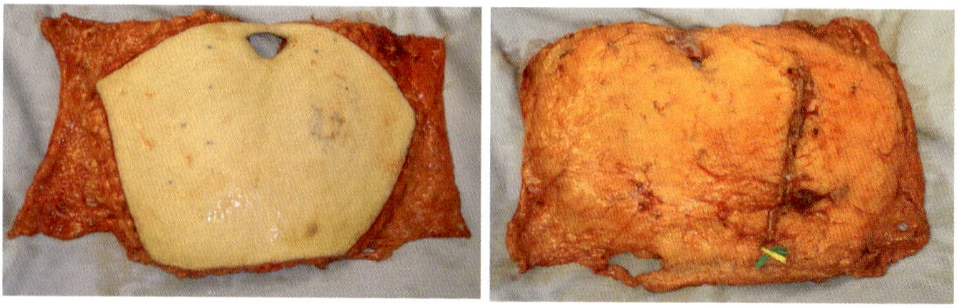

Fig. 20.6 Harvested TRAM flap. *Left*: Skin surface, *Right*: Fat surface with vascular pedicle

20.3 Evaluation

Eventually, the whole region of the flap becomes enhanced in most TRAM flaps. Nevertheless, partial fat necrosis and partial flap loss could still occur. The usefulness of this process depends on the proper evaluation of the effect of the enhancement with ICG. The most effective evaluation is done at the time when the initial diffusion stops or becomes stagnant.

20.4 Results

When only grafting regions which were enhanced before stagnation occurred, there were no complications of the TRAM flaps such as partial fat necrosis or partial flap loss. However, of the 17 cases in which grafts included non-enhanced regions, seven showed partial fat necrosis (Fig. 20.7).

In cases of patients who had mid-abdominal scars, if the patient had a complete midline scar from the cephalad edge to caudal edge, there was no case of the flap in which contralateral region of the vascular pedicle was enhanced. However, the flaps had intact areas a few centimeters from the umbilicus, and the contralateral region of the flap was enhanced in some cases. There was a tendency for the contralateral side of the flap to be enhanced, when the patient had a perforator near the intact area of the midline.

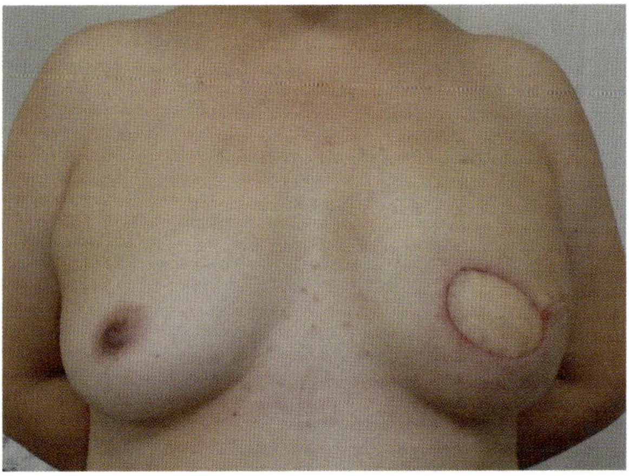

Fig. 20.7 Left reconstructed breast shows symmetric shape without partial fat necrosis

20.5 Discussion

It is useful for the plastic surgeon to use ICG (indocyanine green) for the breast reconstruction surgery, as ICG is also usually used in breast cancer surgery for detecting sentinel lymph nodes.

In the plastic and reconstructive surgery field, Eren et al. [1] describe that ICG fluorescence angiography was useful to evaluate the reliable circulation of the axial pattern flap in rat models. The first clinical report of evaluation of the circulation of the flap with ICG was reported by Still et al. [2] In this report, 18 patients who were burned underwent ICG fluorescence imaging for the evaluation of the circulation of the flap. In one patient, two flaps were evaluated. The entire flaps were enhanced and the whole region survived in 16 flaps. However, in another flap, almost the entire area of the flap was not enhanced and in the end that flap showed almost complete necrosis. In two flaps, un-enhanced regions survived. Holm et al. [3] described the usefulness of ICG fluorescence enhancement for evaluating which regions would survive in 11 axial pattern flaps and four random pattern flaps. Afterward, ICG fluorescence angiography was used to evaluate the free flaps [4, 5].

Partial fat necrosis and partial skin necrosis of flaps are sometimes encountered in breast reconstruction surgery. Neither of them are major complications, but they occasionally influence the shape of the reconstructed breast. It was very difficult for us to detect the partial necrotic area during surgery until the introduction of the ICG navigation surgical system. Since the introduction of the ICG navigation system to breast reconstruction surgery, we have never experienced partial fat necrosis or partial skin necrosis of a TRAM flap which was grafted only from an enhanced region.

Yamaguchi et al. utilized the ICG fluorescence navigation system for breast reconstruction with pedicle TRAM flaps. They mentioned that ICG fluorescence angiography predicted full flap viability [6]. Holm et al. introduced the ICG fluorescence navigation system for SIEA flaps and detected the perfusion area of the superficial epigastric vessels [7]. Newman and Samsom utilized the ICG fluorescence navigation system for detecting the perfusion area of each perforator in the DIEP/TRAM flaps and selected perforators which were included in the flaps [8].

However, almost half of the flaps, which were grafted from non-enhanced regions, revealed partial fat necrosis. The other half of the flaps revealed no complications. The difference of the results depends on how much of the volume of the non-enhanced region is included. On the other hand, there is a gray zone between the intact area and the area of necrosis.

Still et al. reported that non-enhanced regions survived in two cases [2]. Moyer and Lasken also mentioned about "the gray area" of the ICG navigation [9]. Yamaguchi et al. described one of ten cases which showed superficial epitheliolysis and secondary healing developing marginally in the flap, although ICG video-angiography showed no fluorescence defect. The article mentioned that fluorescence intensity seemed to reach a plateau 2–3 min after the ICG intravenous injection [6]. Wu et al. reported that 14 % were underestimated and 14 % were overestimated in random skin flaps and 7 % were underestimated and 7 % were overestimated in perforator flaps. They mentioned that imaging to identify perforators was performed 10 s after dye injection and imaging to assess flap perfusion was usually performed for 2 min separated by an approximately 30 s interval to save the first minute of imaging [10]. Holm et al. [3] and Newman et al. [8] mentioned that all flaps without ICG filling defects survived. However, they did not define the timing of their assessment.

Making a standard of assessment of ICG fluorescence angiography for flaps is important to decrease underestimates and overestimates. In some reports, authors used the time from the start of flap perfusion for assessment [6, 11]. In some reports, they used software for analyzing illumination of the flaps. Neither using the time from the start of perfusion nor using the software to analyze illumination provides a reliable assessment. The flap perfusion time depends on blood pressure or cardiomotility. Illumination of the flap during ICG angiography depends on the brightness or darkness of the operating room. It is impossible to keep the same brightness in the operating room every time. Brightness of the operating room is affected by the number or variety of monitors, even with all of the room lights turned off.

Instead, it's better to note the movement of the enhanced region. By observing at the time when the diffusion of the enhancement stops or stagnates, the viable area of a TRAM flap can be determined. It's necessary to have the operating room dark enough to judge the movement of the enhanced region.

ICG angiography is one of the most useful techniques for decreasing partial fat necrosis and partial flap necrosis in breast reconstruction surgery with TRAM flaps.

20.6 Summary

Free TRAM flaps are frequently used in breast reconstruction. We sometimes experience partial fat necrosis or partial skin necrosis of the TRAM flaps after breast reconstructive surgery. Even if fresh bleeding is confirmed, partial fat necrosis of a part may be encountered. It is very difficult to assess which part of the fat tissue will be necrotic before a flap is grafted. Indocyanine green fluorescence angiography is a useful and reliable method to evaluate the viability of a flap during surgery.

Two milliliters of indocyanine green are injected systemically in the veins. Enhancement of the TRAM flap starts from each perforator individually and linear enhancement extends laterally or radially. Diffuse enhancement starts and extends between the linear enhancement. Then, diffuse enhancement stagnates in 1–2 s. After that, the enhancement region starts to extend again. But, this extension moves slower than the former extension.

Choosing the right time to make your determination of the reliability of an enhanced region is important. In previous reports, some authors used the time from the start of enhancement and other authors used illuminations. However, it is very difficult to determine the reliable enhanced region every time under the fixed conditions. The circulation time of the injected indocyanine green is affected by the patient's blood pressure and other physical conditions. The illumination of the enhanced flap is affected by the brightness of the operating room which in turn depends on the light of surgical monitors, even with the room lights and surgical lights turned off. However, movement of the enhanced region is a reliable guide, because it reflects the physical conditions of the patient. It's necessary for the operating room to be dark enough to judge the movement, and especially to observe the period of stagnation, of the enhanced region.

Previous reports mentioned overestimation and underestimation of the ICG fluorescence angiography which appear in a definite ratio. Overestimation may bring partial fat necrosis after the surgery. We have never experienced partial fat necrosis or partial flap loss in our study. Underestimation depends on the viability of the distal part of the flap which is enhanced after the period of stagnation. The blood circulation is like a reverse flow flap in the region beyond the choked vessels in TRAM flaps. As the reliability of this area is unstable, we don't recommend including it in the area judged to be effective.

References

1. Eren S, Rübben A, Krein R, Larkin G, Hettich R (1995) Assessment of microcirculation of an axial skin flap using indocyanine green fluorescence angiography. Plast Reconstr Surg 96:1636–1649

2. Still J, Law E, Dawson J, Bracci S, Island T, Holtz J (1999) Evaluation of the circulation of reconstructive flaps using laser-induced fluorescence of indocyanine green. Ann Plast Surg 42:266–274
3. Holm C, Mayr M, Höfter E, Becker A, Pfeiffer UJ, Mühlbauer W (2002) Intraoperative evaluation of skin-flap viability using laser-induced fluorescence of indocyanine green. Br J Plast Surg 55:635–644
4. Holm C, Tegeler J, Mayr M, Becker A, Pfeiffer UJ, Mühlbauer W (2002) Monitoring free flaps using laser-induced fluorescence of indocyanine green: a preliminary experience. Microsurgery 22:278–287
5. Pestana IA, Coan B, Erdmann D, Marcus J, Levin LS, Zenn MR (2009) Early experience with fluorescent angiography in free-tissue transfer reconstruction. Plast Reconstr Surg 123:1239–1244
6. Yamaguchi S, De lorenzi F, Petit JY, Rietjen M, Garusi C, Giraldo A, Rey PC, Urban C, Martella S, Bosco R (2004) The "Perfusion Map" of the unipedicle TRAM flap to reduce postoperative partial necrosis. Ann Plast Surg 53:205–209
7. Holm C, Mayr M, Höfter E, Ninkovic M (2007) The versatility of the SIEA flap: a clinical assessment of the vascular territory of the superficial epigastric inferior artery. J Plast Reconstr Aesthet Surg 60:946–951
8. Newman MI, Samson MC (2009) The application of laser-assisted indocyanine green fluorescent dye angiography in microsurgical breast reconstruction. J Reconstr Microsurg 25:21–26
9. Moyer HR, Losken A (2012) Predicting mastectomy skin flap necrosis with indocyanine green angiography: the gray area defined. Plast Reconstr Surg 129:1043–1048
10. Wu C, Kim S, Halvorson EG (2013) Laser-assisted indocyanine green angiography a critical appraisal. Ann Plast Surg 70:613–619
11. Pestana IA, Coan B, Erdman D, Marcus J, Levin LS, Zenn MR (2009) Early experience with fluorescent angiography in free-tissue transfer reconstruction. Plast Reconstr Surg 123:1239–1244

Chapter 21
Intraoperative Evaluation of Flap Circulation by ICG Fluorescence Angiography in the Breast Reconstruction with Pedicled TRAM Frap

Hidekazu Fukamizu, Masao Fujiwara, Takahide Mizukami, and Takeshi Nagata

Abstract Since its introduction, the pedicled transverse rectus abdominis myocutaneous flap (TRAM flap) became a popular procedure for postmastectomy breast reconstruction. Preference for the pedicled TRAM flap was based on its sufficient volume for reconstruction, natural appearing result, acceptable scar of the donor site, and the avoidance of complications caused by the use of implant. However, the perfusion of the pedicled TRAM flap is not as reliable as expected, because this flap has the better blood flow through the inferior epigastric vessels than through the superior epigastric vessels. In general, all the tissue in zone IV of the flap and the parts of the skin in zone II and III tend to be necrotic. When the flap is designed as larger than usual, the inferior epigastric system on the ipsilateral side is prepared for microvascular augmentation.

The traditional methods for evaluating flap circulation, such as examining tissue color, capillary refilling, and dermal bleeding, are based on subjective clinical assessment and can be inaccurate even when used by experienced surgeons. There is still no definitive method of evaluating flap circulation and viability with reasonable objectivity and wide acceptance, instead of several objective techniques. Indocyanine green (ICG) fluorescence angiography is a new method for evaluation of flap circulation. Two ml of 0.25 % ICG solution was injected intravenously, and the fluorescence imaging was obtained by a newly developed near-infrared camera system (PDE, Hamamatsu Photonics K.K. Hamamatsu, Japan). Vascular flow and flap perfusion could be visualized intraoperatively without requiring much time or complexity. The advantages of this method are that real-time information is obtainable and that characteristic fluorescence patterns (such as filling defects, slow filling, and weak fluorescence) are associated with critical flap perfusion deficits, especially in high-risk patients.

H. Fukamizu (✉) • M. Fujiwara • T. Mizukami • T. Nagata
Department of Plastic and Reconstructive Surgery, Hamamatsu University School of Medicine, 1-20-1 Handayama, Higashi-ku, Hamamatsu, Shizuoka 431-3192, Japan
e-mail: fukamizu@hama-med.ac.jp

M. Kusano et al. (eds.), *ICG Fluorescence Imaging and Navigation Surgery*,
DOI 10.1007/978-4-431-55528-5_21

Keywords Breast reconstruction • Pedicled TRAM flap • Indocyanine green • Fluorescence angiography

21.1 Introduction

Patients undergoing mastectomy for breast cancer have many reconstructive options. The pedicled transverse rectus abdominis myocutaneous flap (TRAM flap) remains a common method of postmastectomy restoration when autogenous tissue is required and a free TRAM flap is not desired or is contraindicated [1]. This procedure now accounts for 25–50 % of breast reconstructions performed in the United States [2]. Since its introduction, TRAM flap became a popular procedure for postmastectomy breast reconstruction. Preference for the TRAM flap was based on its sufficient volume for reconstruction, soft and natural appearing result, acceptable scar of the donor site, and the avoidance of complications such as capsular contractures associated with prosthetic implant use. However, the perfusion of superior epigastric vessels which nourish the pedicled TRAM flap is not as reliable as expected, because this flap has the better blood flow through the inferior epigastric vessels than that through the superior epigastric vessels. Therefore, the free TRAM with the deep inferior epigastric artery may be appropriate for the patients who are obese with larger breasts and smokers regardless of longer operative time and the risk of total flap loss due to the microvascular surgery. In Japan the pedicled TRAM flap is an excellent option in many patients because there are less obese patients and smokers. It is important to know, however, that blood flow to the flap is retained through connections between the underlying abdominal muscle and the overlying abdominal fat and skin.

The traditional methods for evaluating flap circulation, such as examining tissue color, capillary refilling, and dermal bleeding, are based on subjective clinical assessment and can be inaccurate even when used by experienced surgeons. There is still no definitive method of evaluating flap circulation and viability with reasonable objectivity and wide acceptance, instead of several objective techniques. In our institution indocyanine green (ICG) fluorescence angiography is always used for evaluation of flap circulation. By using this method, the vascular flow and flap perfusion could be visualized intraoperatively without requiring much time or complexity. The purpose of this text is to introduce the precise procedures of this method in the postmastectomy breast reconstruction with pedicled TRAM flap.

21.2 Vascular Anatomy of TRAM Flap

The rectus abdominis muscle and its overlying skin have the dual blood supply from the deep superior epigastric artery (DSEA) and the deep inferior epigastric artery (DIEA). Both arteries anastomose together above the level of the umbilicus

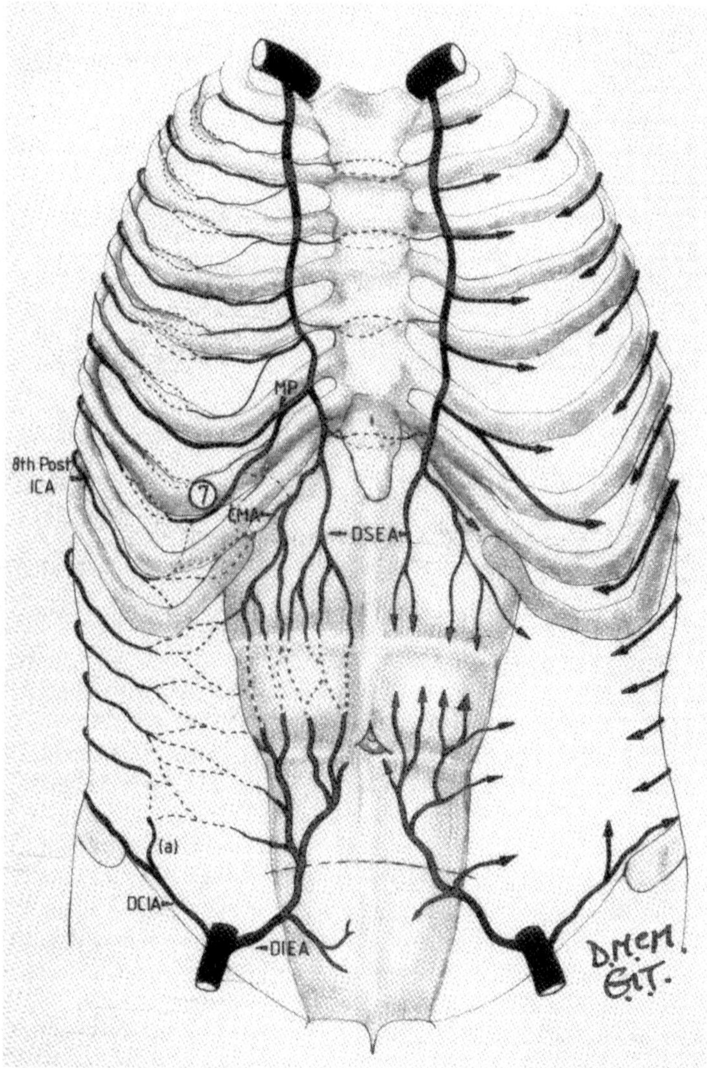

Fig. 21.1 Schematic diagram demonstrates the blood supply of the anterior abdominal wall. Note that the anastomosis between the deep superior epigastric artery (DSEA) and the deep inferior epigastric artery (DIEA) is situated in the segment of the rectus muscle above the umbilicus (From Taylor GI: Plast Reconstr Surg 81:721–724, 1988 [3])

(Fig. 21.1) [3, 4]. There is a large concentration of perforators to supply the overlying fat and skin around the umbilicus. The skin island was originally designed vertically over the primary territory of the rectus muscle. In 1982, Hartrampf et al. [5] reported the flap incorporating a transverse skin island located on the inferior abdominal wall. There is a random portion of the flap across the midline and lateral to the muscle. This type of flap provides a sufficient amount of

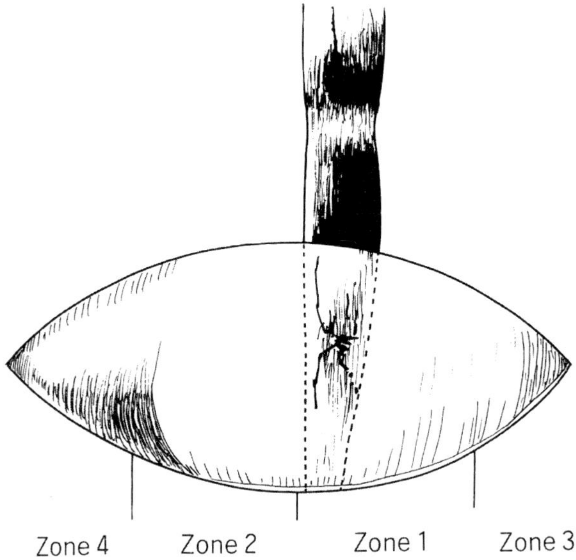

Fig. 21.2 Vascular zones of the conventional pedicled TRAM flap (From Scheflan M, Dinner MI: Ann Plast Surg 10:120–129, 1983 [7])

fatty tissue and the abdominal scar can be low. Furthermore, the longer muscle pedicle is useful for filling in infraclavicular and axillary defects. However, the pedicled lower TRAM flap between the umbilicus and the symphysis pubis is anatomically the most vulnerable design from both an arterial and a venous standpoint.

Scheflan et al. [6, 7] divided the skin island of the flap into four zones, according to the reliability of its circulation and survival (Fig. 21.2). Zone 1 is located directly over the muscle and represents its primary cutaneous territory. Zone 2 is directly across the midline of the abdomen, which extends from the midline of the abdomen to the lateral edge of the contralateral muscle. Zone 2 of the skin island has proved reliable because the circulation is provided by the subdermal and deeper vascular communications of musculocutaneous perforating vessels from the rectus muscle beneath zone 1. Zone 3 is the portion of the skin island lateral to zone 1. Zone 4 is the most distant portion from zone 1 located between the lateral edge of the contralateral rectus sheath and the iliac crest. These two lateral zones, zone 3 and zone 4, are less reliable considering circulation based on one rectus abdominis muscle. In general, most of zone 4 and the lateral aspect of zone 3 are discarded because of inadequate perfusion. In addition the blood flow from the epigastric perforators through DSEA seems to be insufficient for the patients with obesity, heavy cigarette smoking, and advancing age to maintain the viability of the adipose mass of large TRAM flap [8]. Therefore, the microvascularly augmented TRAM flap, which is a superiorly based unipedicled TRAM flap with microvascular anastomosis between either the contralateral or ipsilateral inferior epigastric vascular system and available vessels close to the defect, is usually applied for the breast reconstruction in need of a large volume of soft tissue [9, 10]. Whichever procedure is applied, it is difficult to evaluate how much the circulation can be augmented to the flap.

21.3 Operative Procedures

21.3.1 Preoperative Markings and Preparations

Preoperative markings are completed at the standing position including the vertical midline from the suprasternal notch to the pubis passing through the umbilicus, the inframammary fold of the remaining breast, and its transferred line as a mirror image to the defect side (Fig. 21.3). The skin island of the TRAM flap is marked between the umbilicus and the pubic hair line extending between both anterior iliac spines at the spine position. In general, the superior margin of the

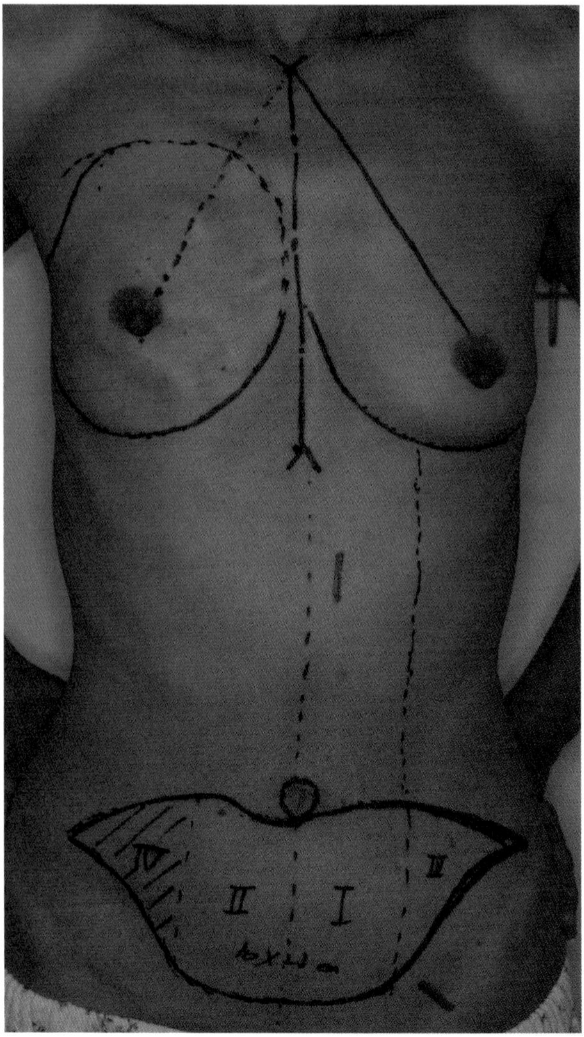

Fig. 21.3 Preoperative markings in the case of secondary breast reconstruction after skin-sparing mastectomy. The conventional pedicled TRAM flap is designed. The *red lines* indicate the location of superior epigastric artery and deep inferior epigastric artery. The *shaded area* indicates zone 4

skin island is located 1 or 2 cm superior to the umbilicus because of a large concentration of perforators to supply the overlying fat and skin around the umbilicus. We always use color Doppler sonography for the mapping of perforators. During surgery, the inferior margin of the skin island may be moved superiorly when direct closure appears difficult or too tight with retraction of the superior abdominal flap.

21.3.2 Elevation of TRAM Flap

The procedure starts with the incision around the umbilicus to allow release of the umbilicus stalk to the midline fascia as described in the text [11]. The superior skin island incision is completed with a bevel of subcutaneous tissue superior to the skin incision to capture as many perforating vessels as possible and to add fatty tissue to the flap for the breast mound reconstruction. The superior abdominal skin and subcutaneous tissue are elevated from the abdominal fascia to the costal margin and to the sternum in the midline to transfer the pedicled TRAM flap through a generous tunnel into the breast area. After the abdominal flap elevation is completed, the superior-based abdominal flap is advanced toward the pubis to make sure that it covers the marked inferior incision for the TRAM skin island without tension. We usually use the contralateral TRAM flap in which the arc of rotation results in less twisting of the muscle below the skin island and in less disruption of the inframammary line. The ipsilateral side (zone 2 and zone 4) of the skin island is first elevated from external oblique and anterior sheath. After that a central strip of anterior rectus sheath is incised to expose the rectus muscle in the contralateral side (zone 1) of the skin island. The exposed muscle is dissected from two parallel incisions located approximately 2 cm lateral to the medial edge of the sheath and 2 cm medial to the lateral edge of the sheath extended to the anterior sheath superior to the skin island.

The skin island is now elevated from the external oblique fascia to the side of the rectus muscle flap and to the midline fascia on the opposite side of the abdomen. DIEA and the paired venae comitantes are dissected as long as possible so that the pedicle can be used to revascularize the flap through microvascular anastomosis on the chest wall when the pedicle of DSEA proves to be inadequate to support the flap. If a TRAM flap is designed as larger than usual, the inferior epigastric system on the ipsilateral side is necessary for microvascular anastomosis just like DIEP flap (Fig. 21.4).

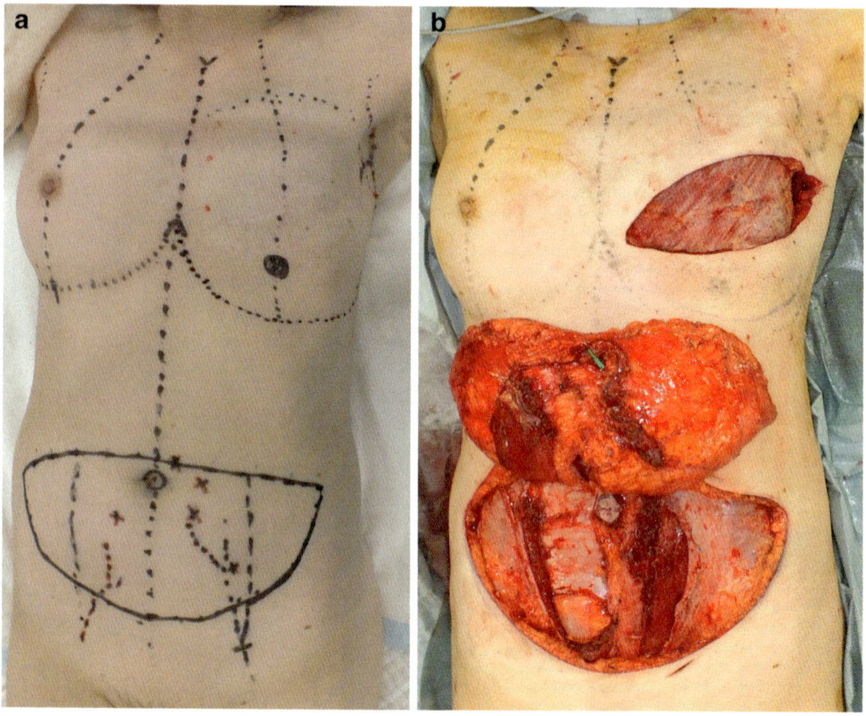

Fig. 21.4 (**a**) Preoperative marking in the case of secondary breast reconstruction. (**b**) The contralateral pedicled TRAM flap with the deep inferior epigastric flap (DIEP flap) on the ipsilateral side for microvascular augmentation is elevated in this case

The contralateral rectus muscle including the skin island is elevated from the posterior rectus sheath based on the superior epigastric system. The pedicled TRAM flap is now passed through tunnel into mastectomy defect. After the contralateral or ipsilateral inferior epigastric vascular pedicles are anastomosed with appropriate recipient vessels when needed, the circulation of the flap is evaluated by indocyanine green (ICG) fluorescence angiography.

21.3.3 Evaluation of Flap Circulation by ICG Fluorescence Angiography

We performed intravenous injection of indocyanine green (ICG) to evaluate perfusion of the flap after the flap transposition and inset. After the injection of 5 mg of ICG (Diagnogreen 0.5 %; Daiichi Pharmaceutical, Tokyo, Japan), fluorescent images were obtained with a newly developed near-infrared camera system (PDE, Hamamatsu Photonics K.K. Hamamatsu, Japan) [12]. After intravenous injection, ICG binds strongly to plasma proteins. In the absence of capillary protein

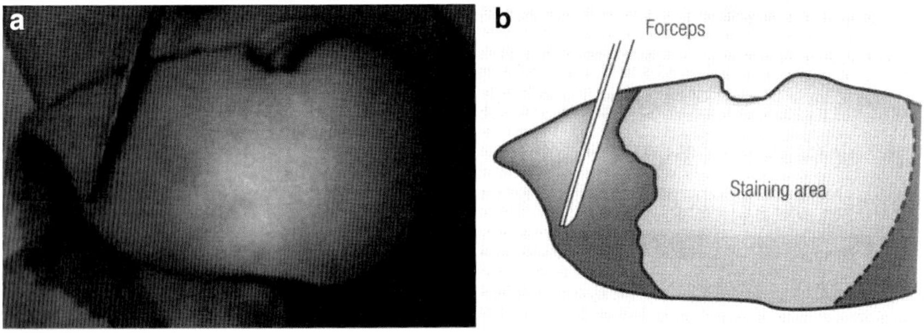

Fig. 21.5 (**a**) ICG angiography of the conventional pedicled TRAM flap. (**b**) A schema showing the staining area. Note that the lateral portion on the *right side* (zone IV) and a part of the *left side* (zone III) of the flap show the poor perfusion compared with zones I and II. Zone IV is removed on the line of forceps

leakage, it is exclusively distributed within the intravascular space [13]. Penetrating deeper into the skin, the excitation light induces fluorescence from blood vessels in the deep dermal plexus and subcutaneous fat, instead of only the superficial dermis [14]. The induced fluorescence is not trapped in the skin and can be recorded by PDE because the skin is relatively transparent to the ICG fluorescence wavelength. In the conventional unipedicled TRAM flap without microvascular augmentation, the arteries in the rectus abdominis muscle showed strong fluorescence about 30 s after the injection of ICG. Some linear fluorescent stains can be seen in the flap about 40 s after the injection followed by diffuse stain of fluorescence. The time taken before the fluorescent stain can be seen in the flap after the injection is decided by blood tension of the patient and the thickness of skin and subcutaneous fat. When the flap has good circulation, it showed homogeneous, rapid filling and strong fluorescence. The area of zone 4 in the conventional pedicled TRAM flap usually showed very weak or no fluorescence, which indicated poor perfusion (Figs. 21.5 and 21.6). Furthermore, the distal portion of zone II and III sometimes reveals weak fluorescence. The area under suspicion of skin and fat necrosis was resected primarily in favor of a smaller final breast volume, and all of the remaining flaps survived without clinically significant skin and fat necrosis. In the case of needing a large volume of soft tissue, we always planned the microvascularly augmented pedicled TRAM flap (Fig. 21.7), which has microvascular anastomosis between either the contralateral or ipsilateral inferior epigastric vascular system and the recipient vessels. The very short half-life of ICG allows sequential monitoring of skin perfusion with short intervals within 30 min between injections [15].

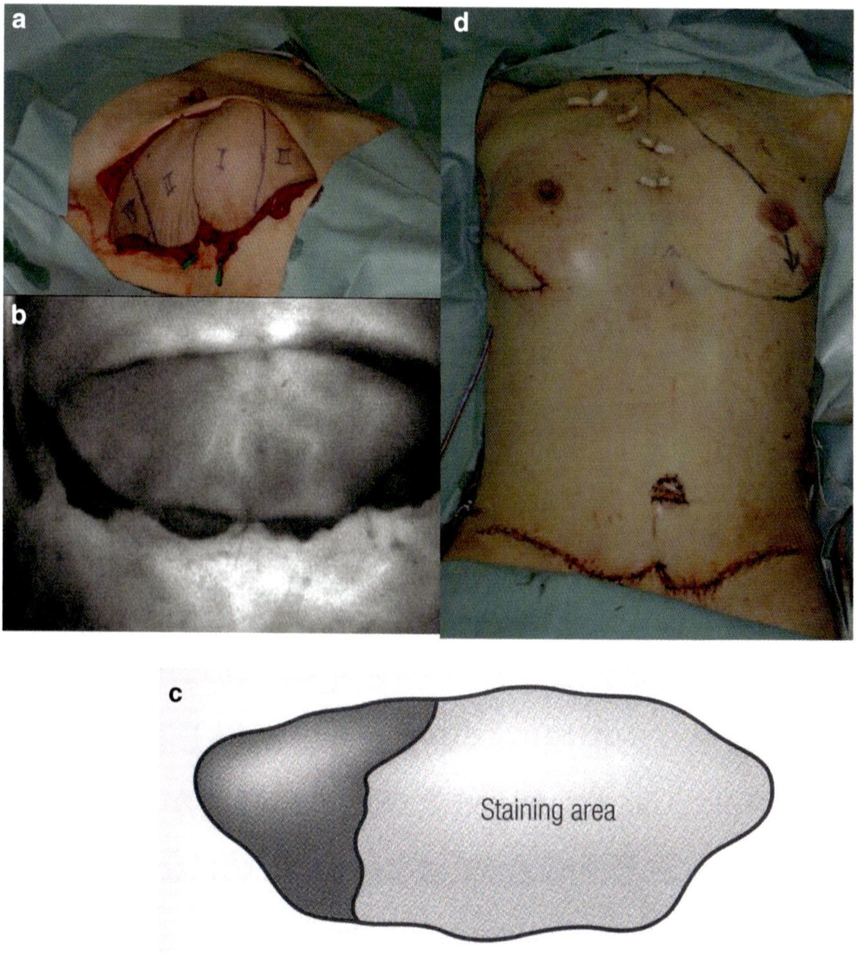

Fig. 21.6 (**a**: *above left*) Intraoperative photographs of the conventional pedicled TRAM flap after passing under the abdominal tunnel. (**b**: *below left*) ICG angiography. (**c**) A schema showing the staining area. (**d**) Immediate postoperative view. In this case a monitoring flap is *left*

21.3.4 Flap Inset and Abdominal Closure

After the flap is passed through a subcutaneous tunnel into the mastectomy defect, it is trimmed and contoured to match the opposite breast mound with the patient in the sitting position. Once the flap is inset and the contralateral or ipsilateral inferior epigastric vascular pedicles are anastomosed with appropriate recipient vessels when needed, attention is turned to the abdominal wall closure. We always incorporate the ipsilateral internal and external oblique fascia with the contralateral anterior rectus sheath. In our institution, we usually do not use artificial mesh. In

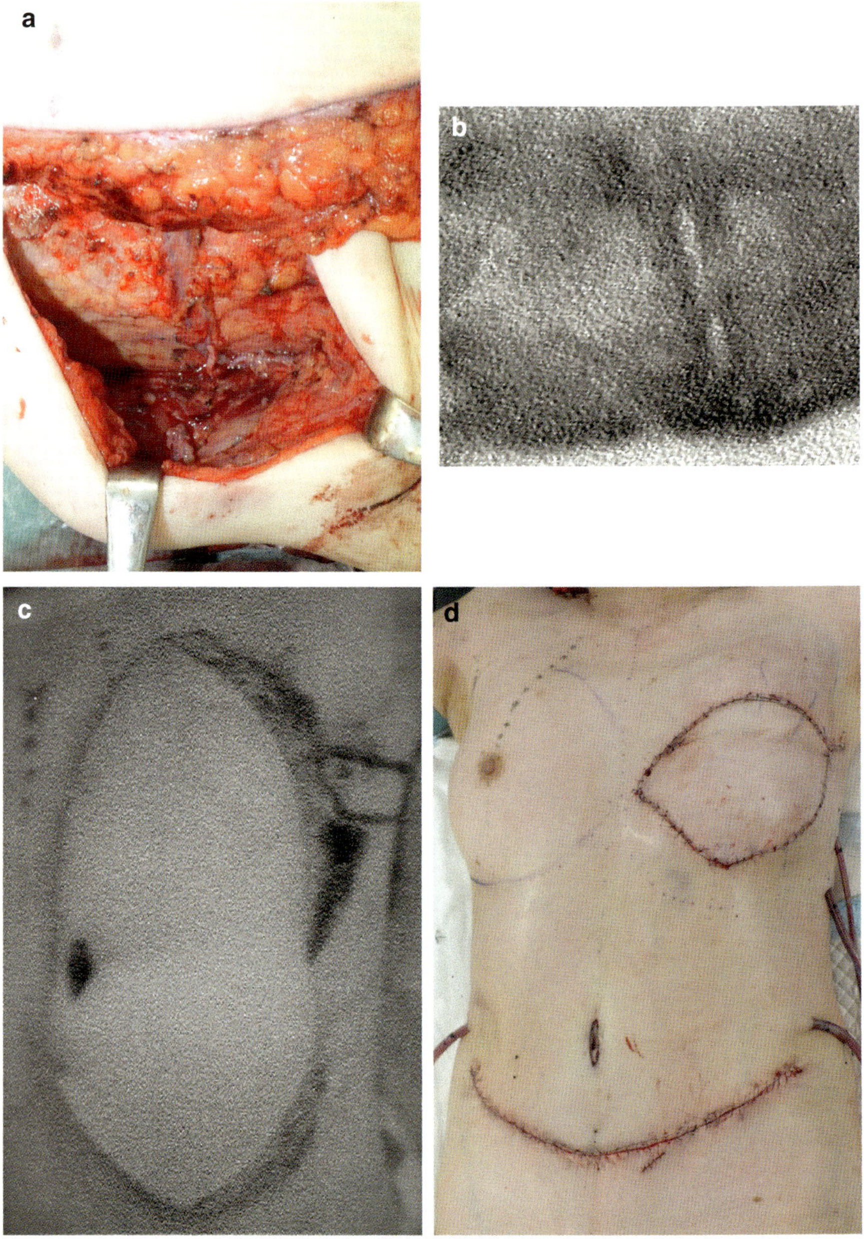

Fig. 21.7 (**a**) The ipsilateral deep inferior epigastric vascular pedicles are anastomosed with the branch of the thoracodorsal vessels. (**b**) ICG angiography showing patency of the anastomosed site. (**c**) ICG angiography of the microvascularly augmented pedicled TRAM flap (Fig. 21.4). Note that all the zones of the flap are stained. (**d**) Immediate postoperative view. No portion of the flap is removed

this final point an additional evaluation of flap circulation by ICG is usually performed to make sure there are no excessive twisting, kinking, and tension. When any part of the flap shows very weak or no fluorescence indicating poor perfusion, we should reconsider whether the flap inset is achieved with an adequate tunnel space and without tension.

21.4 Discussion

ICG angiography is a new method for evaluation of flap circulation. Vascular flow and flap perfusion can be visualized intraoperatively without requiring much time or complexity. The advantages of ICG angiography are that real-time information is obtainable and that characteristic fluorescence patterns (such as filling defects, slow filling, and weak fluorescence) are associated with critical flap perfusion deficits [14, 16]. Familiarity with the technique has resulted in the higher reliability on the initial perfusion scan to assess the skin and fat viability. Because of the reduction in delayed wound healing secondary to skin flap necrosis after breast reconstruction, this technique reduces patient morbidity and the cost of subsequent wound care and diminishes the risk of developing palpable fat necrosis in pedicled TRAM flap reconstruction. Although ICG angiography provides a reliable and rapid intraoperative assessment for the circulation of pedicled TRAM Frap, there are some points to require technological innovation. As the fluorescence is easily interfered by overlying skin, the circulation in the subcutaneous fat layer is difficult to evaluate. There is no data of fluorescence value for an absolute assessment of tissue viability, and it is difficult for the operators to decide which region is surgically resected. Further studies give more clinical effectiveness.

References

1. Davidge KM, Brown M, Morgan P et al (2013) Processes of care in autogenous breast reconstruction with pedicled TRAM flaps: expending postoperative discharge in an ambulatory setting. Plast Reconstr Surg 132:339e–344e
2. Zenn MR (2014) Unipedicled TRAM breast reconstruction. http://emedicine.medscape.com/article/1274334-overview#a0101, Mar 3, 2014
3. Taylor GI (1988) Discussion for Miller LB, Bostwick J, Hartrampf CR, et al: The superiorly based rectus abdominis flap: predicting and enhancing its blood supply based on an anatomic and clinical study. Plast Reconstr Surg 81:721–724
4. Moon HK, Taylor GI (1988) The vascular anatomy of rectus abdominis musculocutaneous flaps based on the deep superior epigastric system. Plast Reconstr Surg 82:815–829
5. Hartrampf CR, Scheflan M, Black PW (1982) Breast reconstruction with a transverse abdominal island flap. Plast Reconstr Surg 69:216–224
6. Scheflan M, Dinner MI (1983) The transverse abdominal island flap: Part I. Indications, contraindications, results, and complications. Ann Plast Surg 10:24–35

7. Scheflan M, Dinner MI (1983) The transverse abdominal island flap: Part II. Surgical technique. Ann Plast Surg 10:120–129
8. Millar LB, Bostwick J, Hartramph CR et al (1988) The superiorly based rectus abdominis flap: predicting and enhancing its blood supply based on an anatomic and clinical study. Plast Reconstr Surg 81:713–720
9. Harashina T, Sone K, Inoue T et al (1987) Augmentation of circulation of pedicled transverse rectus abdominis musculocutaneous flaps by microvascular surgery. Br J Plast Surg 40:367–370
10. Yamamoto Y, Nohira K, Sugihara T et al (1996) Superiority of the microvascularly augmented flap: analysis of 50 transverse rectus abdominis myocutaneous flaps for breast reconstruction. Plast Reconstr Surg 97:79–83
11. Mathes SJ, Lang J (2006) Transverse rectus abdominis musculocutaneous (TRAM) transposition flap. VI Trunk and lower extremity. In: Mathes SJ (ed) Plastic surgery, 2nd edn. Saunders, Philadelphia, pp 712–761
12. Suzuki A, Fujiwara M, Mizukami T et al (2008) Delayed distally based super sural flap: evaluation by indocyanine green fluorescence angiography. J Plast Reconstr Aesthet Surg 61:467–469
13. Ishihara H, Otomo N, Suzuki A et al (1998) Detection of capillary protein leakage by glucose and indocyanine green dilutions during the early post-burn period. Burns 24:525–531
14. Holm C, Mayr M, Hofter E et al (2002) Intraoperative evaluation of skin-flap viability using laser-induced fluorescence of indocyanine green. Br J Plast Surg 55:635–644
15. Krishnan KG, Schackert G, Steinmeier R (2005) The role of near-infrared angiography in the assessment of post-operative venous congestion in random pattern, pedicled island and free flaps. Br J Plast Surg 58:330–338
16. Still J, Law E, Dawson J et al (1999) Evaluation of the circulation of reconstructive flaps using laser-induced fluorescence of indocyanine green. Ann Plast Surg 42:266–274

Chapter 22
Pre- and Intraoperative Identification of Perforator Vessels Using MRA/MDCTA, Doppler Sonography, and ICG Fluorescence Angiography

Toshiyuki Watanabe, Keita Kawai, and Yoshihiro Kimata

Abstract Here, we introduce our method of combined use of magnetic resonance angiography/multidetector-row computed tomography (MRA/MDCTA), Doppler sonography, and indocyanine green (ICG) fluorescence angiography to identify the locations of the perforator vessels of the flaps. This method can be used to accurately confirm perforator vessel location on pre- or intraoperative images. If a detectable perforator is obtained using preoperative MRA/MDCTA and Doppler sonography, we use the term "freestyle perforator-based flap" for propeller or V-Y advancement flaps. In some cases, aggressive perforator dissection is necessary to free these flaps from adhesions and evenly distribute the torsion, and the intraoperative identification of perforator vessels detected by Doppler sonography and ICG fluorescence angiography makes it possible to select perforators of larger caliber and stronger pulsatility without fear of anatomic inconsistencies; furthermore, such identification facilitates the surgical mechanics and shortens the operation time.

Keywords Freestyle perforator flap • Magnetic resonance angiography • Multidetector-row computed tomography angiography • Doppler sonography • Indocyanine green fluorescence angiography

22.1 Introduction

The era of the perforator flap began in 1989 when Koshima and Soeda first described the creation of an inferior epigastric artery skin flap without the use of the rectus abdominis muscle [1]. The use of perforator flaps has become preferred, and many variations have been reported in the literature [2].

T. Watanabe • K. Kawai • Y. Kimata (✉)
Department of Plastic and Reconstructive Surgery, University of Okayama, 2-5-1 Shikata-cho, Okayama 700-8558, Japan
e-mail: kimata@cc.okayama-u.ac.jp

M. Kusano et al. (eds.), *ICG Fluorescence Imaging and Navigation Surgery*,
DOI 10.1007/978-4-431-55528-5_22

In 1987, Taylor and Palmer introduced the angiosome concept, a variation of the cutaneous flap [3, 4]. The anterolateral thigh (ALT), deep inferior epigastric perforator (DIEP), and other flaps have been reported as angiosome and perforasome flaps [5–9]. The freestyle flap concept, introduced by H.C. Wei in 2004, involves the harvesting of skin flaps from any region of the body in which appropriate and detectable perforator vessels are present. However, flap perfusion in some cases of perforator flap use can be difficult to confirm intraoperatively because of anatomical variations [10–13]. Here, we introduce our method of combined use of magnetic resonance angiography/multidetector-row computed tomography (MRA/MDCTA), Doppler sonography, and indocyanine green (ICG) fluorescence angiography to identify the locations of the perforator vessels of the flaps.

22.2 Materials and Methods

Using this method, we created 60 perforator-based flaps (54 perforator flaps, 6 freestyle flaps) for reconstruction at Okayama University Hospital (Okayama, Japan). Here, we describe our combined use of MRA/MDCTA, Doppler sonography, and ICG fluorescence angiography for the pre- and intraoperative identification of perforator vessels.

22.2.1 Preoperative Identification of Perforator Vessels (MRA/MDCTA and Doppler Sonography)

Preoperative imaging of perforator vessels was performed with MRA or MDCTA to identify the perforators. MDCTA was used for 57 flaps, while MRA was used for three flaps. MRA and MDCTA both have advantage and disadvantages. MRI scans were performed on a 3.0 T scanner (Magnetom Verio; Siemens Medical Solutions, Erlangen, Germany) with the administration of intravenous gadolinium using the THRIVE method. A 16-slice MDCT scanner (Aquilion 16; Toshiba Medical System, Tokyo, Japan) was used. A bolus of intravenous contrast agent (Omnipaque 350; GE Healthcare, Chalfont St. Giles, UK) was injected, and the scan was triggered at each point. The obtained 0.5-mm-interval axial images were reformatted and reconstructed into three-dimensional images using the AZE Virtual Place program (AZE Ltd., Tokyo, Japan) [15, 24].

These images can demonstrate anatomic variations as well as the locations, numbers, and diameters of the perforator vessels. In some cases, extremity perforators are not detected on MRA or MDCTA images. One reason is that the axial images are taken at 0.5-mm intervals, which may not detect all perforator vessels.

Another reason is that vasospasms of the perforator vessels might cease during the MDCTA scanning process [14–19].

Based on the angiosome concept and MRA/MDCTA images, Doppler sonography was used to identify the perforator vessels and then mark their plurality for the donor site. At that time, it is important to recognize the differences in body position between MRA/MDCTA scanning and surgery, identify palpable landmarks on the body's surface, and spend sufficient time accurately identifying the perforator vessels [15, 20, 21].

22.2.2 Intraoperative Identification of Perforator Vessels (Doppler Sonography and ICG Fluorescence Angiography)

Doppler sonography and ICG fluorescence angiography through an infrared camera system were used intraoperatively to identify the perforator vessels. Doppler sonography, enclosed in a sterile drape within the surgical field, enabled the identification of the perforators from the subcutaneous underside.

ICG fluorescence angiography enabled identification of the perforator vessels at a depth up to 2 cm from the skin surface through the infrared camera system. We were able to confirm the perforators of the subcutaneous underside through the adjacent adipose tissue. The combined use of these technologies demonstrated marginal or poor flow and perfusion both visually and audibly [20–23].

22.2.3 ICG Fluorescence Dosing Method

ICG fluorescence angiography images were acquired using an infrared camera system (Photodynamic Eye; Hamamatsu Photonics, Hamamatsu, Japan). In all cases, the ICG fluorescent was dissolved in the injectable sterilization water and injected as a bolus infusion through a forearm vein, after which 5 mL of saline was rapidly injected. In the first 50 cases, a total of 10 mg (2 mL) of the ICG fluorescent injected was inserted into a forearm vein, but in 12 cases (24 %) in which the flap thickness was >20 mm, identifying the perforators through the skin and subcutaneous tissue was difficult [24]. We changed the ICG fluorescent dose to 0.3 mg/kg in the most recent nine cases. In two cases, despite a flap thickness >20 mm, we were able to confirm perforator locations on the images. In all cases, the total dose did not exceed 0.5 mg/kg, and no blood vessel spasms or allergic reactions occurred.

22.2.4 *Concrete Method by Flap Type*

22.2.4.1 Freestyle Pedicled Perforator Flap

In the planning of perforator flaps, we confirmed the presence of several perforator vessels around an area of skin loss using MRA/MDCTA and Doppler sonography. When intraoperative skin loss occurred at the time of tumor excision, we designed another perforator flap according to the perforator vessel position, neighboring skin strain, skin loss area shape, and perforasome theory. We mainly created propeller, V-Y advancement, and peninsula flaps. After performing subcutaneous detachment in the area surrounding the perforator vessel, we repeated the ICG fluorescence angiography and Doppler sonography examinations.

By examining the ICG fluorescent contrast, we confirmed the contrasting density area and strong pulse through the skin side while monitoring the perforator vessels on the subcutaneous underside to detect the central continuous perforator vessels. It is important to note that larger perforator flaps require strong pulsatility and a higher caliber of perforator; there are cases in which the perforator vessels of the lower limbs run above or below the fascia for great distances before reaching the skin [20].

We performed perivascular detachment until the flexibility of the perforator flap was ensured. We evaluated flap vascularization; if it was not flexible, we removed the unnecessary blood vessel. We removed the portions lacking acceptable bleeding that were not dyed by examining the ICG fluorescent contrast (Figs. 22.1, 22.2, and 22.3).

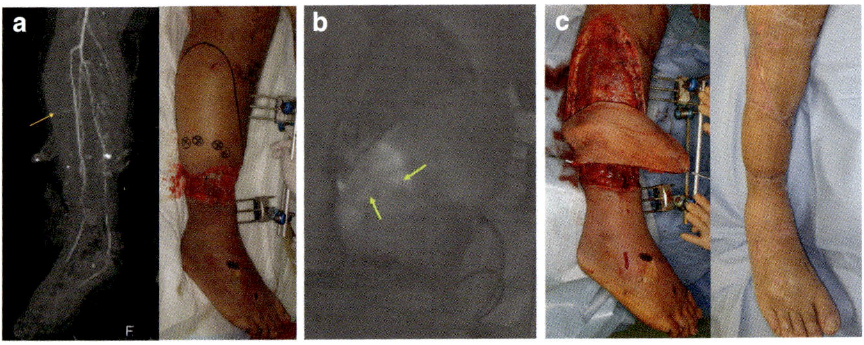

Fig. 22.1 90° Propeller flap
The patient suffered an open tibial and fibula pilon fracture (Gustilo IIIB) in a traffic accident. A propeller perforator flap based on the perforator vessels in the front of the leg was planned
In a preoperative perforator examination, several perforator vessels from the peroneal and anterior tibial artery were confirmed using MDCTA and Doppler sonography. A skin flap harvest was planned on the muscular fascia to match the area of skin loss (**a**) After ICG contrast angiography was performed to ensure flap flexibility, an aggressive perforator dissection was performed, thereby resulting in two dominant perforator vessels (**b**). The flap was then turned 90°. The flap survived completely (**c**)

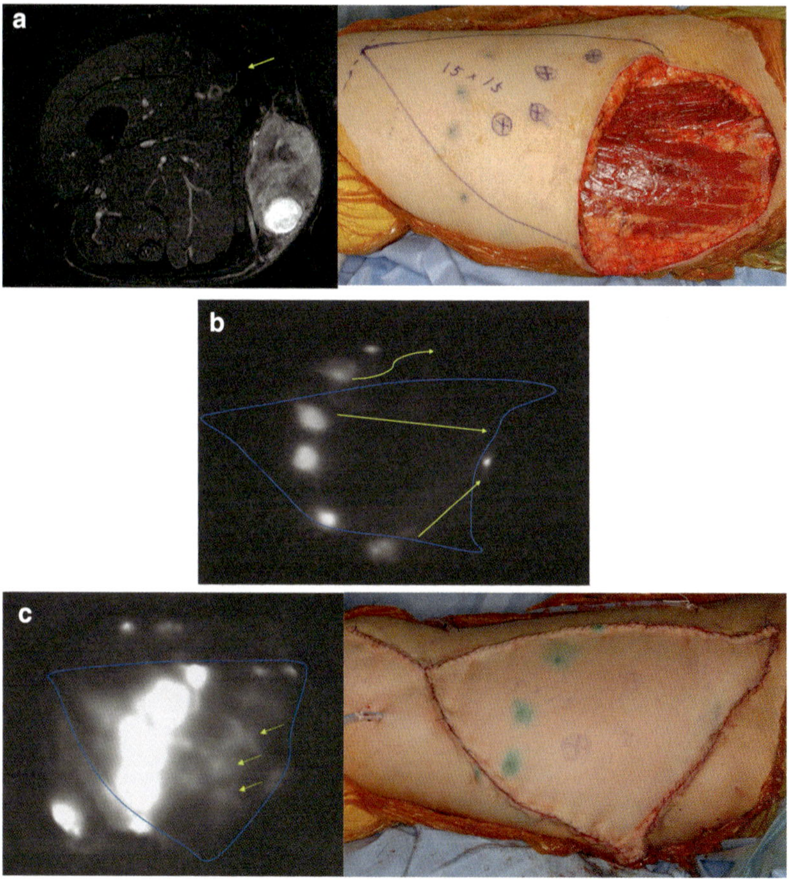

Fig. 22.2 V-Y advancement flap
A wide defect persisted on the right thigh after sarcoma resection. Several perforator vessels were confirmed around the area of skin loss by MRA and Doppler sonography (**a**). The V-Y advancement perforator flap was designed in the direction that would not inhibit the lymph style and where skin tension did not appear. ICG contrast was injected subcutaneously to confirm the lymph style (**b**) ICG fluorescence angiography was performed to identify the blood vessels after perivascular detachment under the muscular fasciae, and several dominant perforator vessels were chosen (**c**). The flexibility of the skin flap was ensured, the flap survived completely, and lymphedema did not develop in the leg

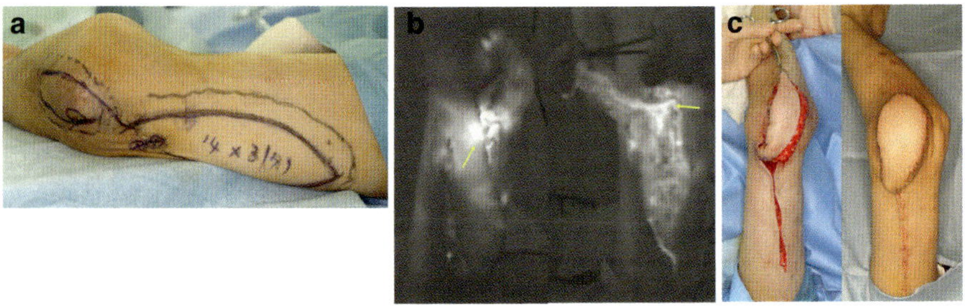

Fig. 22.3 180° Propeller flap
The plate was exposed after bone fixation was performed around the left elbow. Two perforator vessels in the upper arm were identified preoperatively by MDCTA and Doppler sonography (**a**). The skin flap was cut circumferentially under the muscular fasciae to the area of the perforator vessels. After ICG fluorescence angiography was performed to confirm the run of the perivascular branch to penetrate the island skin flap using the Photodynamic Eye (**b**), the perforators were skeletonized to free it from adhesions and turned 180° to cover the loss region. The flap survived completely (**c**)

22.2.4.2 Free Perforator Flap

Free perforator flaps featuring vessel dissection, such as the ALT and DIEP flaps, have been reported to not be subjected to ICG fluorescent contrast examination. We often use this method at the time of the perforasome flap and perforator vessel confirmation during flap defatting (Fig. 22.4).

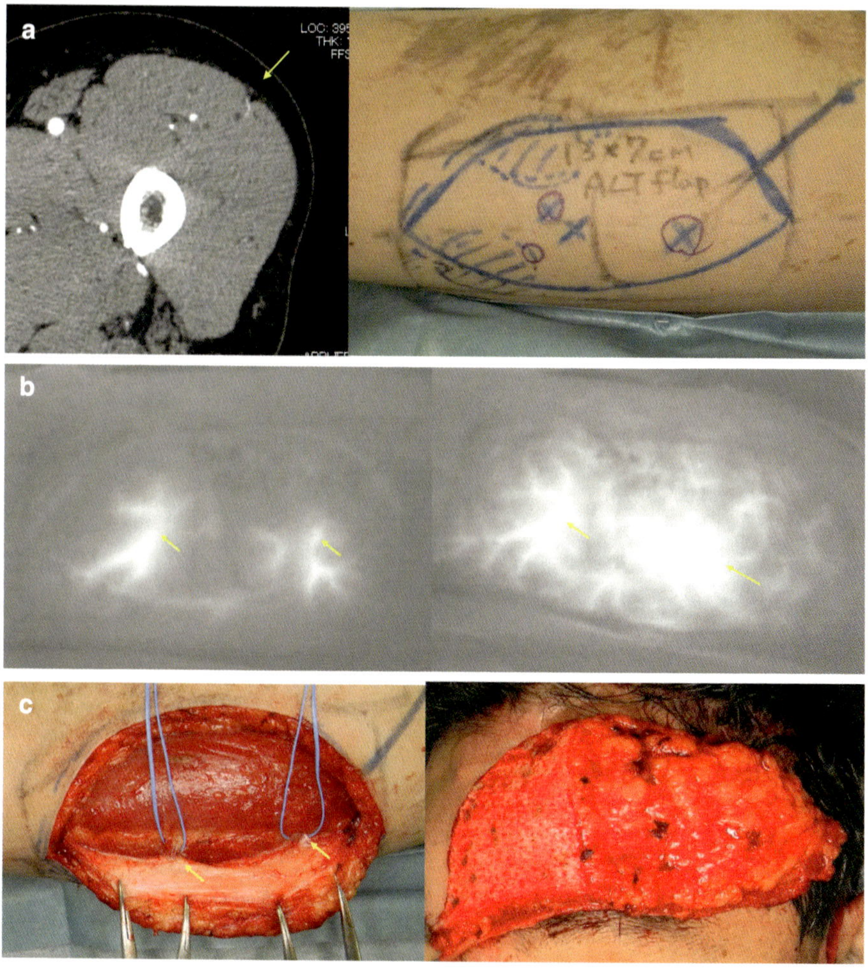

Fig. 22.4 Free ALT flap
Frontal depression was performed after craniotomy. We planned the free ALT flap to include two perforator vessels. The perforator vessels were preoperatively confirmed using MDCTA and Doppler sonography (**a**). Intraoperative ICG fluorescence angiography was performed to confirm the perforator vessels and perforasome in the ALT flap (**b**). Defatting and thinning of the ALT flap were then performed (**c**). The flap survived completely

References

1. Koshima I, Soeda S (1989) Inferior epigastric artery skin flaps without rectus abdominis muscle. Br J Plast Surg 42:645–648
2. Saint-Cyr M, Schaverien M, Rohrich R (2009) Perforator flaps: history, controversies, physiology, anatomy, and use in reconstruction. Plast Reconstr Surg 123:132e–145e
3. Taylor GI, Palmer JH (1987) The vascular territories (angiosomes) of the body: experimental study and clinical application. Br J Plast Surg 40:113e41

4. Taylor GI, Caddy CM, Watterson PA, Crock JG (1990) The venous territories (venosomes) of the human body: experimental study and clinical implications. Plast Reconstr Surg 86:185–213
5. Taylor GI (2003) The angiosomes of the body and their supply to perforator flaps. Clin Plast Surg 30:331e42
6. Saint-Cyr M, Wong C, Schaverien M et al (2009) The perforasome theory: vascular anatomy and clinical implications. Plast Reconstr Surg 124:1529–1544
7. Geddes CR, Morris SF, Neligan PC (2003) Perforator flaps: evolution, classification, and application. Ann Plast Surg 50:90e4
8. Celik N, Wei FC (2003) Technical tips in perforator flap harvest. Clin Plast Surg 30:469e72
9. Blondeel PN, Ali SR (2006) Planning of perforator flaps. In: Blondeel PN, Morris SF, Hallock GG, Neligan PC (eds) Perforator flaps: anatomy, technique, and clinical application, vol I, 1st edn. QMP, St. Louis, p 109e14
10. Mardini S, Tsai FC, Wei FC (2003) The thigh as a model for free style free flaps. Clin Plast Surg 30:473e80
11. Wei FC, Mardini S (2004) Free-style free flaps. Plast Reconstr Surg 114:910e6
12. Morris SF, Neligan PC, Taylor GI (2006) Free-style local perforator flaps. In: Blondeel PN, Morris SF, Hallock GG, Neligan PC (eds) Perforator flaps: anatomy, technique, and clinical application, vol I, 1st edn. QMP, St. Louis, p 948e60
13. Yildirim S, Taylan G, Akoz T (2007) Free-style perforator-based V-Y advancement flap for reconstruction of soft tissue defects at various anatomic regions. Ann Plast Surg 58:501e6
14. Garvey PB, Selber JC, Madewell JE, Bidaut L, Feng L, Yu P (2011) A prospective study of preoperative computed tomographic angiography for head and neck reconstruction with anterolateral thigh flaps. Plast Reconstr Surg 127:1505–1514
15. Satoh T, Kimata Y, Hasegawa K, Namba Y (2011) The utility of multidetector-row computed tomography angiography for evaluating perforators of fibular osteocutaneous flaps. J Reconstr Microsurg 27:29–36
16. Ting JW, Rozen WM, Chubb D, Ferris S, Ashton MW, Grinsell D (2011) Improving the utility and reliability of the deep circumflex iliac artery perforator flap: The use of preoperative planning with CT angiography. Microsurgery 31:603–609
17. Saint-Cyr M, Schaverien M, Arbique G, Hatef D, Brown SA, Rohrich RJ (2008) Three- and four-dimensional computed tomographic angiography and venography for the investigation of the vascular anatomy and perfusion of perforator flaps. Plast Reconstr Surg 121:772–780
18. Schaverien M, Saint-Cyr M, Arbique G, Hatef D, Brown SA, Rohrich RJ (2008) Three- and four-dimensional computed tomographic angiography and venography of the anterolateral thigh perforator flap. Plast Reconstr Surg 121:1685–1696
19. Schaverien MV, Ludman CN, Neil-Dwyer J, Perks GB, Akhtar N, Rodrigues JN, Benetatos K, Raurell A, Rasheed T, McCulley SJ (2011) Contrast-enhanced magnetic resonance angiography for preoperative imaging in DIEP flap breast reconstruction. Plast Reconstr Surg 128:56–62
20. Giunta R, Geisweid A, Feller A (1999) The value of preoperative Doppler sonography for planning free perforator flaps. Plast Reconstr Surg 105:2381–2386
21. Blondeel PN, Beyens G, Verhaeghe R, Van Landuyt K, Tonnard P, Monstrey SJ, Matton G (1998) Doppler flowmetry in the planning of perforator flaps. Br J Plast Surg 51:202–209
22. Liu DZ, Mathes DW, Zenn MR, Neligan PC (2011) The application of indocyanine green fluorescence angiography in plastic surgery. J Reconstr Microsurg 27:355–364
23. Newman MI, Samson MC (2009) The application of laser-assisted indocyanine green fluorescent dye angiography in microsurgical breast reconstruction. J Reconstr Microsurg 25:21–26
24. Onoda S, Azumi S, Hasegawa K, Kimata Y (2013) Preoperative identification of perforator vessels by combining MDCT, Doppler flowmetry, and ICG fluorescent angiography. J Reconstr Microsurg 33:265–269

Chapter 23
Intraoperative Assessment of Intestinal Perfusion Using Indocyanine Green Fluorescence Angiography (ICG-AG) During Pediatric Surgery

Yasushi Iinuma, Yutaka Hirayama, Naoyuki Yokoyama, Tetsuya Otani, Shirou Kuwabara, Hisataka Iida, and Naruki HIgashidate

Abstract We herein report three cases of pediatric surgery in which intraoperative indocyanine green fluorescence angiography (ICG-AG) was performed. A patient with long-gap congenital esophageal atresia underwent gastric transposition for the purpose of esophageal replacement. The good perfusion in mobilized upper esophagus and whole stomach was confirmed with ICG-AG. Subsequently, we could successfully create a gastroesophageal anastomosis, without having to worry about postoperative complications due to perfusion disturbances. In a patient who had undergone massive intestinal resection due to severe intestinal volvulus, the residual region which had been demonstrating abnormal findings by ICG-AG finally developed delayed intestinal stricture.

However, the clinical findings of this region had improved with time in the ICG-AG examination, which had suggested that the intestinal perfusion of this region was preserved. In this case, a perfusion discrepancy between the intestine and the corresponding mesentery was identified, and the presence of this discrepancy was speculated to be the main cause of the delayed intestinal stricture. In a patient with intussusception, the perfusion of the affected region involved in the intussusception had presented long persistent abnormal ICG-AG findings. However, on an empirical basis, it was accepted that the final viability of this affected region would be preserved, in spite of the abnormal ICG-AG findings. We herein demonstrated the feasibility of ICG-AG in pediatric surgical patients, and our findings also suggested that ICG-AG can provide useful information for assessing the intestinal perfusion. However, ICG-AG does not necessarily reflect the mechanism of the patient's specific perfusion disturbance; therefore, when assessing the

Y. Iinuma (✉) • Y. Hirayama • H. Iida • N. HIgashidate
Department of Pediatric Surgery, Niigata City General Hospital, 463-7 Shumoku, Chuo-ku, Niigata 950-1197, Japan
e-mail: iinuma@hosp.niigata.niigata.jp

N. Yokoyama • T. Otani • S. Kuwabara
Department of Digestive Surgery, Niigata City General Hospital, 463-7 Shumoku, Chuo-ku, Niigata 950-1197, Japan

M. Kusano et al. (eds.), *ICG Fluorescence Imaging and Navigation Surgery*,
DOI 10.1007/978-4-431-55528-5_23

intestinal viability with the use of ICG-AG, it is necessary to take into account the possible mechanisms underlying the perfusion disturbances and the individual diseases.

Keywords Indocyanine green fluorescence angiography • Intestinal perfusion • Ischemic injury • Pediatric surgery

23.1 Introduction

In cases of intestinal ischemic injury or digestive surgery in which an intestinal anastomosis is created, the precise assessment of the intestinal viability is necessary to prevent postoperative complications. For the purpose of the intraoperative assessment of the intestinal perfusion, an assessment with the clinical findings of the intestine has been advocated. However, existing methods may provide deceptive findings and are based on the experience of the surgeon. For these reasons, many new techniques for assessing the perfusion of the intestine have been developed.

Recently, the techniques used for the intraoperative assessments of intestinal perfusion have progressed, especially in adult colorectal surgery [1–4]. Among these various techniques, indocyanine green fluorescence angiography (ICG-AG) has been considered to have great potential for clinical use, and the application of this technique has been increasing [3, 4]. However, there have been only a few reports that have described using ICG-AG for pediatric surgical patients [5].

We have used this technique to assess the intestinal perfusion in various pediatric surgical patients since 2011. In this chapter, we present the cases of three pediatric patients in which ICG-AG was performed. We also describe the characteristic points that should be considered, when assessing the intestinal perfusion using this technique in pediatric surgical patients. The details of case 2 and Figs. 23.2a–d and 23.3 have been previously reported [5]. Permission to reuse the contents of that article has been obtained from the publisher.

23.2 The Techniques Used for ICG-AG

ICG-AG was performed according to the method that was previously described in the literature [5]. The photodynamic eye (PDE; Hamamatsu Photonics, Hamamatsu, Japan) fluorescence system was used for the intraoperative imaging. The quantitative changes in the ICG fluorescence intensity over time were analyzed by using an image intensity analysis software program (ROI [region of interest] software; Hamamatsu Photonics K.K.). The various vascular patterns obtained from this intensity analysis software program were classified into four vascular flow patterns, according to the classification described by Matsui et al. [6].

23.3 Case Presentation

23.3.1 Case 1

A 4-month-old male weighing 5,962 g with long-gap congenital esophageal atresia underwent gastric transposition for the purpose of esophageal replacement. After mobilizing the upper esophagus and the whole stomach, ICG-AG was performed to assess the blood perfusion of the esophagus and the whole stomach (Fig. 23.1a). Although the only preserved feeding vessels for the mobilized whole stomach were

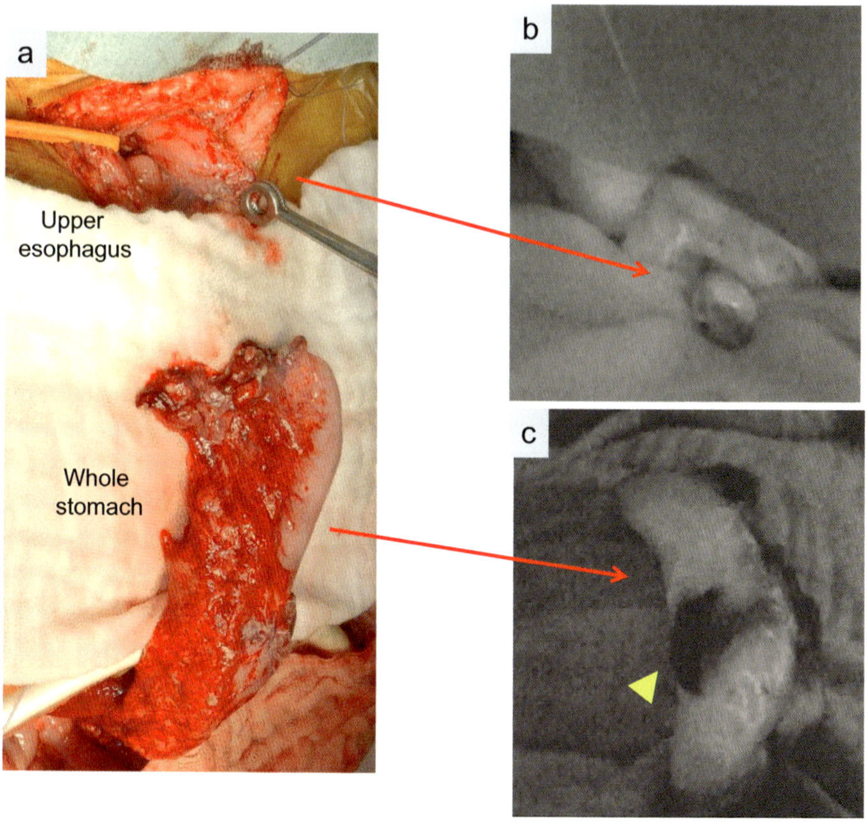

Fig. 23.1 The macroscopic appearance of the mobilized upper esophagus, the whole stomach, and the ICG-AG findings
(**a**): The mobilized upper esophagus and whole stomach of the patient with long-gap congenital esophageal atresia. The only preserved feeding vessels for the mobilized whole stomach were the right gastric and right gastroepiploic arteries. The serosal surface color of both organs showed a normal color
(**b**) and (**c**): The ICG-AG findings obtained immediately following the injection of ICG. The good perfusion was confirmed with ICG-AG in the upper esophagus (**b**) and whole stomach (**c**), except for the small area in which the previous gastrostomy was closed (indicated with an *arrowhead*)

the right gastric and right gastroepiploic arteries, good perfusion in both organs was confirmed with ICG-AG (Figs. 23.1b and c), except for the small area in which the previous gastrostomy was closed (indicated by the arrowhead in Fig. 23.1c). Subsequently, we could successfully create a gastroesophageal anastomosis via the posterior mediastinal route, without having to worry about postoperative complications due to perfusion disturbances, and the postoperative course was uneventful.

23.3.2 Case 2

A 15-year-old male underwent massive intestinal resection due to severe small intestinal volvulus. The residual intestine comprised only 37 cm of proximal jejunum and 7 cm of ileum. The serosal surface color of the distal part of the residual jejunum (DPRJ, the area encircled with the dotted line in Fig. 23.2a) initially showed a slightly darker hue than normal. After several cycles of irrigation of this segment with warm normal saline, the color of the DPRJ improved with time, and the other clinical findings also improved, which was considered to indicate that the perfusion of the DPRJ was preserved. The perfusion of that area was therefore clinically expected to improve with time.

However, the first ICG-AG demonstrated immediate visualization of only a few main trunks of the vasa recta at the DPRJ, which exhibited a slightly darker hue on the serosal surface (Fig. 23.2b and c). Even after the apparent improvement of the color of the DPRJ was obtained, ICG-AG still showed only thin visualization of the vasa recta, including the leading capillary vessels (Fig. 23.2d). Homogeneous visualization of ICG fluorescence was not obtained during this examination. In contrast, in the proximal part of the residual jejunum, the immediate homogenous perfusion of ICG could be observed.

At this time, we finally estimated that the perfusion of the DPRJ was preserved, mainly based on the improvement of the clinical findings of the intestine in spite of the abnormal findings of ICG-AG. The primary anastomosis was performed without additional resection in order to maximize the lengths of the residual intestine. After the initial surgery, the patient developed a delayed partial stricture of the residual intestine, and an additional resection was performed on the 22nd postoperative day. The stricture segment corresponded to the area that presented abnormal findings by ICG-AG at the initial surgery, and this was resected at the second surgery.

The quantitative analysis of changes in the ICG fluorescence intensity over time that was performed on the day after the second surgery showed that the fluorescence intensity at the mesentery gradually increased over time, whereas that observed at the DPRJ demonstrated only a persistent slow increase in intensity and the absence of gradual increases over time (Fig. 23.3). We considered that the pattern of the changes in the ICG fluorescence intensity of the mesentery corresponded to the delayed drainage pattern described by Matsui et al. [6], whereas that of the DPRJ corresponded to the capillary or arterial insufficiency pattern.

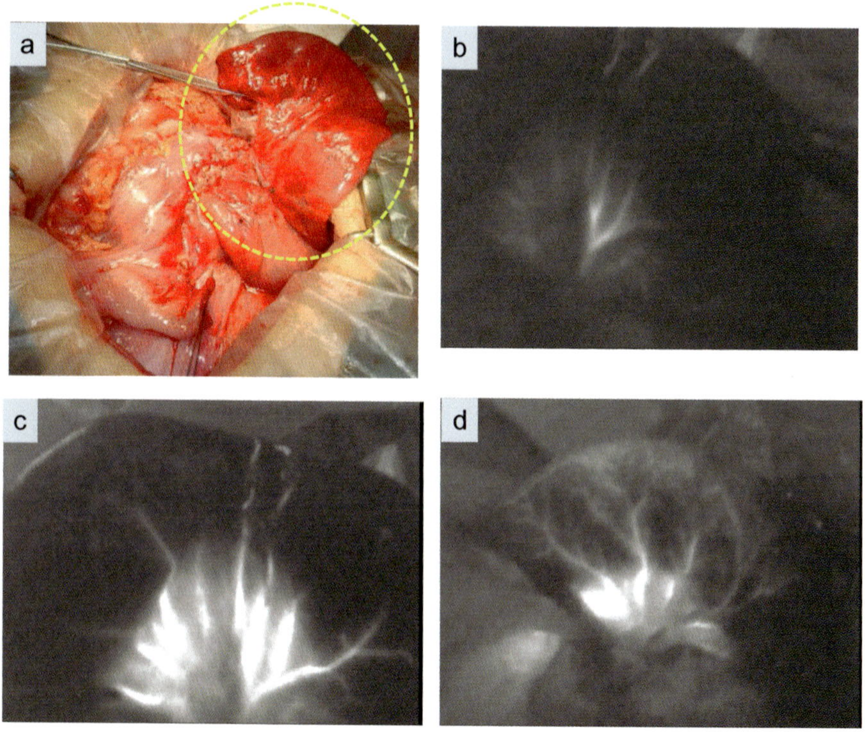

Fig. 23.2 The macroscopic appearance of the residual jejunum following massive intestinal resection and the ICG-AG findings over time
(**a**): The residual jejunum and ileum immediately following massive necrotic intestinal resection. The serosal surface color of the distal part of the residual jejunum (DPRJ, the area encircled with the *dotted line*) showed a slightly darker hue than normal. We considered that the serosal color change shown in (**a**) was caused by transient venous congestion following the release of the intestinal volvulus and could be expected to improve over time
(**b**) and (**c**): These images correspond to the DPRJ in which the serosal surface exhibited a slightly darker hue (indicated with the *encircled dotted line* in (**a**)). Immediate, homogenous visualization of the mesentery was confirmed; however, the same findings were not observed in the intestine except for visualization of only a few main trunks of the vasa recta
(**d**) The findings of ICG-AG about 10 min after the initial intravenous ICG administration at the DPRJ. The capillary vessels communicating with the vasa recta were also gradually visualized

23.3.3 Case 3

A 16-month-old female suffered from ileocecal-type intussusception and underwent surgical reduction at 17 h after the start of the symptoms of the condition. After the reduction, the affected ileocecal regions showed severe congestion and edema, and the serosal surface color of this area showed an apparent darker hue than normal (Fig. 23.4a and b). ICG-AG demonstrated visualization of only a few main trunks of the vasa recta in this area.

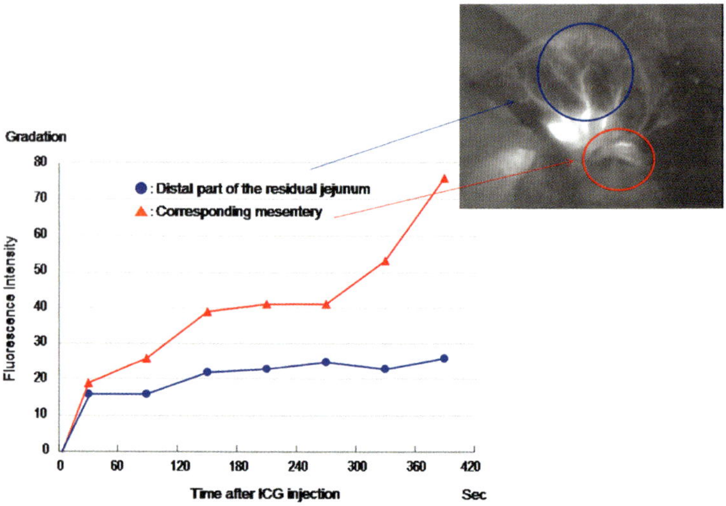

Fig. 23.3 The result of the retrospective quantitative analysis of the changes in the ICG fluorescence intensity at the DPRJ over time after ICG injection at the time of the initial surgery
The fluorescence intensity at the mesentery gradually increased over time, whereas that observed at the DPRJ demonstrated only persistent slow increases in intensity and the absence of gradual increases over time

These findings did not improve for approximately over 10 min, except for the appendix (Fig. 23.4c). Although a quantitative analysis of the changes in the ICG fluorescence intensity over time could not be performed, the ICG fluorescence intensity of the affected ileocecal regions was speculated to correspond to the artificial insufficiency pattern described by Matsui et al. [6].

Based on the ICG-AG vascular pattern exhibited in this region, it would be generally recognized that severe ischemic damage was occurring, and the resection of this region would usually be considered mandatory.

However, in most of the patients with intussusception in which surgical reduction was successful, it is accepted that the perfusion of the affected region will improve with time on an empirical basis. Therefore, additional surgery was not considered to be necessary. The postoperative course was uneventful, and no complications were observed.

23.4 Discussion

In this chapter, we demonstrated that ICG-AG can provide useful real-time information for the assessment of the intestinal perfusion. The feasibility of ICG-AG in pediatric surgical patients was also described.

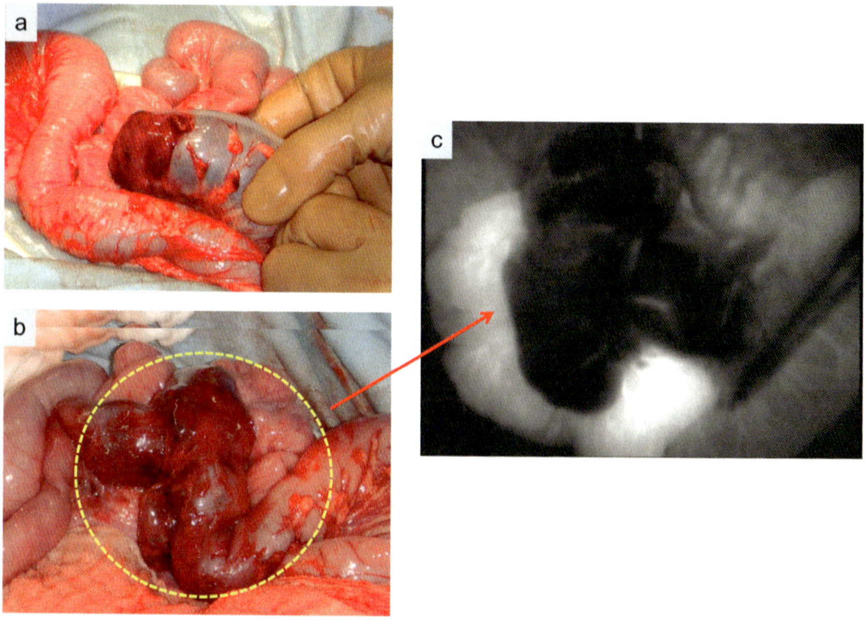

Fig. 23.4 The macroscopic appearance of the ileocecal region in a patient with intussusception and the ICG-AG findings after surgical reduction
(**a**) and (**b**): Panel (**a**) shows the ileocecal region before surgical reduction, and (**b**) shows the same region after surgical reduction (encircled with a *dotted line* in (**b**)). The color of this region after surgical reduction showed a much darker hue than normal
(**c**): ICG-AG demonstrated visualization of only a few main trunks of the vasa recta in this area. These findings did not improve over a period of approximately 10 min. However, on an empirical basis, the additional surgery was not considered to be necessary for this region

In case 1, we could confirm that there was good perfusion even after mobilization of the esophagus and whole stomach. Therefore, we could perform the gastroesophageal anastomosis safely.

Case 2 is considered to be a rare condition that demonstrated the relationship between the results of ICG-AG and the natural final intestinal status in a young human patient. At first, there was a discrepancy between the clinical findings and the results of ICG-AG performed for the assessment of the intestinal perfusion on the affected segment. However, we finally estimated that the perfusion of the DPRJ was preserved, mainly based on the improvement of the clinical findings of the intestine in spite of the abnormal findings of ICG-AG.

From the viewpoint of the final affected intestinal viability, we should have put more weight on the abnormal results of ICG-AG than on the clinical findings.

The findings of that case demonstrated that measurement of the intestinal perfusion based on conventional clinical assessments does not necessarily reflect the precise perfusion status in the intestine.

In this case, the perfusion discrepancy between the affected intestine which developed delayed stricture and the corresponding mesentery was demonstrated at the initial surgery. It is known that 70 % of the mesenteric blood flow is directed to the mucosal and submucosal layers of the bowel, with the reminder supplying the muscle and the serosal layer. Therefore, a vascular flow discrepancy in this region may cause more severe chronic mucosal damage than that affecting the muscle and the serosal layer [7]. Although the precise mechanisms underlying the development of delayed intestinal stricture resulting from intestinal ischemic injury remain unclear, we speculated that the presence of a perfusion discrepancy between the mesentery and corresponding intestine is one of the important causes of delayed intestinal strictures.

In case 3, it was interesting that the persistent abnormal ICG-AG findings did not necessarily reflect the possibility of developing ischemic intestinal injury, in contrast to case 1. Regarding the cause of the persistent abnormal ICG-AG findings in this case, we speculated that this resulted from transient vascular spasm after the reduction of the intussusception [8]. We have not clarified whether these transient vascular spasms were a specific condition that occurs only in patients with intussusception, and further studies are necessary. In contrast to case 1, the clinical course of this case was actually a better predictor of the final outcome than was ICG-AG. We should consider that ICG-AG can only visualize the current status of intestinal perfusion, and it does not necessarily reflect the precise mechanism underlying the vascular perfusion. We should also consider that the discrepancies between the ICG-AG findings and the expected final intestinal viability sometimes exist, especially in pediatric surgical patients.

In conclusion, although further studies are needed to clarify the usefulness of ICG-AG in pediatric surgical patients, our findings suggest that ICG-AG can provide more useful real-time information for the assessment of intestinal perfusion during surgery than can conventional clinical assessment methods. However, when assessing the intestinal viability with this technique, the specific mechanism underlying the perfusion disturbances and the individual diseases should be taken into account. We believe that the routine introduction of this novel technique will reduce the postoperative complication rate after surgery for ischemic intestinal injury in pediatric patients.

Acknowledgment The authors thank Brian Quinn for his critical reading of the manuscript and Tomoharu Mine and Takahiro Irie of IMI Co., Ltd., for their professional assessment of the fluorescence intensity of ICG. The authors also thank Satoshi Takahashi and Kazuhiro Kumagai (Department of Clinical Engineering, Niigata City General Hospital) for their valuable technical assistance.

References

1. Urbanavičius L, Pattyn P, de Putte DV et al (2011) How to assess intestinal viability during surgery: a review of techniques. World J Gastrointest Surg 3:56–69
2. Nachiappan S, Askari A, Am C et al (2014) Intraoperative assessment of colorectal anastomotic integrity: a systemic review. Surg Endosc 28:2513–2530
3. Ris F, Hompes R, Cunningham C et al (2014) Near-infrared (NIR) perfusion angiography in minimally invasive colorectal surgery. Surg Endosc 28:2221–2226
4. Jafari MD, Halabi WJ, Mills SD et al (2013) The use of indocyanine green fluorescence to assess anastomotic perfusion during robotic assisted laparoscopic rectal surgery. Surg Endosc 27:3003–3008
5. Iinuma Y, Hirayama Y, Yokoyama N et al (2013) Intraoperative near-infrared indocyanine green fluorescence angiography (NIR-ICG AG) can predict delayed small bowel stricture after ischemic intestinal injury: report of a case. J Pediatr Surg 48:1123–1128
6. Matsui A, Winer JH, Laurence RG et al (2011) Predicting the survival of experimental ischaemic small bowel using intraoperative near-infrared fluorescence angiography. Br J Surg 98:1725–1734
7. Vollmar B, Menger MD (2011) Intestinal ischemia/reperfusion: microcirculatory pathology and functional consequences. Langenbecks Arch Surg 396:13–29
8. Saltzman DJ, Kerger H, Jimenz JC et al (2013) Microvascular changes following four-hour single arteriole occlusion. Microsurgery 33:207–215

Part XI
Hepato-Pancreatic-Biliary Surgery: Liver

Chapter 24
Basic Aspects of ICG Fluorescence Imaging of the Liver

Mitsuo Kusano, Seiji Ohtsubo, and Shingo Shimada

Abstract ICG itself has long been used for the evaluation of liver function, but the mechanism of the emitted fluorescence following excitation by near-infrared light not only in the liver but also in the lymph nodes remains unclear. In this issue, the kinetics of ICG fluorescent images in hepatocytes in the normal and cirrhotic liver are elucidated macroscopically as well as microscopically using fluorescence microscopy. The time-dependent changes of the fluorescent images of the liver were also investigated using fluorescence microscopy. In the early hepatic phase, examined soon after a systemic injection of ICG, we observed the homogeneous fluorescent image pattern. In the biliary phase, fluorescent cholangiography was demonstrated. Then, in the late hepatic phase, the nodular pattern in the fibrotic or cirrhotic liver and high intense fluorescent illumination were observed several days after the injection of ICG. In fluorescence microscopic observations, the time-dependent transportation of ICG vesicles from the hepatic cytoplasm into bile canaliculi was clearly identified, which provided us valuable microscopic evidence of the time course of the ICG uptake by hepatocytes and the excretion into the bile duct.

Keywords Indocyanine green fluorescence • Cholangiography • Cirrhotic liver • Primary and metastatic liver tumor • Fluorescence microscope

24.1 Introduction

Over the last decade, the clinical applications for the surgical navigation using indocyanine green (ICG) fluorescent images have spread widely [1, 2]. When we were attempting to identify the mesenteric lymph nodes by indocyanine green

M. Kusano (✉)
Department of Surgery, Seiwa Memorial Hospital, 1-5-1-1, Kotoni, Nishi-ku, Sapporo, Hokkaido 063-0811, Japan
e-mail: kusanomitsuo@me.com

S. Ohtsubo • S. Shimada
Department of Oral and Maxillofacial Surgery, Japan Labor Health & Welfare Organization Kushiro Rosai Hospital, Hokkaido, Japan

M. Kusano et al. (eds.), *ICG Fluorescence Imaging and Navigation Surgery*,
DOI 10.1007/978-4-431-55528-5_24

(ICG) fluorescence in animal experiments, we unexpectedly observed that after ICG was injected into the mesenteric fatty tissue, the liver was illuminated by ICG fluorescence. This phenomenon occurred via the ICG flowing into the liver via the portal vein (data not shown). It occurred to us that this unexpected observation might be useful for the identification of liver segments in liver surgery.

We then investigated the use of ICG fluorescence not only for the detection of sentinel nodes of breast and gastrointestinal cancers [1, 2] but also for liver surgery as the "ICG tattooing of liver segments" [3]. Prior to the resection of the liver, we performed the clamping of vessels of the resected liver segment. Immediately after the injection of ICG, no ICG fluorescence could be identified in the vessel-clamped liver segment, but non-clamped liver segments demonstrated bright fluorescence.

Since then, several clinical trials of ICG fluorescent imaging of the liver have been performed such as the detection of liver tumors [4] and the identification of bile leakage [5]. However, it is not clear why ICG emits fluorescence in the liver.

24.2 Fluorescence Images of the Liver After ICG Injected Intravenously

24.2.1 Early Hepatic Phase

At approximately 30 or 40 s after an intravenous injection of ICG, we can identify the fluorescence flow in the hepatic artery (Fig. 24.1a), and several seconds later, we can identify luminal fluorescence flow in the portal vein (Fig. 24.1b). The fluorescence of the collateral portal vein in the portal hypertension was also observed in a cirrhotic patient (Fig. 24.1c).

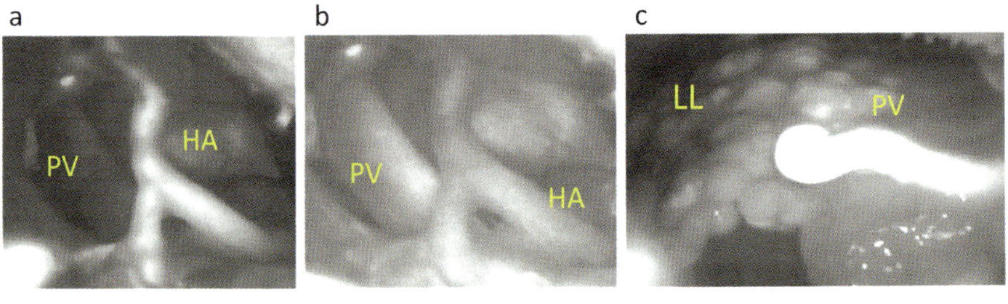

Fig. 24.1 Inflow to the liver. Soon after the injection of ICG, ICG fluorescence flow recognized in common hepatic artery (*HA*) and then in portal vein (*PV*). There was a several-second time lag between the fluorescent image of HA and PV. Pictures of both (**a**) and (**b**) were taken at the operation of pancreaticoduodenectomy. The luminal flow of hepatopetal portal vein was clearly identified with ICG fluorescence (**c**) which was shown in cirrhotic patient. *LL* left lobe

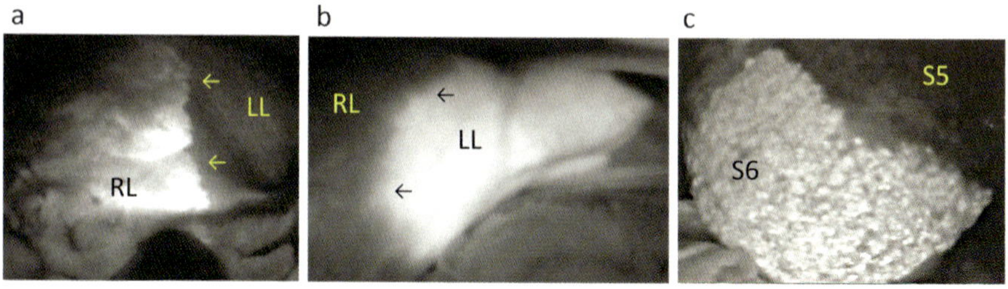

Fig. 24.2 Early hepatic phase. The ICG fluorescence was seen soon after the injection of ICG. These pictures were taken during a hepatectomy ((**a**) left hepatectomy, (**b**) right hepatectomy, and (**c**) S6 segmentectomy). *RL* right lobe, *LL* left lobe, → Cantlie line. The cirrhotic changes are seen in panel (**c**)

After we observed these flows, we saw fluorescence in the entire liver. The fluorescence spread homogeneously throughout the liver within several seconds (Fig. 24.2a–c). During a hepatectomy, the unilateral fluorescent images were seen after clamping the right or left vascular branch of the liver at the hepatic hilum. The tattooing of these hepatic segments was found to be very useful for hepatic surgeries. In addition, the Cantlie line was clearly recognized immediately after the injection of ICG (Fig. 24.2a and b). These findings were very informative for the evaluation of the fluorescence not only in the normal liver but also the cirrhotic liver and tumors in the liver.

The liver began to fluoresce at 40–50 s after the intravenous administration of ICG, which was taken into hepatocytes from the liver sinusoids. The fluorescence then reached a peak for several minutes. This peak was maintained for several hours. At approx. 30 min from the start of the ICG administration, ICG was discharged into the biliary tract via the bile canaliculi. These phenomena reflect the 15-min ICG load test value. The length of time from the uptake of ICG by hepatocytes until the ICG is discharged into the bile duct is relatively short, approx. 10–20 min.

24.2.2 Biliary Phase

One hour after a systemic injection of ICG, we observed the fluorescent images in the biliary tract, which can be described as cholangiography using ICG (Fig. 24.3a, b and c). In an ex vivo experiment, we were also able to detect the fluorescence of a mixture of ICG and bile juice (Fig. 24.3a and b). We evaluated the appropriate dilution ratio of bile juice and ICG solution. The maximum brightness of the ICG fluorescence was observed using the dilution of ICG solution to approx. 100–200-fold.

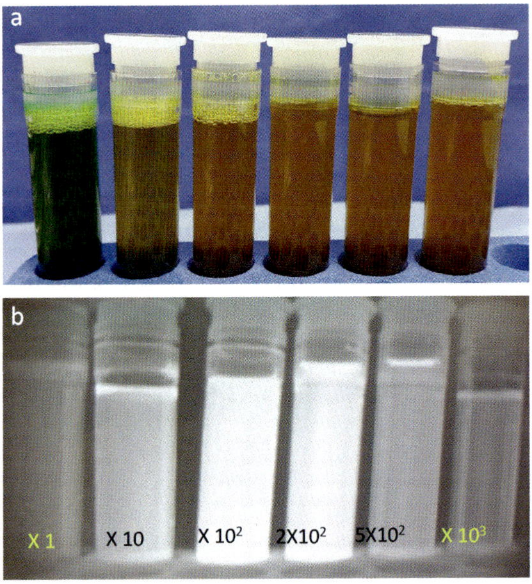

Fig. 24.3 Ex vivo finding of the fluorescence intensity of ICG changes with variations in the ICG concentration. (**a**) Before. (**b**) After excitation by LED: 1 ml of the original ICG solution and 10 ml bile juice combined: the original ICG solution: ICG 25 mg with 10 mL distilled water. The maximum brightness of the ICG fluorescence was observed using the dilution of ICG solution to approx. 100–200-fold. (**c**) Biliary phase. Fluorescent endoscopic picture at the operation of endoscopic cholecystectomy. Around 30 min after injection of ICG, the fluorescence biliary image was obtained, which is applied as the cholangiography at the operation of cholecystectomy

24.2.3 Late Hepatic Phase

ICG can be injected preoperatively as an ICG liver test to provide fluorescent images of liver tumors. We have evaluated the fluorescent images of the noncancerous liver at the late hepatic phase several days after an injection of ICG (Fig. 24.4a and b). In the normal liver, the fluorescence was not seen (Fig. 24.4a), but the retention of fluorescence was observed showing spotty or nodular patterns (Fig. 24.4b).

To detect the tumors and their metastatic lesions in the liver, we injected ICG several days prior to the operation. After a laparotomy, we examined the fluorescent images of the liver using a PDE (photodynamic eye) near-infrared fluorescent imaging system. We found that almost all of the fluorescent images disappeared from the lesions except the fibrotic and cirrhotic lesions, but strong fluorescent images were detected in the cancerous lesions and some types of benign tumors such as small cysts of the liver.

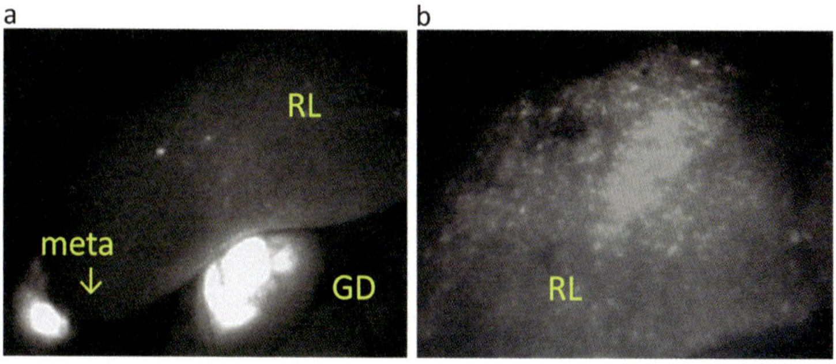

Fig. 24.4 Late hepatic phase. In normal liver, the fluorescent image faded out completely except in the gallbladder (*GB*), metastatic liver tumor (meta), and small cystic lesions (**a**). However, in the fibrotic liver and in the cirrhotic liver, the retention of the fluorescent images was observed in fibrotic or regenerative nodules

24.3 Microscopic Fluorescence Findings of the Liver

To observe fluorescent images in hepatocytes or hepatic tissue, we used a high-performance camera with near-infrared capacity. For the fluorescence observations, we used a Rolera-XR™ digital camera (QImaging, Surrey, BC, Canada) and fluorescence microscope (Eclipse 50i, Nikon, Tokyo). The ORCA-R2 near-infrared camera system (Hamamatsu Photonics, Iwata, Japan) was used for the detection of fluorescence. For the fluorescence microscopy, we used an Eclipse E800 (Nikon). We used an ICG-B-NTE filter set (Opto-Line, Tokyo) with a fluorescent cube for the microscopic observation.

24.3.1 Uptake of ICG in Hepatocytes

We first observed the fluorescence of rat hepatocytes. Immediately after ICG solution was added to the medium, rat hepatocytes fluorescently brightened in the entire cytoplasm of the hepatocyte, but hepatic nuclei did not show fluorescence (Fig. 24.5a). These findings were also observed in hepatocytes that showed a lobular structure in liver tissue (Fig. 24.5b).

We speculate that when ICG is administered intravenously, ICG was taken into hepatocytes through sinusoids into the liver parenchyma by binding to lipoproteins in the blood, and then the hepatocytes were illuminated with fluorescence. The microscopic examination revealed that these early hepatic phase phenomena can be explained as follows: ICG trapped by hepatocytes was transported into the bile canaliculi through the cytoplasm of hepatocytes and then excreted in the bile.

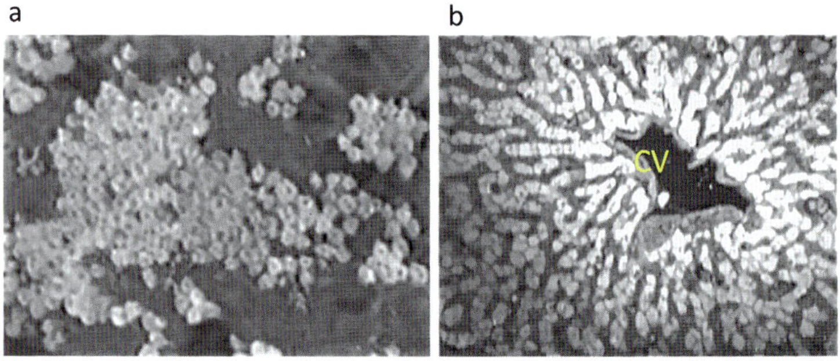

Fig. 24.5 ICG fluorescence in hepatocytes and hepatic lobules. After ICG solution was added to the medium, rat hepatocytes showed fluorescence, but hepatic nuclei did not (**a**). These findings were also observed in the hepatic lobules (**b**)

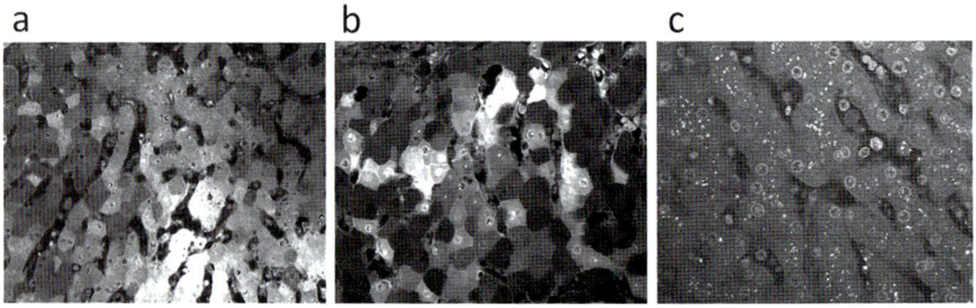

Fig. 24.6 Time-dependent changes of fluorescent images in hepatocytes (porcine liver). The heterogeneity of ICG fluorescent images was observed in biliary (**a**, **b**). After biliary phase, small fluorescent vesicles were seen in the cytoplasm of hepatocytes

24.3.2 *Microscopic Findings of Time-Dependent Changes of Fluorescent Images in Hepatocytes*

Various types of fluorescent illumination were seen in hepatocytes (Fig. 24.6a, b). The fluorescent heterogeneity in hepatocytes may be caused by the difference of timing in the uptake and the excretion of ICG as well as the microvascular differences among hepatocytes. In the early hepatic phase, the time course of the fluorescent images in hepatocytes can be roughly divided into three stages. In the first stage, ICG in the plasma is taken from the sinusoids, and then the entire cytoplasm of the hepatocytes is illuminated with fluorescence. In the second step, small ICG vesicles move from the cytoplasm to bile canaliculi to be excreted into the biliary tract by a vesicle transport mechanism (Fig. 24.7a, b). This can be called the biliary phase.

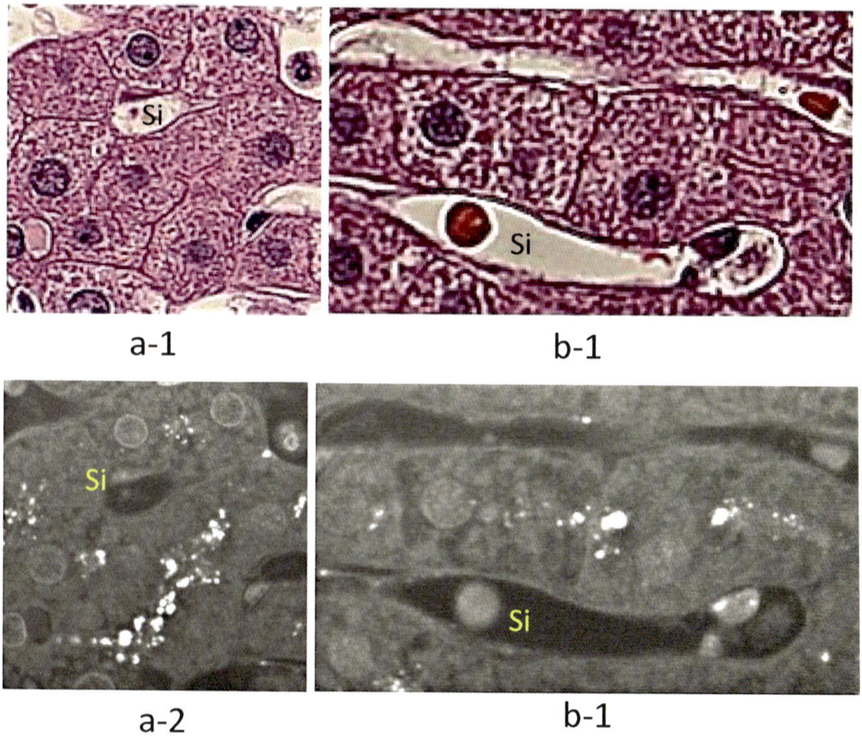

Fig. 24.7 ICG fluorescence vesicles in human hepatocytes. Panels (**a-1**) and (**a-2**) were taken in the same microscopic field, as were panels (**b-1**) and (**b-2**). Panels (**a-1**) and (**b-1**): hematoxylin and eosin stain. Panels (**a-2**) and (**b-2**): fluorescence microscopy. Various types and sizes of ICG vesicles were seen around the biliary surface of the hepatocytes

24.4 Discussion

Our ICG fluorescence findings in the liver in this series were obtained in the process of ICG tattooing or the detection of liver tumors by ICG fluorescent imaging in a clinical setting. Therefore, the timings of ICG administration and of the ICG fluorescent observations were not consistent. However, the evaluation of the fluorescence of the liver works well by the division into three phases (the early hepatic phase, the biliary phase, and the late hepatic phase). In addition, ICG fluorescence of the liver appears to be based on two processes; one is the uptake of ICG into hepatocytes via sinusoids, and the second is the extracellular excretion of ICG into the biliary tract via bile canaliculi which is observed in the early hepatic phase.

The dynamic changes of ICG fluorescence in normal liver in the early phase can be reflected by the plasma clearance of ICG, which was performed as the liver function test. About 90 % of the ICG disappeared from the systemic circulating blood approx. 15 min after the injection of ICG. A delay of ICG clearance was observed in patients with chronic hepatitis and those with cirrhosis. In these patients, we also observed the retention of ICG in fibrotic or regenerative nodules. More intensive ICG fluorescence was seen in hepatocellular carcinoma lesions. We also observed some different ICG fluorescence patterns in the late phase that may reflect the histological degree of differentiation of the tumor in hepatocellular carcinoma and the histological origin of tumors, such as cholangiocellular carcinoma, metastatic cancer, etc.

Clinically, a variety of ICG fluorescent images were observed, but the mechanism underlying the ICG fluorescence in the liver remains to be elucidated. The transportation and behavior of ICG fluorescence particles in hepatocytes are also not well understood. The roles of organelles should be clarified by photochemical investigations, to elucidate the biological behavior of the dynamic fluorescent images not only in the normal liver but also in hepatic tumors.

References

1. Kitai T, Inomoto T, Miwa M, Shikayama T (2005) Fluorescence navigation with indocyanine green for detecting sentinel lymph nodes in breast cancer. Breast Cancer 12:211–215
2. Kusano M, Tajima Y, Yamazaki K, Kato M, Watanabe M, Miwa M (2008) Sentinel node mapping guided by indocyanine green fluorescent imaging: a new method for sentinel node navigation surgery in gastrointestinal cancer. Dig Surg 25(2):103–108
3. Aoki T, Yasuda D, Shimizu Y, Odaira M, Niiya T, Kusano T, Kusano M (2008) Image-guided liver mapping using fluorescence navigation system with indocyanine green for anatomical hepatic resection. World J Surg 32:1763–1767
4. Ishizawa T, Fukushima N, Shibahara MK, Tamura S, Aoki T et al (2009) Real-time identification of liver cancers by using indocyanine green fluorescent imaging. Cancer 115:2491–2504
5. Kaibori M1, Ishizaki M, Matsui K, Kwon AH (2011) Intraoperative indocyanine green fluorescent imaging for prevention of bile leakage after hepatic resection. Surgery 150(1):91–98

Chapter 25
Intraoperative Liver Segmentation Using Indocyanine Green Fluorescence Imaging

Masaki Ueno and Hiroki Yamaue

Abstract Identification of the liver segment during surgery is important for performing anatomical resection. Conventionally, clamping the targeted Glissonian pedicle or dye injection of the targeted Glissonian pedicle has been used to identify the liver segment. Although these methods are simple procedures, they do not depict the intrahepatic segmental plane. Also, dye stain color is transitional and cannot be observed during surgery. Recently, near-infrared fluorescence (NIRF) imaging with indocyanine green (ICG) has been developed as a novel imaging system. In the field of liver surgery, this technique is clinically used for tumor identification, bile leak test, and novel anatomical segmentation during surgery. In this chapter, counterperfusion and direct perfusion methods using NIRF images are proposed to perform intraoperative hepatic segmentation. With these techniques, we can clearly and continuously depict liver segmentation not only on the surface of the liver but also on the intrahepatic segmental plane.

Keywords Hepatic segment • Anatomical resection • Indocyanine green • Near infrared • Hepatocellular carcinoma

25.1 Introduction

25.1.1 Anatomical Liver Resection

In performing hepatic resection, there are two types of procedures. One is anatomical resection and the other is nonanatomical resection. Anatomical resection entails systematic removal of a hepatic segment including the tumor-bearing portal branches and their associated liver parenchyma with tumor. Because hepatocellular carcinoma (HCC) tends to invade into a portal vein and metastasizes the perfusion area of the invaded portal vein, this portal vein-oriented anatomical resection has been theoretically considered oncological resection [1–4].

M. Ueno (✉) • H. Yamaue
Second Department of Surgery, Wakayama Medical University, 811-1 Kimiidera, Wakayama 641-8510, Japan
e-mail: ma@wakayama-med.ac.jp

M. Kusano et al. (eds.), *ICG Fluorescence Imaging and Navigation Surgery*,
DOI 10.1007/978-4-431-55528-5_25

In addition, anatomical resection is preferred because it reduces intraoperative bleeding and rates of postoperative complications because of the preservation of the vascular and biliary structures of the remnant liver [5].

During anatomical liver resection, identification of the hepatic segment is important. Various procedures have been developed to identify the hepatic segment [6, 7]. Although these procedures have been useful, there are some shortcomings. To overcome these shortcomings, a new procedure using indocyanine green (ICG) and its near-infrared fluorescence (NIRF) imaging was developed.

25.1.2 Conventional Procedures for Hepatic Segmentation

The Glissonian approach is one conventional procedure for hepatic segmentation [7]. This technique consists of dissection of the Glissonian sheath from the liver parenchyma toward the targeted Glissonian pedicle (the tumor-bearing area). By clamping the targeted Glissonian pedicle, the planned resection area is outlined as an ischemic area. Although this technique is simple and needs no special equipment, it is technically difficult for some patients needing resection of segment V, VI, VII, or VIII.

Another conventional procedure is a dye staining method involving intraoperative ultrasonography (IOUS) [6]. According to this technique, the tumor-bearing portal pedicle is punctured under IOUS guidance, and then 5 mL of indigo carmine dye is injected into that branch. The stained area becomes evident on the liver surface and guides the appropriate anatomical resection plane. This procedure is also simple. However, this staining is transient and disappears after a short time.

25.1.3 A Novel Method for Hepatic Segmentation Using ICG and NIRF

Optical imaging using NIRF with ICG injection has been recently recognized as a novel technique for intraoperative and real-time imaging diagnosis for various surgical procedures, such as sentinel node navigation for foregut and breast cancer [8–10], checking intraoperative vascular flow of neurovascular surgery [11] and checking graft patency of cardiovascular surgery [12] and liver surgery [13–18].

For liver surgery, there are three ways to use intraoperative NIRF imaging with ICG. One is detection of small metastatic nodules on the liver surface [13–15]; another is liver mapping [16, 17]; and the other is checking bile leakage [18].

In this chapter, we show a novel intraoperative technique for identifying the hepatic segment using NIRF imaging with ICG injection and discuss the usefulness of this technique.

25.2 Materials and Methods

25.2.1 ICG as a Fluorescent Agent

ICG has been widely used in estimating liver functional reserve. ICG features very low toxicity and is thought to shift approximately 90 % of the dose of injected ICG from the vessel into hepatocyte, if the liver functional reserve is normally maintained.

Also, ICG is recognized as a fluorescent agent and has been used in ophthalmology for imaging retinal blood vessels [19]. The absorption and fluorescence spectrum of ICG are in the near-infrared wavelength. Its maximum excitation and emission peaks are at wavelengths 760 nm and 830 nm, respectively, in blood.

25.2.2 NIRF Imaging System

When observing ICG fluorescence, a special near-infrared (NIR) imaging camera is needed. In this chapter, we describe the use of two NIRF imaging systems for open liver surgery: photodynamic eye (PDE; Hamamatsu Photonics, Hamamatsu, Japan) (Fig. 25.1a) and HyperEye Medical System (HEMS; Mizuho Medical, Tokyo, Japan) (Fig. 25.1b).

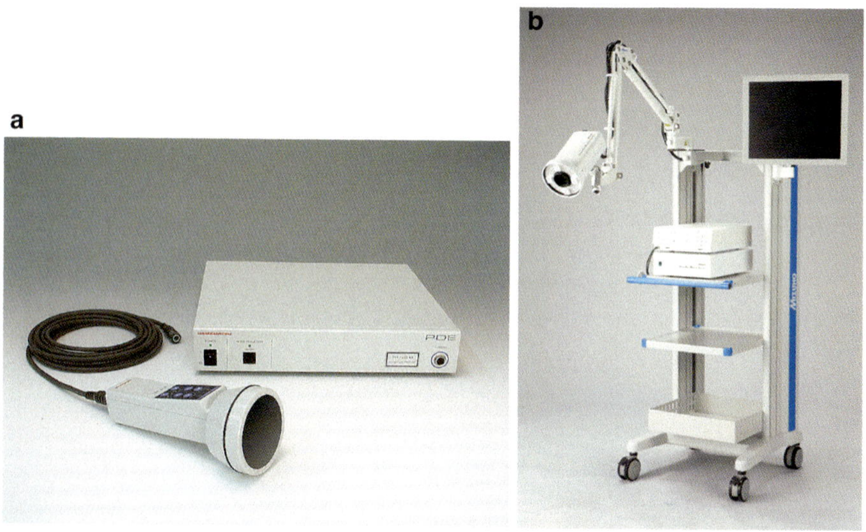

Fig. 25.1 Near-infrared fluorescence imaging system. Photodynamic eye has a single monochrome charge-coupled device (CCD) and outputs gray-scale images (**a**). HyperEye Medical System has a single CCD that has *red*, *green*, *blue*, and infrared filters and can output gray-scale and color plus infrared images (**b**)

PDE irradiates the NIR wavelength of 760 nm by using a red light-emitting diode (LED) and band-pass filter, and the emission peak at the wavelength of 830 nm is observed through the long-wave pass filter and a single monochrome charge-coupled device (CCD) with high sensitivity in NIR waves.

HEMS also irradiates the NIR wavelengths of 760 nm and detects the NIR wavelengths of 830 nm as well as the PDE does. Different from the PDE, HEMS has a single special CCD image sensor that has red, green, and blue filters and also an infrared filter that enables detection of both visible and NIR radiation simultaneously and outputs real-time color and NIR imaging.

25.3 Techniques of ICG Injection for Intraoperative Liver Segmentation

There are two ways to perform ICG injection for intraoperative liver segmentation. One is the counterperfusion method and the other is the direct perfusion method.

25.3.1 *Counterperfusion Method*

The counterperfusion method is based on the Glissonian approach [7]. The procedure of the counterperfusion method is as follows. First, the Glissonian sheath is dissected from the liver parenchyma toward the tumor-bearing Glissonian pedicle from the hilar plate and encircling the Glissonian pedicle (Fig. 25.2a). Next, ligation is performed or a tourniquet is placed, and blood inflow of the planned resection area is occluded (Fig. 25.2b). After that, the surface of the inflow-occluded area becomes ischemic. However, when a patient has a cirrhotic liver, the ischemic change is sometimes unclear (Fig. 25.2c). Then, ICG water solution (1 mL of 2.5 mg/mL) is intravenously injected. The NIRF imaging can be observed approximately 20 s after ICG injection. The blood perfusion area, namely, the remnant hepatic segment, gradually emits ICG fluorescence. Therefore, the planned resection area, where the inflow is occluded, is observed as the nonfluorescent area (Fig. 25.2d).

25.3.2 *Direct Perfusion Method*

The direct perfusion method is performed in the same way as the indigo carmine dye staining method [6]. If a targeted Glissonian pedicle is far from the hilar plate and the counterperfusion method is technically difficult, then this procedure is applied. The procedure is as follows: directly puncture the target portal vein pedicle

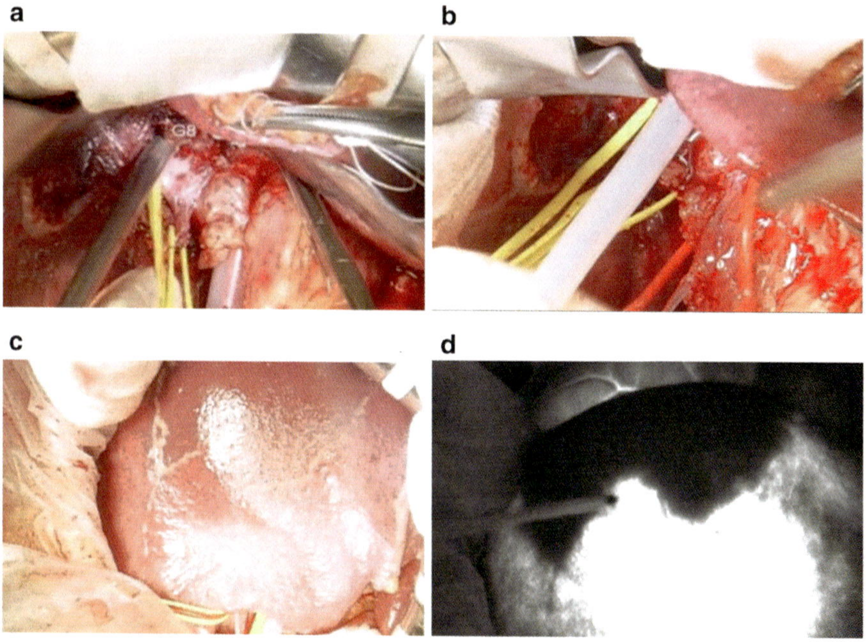

Fig. 25.2 The procedures of counterperfusion method are shown (a case of segment VIII resection). The Glissonian branch of segment VIII (G8) was dissected from the hilar plate (**a**). G8 pedicle was clamped (**b**). Segment VIII became ischemic, but it is not clearly visible (**c**). After peripheral venous injection of 1 mL ICG water solution (2.5 mg/mL), segment VIII was clearly depicted by NIRF imaging (**d**)

with a 23- or 21-gauge needle under IOUS guidance. We puncture approximately 1 cm distal from the target Glissonian pedicle to avoid ICG from straying to some other portal vein branches. Next, 1 mL of 5 mg/mL ICG water solution is injected slowly [16]. Immediately after the ICG injection, the Pringle maneuver is performed to prevent ICG from going away from the liver parenchyma. After that, the NIRF image is observed. In this method, contrary to the perfusion method, the planned resection area shows fluorescence of ICG (Fig. 25.3).

25.4 Imaging Results

25.4.1 Images of the Counterperfusion Method During Liver Resection

We show images of right anterior sectionectomy using this counterperfusion method with the HEMS camera system (Fig. 25.4a–d). After completion of the Pringle maneuver and the Glissonian approach, the Glissonian pedicle of segments

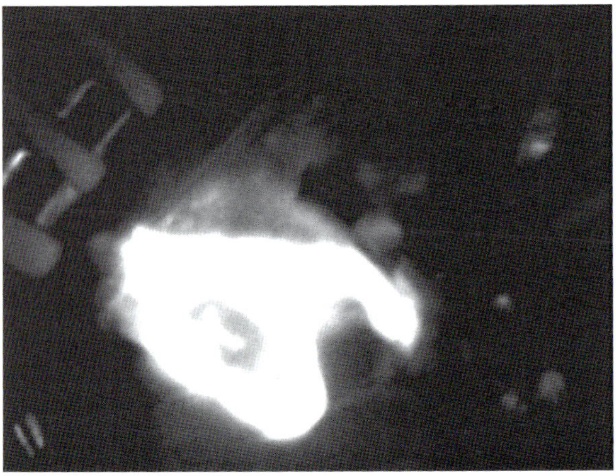

Fig. 25.3 The fluorescent image of direct perfusion method is shown (a case of segment VI resection). Immediately after direct injection of 1 mL ICG water solution (5 mg/mL) to the target portal vein, the planned resection area showed fluorescence

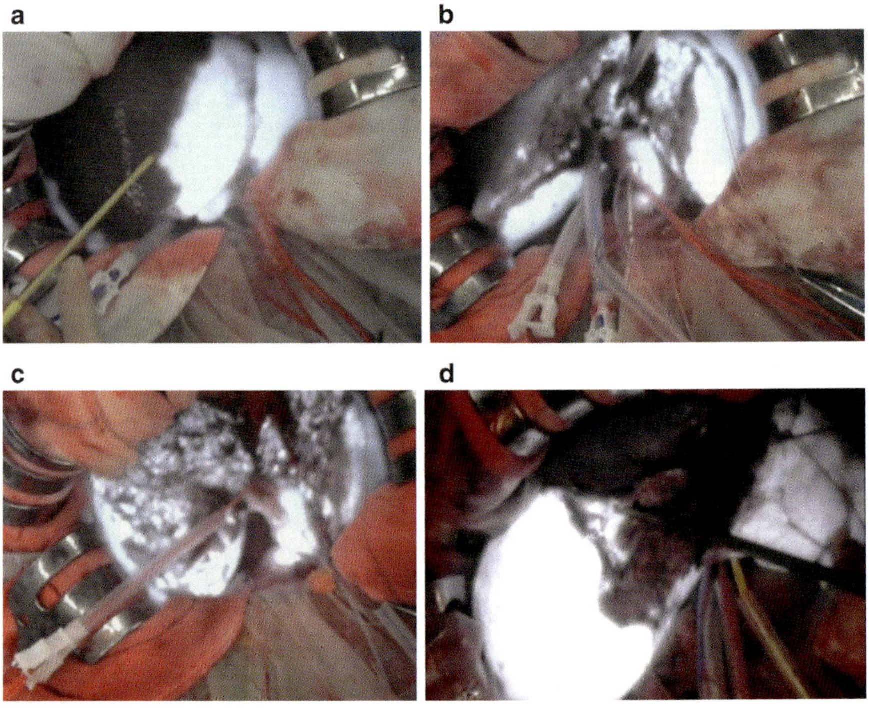

Fig. 25.4 Images of right anterior sectionectomy are shown. The right anterior section was shown as the nonfluorescent area (**a**). During parenchymal resection, the fluorescence was maintained (**b**). If resection is performed as planned, then the fluorescence can be observed on the cut surface (**c**). If not, then the nonfluorescent portion would remain on the cut surface (**d**)

V and VIII was encircled and clamped during the entire surgery. After 1 mL of 2.5 mg/dL ICG water solution was injected intravenously, the NIRF images were observed by using the HEMS camera system. Approximately 60 s after injection, fluorescence had maximum intensity and clearly depicted the planned resection area (Fig. 25.4a). Based on this fluorescent borderline, liver resection was performed. During liver resection, the NIRF image was observed repeatedly, and the resection line or transection plane could be visually checked (Fig. 25.4b). After resection, we could confirm that the resection was performed as planned by observing fluorescence on the cut surface (Fig. 25.4c). When there is a part that does not show fluorescence on the cut surface, then this indicates that the resection might not have been performed as planned, because the nonfluorescent lesion would be a part of a planned resection area (Fig. 25.4d).

25.4.2 Images of the Direct Staining Method During Liver Resection

An image of the segment VI resection using direct perfusion method is shown (Fig. 25.5). Immediately after ICG injection, segment VI emitted strong fluorescence. Because blood inflow was occulted by the Pringle maneuver, ICG remained in segment VI and maintained fluorescence during the Pringle maneuver. Under this Pringle maneuver, we could resect the liver parenchyma while observing fluorescence on the cut surface of the removal side.

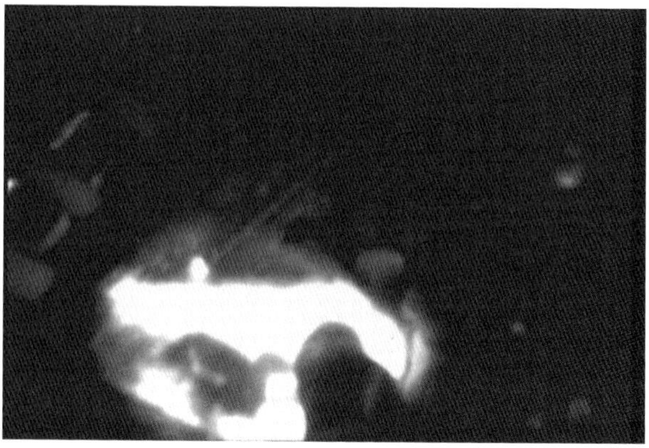

Fig. 25.5 A fluorescent image of segment VI resection using direct perfusion method is shown. Segment VI was depicted as the fluorescent area. Under the Pringle maneuver, the area of segment VI was marked using electrocautery and resected.

25.5 Discussion

Liver anatomy that divides the hepatic parenchyma into segments I to VIII based on the branching form of the Glissonian pedicle is familiar worldwide and is recognized as Couinaud's segmentation. Using Couinaud's segmentation, liver surgeons visualize the existing tumor area and proposed anatomical resection. In addition, because three-dimensional intrahepatic vascular anatomy reconstructed by contrast-enhanced multi-detector row CT images has been easily acquired, precise simulation of anatomical resection could be achieved [20, 21].

In this chapter, we present counterperfusion and direct perfusion methods using novel NIRF imaging with ICG injection for detecting liver segmentation intraoperatively. Hemihepatectomy or left lateral sectionectomy will not always need this NIRF imaging because of its simple cut plane. However, right anterior, right posterior, and left medial sectionectomy, segmentectomy, and anatomical resection less than segmentectomy, which are sometimes complicated in the cut plane, will benefit from these novel methods. Because the counterperfusion method requires dissection of the hilar plate, right anterior, right posterior, and left medial sectionectomy would be suitable for this method. However, resection of segment V, VI, VII, or VIII, during which it is sometimes technically difficult to encircle the root of the Glissonian pedicle, will be favorable for the direct perfusion method.

Conventionally, the Glissonian approach and dye staining method have been useful for detecting segments of the surface of liver parenchyma [7, 6]. Although surgical approaches for these conventional methods are similar to those of our novel methods, imaging results are completely different.

First, we can point out good coloring or fluorescence with ICG-NIRF imaging. In repeat hepatectomy or in cirrhotic liver parenchyma, conventional methods are sometimes not so clear, and it is difficult to depict the resection line. However, in such a situation, ICG-NIRF imaging can provide clear visualization [22]. Additionally, the dye staining method requires hepatic artery clamping to obtain clear coloring [6]. However, the direct perfusion method using ICG does not require clamping of the hepatic artery.

Second, ICG-NIRF imaging can show the intrahepatic transection plane during surgery, which is impossible with conventional methods. This will provide a stable transecting line to the deeper side and will prevent uncertainty during parenchymal resection. This image can be easily obtained by the counterperfusion method. When liver function is well preserved, most of the ICG is taken into hepatocytes 15 min after venous injection; therefore, the remnant liver parenchyma retains the fluorescence during surgery. However, the planned resection area remains a nonfluorescent area.

Recently, the laparoscopic procedure of liver resection has become popular [23]. Along with it, an NIR imaging camera with a laparoscope mounting has been developed and clinically used. Several papers have already reported clinical usage of laparoscopic NIRF imaging. Therefore, our procedures should also be performed laparoscopically in the future [24, 25].

In conclusion, intraoperative identification of the hepatic segment using NIRF imaging with ICG is a novel procedure that should overcome the weaknesses of conventional methods. This method should be applied to navigation surgery of the liver and will be helpful for laparoscopic anatomical resection in the future.

References

1. Eguchi S, Kanematsu T, Arii S, Okazaki M, Okita K, Omata M, Ikai I, Kudo M, Kojiro M, Makuuchi M, Monden M, Matsuyama Y, Nakanuma Y, Takayasu K (2008) Comparison of the outcomes between an anatomical subsegmentectomy and a non-anatomical minor hepatectomy for single hepatocellular carcinomas based on a Japanese nationwide survey. Surgery 143 (4):469–475. doi:10.1016/j.surg.2007.12.003, S0039-6060(08)00082-2 [pii]
2. Agrawal S, Belghiti J (2011) Oncologic resection for malignant tumors of the liver. Ann Surg 253(4):656–665. doi:10.1097/SLA.0b013e3181fc08ca, 00000658-201104000-00005 [pii]
3. Hasegawa K, Kokudo N, Imamura H, Matsuyama Y, Aoki T, Minagawa M, Sano K, Sugawara Y, Takayama T, Makuuchi M (2005) Prognostic impact of anatomic resection for hepatocellular carcinoma. Ann Surg 242(2):252–259, doi:00000658-200508000-00014 [pii]
4. Ahn KS, Kang KJ, Park TJ, Kim YH, Lim TJ, Kwon JH (2013) Benefit of systematic segmentectomy of the hepatocellular carcinoma: revisiting the dye injection method for various portal vein branches. Ann Surg 258(6):1014–1021. doi:10.1097/SLA.0b013e318281eda3
5. Billingsley KG, Jarnagin WR, Fong Y, Blumgart LH (1998) Segment-oriented hepatic resection in the management of malignant neoplasms of the liver. J Am Coll Surg 187(5):471–481
6. Makuuchi M, Hasegawa H, Yamazaki S (1985) Ultrasonically guided subsegmentectomy. Surg Gynecol Obstet 161(4):346–350
7. Takasaki K, Kobayashi S, Tanaka S, Saito A, Yamamoto M, Hanyu F (1990) Highly anatomically systematized hepatic resection with Glissonean sheath code transection at the hepatic hilus. Int Surg 75(2):73–77
8. Kusano M, Tajima Y, Yamazaki K, Kato M, Watanabe M, Miwa M (2008) Sentinel node mapping guided by indocyanine green fluorescence imaging: a new method for sentinel node navigation surgery in gastrointestinal cancer. Dig Surg 25(2):103–108, doi: 000121905 [pii]
9. Troyan SL, Kianzad V, Gibbs-Strauss SL, Gioux S, Matsui A, Oketokoun R, Ngo L, Khamene A, Azar F, Frangioni JV (2009) The FLARE intraoperative near-infrared fluorescence imaging system: a first-in-human clinical trial in breast cancer sentinel lymph node mapping. Ann Surg Oncol 16(10):2943–2952. doi:10.1245/s10434-009-0594-2
10. Hirono S, Tani M, Kawai M, Okada K, Miyazawa M, Shimizu A, Uchiyama K, Yamaue H (2012) Identification of the lymphatic drainage pathways from the pancreatic head guided by indocyanine green fluorescence imaging during pancreaticoduodenectomy. Dig Surg 29 (2):132–139. doi:10.1159/000337306, 000337306 [pii]
11. Raabe A, Beck J, Gerlach R, Zimmermann M, Seifert V (2003) Near-infrared indocyanine green video angiography: a new method for intraoperative assessment of vascular flow. Neurosurgery 52(1):132–139, discussion 139
12. Rubens FD, Ruel M, Fremes SE (2002) A new and simplified method for coronary and graft imaging during CABG. Heart Surg Forum 5(2):141–144
13. Gotoh K, Yamada T, Ishikawa O, Takahashi H, Eguchi H, Yano M, Ohigashi H, Tomita Y, Miyamoto Y, Imaoka S (2009) A novel image-guided surgery of hepatocellular carcinoma by indocyanine green fluorescence imaging navigation. J Surg Oncol 100(1):75–79. doi:10.1002/jso.21272

14. Ishizawa T, Fukushima N, Shibahara J, Masuda K, Tamura S, Aoki T, Hasegawa K, Beck Y, Fukayama M, Kokudo N (2009) Real-time identification of liver cancers by using indocyanine green fluorescent imaging. Cancer 115(11):2491–2504. doi:10.1002/cncr.24291
15. Morita Y, Sakaguchi T, Unno N, Shibasaki Y, Suzuki A, Fukumoto K, Inaba K, Baba S, Takehara Y, Suzuki S, Konno H (2013) Detection of hepatocellular carcinomas with near-infrared fluorescence imaging using indocyanine green: its usefulness and limitation. Int J Clin Oncol 18(2):232–241. doi:10.1007/s10147-011-0367-3
16. Aoki T, Yasuda D, Shimizu Y, Odaira M, Niiya T, Kusano T, Mitamura K, Hayashi K, Murai N, Koizumi T, Kato H, Enami Y, Miwa M, Kusano M (2008) Image-guided liver mapping using fluorescence navigation system with indocyanine green for anatomical hepatic resection. World J Surg 32(8):1763–1767. doi:10.1007/s00268-008-9620-y
17. Uchiyama K, Ueno M, Ozawa S, Kiriyama S, Shigekawa Y, Hirono S, Kawai M, Tani M, Yamaue H (2011) Combined intraoperative use of contrast-enhanced ultrasonography imaging using a sonazoid and fluorescence navigation system with indocyanine green during anatomical hepatectomy. Langenbecks Arch Surg 396(7):1101–1107. doi:10.1007/s00423-011-0778-7
18. Kaibori M, Ishizaki M, Matsui K, Kwon AH (2011) Intraoperative indocyanine green fluorescent imaging for prevention of bile leakage after hepatic resection. Surgery 150(1):91–98. doi:10.1016/j.surg.2011.02.011, S0039-6060(11)00067-5 [pii]
19. Craandijk A, Van Beek CA (1976) Indocyanine green fluorescence angiography of the choroid. Br J Ophthalmol 60(5):377–385
20. Saito S, Yamanaka J, Miura K, Nakao N, Nagao T, Sugimoto T, Hirano T, Kuroda N, Iimuro Y, Fujimoto J (2005) A novel 3D hepatectomy simulation based on liver circulation: application to liver resection and transplantation. Hepatology 41(6):1297–1304. doi:10.1002/hep.20684
21. Takamoto T, Hashimoto T, Ogata S, Inoue K, Maruyama Y, Miyazaki A, Makuuchi M (2013) Planning of anatomical liver segmentectomy and subsegmentectomy with 3-dimensional simulation software. Am J Surg 206(4):530–538. doi:10.1016/j.amjsurg.2013.01.041, S0002-9610(13)00291-2 [pii]
22. Inoue Y, Arita J, Sakamoto T, Ono Y, Takahashi M, Takahashi Y, Kokudo N, Saiura A (2014) Anatomical Liver Resections Guided by 3-Dimensional Parenchymal Staining Using Fusion Indocyanine Green Fluorescence Imaging. Ann Surg. doi:10.1097/SLA.0000000000000775
23. Buell JF, Cherqui D, Geller DA, O'Rourke N, Iannitti D, Dagher I, Koffron AJ, Thomas M, Gayet B, Han HS, Wakabayashi G, Belli G, Kaneko H, Ker CG, Scatton O, Laurent A, Abdalla EK, Chaudhury P, Dutson E, Gamblin C, D'Angelica M, Nagorney D, Testa G, Labow D, Manas D, Poon RT, Nelson H, Martin R, Clary B, Pinson WC, Martinie J, Vauthey JN, Goldstein R, Roayaie S, Barlet D, Espat J, Abecassis M, Rees M, Fong Y, McMasters KM, Broelsch C, Busuttil R, Belghiti J, Strasberg S, Chari RS (2009) The international position on laparoscopic liver surgery: the Louisville Statement, 2008. Ann Surg 250(5):825–830
24. Jafari MD, Lee KH, Halabi WJ, Mills SD, Carmichael JC, Stamos MJ, Pigazzi A (2013) The use of indocyanine green fluorescence to assess anastomotic perfusion during robotic assisted laparoscopic rectal surgery. Surg Endosc 27(8):3003–3008. doi:10.1007/s00464-013-2832-8
25. Cahill RA, Anderson M, Wang LM, Lindsey I, Cunningham C, Mortensen NJ (2012) Near-infrared (NIR) laparoscopy for intraoperative lymphatic road-mapping and sentinel node identification during definitive surgical resection of early-stage colorectal neoplasia. Surg Endosc 26(1):197–204. doi:10.1007/s00464-011-1854-3

Chapter 26
Liver Parenchymal Staining Using Fusion ICG Fluorescence Imaging

Yosuke Inoue, Takeaki Ishizawa, and Akio Saiura

Abstract Anatomic liver resection is established in treating hepatocellular carcinoma or other malignancies to achieve curability and functional preservation. However, the conventional demarcation technique marks only the organ surface and sometimes fails to execute a completely valid demarcation. In this chapter, we describe the efficacy of anatomical liver resection guided by fused images comprising a macroscopic view and indocyanine green fluorescence imaging (IGFI). This method called as fusion IGFI employs a fluorescence imaging system (HyperEye Medical System, Mizuho Ikakogyo Co., LTD, Japan) able to fuse images from the macroscopic and near-infrared ray views on a single monitor. Fusion IGFI includes three approaches of staining, i.e., IV method, PV method, and vein-oriented method, and is a safe imaging technique for anatomic liver resection that attained valid three-dimensional parenchymal demarcation with better feasibility and clearer demarcation than conventional demarcation technique.

Keywords Indocyanine green fluorescence imaging • Anatomical liver resection • Intraoperative diagnosis

Abbreviations

HCC	Hepatocellular carcinoma
IGFI	Indocyanine green fluorescence imaging
HEMS	HyperEye Medical System
ICG	Indocyanine green
IOUS	Intraoperative ultrasonography
CE	Contrast enhanced

Y. Inoue, M.D., Ph.D. (✉) • T. Ishizawa, M.D., Ph.D. • A. Saiura, M.D., Ph.D.
Department of Gastrointestinal Surgery, Cancer Institute Hospital, Japanese Foundation for Cancer Research, 3-8-31 Ariake, Koto-ku, Tokyo 135-8550, Japan
e-mail: inouey-tky@umin.ac.jp

M. Kusano et al. (eds.), *ICG Fluorescence Imaging and Navigation Surgery*,
DOI 10.1007/978-4-431-55528-5_26

26.1 Background

Liver resection requires a precise understanding of the relevant anatomy and real-time navigation of parenchymal dissection. Anatomical resections guided by a demarcation line after portal staining [1–3] or inflow clamping of the target territory [4] are established methods for the curative treatment of hepatocellular carcinoma (HCC) [5, 6], and then subsequently applied to other malignancies. However, these techniques rely on marking of the liver surface to recognize the target territory, and thus surgeons have to determine the three-dimensional resection plane based on the landmark vessels and educated guesswork.

Indocyanine green fluorescence imaging (IGFI) has been reported to be useful in enhancing tumorous lesions, the biliary system, and vessels during upper abdominal surgeries [7–10]. Fusion of IGFI and macroscopic views on a single screen (fusion IGFI) has also allowed clear delineation of arterial flow and biliary anatomy [11].

In this chapter, we describe our experiences of fusion IGFI applied to anatomical liver resections with persistent, three-dimensional parenchymal staining of the target territory [3, 12].

26.2 Methods

26.2.1 Instruments

For fusion IGFI, we used a fluorescence imaging system (HEMS, HyperEye Medical System; Mizuho Ikakogyo Co., Ltd., Japan), which could fuse images from the macroscopic view and the near-infrared ray view on a single monitor (Fig. 26.1a). By this instrument, we could visualize the IGFI image as it would appear in the macroscopic view (Fig. 26.1b, c) [11, 13]. The mode of monitoring could be switched instantly between fusion IGFI and normal macroscopic imaging by turning on or off the near-infrared ray with one button.

26.2.2 Surgical Technique

Terminology surrounding the liver anatomy and resection is defined according to the International Hepato-Pancreato-Biliary Association, Brisbane, classification [14].

The indocyanine green (ICG) staining technique involved either systemic venous injection of a dye after clamping the inflow to the target vessels (IV method), portal puncture and direct injection (PV method), and systemic venous injection after clamping the outflow to the target major hepatic vein

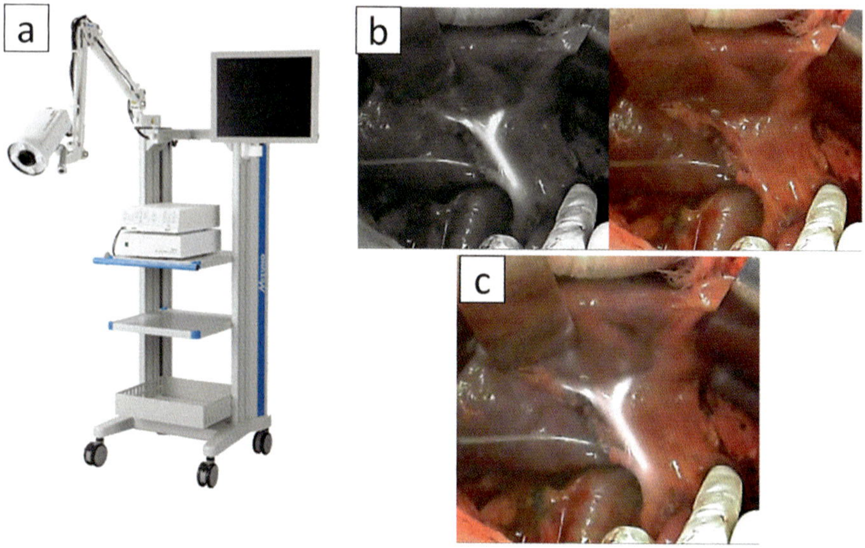

Fig. 26.1 (**a**) External view of HyperEye Medical System
(**b**) The conventional mode of IGFI (*left side*) and macroscopic view (*right side*) of intraoperative cholangiography
(**c**) The fusion IGFI mode. The IGFI image is fused to macroscopic image in a single monitor

(vein-oriented staining method). Macroscopic observation under surgical lights was used to conduct the conventional demarcation technique.

Following a laparotomy with an inverted L-shaped incision, the liver was mobilized adequately according to the planned resection type. With the PV method, intraoperative ultrasonography (IOUS) was performed to confirm the tumor location and tumor-bearing portal branch.

26.2.3 IV Method

After dissection of the hepatic hilum, arterial and portal branches of the future resected hemiliver, section, or segment were exposed and taped. These inflow vessels were first temporarily clamped to confirm the demarcation line and intrahepatic blood flow by US, and then ligated and divided for a subsequent bolus intravenous injection of 2.5 mg ICG. Ten to twenty seconds after ICG injections, the splanchnic arteries and veins appeared enhanced on fusion IGFI, and ICG fluorescence was accumulated in the future remnant territory as counterstaining.

26.2.4 PV Method

After the puncture of the target portal branch, a mixture of 5 ml indigo carmine, 2.5 mg ICG, and 0.5 ml perflubutane suspension (Sonazoid; GE Healthcare, Oslo, Norway) was injected into the branch under contrast-enhanced (CE) IOUS guidance with the hepatic artery clamped. Under harmonic-imaging US guidance, we adjusted the injection speed according to the injection flow visualized in the portal vein to minimize the regurgitation or spillover into the non-eligible branches. The stained region was confirmed by macroscopic inspection, fusion IGFI, and CE-IOUS.

26.2.5 Vein-Oriented Staining

After full mobilization of the future resected liver, the target major hepatic vein was encircled and clamped at its root and 2.5 mg ICG was administered via bolus intravenous injection. After 3–4 min, the ICG had gradually accumulated in the non-veno-occlusive area, i.e., future remnant areas visible by counterstaining.

26.2.6 Acquisition of Fusion IGFI Images

After injection of a dye agent including ICG, video fluorescence images of the liver were recorded with the fusion IGFI camera positioned 40 cm above the subject surface and without surgical lights. Still fusion IGFI images could also be collected using the capture function of HEMS.

26.2.7 Acquisition of Conventional Demarcation Images

To gain conventional demarcation images, the near-infrared ray was turned off and macroscopic images were captured with the same function or with a digital camera under surgical lights.

26.3 Case Presentations

26.3.1 Case 1: IV Method

A 54-year-old woman developed intrahepatic cholangiocellular carcinoma located in the center of left lateral segment invading the umbilical portion, and we planned anatomical resection of left hemiliver.

We performed IV method to gain the counterstaining of left hemiliver. After full mobilization of the left liver, hepatic hilum was dissected, and left hepatic artery and left portal vein were taped, respectively. IOUS was performed and inflow occlusion of left hemiliver was confirmed with selective clamp of both vessels. After ligation and division of these vessels, we administered 2.5 mg ICG intravenously. In 5 min, ICG was well accumulated in the remnant sections as counterstain, and clear demarcation appeared on the liver surface (Fig. 26.2a). Under Pringle maneuver, we performed parenchymal dissection using clamp crashing

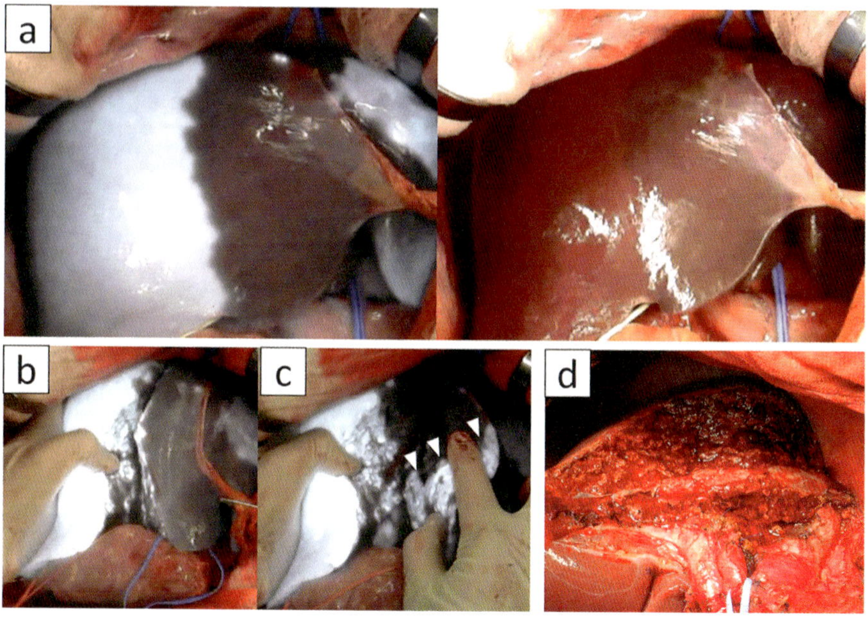

Fig. 26.2 Intrahepatic cholangiocellular carcinoma located in segment 3
(**a**) Fusion IGFI during counterstaining of left hemiliver using IV method (*left side*). The stained area is demarcated clearer than conventional demarcation method by vascular clamping (*right side*)
(**b**) Fusion IGFI during parenchymal dissection. The dissection plane is represented as contour of ICG uptake
(**c**) The deposit of ICG in specimen side (*white arrowheads*) indicates the dissection plane slightly extends toward the segment 5
(**d**) Macroscopic view after resection. The middle hepatic vein is longitudinally exposed as a landmark

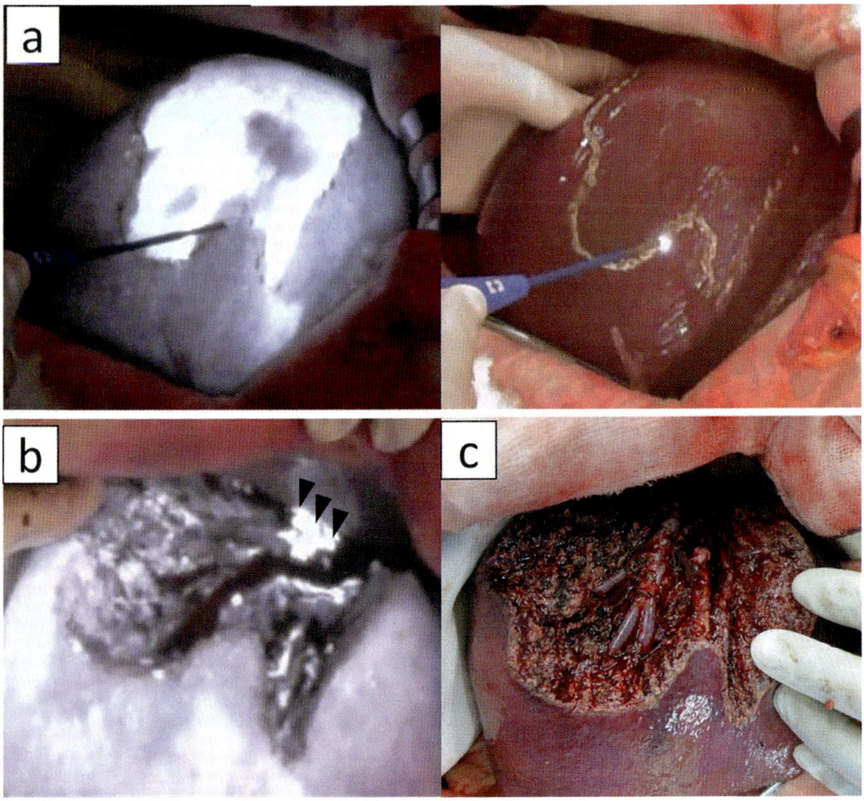

Fig. 26.3 Hepatitis C-related hepatocellular carcinoma located in segment 8
(**a**) Fusion IGFI of parenchymal staining of segment 8 using PV method (*left side*). The stained area is demarcated clearer than conventional indigo carmine staining (*right side*)
(**b**) After resection of segment 8. Fusion ICG indicates the small portion of dorsal area of segment 8 is remnant (*arrowheads*)
(**c**) Macroscopic view after resection. The right and middle hepatic vein is longitudinally exposed as a landmark of intersegmental plane

method. During parenchymal dissection, IGFI showed the intersegmental plane as the contour of parenchymal ICG uptake. During and after parenchymal dissection, we referred fusion IGFI monitor occasionally, judging whether ongoing dissection line is adequate or not (Fig. 26.2b, c, and d).

26.3.2 Case 2: PV Method

A 52-year-old man developed hepatitis C-related HCC located in segment 8 and underwent anatomical resection of this segment.

After mobilization of the liver, intraoperative ultrasonography (IOUS) was performed, and each branch of portal pedicle in segment 8 was identified. We performed PV method targeting the main trunk of segment 8. In this case, the liver surface was poorly stained by conventional method, whereas fusion IGFI showed a clearer stained area than that of the macroscopic indigo carmine stain (Fig. 26.3a) and exactly corresponded to the demarcation line identified in the CE-IOUS and preoperative simulation.

During parenchymal dissection, IGFI showed the intersegmental plane as the contour of parenchymal ICG uptake. After resection, we could evaluate the achievement of the anatomical resection by observing whether or not ICG fluorescence remained in the cut surface of the remnant liver (Fig. 26.3b, c).

26.3.3 Case 3: Vein-Oriented Staining Method

A 51-year-old man had developed synchronous multiple liver metastases from cecal cancer. Synchronous resection of primary lesion and liver metastases was considered. Preoperative and intraoperative imaging analysis showed 16 metastatic tumors located across the liver. Among them, 13 nodules were located within the watershed of the right hepatic vein (RHV). Volumetric analysis indicated that the veno-occlusive area of RHV corresponded to 40 % of total liver, and the liver functional reserve was well maintained. Thus, anatomical resection of the RHV watershed combined with limited resections in left liver was considered to be acceptable. After full mobilization of the right liver, the RHV was encircled and clamped at its root and 2.5 mg ICG was administered via bolus intravenous injection. After 3 min, the ICG had gradually accumulated in the non-veno-occlusive area, i.e., future remnant areas visible by counterstaining (Fig. 26.4a). We conducted parenchymal dissection according to the persistent and three-dimensional staining of the parenchymal border sacrificing the dorsal and lateral branches of segment 8 while preserving the ventral and medial branches, also extending to the segment 5 to clear the tumor margin (Fig. 26.4b). After resection, the watershed of RHV as well as segment 5 was extirpated completely, preserving the territory of ventral area in segment 8 (Fig. 26.4c).

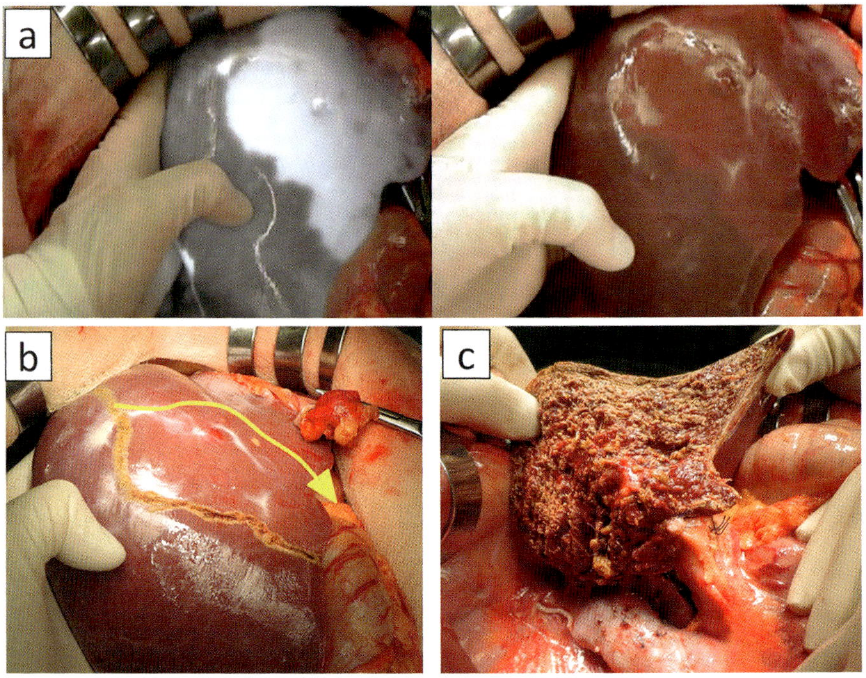

Fig. 26.4 Multiple liver metastases from cecal cancer
(**a**) Fusion IGFI during staining of watershed of the right hepatic vein (RHV) using vein-oriented staining method (*left side*). The stained area is demarcated clearer than conventional demarcation method by simultaneously clamping the RHV and the hepatic artery (*right side*)
(**b**) The actual dissection line is modified to include the nodules in segment 5 (*yellow line*)
(**c**) Macroscopic view after resection. After resection, the watershed of RHV as well as segment 5 was extirpated completely, preserving the territory of ventral area in segment 8

26.4 Comment

In this chapter, we reported novel applications of fusion IGFI to the three-dimensional staining of liver territories. With HEMS, we could safely obtain more precise and clearer navigation of anatomical resection and also record and share objective images among participants.

Anatomical liver resection is traditionally done according to superficial markings generated by dye staining of the portal branch [1, 2] or by shutting off the blood supply of future resection territory [4]. However, these methods have some limitations. First, the dying agent, commonly indigo carmine or methylene blue, may be rapidly washed out resulting in loss of the staining area. Second, in difficult settings such as the bumpy surface of cirrhotic liver or an irregular surface after adhesionectomy, visualizing a clear contour pattern using conventional dying or blood supply-oriented demarcation can be problematic. Third, the direction of parenchymal dissection is dependent on the surgeon's interpretation of the demarcation using landmark vessels, although three-dimensional simulation analysis has shown that the intersegmental plane is not always flat [15].

Despite these limitations, the feasibility of liver demarcation techniques is rarely discussed. Inoue et al. documented the feasibility and usefulness of HEMS in staining the liver territories, comparing the success rate and quantified contrast between HEMS staining and conventional staining. In the report, fusion IGFI using HEMS provided valid and persistent demarcation for almost all cases. On the other hand, conventional techniques achieved valid demarcation in only 41.7 % of patients. Moreover, if the demarcation line is completely invisible, precise anatomical resection remains very difficult. Recently, repeat resection for recurrent HCC [16, 17] or metastasis [18, 19] as well as two-staged hepatectomy for bilobar multiple liver metastasis [20] was reported to improve long-term survival, and in such cases, HEMS could provide robust and clear demarcation.

There are some knacks in staining the target territory by PV method. Minimizing regurgitation into the non-eligible branches is essential to avoid misunderstanding of eligible liver territories, particularly with strongly contrasted demarcation techniques such as IGFI staining. For this purpose and for segmental validation, we injected a mixture of three dye agents in this study: ICG, indigo carmine, and Sonazoid. Under Sonazoid US guidance, we could clearly visualize the injection flow in the portal vein and adjust the optimal injection speed accordingly [21]. Moreover, ICG remained in the area longer than indigo carmine, allowing slow and careful injection. By this method, the target parenchyma could be visualized three-dimensionally also on CE-IOUS, helping us to adjust the dissection direction. However, Sonazoid staining was easily affected by the parenchymal dissection procedure used and the B-mode IOUS, and the staining effect did not last throughout the resection.

Another strong point of fusion IGFI is three-dimensional staining of liver parenchyma as well as strong contrast visible on the liver surface. Watching the IGFI monitor, we could dissect the parenchyma according to the ICG-stained border on the ongoing dissection plane, adjusting the dissection direction toward future specimen or remnant liver, according to the required safety margin or parenchymal preservation [3]. Liver segment mapping with IGFI using a conventional infrared-based navigation system achieved a high success rate in segmental identification [22]. HEMS thus allows a quicker and more direct understanding of the three-dimensional stained area, without the surgeon having to integrate the two separate images in their brain to clearly appreciate the anatomy.

Based on the current results, we advocate using fusion IGFI for open anatomical resections due to the three-dimensional staining ability and clearer demarcation attained by this method compared to a conventional technique. Moreover, we consider the most optimal environment for this method is laparoscopic setting. Anatomical liver segmentectomy [23] or segment staining using IGFI in laparoscopic surgery [24] has recently been reported, although fusion IGFI-guided liver resection has never been reported for laparoscopic liver surgery. Laparoscopic surgery is performed throughout the TV monitor and therefore if the fusion IGFI system could be mounted on the laparoscopic monitoring system, surgeons could view the ordinal and fusion IGFI images in turn via a simple switch without averting one's gaze. Future innovation in interfacing and image resolution would achieve this perspective.

In conclusion, fusion IGFI was applied safely and successfully to anatomical liver resection. Further application of this method must include laparoscopic liver surgery.

References

1. Makuuchi M, Hasegawa H, Yamazaki S (1985) Ultrasonically guided subsegmentectomy. Surg Gynecol Obstet 161(4):346–350
2. Takayama T, Makuuchi M, Watanabe K, Kosuge T, Takayasu K, Yamazaki S, Hasegawa H (1991) A new method for mapping hepatic subsegment: counterstaining identification technique. Surgery 109(2):226–229
3. Inoue Y, Arita J, Sakamoto T, Ono Y, Takahashi M, Takahashi Y, Kokudo N, Saiura A (2014) Anatomical liver resections guided by 3-dimensional parenchymal staining using fusion indocyanine green fluorescence imaging. Ann Surg 262(1):105–111. doi:10.1097/SLA.0000000000000775
4. Takasaki K (1998) Glissonean pedicle transection method for hepatic resection: a new concept of liver segmentation. J Hepatobiliary Pancreat Surg 5(3):286–291
5. Hasegawa K, Kokudo N, Imamura H, Matsuyama Y, Aoki T, Minagawa M, Sano K, Sugawara Y, Takayama T, Makuuchi M (2005) Prognostic impact of anatomic resection for hepatocellular carcinoma. Ann Surg 242(2):252–259. doi:00000658-200508000-00014 [pii]
6. Eguchi S, Kanematsu T, Arii S, Okazaki M, Okita K, Omata M, Ikai I, Kudo M, Kojiro M, Makuuchi M, Monden M, Matsuyama Y, Nakanuma Y, Takayasu K (2008) Comparison of the outcomes between an anatomical subsegmentectomy and a non-anatomical minor hepatectomy for single hepatocellular carcinomas based on a Japanese nationwide survey. Surgery 143 (4):469–475. doi: S0039-6060(08)00082-2 [pii] 10.1016/j.surg.2007.12.003
7. Gotoh K, Yamada T, Ishikawa O, Takahashi H, Eguchi H, Yano M, Ohigashi H, Tomita Y, Miyamoto Y, Imaoka S (2009) A novel image-guided surgery of hepatocellular carcinoma by indocyanine green fluorescence imaging navigation. J Surg Oncol 100(1):75–79. doi:10.1002/jso.21272
8. Ishizawa T, Fukushima N, Shibahara J, Masuda K, Tamura S, Aoki T, Hasegawa K, Beck Y, Fukayama M, Kokudo N (2009) Real-time identification of liver cancers by using indocyanine green fluorescent imaging. Cancer 115(11):2491–2504. doi:10.1002/cncr.24291
9. Ishizawa T, Tamura S, Masuda K, Aoki T, Hasegawa K, Imamura H, Beck Y, Kokudo N (2009) Intraoperative fluorescent cholangiography using indocyanine green: a biliary road map for safe surgery. J Am Coll Surg 208(1):e1–4. doi: S1072-7515(08)01445-2 [pii] 10.1016/j.jamcollsurg.2008.09.024
10. Satou S, Ishizawa T, Masuda K, Kaneko J, Aoki T, Sakamoto Y, Hasegawa K, Sugawara Y, Kokudo N (2012) Indocyanine green fluorescent imaging for detecting extrahepatic metastasis of hepatocellular carcinoma. J Gastroenterol. doi:10.1007/s00535-012-0709-6
11. Kawaguchi Y, Ishizawa T, Masuda K, Sato S, Kaneko J, Aoki T, Beck Y, Sugawara Y, Hasegawa K, Kokudo N (2011) Hepatobiliary surgery guided by a novel fluorescent imaging technique for visualizing hepatic arteries, bile ducts, and liver cancers on color images. J Am Coll Surg 212(6):e33–39. doi: S1072-7515(11)00186-4 [pii] 10.1016/j.jamcollsurg.2011.03.006

12. Inoue Y, Saiura A, Arita J, Takahashi Y (2014) Hepatic vein-oriented liver resection using fusion indocyanine green fluorescence imaging. Ann Surg 14. doi: 10.1097/SLA.0000000000000833
13. Handa T, Katare RG, Nishimori H, Wariishi S, Fukutomi T, Yamamoto M, Sasaguri S, Sato T (2010) New device for intraoperative graft assessment: HyperEye charge-coupled device camera system. Gen Thorac Cardiovasc Surg 58(2):68–77. doi:10.1007/s11748-009-0536-8
14. Strasberg SM (2005) Nomenclature of hepatic anatomy and resections: a review of the Brisbane 2000 system. J Hepatobiliary Pancreat Surg 12(5):351–355. doi:10.1007/s00534-005-0999-7
15. Shindoh J, Mise Y, Satou S, Sugawara Y, Kokudo N (2011) The intersegmental plane of the liver is not always flat--tricks for anatomical liver resection. Ann Surg 251(5):917–922. doi:10.1097/SLA.0b013e3181d773ae
16. Shimada M, Matsumata T, Taketomi A, Yamamoto K, Itasaka H, Sugimachi K (1994) Repeat hepatectomy for recurrent hepatocellular carcinoma. Surgery 115(6):703–706
17. Minagawa M, Makuuchi M, Takayama T, Kokudo N (2003) Selection criteria for repeat hepatectomy in patients with recurrent hepatocellular carcinoma. Ann Surg 238(5):703–710. doi: 10.1097/01.sla.0000094549.11754.e6 00000658-200311000-00011 [pii]
18. Andreou A, Brouquet A, Abdalla EK, Aloia TA, Curley SA, Vauthey JN (2011) Repeat hepatectomy for recurrent colorectal liver metastases is associated with a high survival rate. HPB (Oxford) 13(11):774–782. doi:10.1111/j.1477-2574.2011.00370.x
19. Wicherts DA, de Haas RJ, Salloum C, Andreani P, Pascal G, Sotirov D, Adam R, Castaing D, Azoulay D (2013) Repeat hepatectomy for recurrent colorectal metastases. Br J Surg 100 (6):808–818. doi:10.1002/bjs.9088
20. Adam R, Laurent A, Azoulay D, Castaing D, Bismuth H (2000) Two-stage hepatectomy: a planned strategy to treat irresectable liver tumors. Ann Surg 232(6):777–785
21. Shindoh J, Seyama Y, Umekita N (2012) Three-dimensional staining of liver segments with an ultrasound contrast agent as an aid to anatomic liver resection. J Am Coll Surg 215(2):e5–10. doi: S1072-7515(12)00405-X [pii] 10.1016/j.jamcollsurg.2012.05.017
22. Aoki T, Yasuda D, Shimizu Y, Odaira M, Niiya T, Kusano T, Mitamura K, Hayashi K, Murai N, Koizumi T, Kato H, Enami Y, Miwa M, Kusano M (2008) Image-guided liver mapping using fluorescence navigation system with indocyanine green for anatomical hepatic resection. World J Surg 32(8):1763–1767. doi:10.1007/s00268-008-9620-y
23. Ishizawa T, Gumbs AA, Kokudo N, Gayet B (2012) Laparoscopic segmentectomy of the liver: from segment I to VIII. Ann Surg 256(6):959–964. doi:10.1097/SLA.0b013e31825ffed3
24. Ishizawa T, Zuker NB, Kokudo N, Gayet B (2012) Positive and negative staining of hepatic segments by use of fluorescent imaging techniques during laparoscopic hepatectomy. Arch Surg 147(4):393–394. doi:147/4/393 [pii]

Part XII
Hepato-Pancreatic-Biliary Surgery: Liver Tumors

Chapter 27
Anatomical Hepatectomy Using Indocyanine Green Fluorescent Imaging and Needle-Guiding Technique

Toshiya Kamiyama, Tatsuhiko Kakisaka, Hideki Yokoo, Tatsuya Orimo, Kenji Wakayama, Hirofumi Kamachi, Yosuke Tsuruga, and Akinobu Taketomi

Abstract Anatomical hepatectomy using indocyanine green (ICG) fluorescent imaging and the needle-guiding technique is described in this chapter. Using this procedure, the root of the portal vein of the segment including the hepatocellular carcinoma is punctured with a 22 G Cattelan needle under ultrasonography (US). After backflow is confirmed, 1 mL of diluted (twofold) ICG solution is injected into the branch of the portal vein and monitored by US. The surface of the liver is observed with the ICG fluorescent imaging system. This novel operative procedure using ICG fluorescent imaging is able to clearly visualize the margins between the liver segments. However, this method cannot be used to guide to the root of the relevant portal vein. In order to overcome this disadvantage, an indwelling needle (18 G/65 mm) is used to puncture the outside of the margin of the stained segments under US, and the tip of the outer needle is placed in close proximity of the portal vein. This needle-guiding technique can accurately be used to guide toward the root of the portal vein to be ligated. Moreover, counterstaining with ICG fluorescent imaging defines the avascular segment to be resected as the nonstaining area, and thus, the liver fed by the tumor-bearing portal vein can be successfully resected. Using the ICG fluorescent imaging and needle-guiding technique, anatomical hepatectomy can be performed correctly and safely.

Keywords ICG • Fluorescent image • Hepatectomy • Segmentectomy

---

T. Kamiyama, M.D., F.A.C.S. (✉) • T. Kakisaka, M.D. • H. Yokoo, M.D. • T. Orimo, M.D. • K. Wakayama, M.D. • H. Kamachi, M.D. • Y. Tsuruga, M.D. • A. Taketomi, M.D., F.A.C.S.
Department of Gastroenterological Surgery I, Hokkaido University Graduate School of Medicine, North 15, West 7, Kita-ku, Sapporo, Hokkaido 060-8638, Japan
e-mail: t-kamiya@med.hokudai.ac.jp

M. Kusano et al. (eds.), *ICG Fluorescence Imaging and Navigation Surgery*,
DOI 10.1007/978-4-431-55528-5_27

27.1 Anatomical Resection for Hepatocellular Carcinoma

Liver resection for hepatocellular carcinoma (HCC) has the highest local controllability among all local treatments and results in good survival rates [1, 2]. However, the recurrence rates of HCC continue to remain high even after curative hepatectomy [3]. Many factors related to the prognosis and recurrence of HCC have been reported. Vascular invasion to the portal vein and/or hepatic vein and intrahepatic metastasis are important factors that influence the outcome of hepatic resection [4, 5]. Tumor recurrence in the remnant liver after liver resection is recognized as an intrahepatic metastasis caused by the dissemination of cells in the portal vein or by metachronous multicentric hepatocarcinogenesis [6]. It has been reported that multinodular recurrences are mainly caused by metastatic recurrence from the main tumor via the portal system [7]. HCC invades the portal vein and forms tumor thrombus even when the tumor size is small [8]. On the other hand, since the hepatic segment fed by the portal vein is completely removed by anatomical resection, intrahepatic metastasis caused by disseminated cells in the tumor-bearing portal vein can theoretically be eradicated [9]. A recent report recommended that an anatomical segmentectomy be performed when the size of a single HCC ranges from 2 to 5 cm [10]. We have also reported that anatomical resection improved the surgical outcome of patients with HCC meeting the Milan criteria [11]. Anatomical resection is defined as a resection in which lesion(s) is completely removed anatomically on the basis of Couinaud's classification (segmentectomy, sectionectomy, hemihepatectomy, or more). Sectionectomy and hemihepatectomy can be performed with vascular dissection at the hepatic hilar area using either the individual or Glissonian approach (extrafascial approach). There are two main methods of segmentectomy. The first method uses vascular dissection at the hepatic hilar area using the Glissonian approach (extrafascial approach), and the second uses intraoperative ultrasonography (US) and injection of a dye to distinguish the relevant portal vein; thus, the portal vein is punctured and indigo dye is injected directly in situ [12]. However, segmentectomy is sometimes very difficult to perform using the Glissonian approach alone. It has been reported that segmentectomy can be successfully performed together with vascular dissection at the hepatic hilar area using the Glissonian approach (extrafascial approach) [13]. Although the indigo staining method is effective for determining the segment on the liver surface, it cannot always distinguish the boundary of the segment when hepatitis becomes chronic or cirrhosis develops because the color of the liver is darkened. Also, this method cannot be used to guide to the root of the relevant portal vein or to indicate the cut surface. Herein, we introduce a novel operative procedure using ICG fluorescent imaging and a needle-guiding technique.

27.2 Fluorescent Imaging System

The ICG fluorescent imaging system is described in detail in the paper by Aoki et al. [14]. Briefly, ICG binds to plasma proteins, and protein-bound ICG emits light with a peak wavelength of around 830 nm when exposed to near-infrared light. The fluorescent imaging system used in this study (PDE-neo, PDE-neo C10935-20; Hamamatsu Photonics, Hamamatsu, Japan) captures protein-bound ICG fluorescence when exposed to near-infrared light. The imaging system consists of a light source, a light-emitting diode (LED), which emits light at a wavelength of 760 nm, and a detector consisting of charge-coupled device (CCD) camera, which subsequently filters light with a wavelength of 820 nm. In particular, the sensor is composed of a CCD camera surrounded by 36 LEDs on a small head unit. The captured fluorescence signals are sent to a digital video processor or control unit, which is connected to a computer monitor for immediate visualization [14].

27.3 ICG Staining

Our segmentectomy method is shown in Fig. 27.1. ICG staining is performed intraoperatively using US. Preoperative image examination, in particular, three-dimensional computed tomography (3D-CT), is essential in anatomical resection given the amount of information about the vascular anatomical and tumor location that it provides to the surgeon [15].

Case: The patient presented a HCC of 3 cm in subsegment S8ab of the liver. Preoperative enhanced CT demonstrated the tumor in the segment fed by the portal vein (P8ab) (Fig. 27.2a). The 3D image reconstructed from a 2D-CT image indicated the root of the P8ab (Fig. 27.2b). Subsequently, laparotomy, cholecystectomy, and intraoperative cholangiography were performed to map the bile duct. The right lobe was removed using the Kocher maneuver to visually expose the boundary between the anterior and posterior sections. The whole liver was examined by intraoperative US to detect the intrahepatic metastasis and to confirm the anatomical structures (i.e., of the branches of the hepatic vein and portal vein). For the occlusion of inflow, the hepatoduodenal ligament was encircled by two elastic tapes. Next, the root of the portal vein (P8ab) feeding segment S8ab was punctured with a 22 G Cattelan needle under US. After backflow was confirmed, 1 mL of diluted (2-fold) ICG solution was injected into the branch of the P8ab while monitored by US. The influx of the ICG solution could be observed by US. If the ICG solution overflowed to the nontargeted portal branches, the injection speed was slowed. Following injection of the ICG solution, the inflow to the liver was successively interrupted by occlusion of the hepatoduodenal ligament to prevent the washout of ICG solution. After dimming of the surgical lights, the surface of the liver was observed with the PDE-neo imaging system. The margin of the S8ab became evident and was marked with an electric scalpel (Fig. 27.3a).

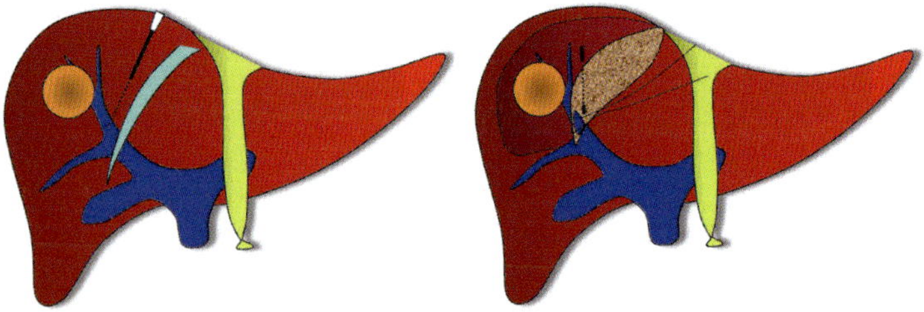

Fig. 27.1 The root of the portal vein (P8ab) feeding segment S8ab was punctured with a 22 G Cattelan needle under ultrasonography (US). After the backflow was confirmed, 1 mL of indocyanine green (ICG) solution (diluted twofold) was injected into the branch of the P8ab under monitoring by US. The indwelling needle 18 G/65 mm then was used to puncture the outside margins of the stained segments under US, and the tip of the outer needle was placed in close proximity of the P8ab

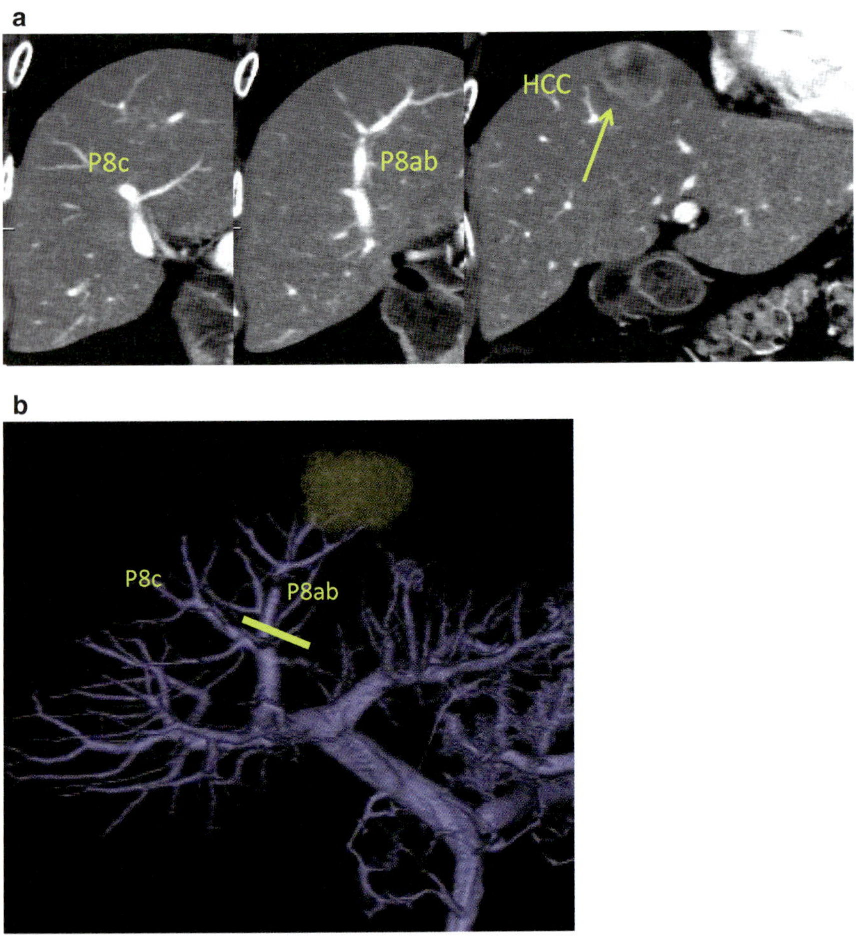

Fig. 27.2 (**a**) Enhanced computed tomography (CT) demonstrated the tumor in the S8ab subsegment. (**b**) Three-dimensional (3D)-CT revealed the P8ab was the tumor-bearing portal vein

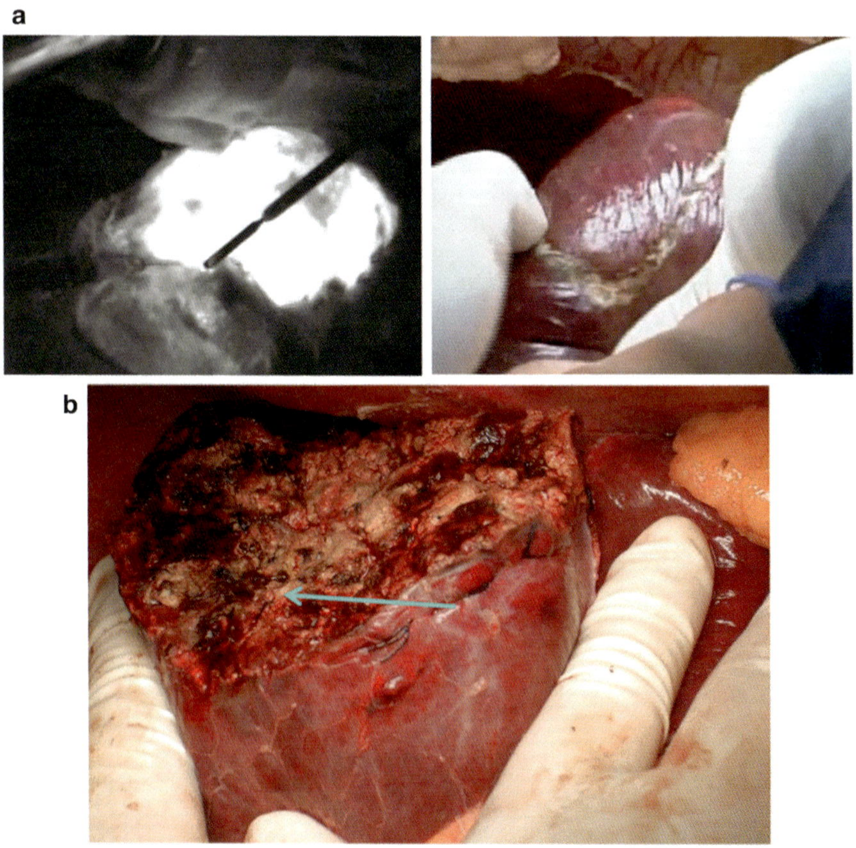

Fig. 27.3 (a) After the injection of the indocyanine green (ICG) solution, the surface of the liver was observed with the PDE-neo imaging system. The boundary of the S8ab could be distinguished and was marked with an electric scalpel. (**b**) The parenchyma dissection was completed along the boundary of the S8ab marked with an electric scalpel. The root of P8ab is indicated by the *arrow*

27.4 Needle-Guiding Technique

Although this method of staining with ICG solution can effectively distinguish segments on the liver surface, it cannot correctly guide to the root of the relevant portal vein and the cut surface. Therefore, to overcome these disadvantages, the indwelling 18 G/65 mm needle is used to puncture the outside of the margin of the stained segments under US, and the tip of the outer needle is placed in close proximity to the P8ab segment (i.e., the needle-guiding technique). This needle is then ligated with a 4-0 silk thread and fixed onto the surface of the liver (Fig. 27.1).

27.5 Hepatectomy

Our standard transection technique of the liver parenchyma is performed using the hook spatula of an ultrasonic harmonic scalpel (Ethicon Endo-Surgery) and a TissueLink DS3.0 monopolar sealer (Classy Med) with soft coagulation mode of VIO300S (ERBE). Vessels are carefully exposed with the hook spatula. Vessels less than 2 mm in diameter are coagulated with the DS3.0 and cut with the hook spatula. Vessels greater than 2 mm in diameter are ligated. Inflow occlusion is applied in an intermittent manner, with 15 min of occlusion alternating with 5 min of reperfusion. During transection of the liver parenchyma, the central venous pressure is maintained below 5 cm H_2O to prevent venous hemorrhage.

In the case described above, after the segmentectomy of the S8ab using ICG staining and the needle-guiding technique, the parenchyma was then dissected near the puncture point. After an initial small dissection of the parenchyma, the outer needle was exposed, and the parenchyma was continuously dissected guided by this outer needle. After the cut surface reached the tip of the outer needle, the Glisson of segment S8ab was located and ligated. The parenchyma dissection was completed along the boundary of the S8ab marked with an electric scalpel (Fig. 27.3b).

27.6 ICG Counterstaining

If the puncture of the tumor-bearing portal branch is difficult, a counterstaining identification technique can be used to puncture the adjacent portal branches [12]. Takayama et al. [16] described how under ultrasonic guidance each of the neighboring portal units can be sequentially stained, thus defining the avascular subsegment to be resected as the nonstaining area for the HCC, in which hepatic arterial and portal venous embolizations were already performed.

In our patient, HCC was located in the S6 (Fig. 27.4a, b). This tumor was treated with transarterial chemoembolization (TACE) three times. Due to the cirrhosis present in the noncancerous liver of this patient, the resectable volume of the liver was limited, and because this tumor-bearing portal vein was narrowed, the US-guiding puncture was very difficult to perform. As a result, the two neighboring portal vein branches were punctured, injected with ICG solution, and the surface of the liver was observed using the PDE-neo imaging system. This counterstaining with ICG fluorescent imaging defined the avascular segment to be resected as the nonstaining area and clearly identified the margins between these two areas (Fig. 27.5a, b). The liver fed by the tumor-bearing portal vein was successfully resected.

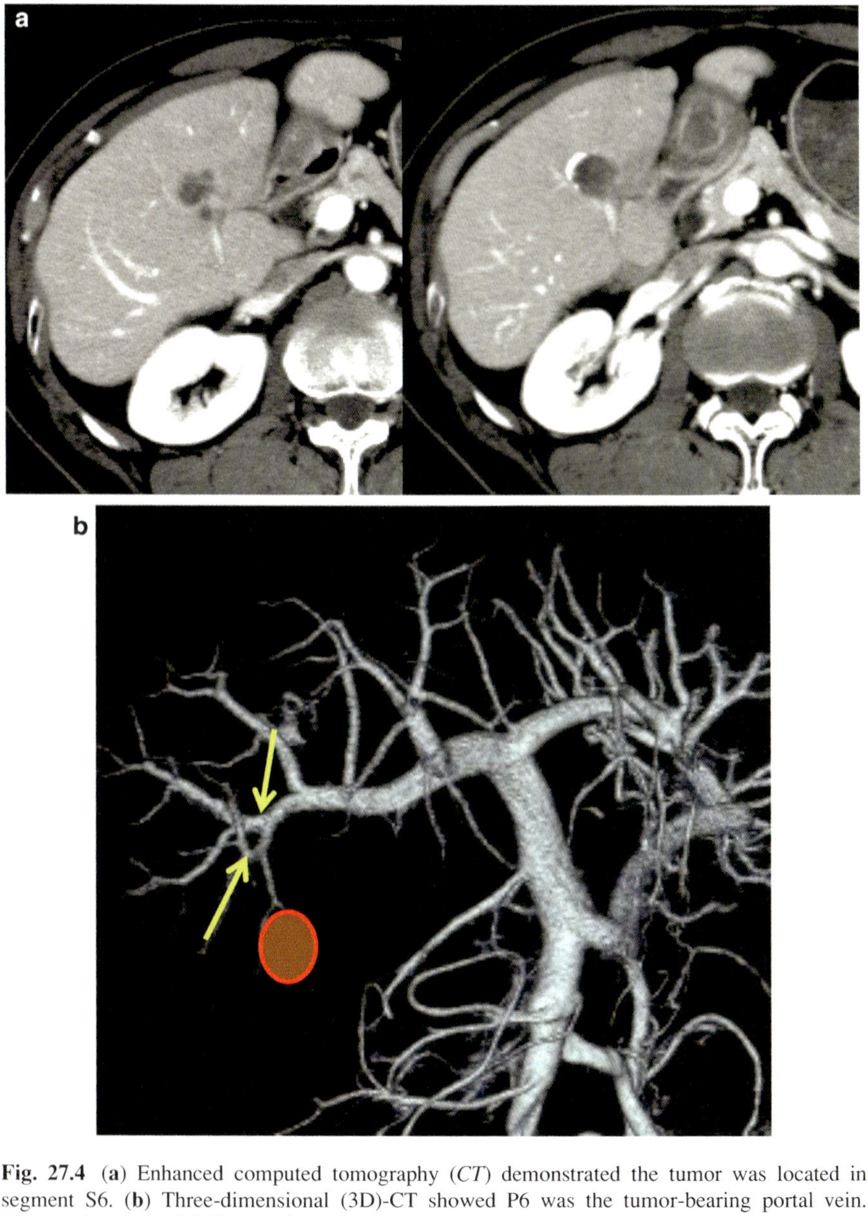

Fig. 27.4 (a) Enhanced computed tomography (*CT*) demonstrated the tumor was located in segment S6. (b) Three-dimensional (3D)-CT showed P6 was the tumor-bearing portal vein. Indocyanine green (*ICG*) was injected into the two points indicated by the *arrows*

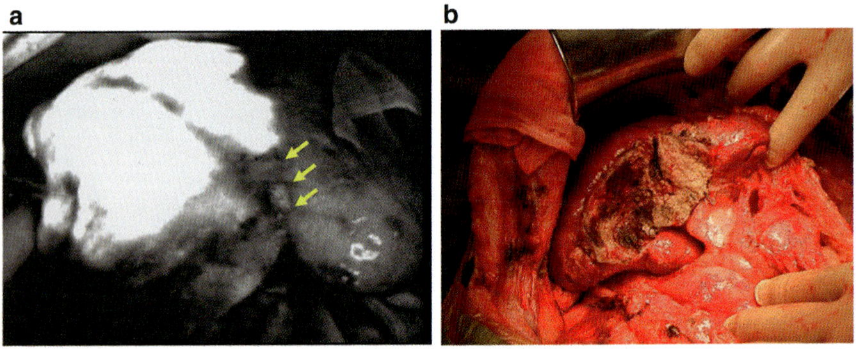

Fig. 27.5 (a) This counterstain with indocyanine green (ICG) fluorescent imaging defined the avascular segment to be resected as the nonstaining area. The margin between segments S5 and S6 is indicated by the *arrows*. (**b**) The parenchyma dissection was completed along the boundary of the S6 segment marked with an electric scalpel

27.7 Conclusion

Although staining with indigo dye is an effective technique for determining segmentation on the surface of the liver, it cannot always distinguish the margins of the segment clearly if the liver develops chronic hepatitis or cirrhosis because the liver darkens in color. Moreover, this method cannot correctly guide to the root of the relevant portal vein and the cut surface. However, the novel procedure reported here using ICG fluorescent imaging is able to clearly visualize the boundary between the segments. Furthermore, coupling imaging with the needle-guiding technique can accurately guide to the root of the portal vein to be ligated.

References

1. Bismuth H, Majno PE, Adam R (1999) Liver transplantation for hepatocellular carcinoma. Semin Liver Dis 19(3):311–322. doi:10.1055/s-2007-1007120
2. Fan ST, Cheung ST, Lo CM (2000) Indications for liver transplantation in patients with chronic hepatitis B and C virus infection and hepatocellular carcinoma. J Gastroenterol Hepatol 15(Suppl):E181–E186
3. Llovet JM, Fuster J, Bruix J (1999) Intention-to-treat analysis of surgical treatment for early hepatocellular carcinoma: resection versus transplantation. Hepatology (Baltimore, MD) 30 (6):1434–1440. doi:10.1002/hep.510300629
4. Margarit C, Escartin A, Castells L, Vargas V, Allende E, Bilbao I (2005) Resection for hepatocellular carcinoma is a good option in Child-Turcotte-Pugh class A patients with cirrhosis who are eligible for liver transplantation. Liver Transplant 11(10):1242–1251. doi:10.1002/lt.20398
5. Poon RT, Fan ST, Lo CM, Liu CL, Wong J (2002) Long-term survival and pattern of recurrence after resection of small hepatocellular carcinoma in patients with preserved liver function: implications for a strategy of salvage transplantation. Ann Surg 235(3):373–382

6. Adachi E, Maeda T, Matsumata T, Shirabe K, Kinukawa N, Sugimachi K, Tsuneyoshi M (1995) Risk factors for intrahepatic recurrence in human small hepatocellular carcinoma. Gastroenterology 108(3):768–775
7. Adachi E, Maehara S, Tsujita E, Taguchi K, Aishima S, Rikimaru T, Yamashita Y, Tanaka S (2002) Clinicopathologic risk factors for recurrence after a curative hepatic resection for hepatocellular carcinoma. Surgery 131(1 Suppl):S148–S152
8. Ikai I, Arii S, Ichida T, Okita K, Omata M, Kojiro M, Takayasu K, Nakanuma Y, Makuuchi M, Matsuyama Y, Yamaoka Y (2005) Report of the 16th follow-up survey of primary liver cancer. Hepatol Res 32(3):163–172. doi:10.1016/j.hepres.2005.04.005
9. Makuuchi M, Hasegawa H, Yamazaki S (1985) Ultrasonically guided subsegmentectomy. Surg Gynecol Obstet 161(4):346–350
10. Eguchi S, Kanematsu T, Arii S, Okazaki M, Okita K, Omata M, Ikai I, Kudo M, Kojiro M, Makuuchi M, Monden M, Matsuyama Y, Nakanuma Y, Takayasu K (2008) Comparison of the outcomes between an anatomical subsegmentectomy and a non-anatomical minor hepatectomy for single hepatocellular carcinomas based on a Japanese nationwide survey. Surgery 143 (4):469–475. doi:10.1016/j.surg.2007.12.003
11. Kamiyama T, Nakanishi K, Yokoo H, Kamachi H, Matsushita M, Todo S (2010) The impact of anatomical resection for hepatocellular carcinoma that meets the Milan criteria. J Surg Oncol 101(1):54–60. doi:10.1002/jso.21414
12. Kishi Y, Hasegawa K, Kaneko J, Aoki T, Beck Y, Sugawara Y, Makuuchi M, Kokudo N (2012) Resection of segment VIII for hepatocellular carcinoma. Br J Surg 99(8):1105–1112. doi:10.1002/bjs.8790
13. Yamamoto M, Katagiri S, Ariizumi S, Kotera Y, Takahashi Y, Egawa H (2014) Tips for anatomical hepatectomy for hepatocellular carcinoma by the Glissonean pedicle approach (with videos). J Hepato-biliary-Pancreat Sci 21(8):E53–E56. doi:10.1002/jhbp.117
14. Aoki T, Yasuda D, Shimizu Y, Odaira M, Niiya T, Kusano T, Mitamura K, Hayashi K, Murai N, Koizumi T, Kato H, Enami Y, Miwa M, Kusano M (2008) Image-guided liver mapping using fluorescence navigation system with indocyanine green for anatomical hepatic resection. World J Surg 32(8):1763–1767. doi:10.1007/s00268-008-9620-y
15. Kamiyama T, Nakagawa T, Nakanishi K, Kamachi H, Onodera Y, Matsushita M, Todo S (2006) Preoperative evaluation of hepatic vasculature by three-dimensional computed tomography in patients undergoing hepatectomy. World J Surg 30(3):400–409. doi:10.1007/s00268-005-0383-4
16. Takayama T, Makuuchi M, Watanabe K, Kosuge T, Takayasu K, Yamazaki S, Hasegawa H (1991) A new method for mapping hepatic subsegment: counterstaining identification technique. Surgery 109(2):226–229

Chapter 28
Microscopic Findings of Fluorescence of Liver Cancers

Shingo Shimada, Seiji Ohtsubo, and Mitsuo Kusano

Abstract Reports detailing microscopic observations of indocyanine green (ICG) fluorescence imaging (IFI) in hepatocellular carcinoma (HCC) and metastatic liver cancer are rare. We were able to perform microscopic IFI results in postoperative paraffin-embedded tissue samples from liver tumors. Methods: Between April 2010 and March 2014, 19 patients with HCC or liver metastases of colorectal tumors underwent liver resection. ICG solution was injected into the peripheral vein from 14 to 2 days prior to operation. After operation, we microscopically performed tissue section IFI using a fluorescence microscope with a near-infrared cube. Results: We observed that IFI characteristics depended on tumor type microscopically. In normal liver tissue, fluorescence consistent with a capillary bile cavity was observed. HCC generally had heterogeneous IFI. Well- or moderately differentiated HCC showed cytoplasmic fluorescence as observed by ICG fluorescence microscopy. Furthermore, poorly and unknown differentiated HCC except one case showed nuclear fluorescence in cancer cells and cytoplasmic fluorescence in the surrounding noncancer cells. In metastatic carcinoma, we observed that non-tumor cells in the marginal region and tumor cells in the central region did not fluoresce. Conclusions: We suggest that the variations in ICG fluorescence imaging patterns may reflect different tumor characteristics. ICG fluorescence in paraffin-embedded tissue samples is preserved in the long term.

Keywords Fluorescence imaging • Hepatocellular carcinoma • Metastatic liver cancer • Microscopic findings

S. Shimada, M.D., Ph.D. (✉)
Department of Surgery, Japan Labor Health & Welfare Organization, Kushiro Rosai Hospital, 13-23 Nakazono-cho, Kushiro, Hokkaido 085-8533, Japan
e-mail: shingoshimada1979@true.ocn.ne.jp

S. Ohtsubo, M.D., Ph.D.
Department of Oral and Maxillofacial Surgery, Japan Labor Health & Welfare Organization, Kushiro Rosai Hospital, 13-23 Nakazono-cho, Kushiro, Hokkaido 085-8533, Japan

M. Kusano, M.D., Ph.D.
Department of Surgery, Seiwa Memorial Hospital, 1-5-1-1, Kotoni, Nishi-ku, Sapporo, Hokkaido 063-0811, Japan

M. Kusano et al. (eds.), *ICG Fluorescence Imaging and Navigation Surgery*,
DOI 10.1007/978-4-431-55528-5_28

28.1 Introduction

Indocyanine green (ICG) combines with serum proteins in vivo and produces a fluorescence signal [1]. ICG fluorescence imaging (IFI) is increasingly being used in fluorescence-guided surgery; i.e., in breast [2], gastric [3, 4], and esophageal cancer [5] surgeries and vascular surgery [6]. Applications of IFI, including tattooing of liver segments [7, 8] and providing biliary tract contrast [9], have been reported in the liver surgery field. Some institutions have recently reported IFI macroscopic features in hepatocellular carcinoma (HCC) and metastatic liver tumors [10–13]. Liver tumors can be observed using fluorescence imaging and generally have heterogeneous fluorescence in the central region of the HCC [10, 11]. In contrast, metastatic liver tumors have a corona-like fluorescence pattern in the marginal region of the tumor [10, 12, 13]. Then, IFI can be used for intraoperative tumor detection. However, there are few reports focused on postoperative IFI samples. Particularly, reports detailing microscopic IFI observations in HCC and metastatic liver tumors are not so many.

In this study, we observed microscopic IFI characteristics in liver tumors using postoperative paraffin-embedded tissue. Therefore, we described the following results.

28.2 Materials and Methods

Between April 2010 and March 2014, 19 patients with liver tumors underwent liver resection at the Japan Labor Health and Welfare Organization, Kushiro Rosai Hospital, Department of Surgery in Kushiro, Japan. This study was approved by the Ethics Committee of the Kushiro Rosai Hospital and performed according to the Helsinki Declaration guidelines.

ICG solution was injected into the peripheral vein from 14 to 2 days prior to the operation.

To evaluate the liver tissue, we also performed intraoperative ICG injection in several cases.

The ICG injection dose was 0.5 mg/kg. IFI in resected liver sections were observed by using a photodynamic emission (PDE) camera (Hamamatsu Photonics, Hamamatsu). After operation, we microscopically observed paraffin-embedded tissue section IFI using a fluorescence microscope with a near-infrared cube (Opto-Line, Tokyo).

28.3 Results

28.3.1 Clinicopathological Characteristics

A total of 19 patients were observed in this study. Of these patients, 12 patients had hepatocellular carcinoma, while seven patients had liver metastases of colorectal cancer (CRC). In HCC patients, the number of males and females was 8 and 4, respectively. Two cases were well differentiated; four cases had moderate differentiation, and five cases had poor differentiation. One case had unknown differentiation. As for noncancerous liver, two cases had normal livers (NL), one case had chronic hepatitis (CH), four cases had liver fibrosis (LF), and five cases had liver cirrhosis (LC). In metastatic liver tumor cases, all patients were male and had no cirrhosis and fibrosis (Table 28.1).

28.3.2 Macroscopic Findings of Fluorescence: Liver Sections

Six HCC cases had total tumor fluorescence emission (total tumor type), four cases had partial tumor fluorescence emission (partial tumor type), and two cases had rim-like fluorescence (rim type) in the liver sections. All cases of well- or moderately differentiated tumors had total tumor-type fluorescence. In five cases with poorly differentiated HCC, there were no tumors with total tumor-type fluorescence, four cases with partial tumor-type fluorescence, and one case (case 9) with rim-type fluorescence. Case 12, which had an unknown HCC differentiation classification, had rim-type fluorescence. In cases of metastatic liver tumors derived from CRC, all cases had rim-like fluorescence at the marginal region of the tumor in the liver sections (Table 28.1).

28.3.3 Microscopic Findings of Fluorescence

Hepatocytes from cirrhotic livers had stronger IFI values than those from non-cirrhotic livers. While hepatocyte IFI values in non-cirrhotic livers were weaker than cirrhotic livers, the IFI values in the sinusoidal lacuna in non-cirrhotic livers were higher than those in cirrhotic livers (Table 28.1, Fig. 28.1a, b).

In hepatocellular carcinoma cases, tumor cells had heterogeneous fluorescence. Well- or moderately differentiated HCC showed cytoplasmic fluorescence as observed by ICG fluorescence microscopy (Table 28.1, Fig. 28.1c, d). Furthermore, poorly and unknown differentiated HCC except one case showed nuclear

Table 28.1 Clinicopathological characteristics and observations of IFI

Case	Age	Sex	Diagnosis	Pathology and differentiation	Noncancerous liver	IFI of section	IFI of microscopy
1	66	F	HCC	Hepatocellular carcinoma-well	LC	Total, heterogeneously	Cytosol of cancer cell
2	79	F	HCC	Hepatocellular carcinoma-well	LF	Total, heterogeneously	Cytosol of cancer cell
3	71	M	HCC	Hepatocellular carcinoma-mod	NL	Total, heterogeneously	Cytosol of cancer cell
4	49	M	HCC	Hepatocellular carcinoma-mod	LC	Total, heterogeneously	Cytosol of cancer cell
5	54	M	HCC	Hepatocellular carcinoma-mod	LC	Total, heterogeneously	Cytosol of cancer cell
6	75	M	HCC	Hepatocellular carcinoma-mod	LF	Total, heterogeneously	Cytosol of cancer cell
7	80	F	HCC	Hepatocellular carcinoma-por	CH	Partial, heterogeneously	Nuclei of cancer cell and cytosol of noncancer cell
8	78	M	HCC	Hepatocellular carcinoma-por	LF	Partial, heterogeneously	Nuclei of cancer cell and cytosol of noncancer cell
9	65	M	HCC	Hepatocellular carcinoma-por	LF	Rim	Nuclei of cancer cell and cytosol of noncancer cell
10	74	M	HCC	Hepatocellular carcinoma-por	LC	Partial, heterogeneously	Cytosol of cancer cell
11	61	M	HCC	Hepatocellular carcinoma-por	LC	Partial, heterogeneously	Nuclei of cancer cell and cytosol of noncancer cell
12	32	F	HCC	Hepatocellular carcinoma-unknown	NL	Rim	Nuclei of cancer cell and cytosol of noncancer cell

13	66	M	Metastasis of CRC	Adenocarcinoma-mod	NL	Rim	Cytosol of noncancer cell
14	70	M	Metastasis of CRC	Adenocarcinoma-mod	NL	Rim	Cytosol of noncancer cell
15	72	M	Metastasis of CRC	Adenocarcinoma-mod	NL	Rim	Cytosol of noncancer cell
16	58	M	Metastasis of CRC	Adenocarcinoma-mod	NL	Rim	Cytosol of noncancer cell
17	45	M	Metastasis of CRC	Adenocarcinoma-mod	NL	Rim	Cytosol of noncancer cell
18	74	M	Metastasis of CRC	Adenocarcinoma-mod	NL	Rim	Cytosol of noncancer cell
19	66	M	Metastasis of CRC	Adenocarcinoma-muc	NL	Rim	Cytosol of noncancer cell

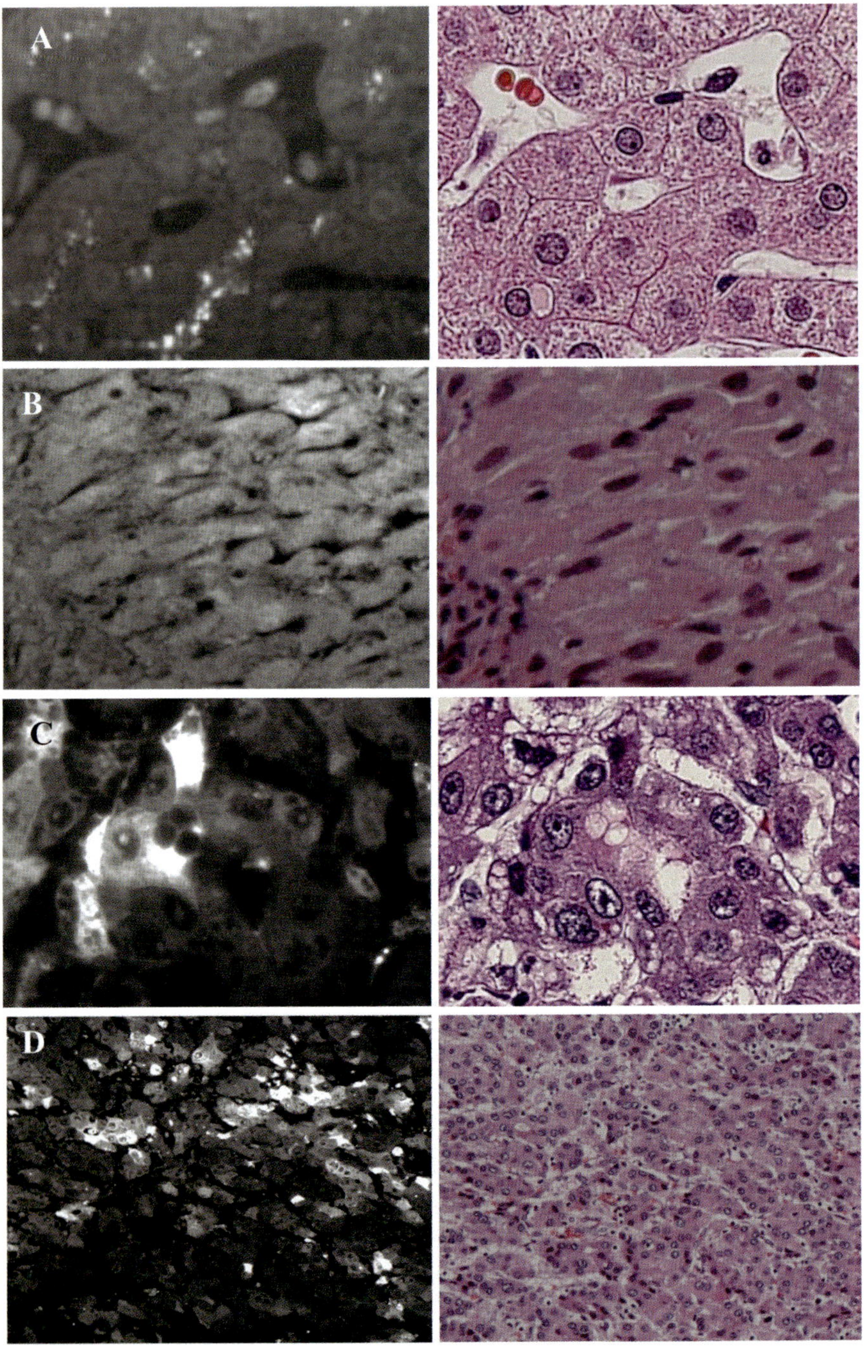

Fig. 28.1 (continued)

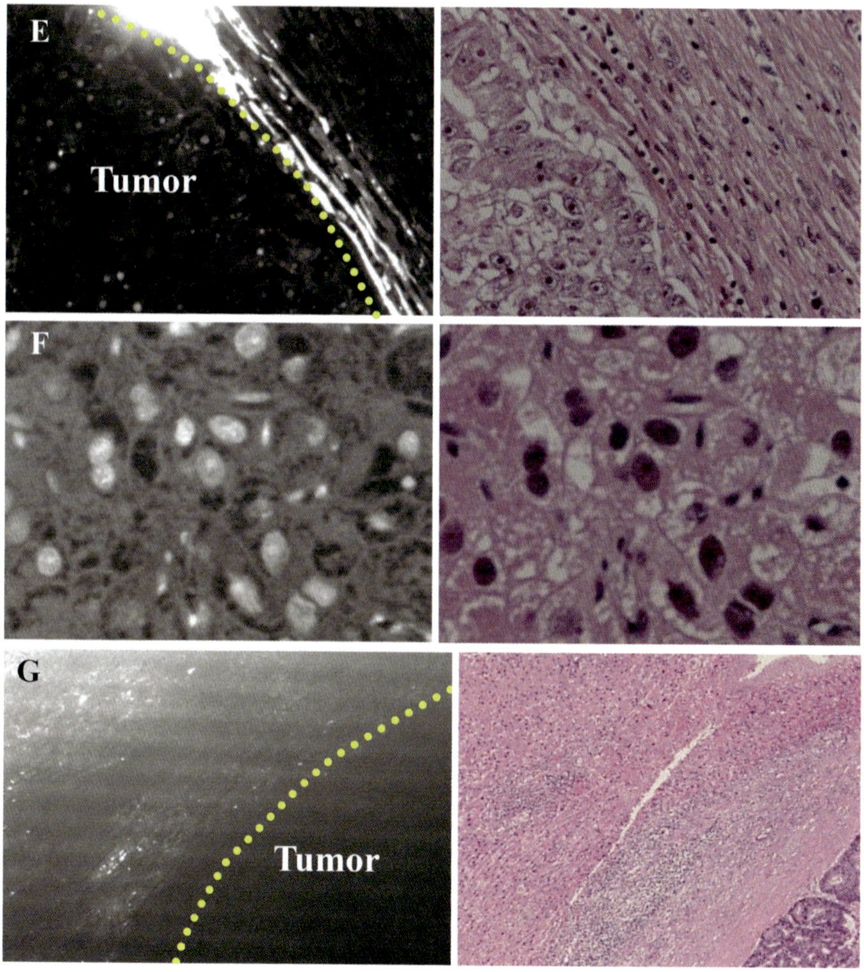

Fig. 28.1 Microscopic findings from ICG fluorescence imaging (IFI) in tissue sections using a fluorescence microscope with a near-infrared cube. (**a**) Normal liver: hepatocyte IFI was not strong; IFI in the sinusoidal lacuna exhibited increased strength (case 3). (**b**) Cirrhotic livers: hepatocytes had stronger IFI than normal livers (case 5). (**c**) IFI was observed in the cytoplasm of cancer cells (case 9). (**d**) IFI was observed in the cytoplasm of cancer cells (case 4). (**e**) Tumor cells had heterogeneous fluorescence. We observed the IFI of cancer cells and of noncancer cells surrounding cancer cells (case 12). (**f**) Nuclear IFI in cancer cells was observed (case 12). (**g**) IFI existed in the cytoplasm of noncancer cells surrounding cancer cells (case 14)

fluorescence in cancer cells and cytoplasmic fluorescence in the surrounding noncancer cells (Table 28.1, Fig. 28.1e, f).

Metastatic liver cancers showed that cytoplasmic IFI in noncancer cells surrounding cancer cells (N) (Fig. 28.1g).

28.4 Discussion

In this study, we were able to observe the microscopic characteristics of different tumor types using ICG fluorescence imaging (IFI). In normal hepatocytes, fluorescence consistent with a capillary bile cavity was observed. In hepatocellular carcinoma, the IFI was heterogeneous and exhibited various patterns. In metastatic carcinoma, we observed that non-tumor cells in the marginal region and tumor cells in the central region did not fluoresce.

ICG is generally used as a liver function assay [14]. Moreover, ICG, which is approved by the Food and Drug Administration, is safe and comparatively economical. ICG combines with serum proteins in vivo and fluoresces under excitation at 760–820 nm [1].

In animal experiments, ICG that was injected into the peripheral vein accumulated in the liver [15] demonstrating that ICG has a high affinity for the liver. OATP1B3 and NTCP have been demonstrated to transport ICG [16]. Eisai rats that lack functional MRP2 revealed that biliary ICG excretion is mediated by MRP2 [17].

Ishizawa et al. reported that well- or moderately differentiated HCC mostly displayed uniform or partial type fluorescence, poorly differentiated HCC mostly displayed rim-type fluorescence, and metastatic tumors mostly displayed rim-type fluorescence [10] in part because the degree of NTCP and OATP8 expression varied according to tumor differentiation [18]. The results of this study also showed similar pattern. They also reported that HCC of the total or partial tumor type exhibited fluorescence within the cytoplasm and pseudoglands under ICG fluorescence imaging. Additionally, HCC or metastatic cancer with the rim type had ICG fluorescence in noncancer cells surrounding cancer cells [18]. They suggested that the cause was the following: While ICG portal uptake ability was preserved, biliary excretion ability was reduced in differentiated HCC [18]. The biliary excretion ability of normal hepatocytes declined due to compression from the tumor in poorly differentiated HCC or metastatic cancer. Consistent with these reports, in the present study, it was observed that the differentiated HCC exhibited fluorescence cytoplasmic signal under ICG fluorescence microscopy, and metastatic cancers exhibited ICG fluorescence in noncancer cells surrounding the cancer cells. In some cases that exhibited rim IFI in poorly differentiated HCC or HCC of unknown differentiation status, there was nuclear IFI in cancer cells and cytoplasmic IFI in noncancer cells surrounding the cancer cells. Cancer cells may not fluoresce in metastatic liver cancer cases because of the following: Cancer cells do not have the characteristics of hepatocytes.

Macroscopic observations between metastatic liver cancer and HCC with the rim type were the same; however, microscopic observations between metastatic liver cancer and HCC with the rim type were somewhat disparate. While cancer cells did not exhibit IFI in metastatic liver cancers, the cancer cells exhibited IFI in different regions in poorly differentiated HCC or HCC of unknown differentiation status compared with other types. The exact cause of this phenomenon is elusive, but may be related to the tumor characteristics derived from differentiation. Further investigation is necessary to clarify these observations.

In noncancerous liver tissue, hepatocytes in cirrhotic livers had stronger IFI values than non-cirrhotic livers. However, there were stronger IFI values in the sinusoidal lacuna in non-cirrhotic livers than cirrhotic livers. This result may be due to the early washout of ICG resulting from the preserved ICG excretion ability of hepatocytes. After ICG injection, we observed immediate emission and early washout in the normal liver. Conversely, we observed late emission and late washout in cirrhotic livers as an aggravation of cirrhosis.

In this study, we successfully observed IFI at the cellular level using fluorescence microscopy with a near-infrared cube. This type of research is rare and is a useful method for progressing ICG fluorescence method research.

In conclusion, we suggest that variations in ICG fluorescence imaging reflect different tumor characteristics. However, further investigations are needed to clarify these mechanisms.

References

1. Tanaka E, Choi HS, Fujii H, Bawendi MG, Frangioni JV (2006) Image-guided oncologic surgery using invisible light: completed pre-clinical development for sentinel lymph node mapping. Ann Surg Oncol 13:1671–1681
2. Kitai T, Inamoto T, Miwa M, Shikayama T (2005) Fluorescence navigation with indocyanine green for detecting sentinel lymph nodes in breast cancer patients. Breast Cancer 12:211–215
3. Kusano M, Tajima Y, Yamazaki K, Kato M, Watanabe M, Miwa M (2008) Sentinel nodemapping guided by indocyanine green fluorescence imaging: a new method for sentinel node navigation surgery in gastrointestinal cancer. Dig Surg 25:103–108
4. Tajima Y, Yamazaki K, Masuda Y et al (2009) Sentinel node mapping guided by indocyanine green fluorescence imaging in gastric cancer. Ann Surg 249:58–62
5. Parungo CP, Ohnishi S, Kimu SW et al (2005) Intraoperative identification of esophageal sentinel lymph nodes with near-infrared fluorescence imaging. J Thorac Cardiovasc Surg 129:844–850
6. Rubens FD, Ruel M, Fremes SE (2002) A new and simplified method for coronary and graft imaging during CABG. Heart Surg Forum 5:141–144
7. Aoki T, Yasuda D, Shimizu Y et al (2008) Image-guided liver mapping using fluorescence navigation system with indocyanine green for anatomical hepatic resection. World J Surg 32:1763–1767
8. Uchiyama K, Ueno M, Ozawa S et al (2011) Combined intraoperative use of contrast-enhanced ultrasonography imaging using a sonazoid and fluorescence navigation system with indocyanine green during anatomical hepatectomy. Langenbecks Arch Surg 396:1101–1107
9. Ishizawa T, Tamura S, Masuda K et al (2009) Intraoperative fluorescent cholangiography using indocyanine green: a biliary road map for safe surgery. J Am Coll Surg 208:e1–e4
10. Ishizawa T, Fukushima N, Shibahara J et al (2009) Real-time identification of liver cancers by using indocyanine green fluorescent imaging. Cancer 115:2491–2504
11. Morita Y, Sakaguchi T, Unno N et al (2013) Detection of hepatocellular carcinomas with near-infrared fluorescence imaging using indocyanine green: its usefulness and limitation. Int J Clin Oncol 18:232–241

12. Yokoyama N, Otani T, Hashidate H et al (2012) Real-time detection of hepatic micrometastases from pancreatic cancer by intraoperative fluorescence imaging. Cancer 118:2813–2819
13. van der Vorst JR, Schaafsma BE, Hutteman M et al (2013) Near-infrared fluorescence-guided resection of colorectal liver metastases. Cancer 119:3411–3418
14. Kanematsu T, Furui J, Yanaga K, Okudaira S, Shimada M, Shirabe K (2002) A 16-year experience in performing hepatic resection in 303 patients with hepatocellular carcinoma: 1985–2000. Surgery 131:s153–s158
15. Yaseen MA, Yu J, Wong MS, Anvari B (2008) In-vivo fluorescence imaging of mammalian organs using charge-assembled mesocapsule constructs containing indocyanine green. Opt Express 16:20577–20587
16. Stieger B, Heger M, Graaf W, Paumgartner G, Gulik T (2012) The emerging role of transport systems in liver function tests. Eur J Pharmacol 675:1–5
17. Sathirakul K, Suzuki H, Yasuda K et al (1993) Kinetic analysis of hepatobiliary transport of organic anions in Eisai hyperbilirubinemic mutant rats. J Pharmacol Exp Ther 265:1301–1312
18. Ishizawa T, Masuda K, Urano Y et al (2014) Mechanistic background and clinical applications of indocyanine green fluorescence imaging of hepatocellular carcinoma. Ann Surg Oncol 21:440–448

Chapter 29
Intraoperative Detection of Hepatocellular Carcinoma Using Indocyanine Green Fluorescence Imaging

Kunihito Gotoh, Shogo Kobayashi, Shigeru Marubashi, Terumasa Yamada, Hirofumi Akita, Hidenori Takahashi, Masahiko Yano, Osamu Ishikawa, and Masato Sakon

Abstract Indocyanine green (ICG)-based fluorescence imaging has been recently applied to liver surgery to detect hepatocellular carcinoma (HCC). This technique is quite safe and simple. Briefly, ICG is intravenously injected at a dose of 0.5 mg/kg body weight as a routine preoperative liver function test before surgery. On the day of surgery, after laparotomy, the liver surface is examined by a commercially available near-infrared (NIR) camera system with the surgical lights turned off. HCC nodules are usually detected as intense fluorescent signals by this method. In this chapter, we introduce the clinical applications of ICG fluorescence imaging in HCC surgery and review the clinical study literature to date. This technique is highly sensitive and complementary to conventional modalities for the detection of HCC. Although there are some limitations, such as the low penetration depth and the detection of false-positive lesions, this technique is expected to be indispensable for the diagnosis and treatment of HCC in the near future, with further developments in basic research and improvements of the devices.

Keywords Indocyanine green (ICG) • Hepatocellular carcinoma (HCC) • Near infrared (NIR)

K. Gotoh (✉)
Department of Surgery, Osaka Medical Center for Cancer and Cardiovascular Diseases, 1-3-3 Nakamichi, Higashinari-ku, Osaka 537-8511, Japan

Department of Surgery, Osaka University, Osaka, Japan
e-mail: kgotou@gesurg.med.osaka-u.ac.jp

S. Kobayashi • H. Akita • H. Takahashi • M. Yano • O. Ishikawa • M. Sakon
Department of Surgery, Osaka Medical Center for Cancer and Cardiovascular Diseases, 1-3-3 Nakamichi, Higashinari-ku, Osaka 537-8511, Japan

S. Marubashi
Department of Surgery, Osaka University, Osaka, Japan

T. Yamada
Department of Surgery, Higashiosaka City General Hospital, Osaka, Japan

M. Kusano et al. (eds.), *ICG Fluorescence Imaging and Navigation Surgery*,
DOI 10.1007/978-4-431-55528-5_29

29.1 Introduction

Hepatocellular carcinoma (HCC) is one of the most common malignancies worldwide. Following improvements in surgical techniques and preoperative imaging modalities, long-term survival has been achieved in some patients treated with hepatic resection [1]. However, even when curative resection is performed, 70–80 % of patients experience tumor recurrence within 5 years postoperatively [2–4]. A possible explanation for this high early recurrence rate is the presence of small metastatic lesions that are missed using current preoperative and intraoperative detection methods [5, 6]. Therefore, conducting a more sensitive and accurate intrahepatic imaging evaluation of these types of lesions is essential for determining the extent of hepatic resection.

Recently, intraoperative imaging using near-infrared (NIR) fluorescence light has been applied to various surgeries. Indocyanine green (ICG) is a NIR fluorescent dye approved by the Food and Drug Administration for use in cardiocirculatory and liver function diagnostic procedures. Several studies have reported the usefulness of ICG intraoperative fluorescence imaging for detecting sentinel nodes in cases of breast, gastric, and colon cancer [7–9]. In 2007, we incidentally found that HCC tumors show very intense fluorescent signals using this method in patients given with ICG several days prior to surgery as a routine preoperative liver function test. [10] This technique provides not only real-time visualization of HCC nodules but also highly sensitive identification of small and grossly unidentifiable HCC nodules, enhancing the accuracy of liver resection.

This review describes the techniques, current applications, and future perspectives regarding ICG fluorescence imaging for HCC.

29.2 Technique of ICG Fluorescence Imaging for HCC Detection

The technique for ICG fluorescence imaging of HCC is quite safe and simple. The patient is administered with ICG (Diagnogreen Inj., Daiichi Pharmaceutical, Tokyo, Japan) intravenously at a dose of 0.5 mg/kg body weight as a routine preoperative liver function test prior to undergoing surgery [11]. The interval between ICG injection and surgery is usually within 14 days in HCC patients. On the day of surgery, after laparotomy, the liver surface is observed using a commercially available near-infrared (NIR) camera system with the surgical lights turned off. This system activates ICG with emitted light at a wavelength of 760 nm and filters out light with a wavelength below 820 nm. The light source is a light-emitting diode (LED), and the detector is a charge-coupled device (CCD) camera. The camera unit of the device is handled directly, and real-time fluorescence images are obtained on the monitor in the operating room.

29.3 Detection of HCC Nodules Using ICG Fluorescence Imaging

HCC nodules are usually detected as intense fluorescent signals using intraoperative ICG fluorescence imaging (Fig. 29.1). In a preliminary study, we reported that ten primary HCC nodules showed intense fluorescent signals and were easily detected using this method [10]. At the same time, Ishizawa et al. reported detecting 63 primary HCC nodules using the same technique [12]. Previously published studies of HCC detection are summarized in Table 29.1 [10, 12–14]. The rate of HCC detection on intraoperative fluorescence imaging is reported to be 52–100 % and is strongly dependent on the distance from the liver surface to the tumor. There is a technical limitation in that the tissue penetration depth of the fluorescence emitted by ICG is only 5–10 mm. Morita et al. demonstrated that the average distance from the liver surface to tumors unidentified on intraoperative fluorescence imaging is 10.4 (0–27) mm [13]. In that study, 26 tumors unidentified on intraoperative fluorescence imaging were identified in the sectioned specimens using ex vivo fluorescence imaging. Van der Vorst et al. reported that, in their study, 71 liver metastases, all of which were ≤6.2 mm from the liver surface, were

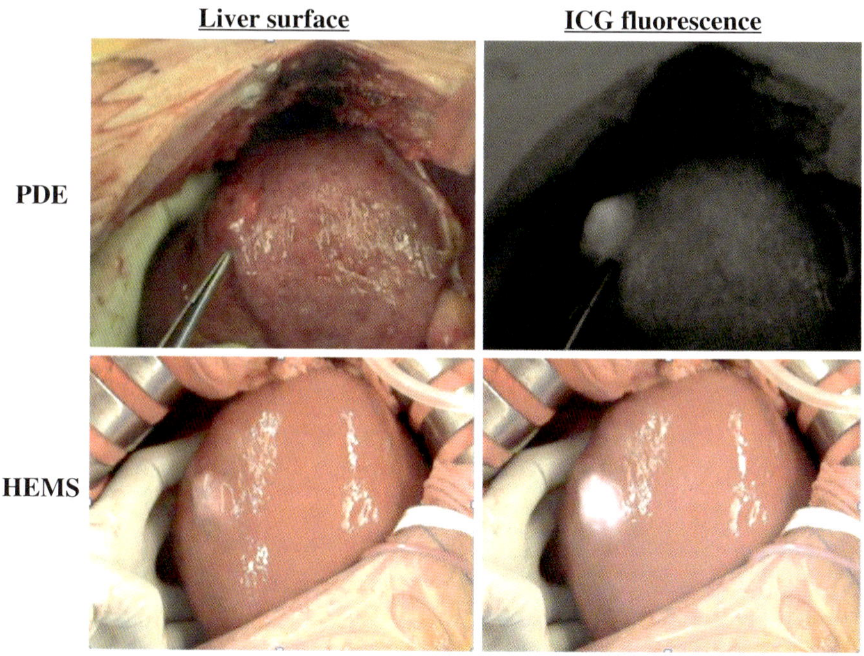

Fig. 29.1 ICG fluorescence imaging for primary HCC. Gross appearance (*left*) and intraoperative ICG fluorescence imaging (*right*) of liver surfaces. Fluorescence imaging by using a commercially available near-infrared (NIR) camera system (**a**) Photodynamic Eye (PDE; Hamamatsu Photonics K.K., Hamamatsu, Japan) and (**b**) HyperEye Medical System (HEMS, Mizuho Co., Tokyo, Japan)

Table 29.1 HCC detection using ICG fluorescence imaging

Author	Year	Number of patients	Time between injection and surgery (days)	HCC detection rate by intraoperative imaging (%)	HCC detection rate by ex vivo imaging (%)	Newly detected lesions	Newly detected HCC
Gotoh	2009	10	1–8	100 (10/10)	100 (10/10)	8	4
Ishizawa	2009	37	1–7	51 (21/41)	100 (63/63)	13	8
Morita	2011	58	3–28	62 (47/76)	96 (73/76)	35	6
Ishizawa	2013	170	1–52	NA	99 (273/276)	37	21

HCC hepatocellular carcinoma, *NA* not available

detected on intraoperative ICG fluorescence imaging, whereas 26 liver metastases identified on conventional imaging could not be detected using intraoperative ICG fluorescence imaging, all of which were deeper than 8 mm from the liver surface [15]. Therefore, this technique is expected to improve the performance of imaging devices in terms of achieving deeper visualization.

Following resection and sectioning, all liver tumors are examined using ICG fluorescence imaging *ex vivo*. The detection rate is reported to be almost 100 % [10, 12–14]. Ishizawa et al. reported that, in false-negative cases of ICG fluorescence imaging, the interval between the intravenous injection of ICG and surgery is exceptionally long compared with that seen in the remaining identified patients [14]. On the other hand, they found that the signal intensity of the noncancerous liver parenchyma was higher especially in patients with advanced cirrhosis who had received the ICG injection within 24 h before surgery [12]. A previously performed study in rats showed an optimal cancer-to-liver contrast in the group where ICG was administered at 72 h prior to surgery [16]. Further studies are needed to determine the optimal interval between ICG injection and surgery for obtaining good cancer-to-liver contrast.

29.4 Correlation Between the ICG Fluorescence Pattern and HCC Differentiation

The fluorescence patterns observed under NIR are classified into three groups: total fluorescent type, partial fluorescent type, and rim fluorescent type (Fig. 29.2). Several studies have reported a significant correlation between HCC differentiation and the fluorescence pattern [13, 14]. Combining these studies, a total of 346 patients were included (total type ($n = 150$), partial type ($n = 145$), and rim type ($n = 51$)). Among the rim fluorescent-type patients, three cases (6 %) were classified as well-differentiated carcinoma, and 22 cases (43 %) were classified as poorly differentiated carcinoma. On the other hand, in the other fluorescent-type groups (total and partial), 85 cases (29 %) involved well-differentiated carcinoma,

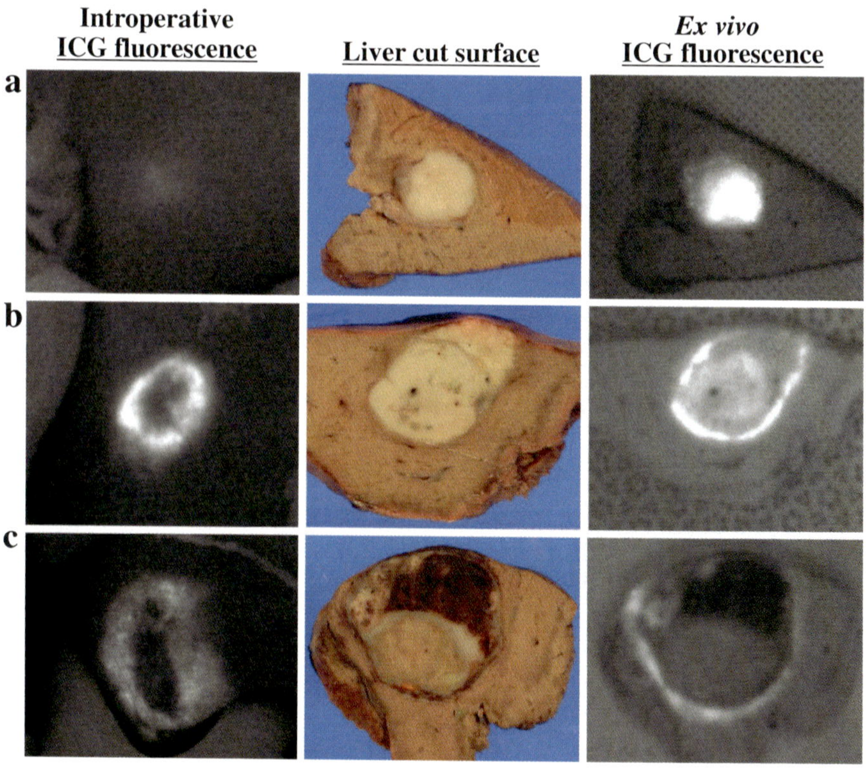

Fig. 29.2 ICG fluorescence patterns of HCC. Intraoperative ICG fluorescence imaging (*left*), gross appearance (*middle*), and postoperative ICG fluorescence imaging (*right*) of liver cut surfaces. (**a**) Total fluorescence type. (**b**) Partial fluorescence type. (**c**) Rim fluorescence type

and five cases (2 %) involved poorly differentiated carcinoma. These results suggest that the rate of the rim fluorescent type is significantly lower among cases of well-differentiated carcinoma and higher among cases of poorly differentiated carcinoma compared to that of the other fluorescent types. It is hypothesized that the mechanisms of ICG accumulation in HCC nodules are associated with ICG transporter expression levels. Ishizawa et al. reported the expression of Na^{+}/taurocholate cotransporting polypeptide (NTCP) and organic anion-transporting polypeptide 8 (OATP8), the major uptake transporters for ICG [17], in the cancerous tissues of HCC lesions showing total and partial fluorescence patterns, but not lesions showing rim-type fluorescence, according to a gene expression and immunostaining analysis [14]. These results suggest that, in differentiated HCC tissues, the portal uptake function is preserved, whereas the biliary excretion of ICG is likely impaired. It has also been suggested that most poorly differentiated HCCs exhibit rim-type fluorescence on ICG fluorescence images as a result of an impaired portal uptake function in cancerous tissues. However, further research is needed to confirm the mechanism and pattern of ICG accumulation in HCC nodules.

29.5 Newly Detected Lesions on ICG Fluorescence Imaging

ICG fluorescence imaging technique can be used to achieve the enhanced detection of small HCC nodules undetectable with conventional detection methods, including preoperative CT, intraoperative ultrasound (IOUS), palpation, and visual inspection (Fig. 29.3). Previously published studies of newly detected HCC nodules are also summarized in Table 29.1 [10, 12–14]. The detection rate of new HCC lesions on intraoperative ICG fluorescence imaging is reported to be 10–40 %. Despite recent advances in preoperative imaging modalities, this technique detected new HCC nodules in 40 % of the patients in our preliminary study. Because most small HCC nodules (<10 mm in diameter) are pathologically well differentiated [18], lack typical imaging patterns for HCC, and are not always hypervascular [19], it is sometimes very difficult to diagnose these lesions as HCC preoperatively. In fact, all of the new HCC nodules detected in our study were very small (3–6 mm), and most of them were diagnosed as well-differentiated HCC. Sahani et al. reported that one of the main limitations of IOUS is the hampered detection of superficial and small tumors [20]. ICG fluorescence imaging performs well in cases of superficial and small tumors, although it is unable to visualize deeper tumors. Therefore, intraoperative ICG fluorescence imaging should be viewed as a complementary adjuvant to conventional imaging techniques for the preoperative and intraoperative detection of HCC.

On the other hand, previous studies have demonstrated that nonmalignant lesions (regenerative nodules, dysplastic nodules, bile duct proliferation, cysts, fibrosis, and normal liver parenchyma) display ICG uptake [10, 12–14]. The false-positive rate on intraoperative ICG fluorescence imaging is reported to be 38–83 % (Table 29.1). Since ICG is not a cancer-specific dye, it is difficult to distinguish HCC from benign lesions using ICG fluorescence imaging. Therefore, further basic studies, including molecular, genetic, and immunohistochemical research, are needed to clarify the mechanisms and patterns of ICG accumulation in HCC nodules.

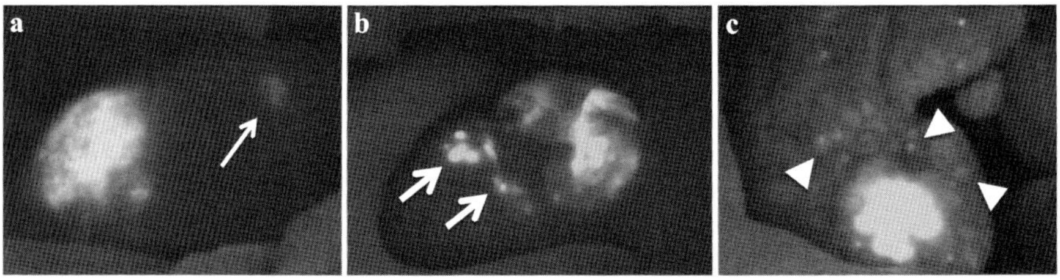

Fig. 29.3 Newly detected HCC under ICG fluorescence imaging. (**a**) New single HCC (*thin arrow*) was detected in a different hepatic segment from main tumor. (**b**) Small newly HCCs (*thick arrows*) were detected around the main tumor. (**c**) Tiny newly HCCs (*arrowheads*) were scattered around the main tumor

29.6 Detection of Extrahepatic HCC Tumors Using ICG Fluorescence Imaging

HCC tumors are sometimes found outside the liver, in cases of extrahepatic metastasis or ectopic HCC, a rare clinical entity defined as HCC arising from extrahepatic liver tissue. Extrahepatic HCC tumors also demonstrate ICG uptake and emit fluorescence when illuminated by NIR light. We experienced two rare cases of HCC metastasis. The first case involved solitary and metachronous metastasis to the appendix arising from HCC [21], while the second case comprised abdominal wall metastasis of HCC. The tumors showed intense fluorescent signals on intraoperative ICG fluorescence imaging (Fig. 29.4a, b). In particular, in the

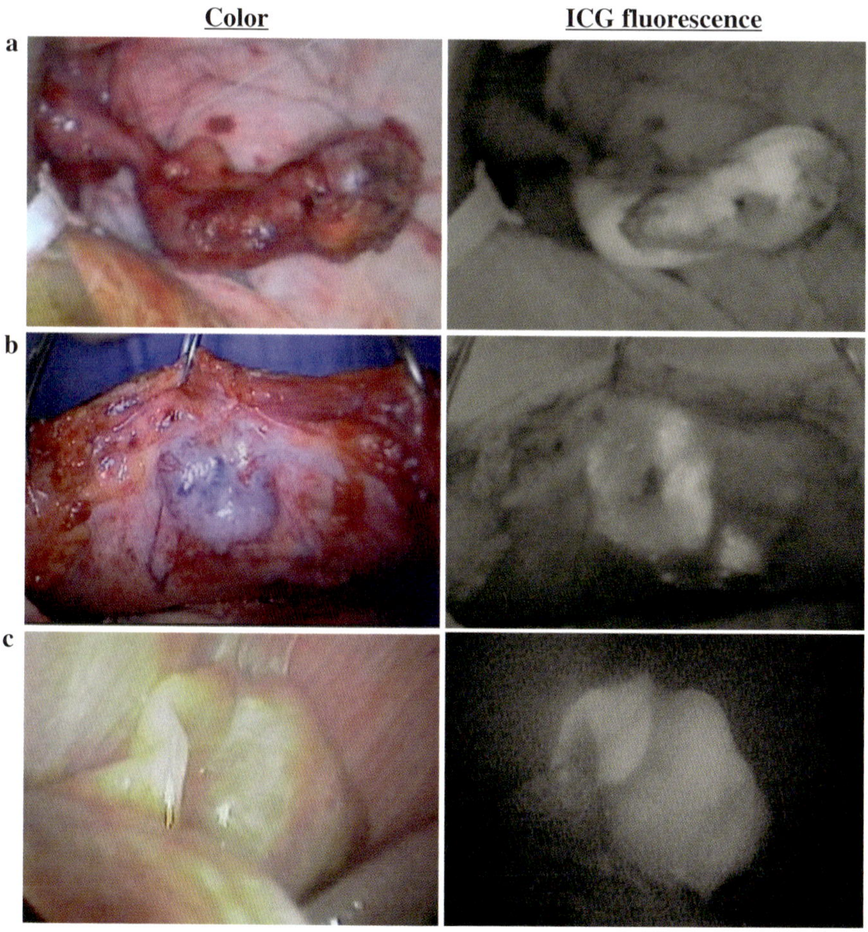

Fig. 29.4 ICG fluorescence imaging for extrahepatic HCC. Gross appearance (*left*) and intraoperative ICG fluorescence imaging (*right*). (**a**) HCC metastasis to the appendix. (**b**) HCC metastasis to the abdominal wall. (**c**) Ectopic HCC arising in the left triangular ligament of the liver

second case, small metastasis lesions were observed around the main tumor on ICG fluorescence imaging and were completely resected with negative margins under guidance with this system. We also previously reported the usefulness of ICG fluorescence imaging for detecting ectopic HCC arising in the left triangular ligament of the liver [22]. In that report, the tumor was examined using a prototype laparoscopic near-infrared camera system (Hamamatsu Photonics K.K., Hamamatsu, Japan) and was found to show bright fluorescent signals (Fig. 29.4c). The tumor was subsequently resected with an adequate margin under guidance with the above system. Satou et al. reported that, of 28 lesions for which ICG fluorescence was performed intraoperatively, 24 lesions exhibited fluorescence and were proven to be HCC metastases pathologically [23]. Five of these lesions were newly identified on ICG fluorescent imaging. Therefore, ICG fluorescence imaging is also a useful tool for intraoperatively detecting HCC tumors outside the liver.

29.7 Future Perspectives

As described above, there are two major challenges when identifying HCC using ICG fluorescent imaging: the low tissue penetration depth and the detection of false-positive lesions. The available literature currently reports a penetration depth ranging from approximately 5–10 mm. The ability to visualize tumors located in deeper regions would provide further improvements in the accuracy of resection of HCC lesions. In particular, ICG fluorescence imaging may be of great value in laparoscopic and robotic liver surgery, as it is not possible to palpate the liver. Moreover, modifying the ICG with a cancer-specific antibody would not only enhance the accuracy of this technique for tumor diagnosis and localization but also provide a novel photosensitive substance for use in photodynamic therapy. Since ICG is also a photosensitive substance, the development of novel photodynamic therapy that takes advantage of this property and the accumulation of ICG in HCC tumor may be possible [24]. Therefore, further improvements in camera systems and fluorophores are needed for ICG fluorescence imaging to become an indispensable technique for the diagnosis and treatment of HCC.

29.8 Conclusion

ICG fluorescence imaging for HCC detection is already useful in clinical settings for hepatic surgeons. With further developments in basic research and improvements of the devices, this technique is expected to be indispensable for the diagnosis and treatment in HCC surgery.

Acknowledgment This work was supported in part by a grant from Osaka foundation for the prevention of cancer and cardiovascular diseases and by a grant from the Otsuka Research Fund.

References

1. Poon RT, Fan ST, Lo CM et al (2001) Improving survival results after resection of hepatocellular carcinoma: a prospective study of 377 patients over 10 years. Ann Surg 234:63–70
2. Llovet JM, Fuster J, Bruix J (1999) Intention-to-treat analysis of surgical treatment for early hepatocellular carcinoma: resection versus transplantation. Hepatology 30:1434–1440
3. Sasaki Y, Yamada T, Tanaka H et al (2006) Risk of recurrence in a long-term follow-up after surgery in 417 patients with hepatitis B- or hepatitis C-related hepatocellular carcinoma. Ann Surg 244:771–780
4. Katz SC, Shia J, Liau KH et al (2009) Operative blood loss independently predicts recurrence and survival after resection of hepatocellular carcinoma. Ann Surg 249:617–623
5. Sakon M, Umeshita K, Nagano H et al (2000) Clinical significance of hepatic resection in hepatocellular carcinoma: analysis by disease-free survival curves. Arch Surg 135:1456–1459
6. Shimada M, Takenaka K, Taguchi K et al (1998) Prognostic factors after repeat hepatectomy for recurrent hepatocellular carcinoma. Ann Surg 227:80–85
7. Kitai T, Inomoto T, Miwa M, Shikayama T (2005) Fluorescence navigation with indocyanine green for detecting sentinel lymph nodes in breast cancer. Breast Cancer 12:211–215
8. Miyashiro I, Miyoshi N, Hiratsuka M et al (2008) Detection of sentinel node in gastric cancer surgery by indocyanine green fluorescence imaging: comparison with infrared imaging. Ann Surg Oncol 15:1640–1643
9. Noura S, Ohue M, Seki Y et al (2008) Evaluation of the lateral sentinel node by indocyanine green for rectal cancer based on micrometastasis determined by reverse transcriptase-polymerase chain reaction. Oncol Rep 20:745–750
10. Gotoh K, Yamada T, Ishikawa O et al (2009) A novel image-guided surgery of hepatocellular carcinoma by indocyanine green fluorescence imaging navigation. J Surg Oncol 100:75–79
11. Makuuchi M, Kosuge T, Takayama T et al (1993) Surgery for small liver cancers. Semin Surg Oncol 9:298–304
12. Ishizawa T, Fukushima N, Shibahara J et al (2009) Real-time identification of liver cancers by using indocyanine green fluorescent imaging. Cancer 115:2491–2504
13. Morita Y, Sakaguchi T, Unno N et al (2013) Detection of hepatocellular carcinomas with near-infrared fluorescence imaging using indocyanine green: its usefulness and limitation. Int J Clin Oncol 18:232–241
14. Ishizawa T, Masuda K, Urano Y et al (2014) Mechanistic background and clinical applications of indocyanine green fluorescence imaging of hepatocellular carcinoma. Ann Surg Oncol 21:440–448
15. van der Vorst JR, Schaafsma BE, Hutteman M et al (2013) Near-infrared fluorescence-guided resection of colorectal liver metastases. Cancer 119:3411–3418
16. van der Vorst JR, Hutteman M, Mieog JS et al (2012) Near-infrared fluorescence imaging of liver metastases in rats using indocyanine green. J Surg Res 174:266–271
17. de Graaf W, Hausler S, Heger M et al (2011) Transporters involved in the hepatic uptake of (99m) Tc-mebrofenin and indocyanine green. J Hepatol 54:738–745
18. Kenmochi K, Sugihara S, Kojiro M (1987) Relationship of histologic grade of hepatocellular carcinoma (HCC) to tumor size, and demonstration of tumor cells of multiple different grades in single small HCC. Liver 7:18–26
19. Takayasu K, Muramatsu Y, Mizuguchi Y et al (2004) Imaging of early hepatocellular carcinoma and adenomatous hyperplasia (dysplastic nodules) with dynamic ct and a combination of CT and angiography: experience with resected liver specimens. Intervirology 47:199–208
20. Sahani DV, Kalva SP, Tanabe KK et al (2004) Intraoperative US in patients undergoing surgery for liver neoplasms: comparison with MR imaging. Radiology 232:810–814
21. Imada S, Noura S, Ohue M et al (2013) Recurrence of hepatocellular carcinoma presenting as an asymptomatic appendiceal tumor: report of a case. Surg Today 43:685–689

22. Kanzaki R, Yamada T, Gotoh K et al (2010) Ectopic Hepatocellular Carcinoma Arising in the Left Triangular Ligament of the Liver. Case Rep Gastroenterol 4:138–143
23. Satou S, Ishizawa T, Masuda K et al (2013) Indocyanine green fluorescent imaging for detecting extrahepatic metastasis of hepatocellular carcinoma. J Gastroenterol 48:1136–1143
24. Kaneko J, Inagaki Y, Ishizawa T et al (2014) Photodynamic therapy for human hepatoma-cell-line tumors utilizing biliary excretion properties of indocyanine green. J Gastroenterol 49:110–116

Chapter 30
Laparoscopic Intraoperative Identification of Liver Tumors by Fluorescence Imaging

Masaki Kaibori, Kosuke Matsui, Hiroya Iida, Morihiko Ishizaki, and Masanori Kon

Abstract Fluorescence imaging using indocyanine green (ICG) has recently been applied to laparoscopic surgery to identify cancerous tissues, lymph nodes, and vascular anatomy. Here, we report the use of ICG fluorescence imaging to visualize liver tumors and cysts during laparoscopic liver resection. Our results show that ICG fluorescence imaging is safe and feasible, with many applications in laparoscopic liver surgery.

Keywords Laparoscopic liver navigation • Indocyanine green • Fluorescence imaging • Liver tumor • Liver cyst

30.1 Introduction

Indocyanine green (ICG) binds to plasma proteins and these protein-bound ICG complexes emit near-infrared light [1, 2]. In our department, ICG is intravenously administered preoperatively to all surgical patients to estimate the maximum hepatic volume that can be resected safely, based on measurement of the ICG retention rate at 15 min (ICGR15) [3]. Human bile also contains proteins that bind ICG [4]. In a recent report, we showed that ICG fluorescence cholangiography can detect insufficiently closed bile duct stumps that could not be identified using a standard bile leak test [5]. In addition, ICG fluorescence imaging of liver tumors has been used for their intraoperative navigation [6]. Our experience suggests that liver cancer can be identified by fluorescence imaging, based on the visualization of the ICG remaining in the cancerous tissues and/or in the surrounding liver tissues after preoperative intravenous injection.

The role of laparoscopic hepatectomy in the surgical treatment of liver tumors has expanded [7, 8]. Kaneko et al. reported that laparoscopic hepatectomy improved patients' quality of life postoperatively, with no reduction in the

M. Kaibori (✉) • K. Matsui • H. Iida • M. Ishizaki • M. Kon
Department of Surgery, Hirakata Hospital, Kansai Medical University, 2-3-1 Shinmachi, Hirakata, Osaka 573-1191, Japan
e-mail: kaibori@hirakata.kmu.ac.jp

M. Kusano et al. (eds.), *ICG Fluorescence Imaging and Navigation Surgery*,
DOI 10.1007/978-4-431-55528-5_30

curability of the disease [9, 10]. Laparoscopic fluorescence imaging systems became commercially available in 2011 and are now also being used during laparoscopic hepatectomy. The aim of this study was to evaluate the role of laparoscopic ICG fluorescence imaging in the intraoperative identification of liver tumors and liver cysts based on their fluorescence patterns.

30.2 Materials

The laparoscopic system was from Karl Storz GmbH (Tuttlingen, Germany). Images were generated using the high-end full high-definition camera system (Image 1 Spies, Karl Storz) connected to a laparoscope with a 30° viewing direction and 10-mm diameter. The laparoscope is equipped with a specific filter for the optimal detection of near-infrared (NIR) fluorescence and white light without manual switching between the two. The system's powerful xenon light source (D-Light P SCB, Karl Storz) provides both visible and NIR excitation light. Switching from standard light to NIR is controlled by the surgeon by means of a pedal. Visualization both under standard and NIR light is improved by an image enhancement system (Image 1 Spies, Karl Storz) that offers adjustable visualization modalities that can be selected according to the surgeon's preferences. The fluorescent source was ICG (Diagnogreen, Daiichi Sankyo, Tokyo, Japan), injected at a rate of 0.5 mg/kg i.v. 1–8 weeks prior to surgery, except in patients undergoing surgery for liver cysts (see below).

30.3 Evaluation of ICG Fluorescence Imaging During Laparoscopic Liver Navigation

30.3.1 Hepatocellular Carcinoma

We retrospectively reviewed 34 patients with hepatocellular carcinoma (HCC) who underwent laparoscopic hepatic resection at our institution between January 2014 and March 2015. Intraoperative ICG fluorescence images of the tumors were used to classify the tumors into the following three groups according to the intensity of the fluorescence in the tumor region: whole (Fig. 30.1a–c), partial (Fig. 30.1d–f), and ring (Fig. 30.1g–i) types. The fluorescence intensity of the tumor region significantly differed between the three groups, as did the fluorescence ratios of the cancerous/noncancerous regions. Histological evaluation showed that cirrhosis was significantly more common in the whole type than in the partial and ring types

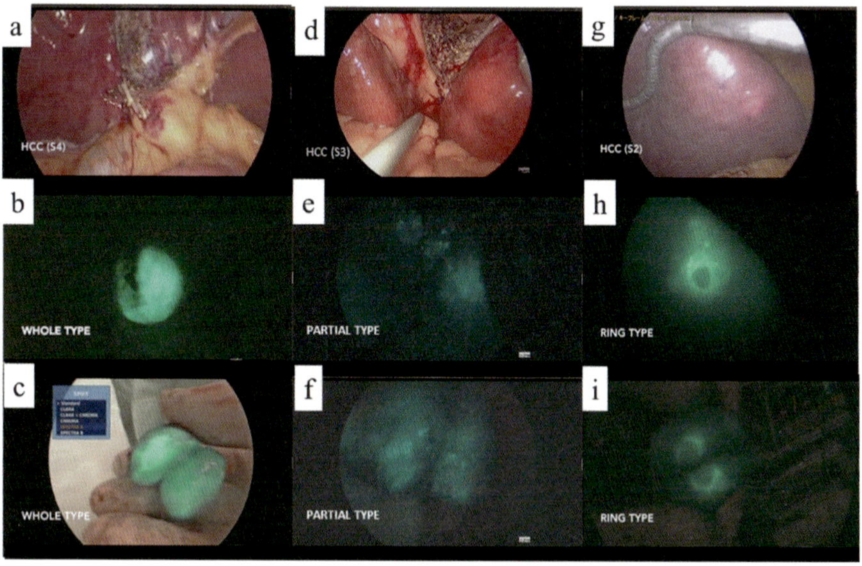

Fig. 30.1 Three types of hepatocellular carcinoma (HCC) as determined by intraoperative laparoscopic indocyanine green (ICG) fluorescence imaging. (**a**) Laparoscopic view using standard light. (**b**) Whole positive fluorescence in the cancerous region. (**c**) The incised lesion also showed whole positive fluorescence in the cancerous region, which was diagnosed as HCC. (**d**) Laparoscopic view using standard light. (**e**) Partial positive fluorescence in the cancerous region. (**f**) The incised lesion also showed partial positive fluorescence in the cancerous region, which was diagnosed as HCC. (**g**) Laparoscopic view using standard light. (**h**) Ring positive fluorescence in the cancerous region. (**i**) The incised lesion also showed ring positive fluorescence in the cancerous region, which was diagnosed as HCC

of tumors (data not shown). The percentage of cases of well-differentiated HCC was higher in the partial type than in the other types, whereas the percentage of poorly differentiated HCC cases was highest in the ring type (data not shown). Thus, ICG fluorescence imaging in HCC is presumably sensitive to both tumor differentiation and fibrosis in the noncancerous liver parenchyma.

In recurrent HCC, detection of the tumor margins, whether by visual inspection, palpation, or intraoperative ultrasound, is challenging in patients previously treated with transarterial chemoembolization (TACE) or radiofrequency ablation. Using ICG fluorescence imaging, viable cancer could be clearly distinguished from necrotic liver tissue following TACE (Fig. 30.2).

30.3.2 Intrahepatic Cholangiocellular Carcinoma

ICG fluorescence imaging of the liver surface clearly identified regions of cholestasis caused by tumor invasion of the bile duct or by thrombi.

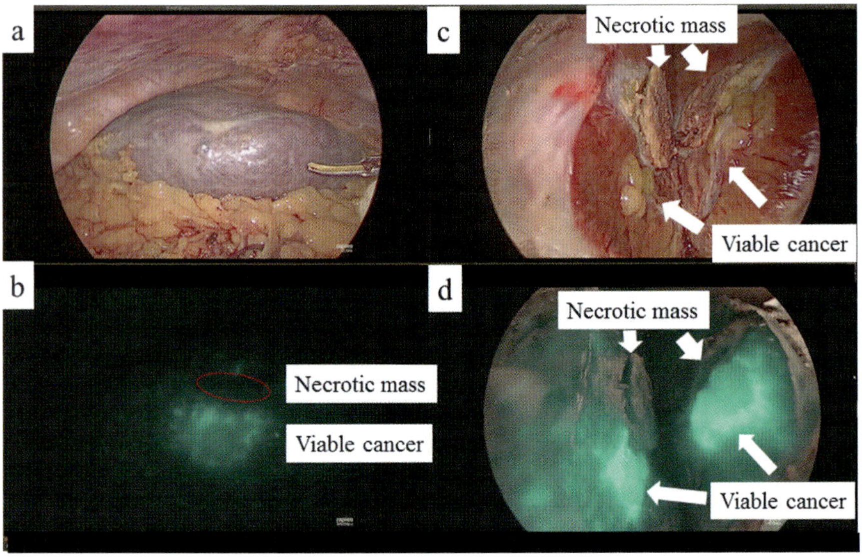

Fig. 30.2 Detection of the tumor margin in recurrent hepatocellular carcinoma (HCC) using laparoscopic indocyanine green (ICG) fluorescence imaging. (**a**) Laparoscopic view using standard light. (**b**) ICG-positive and ICG-negative fluorescence on the surface of the liver. (**c**) The area of positive fluorescence was diagnosed as HCC and the area of negative fluorescence as necrosis. (**d**) ICG-positive and ICG-negative fluorescence of the incised lesion

In open laparotomy, fluorescence images of the liver surface were obtained intraoperatively with a fluorescence imaging system (PDE; Hamamatsu Photonics, Hamamatsu, Japan) composed of a charge-coupled device camera that excluded light with wavelengths of less than 820 nm and 36 light-emitting diodes with a wavelength of 760 nm [1, 4]. The cholestatic regions on the surface of the liver were clearly delineated with fluorescence imaging (Fig. 30.3), whereas using a laparoscopic system fluorescence in the same regions was relatively weak (Fig. 30.4). The latter result reflects the fact that, in the laparoscopic system, the fluorescence strength cannot be adjusted.

30.3.3 Liver Cyst

Laparoscopic resection of symptomatic nonparasitic liver cysts is a feasible and effective method to relieve symptoms using a minimally invasive surgical procedure. Laparoscopic deroofing, as a standard approach to the surgical treatment of

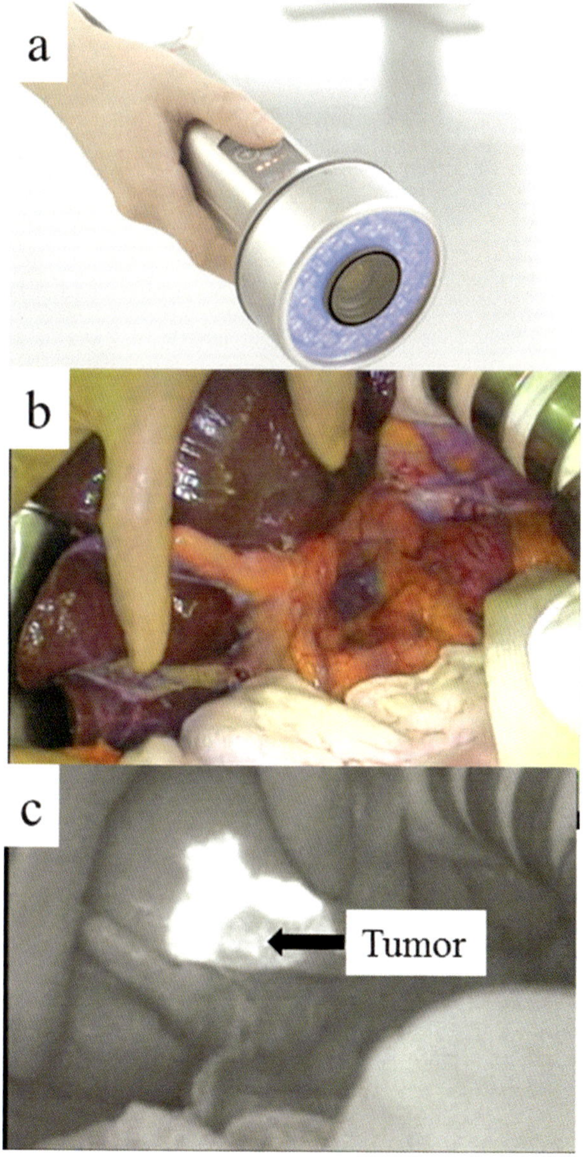

Fig. 30.3 Fluorescence imaging of intrahepatic cholangiocellular carcinoma (ICC). (**a**) The fluorescence imaging system (PDE; Hamamatsu Photonics, Hamamatsu, Shizuoka) consisted of a charge-coupled device camera that filtered out light with wavelengths less than 820 nm and 36 light-emitting diodes with a wavelength of 760 nm. (**b**) Operative view using a standard light. (**c**) Intraoperative fluorescence imaging of cholestatic regions in ICC

liver cysts, is well established [11, 12]. However, postoperative bile leakage is one of the most severe complications after deroofing [13]. Moreover, care must be taken to avoid resection of the hepatic parenchyma, because transected bile ducts may lead to postoperative bile leaks. Carrying out a laparoscopic cholangiogram during

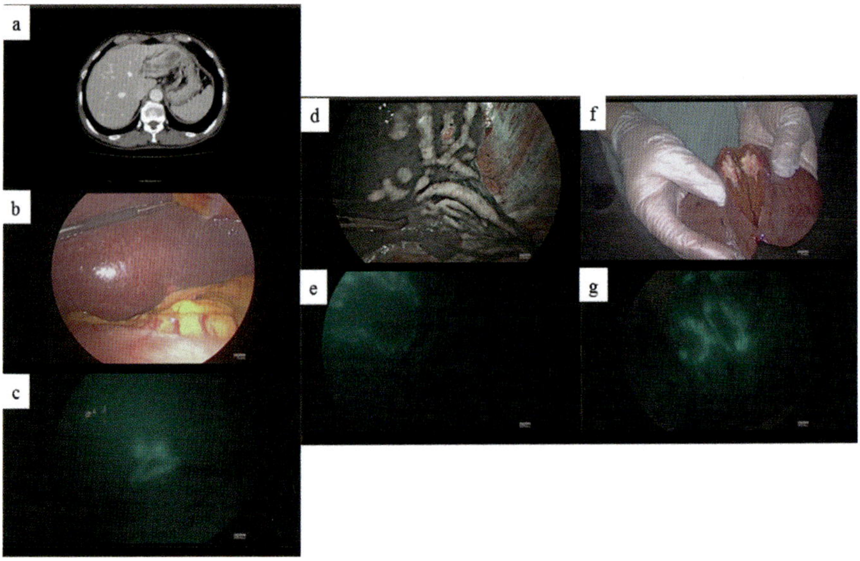

Fig. 30.4 Laparoscopic fluorescence imaging of intrahepatic cholangiocellular carcinoma (ICC). (**a**) Preoperative contrast-enhanced computed tomography in a patient with ICC and a dilated bile duct in the left liver. (**b**) Laparoscopic view using standard light. (**c**) Ring positive indocyanine green (ICG) fluorescence in the cancerous region. (**d**) Laparoscopic view using standard light shows the dilated bile duct in the left liver. (**e**) Fluorescence imaging of the dilated bile duct. (**f**) The incised lesion as seen using standard light. (**g**) The incised lesion also showed ring positive fluorescence in the cancerous region, which was diagnosed as ICC

laparoscopic surgery is challenging when the cystic contents suggest a biliary communication and bile leakage has occurred intraoperatively. ICG, once injected, concentrates in bile and thus outlines the anatomy of the biliary tree, especially Calot's triangle, which can then be visualized under NIR light during laparoscopic cholecystectomy [14]. The ICG solution (2.5 mg/ml; 1 ml) is injected intravenously 3 h before surgery to allow the dye to concentrate in the intrahepatic bile ducts. Most of our patients with liver cysts undergo a preoperative CT scan and magnetic resonance cholangiopancreatography (Fig. 30.5a, b). This allows an anatomic examination of the junction of the cystic and common bile ducts (Fig. 30.5d, e). After partial deroofing, ICG fluorescence imaging provides a clear view of the intrahepatic bile ducts (Fig. 30.5f, g). In the case shown in Fig. 30.5, using the technique described herein, only the cyst wall was resected, and postoperative bile leaks were avoided.

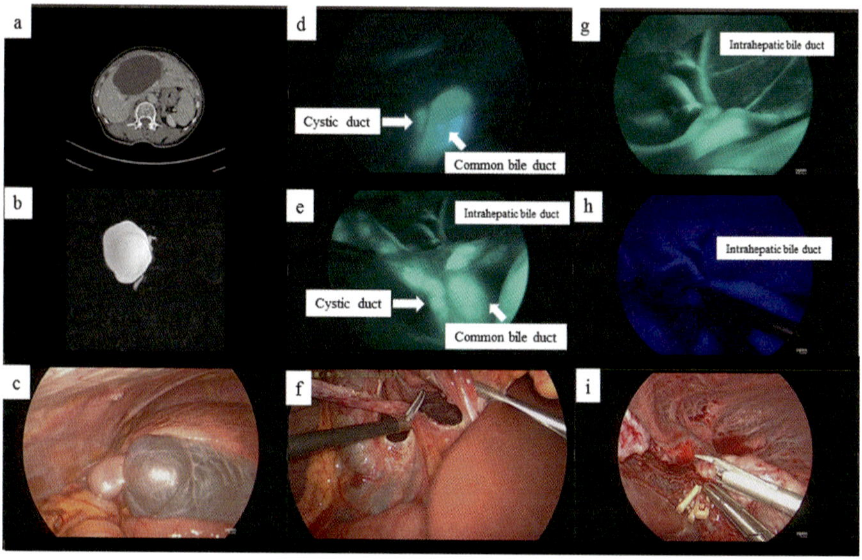

Fig. 30.5 Laparoscopic fluorescence imaging of a liver cyst. (**a**) Preoperative enhanced computed tomography and (**b**) preoperative magnetic resonance cholangiopancreatography in a patient with a large liver cyst. (**c**) Laparoscopic view using standard light. (**d**, **e**) Identification of the anatomy of the junction of the cystic duct and common bile duct using laparoscopic fluorescence imaging. (**f**) Laparoscopic deroofing. (**g**) Identification of the intrahepatic bile duct using laparoscopic fluorescence imaging. (**h**) The injured bile duct was closed using a metallic clip, seen on the fluorescence image. (**i**) Laparoscopic view using standard light

References

1. Landsman ML, Kwant G, Mook GA, Zijlstra WG (1976) Light-absorbing properties, stability, and spectral stabilization of indocyanine green. J Appl Physiol 40:575–583
2. Mordon S, Devoisselle JM, Soulie-Begu S, Desmettre T (1998) Indocyanine green: physicochemical factors affecting its fluorescence in vivo. Microvasc Res 55:146–152
3. Hasegawa K, Kokudo N, Imamura H, Matsuyama Y, Aoki T, Minagawa M, Sano K, Sugawara Y, Takayama T, Makuuchi M (2005) Prognostic impact of anatomic resection for hepatocellular carcinoma. Ann Surg 242:252–259
4. Mulllock BM, Shaw LJ, Fitzharris B, Peppard J, Hamilton MJ, Simpson MT et al (1985) Sources of proteins in human bile. Gut 26:500–509
5. Kaibori M, Ishizaki M, Matsui K, Kwon AH (2011) Intraoperative indocyanine green fluorescent imaging for prevention of bile leakage after hepatic resection. Surgery 150:91–98
6. Ishizawa T, Fukushima N, Shibahara J, Masuda K, Tamura S, Aoki T, Hasegawa K, Beck Y, Fukayama M, Kokudo N (2009) Real-time identification of liver cancers by using indocyanine green fluorescent imaging. Cancer 115:2491–2504
7. Buell JF, Cherqui D, Geller DA, O'Rourke N, Iannitti D, Dagher I et al (2009) The international position on laparoscopic liver surgery: the Louisville Statement, 2008. Ann Surg 250:825–830
8. Edwin B, Nordin A, Kazaryan AM (2011) Laparoscopic liver surgery: new frontiers. Scand J Surg 100:54–65

9. Kaneko H, Takagi S, Shiba T (1996) Laparoscopic partial hepatectomy and left lateral segmentectomy: technique and results of a clinical series. Surgery 120:468–475
10. Kaneko H, Takagi S, Otsuka Y, Tsuchiya M, Tamura A, Katagiri T et al (2005) Laparoscopic liver resection of hepatocellular carcinoma. Am J Surg 189:190–194
11. Szabó LS, Takács I, Arkosy P, Sápy P, Szentkereszty Z (2006) Laparoscopic treatment of nonparasitic hepatic cysts. Surg Endosc 20:595–597
12. Treckmann JW, Paul A, Sgourakis G, Heuer M, Wandelt M, Sotiropoulos GC (2010) Surgical treatment of nonparasitic cysts of the liver: open versus laparoscopic treatment. Am J Surg 199:776–781
13. Mazza OM, Fernandez DL, Pekolj J, Pfaffen G, Sanchez Clariá R, Molmenti EP et al (2009) Management of nonparasitic hepatic cysts. J Am Coll Surg 209:733–739
14. Boni L, David G, Mangano A, Dionigi G, Rausei S, Spampatti S et al. Clinical applications of indocyanine green (ICG) enhanced fluorescence in laparoscopic surgery. Surg Endosc, 2014 Oct 11. [Epub ahead of print]

Chapter 31
Application of Indocyanine Green Fluorescence Imaging to Pediatric Hepatoblastoma Surgery

Norihiko Kitagawa

Abstract We will elaborate on navigation surgery using indocyanine green (ICG) fluorescence imaging in pediatric hepatoblastoma. Chemotherapy is effective against hepatoblastoma, and while complete surgical resection of the primary lesion can often result in recovery, prognosis in patients with distant metastases is poor. In recent years, the importance of proactively resecting lung metastases has been highlighted. Previously, metastases discovered during visual inspection and palpation were resected; however, this approach lacked objectivity and was subject to the skill of the surgeon. Using ICG fluorescence method has facilitated the intraoperative discovery of micrometastases. In ten patients in which lung metastases were detected, we used ICG fluorescence imaging and resected a total of 250 fluorescence-positive masses. The smallest metastasis had a diameter of 62 μm. Twenty-nine masses were false-positives; these were concentrated in two patients. When observing biopsy samples of the false-positive masses under a fluorescence microscope, luminescent thrombi and granulomas were apparent. The reason for the fluorescence is unknown, although it is possible that the masses contained micrometastases with diameters that were too small to be histopathologically identified. There were no false-negatives. ICG fluorescence imaging was also demonstrated to be an effective method for identifying metastases in the lymph nodes and peritonea. Additionally, as in surgery for hepatocellular carcinoma in adults, ICG fluorescence imaging was useful for hepatoblastoma, in terms of identifying tumors during primary liver tumor resection, and for intraoperative cholangiography.

Keywords Hepatoblastoma • Pediatric • Surgery • Indocyanine green

---

N. Kitagawa (✉)
Department of Surgery, Kanagawa Children's Medical Center, 2-138-4 Mutsukawa, Minami-ku, Yokohama, Kanagawa 232-8555, Japan
e-mail: norihikok@nifty.com

M. Kusano et al. (eds.), *ICG Fluorescence Imaging and Navigation Surgery*,
DOI 10.1007/978-4-431-55528-5_31

31.1 Introduction

Hepatoblastoma is the most prevalent malignant liver tumor in children [1]. Chemotherapy is effective, and recovery can often be achieved following complete surgical resection of the primary tumor [2]. According to the results of the Japanese Study Group for Pediatric Liver Tumor (JPLT-2), the 5-year survival rate for those with no distant metastases was good (88.6 %). However, the prognosis for cases where distant metastases are present remains poor, with a JPLT-2 5-year survival rate of 43.9 % [3]. Metastases from a hepatoblastoma are found primarily in the lungs; in recent years, the importance of proactively resecting metastases has been highlighted [4–8], and as such, we proactively resect lung metastases. In the past, surgery for lung metastases consisted of resecting lesions found during visual inspection and palpation by the surgeon. However, this method is reliant on the skill of the surgeon and lacks objectivity. With the introduction of navigation surgery using indocyanine green (ICG) fluorescence imaging, the discovery and resection of lung micrometastases have become very easy. Additionally, as in surgery for hepatocellular carcinoma in adults, ICG fluorescence imaging is also useful in hepatoblastoma surgery, in terms of identifying tumors during surgery on the primary liver tumor, and for intraoperative cholangiography. In this manuscript, we will describe applications of this method during surgery for primary hepatoblastoma and associated metastases.

31.2 Clinical Applications

The use of ICG fluorescence imaging in surgery for hepatoblastoma is classified into two methods. The first is similar to that employed during surgery for hepatocellular carcinoma and utilizes the fact that the ability of hepatoblastoma cells to metabolize bile is inferior to that of healthy liver cells [9]. This method requires intravenous injection of ICG, which resides for a long time within the cell. The second method is to image mainly the biliary tract, using ICG as a nonradioactive contrast agent. Below, we discuss both primary liver tumors and metastases and cover the use of these two ICG methods.

31.2.1 Primary Lesions

When using ICG fluorescence during hepatectomy or liver transplant surgery, we normally intravenously inject 0.5 mg/kg of ICG (Diagnogreen, Daiichi-Sankyo, Tokyo) 48–72 h prior to surgery [9, 10]; this is earlier than the administration of ICG used in lung metastases surgeries. Since ICG remains even in healthy livers, it provides good contrast with the tumor during surgery. For intraoperative infrared radiation and fluorescence detection, we use PDE-neo (Photodynamic Eye, Hamamatsu Photonics, Hamamatsu, Japan).

31.2.1.1 Evaluation of Residual Tumors

The most meaningful use of ICG fluorescence during hepatectomy is to provide confirmation that there is no residual tumor in the remaining liver. In hepatoblastoma, because the tumor is often large, it is common for the tumor to be immediately adjacent to the hepatic vein and/or other hepatic vessels, even after achieving tumor shrinkage with chemotherapy. In such cases, it is common that sufficient margins cannot be taken from the remaining liver and/or tumor. Historically, this was confirmed with intraoperative rapid pathological diagnosis; however, employing the ICG fluorescence method enables the presence of residual tumors to be confirmed in real time. It is possible to capture nearly everything as residual tumors in the hepatic radial margin are present on a surface 1 cm deep or less, within the detectable depth of this method [11].

31.2.1.2 Intraoperative Cholangiography

During a hepatectomy or liver transplant, imaging of the bile duct to confirm the bile duct course and inspecting for bile leakage in the hepatic radial margin after completion of the resection are normally conducted using X-ray. However, in order to obtain results in real time, a large-scale fluoroscopy X-ray system must be used, raising the problem of radiation exposure for the patient and medical staff. These issues can be resolved using the ICG fluorescence method [12, 13]. In this case, the concentration of ICG would differ from that observed during intravenous injection, and 2.5 mg/ml would be injected into the bile duct during surgery [12].

31.2.1.3 Evaluation of Extrahepatic Spreading of the Tumor

In order to lead the management of hepatoblastoma with chemotherapy, it is common to diagnose the histology based on a biopsy taken during initial examination. Therefore, during hepatectomy or liver transplantation, peritoneal adhesion to the tumor of the biopsy site is common. In such cases, there is a risk that the tumor has infiltrated into the peritoneum, necessitating that a section of the peritoneum is also resected. While confirmation is difficult with the naked eye, the infiltration range of the tumor can be identified using the ICG method, resolving this problem. In addition, it is not uncommon for a hepatoblastoma to rupture; in these cases there is also a concern of peritoneal dissemination, which can be confirmed with this method.

31.2.2 Metastatic Lesions

In the use of ICG fluorescence during surgery for hepatoblastoma, the area that this method exhibits its greatest power is in the detection of metastases. The lung is the most common site of metastatic lesions, although in rare cases hepatoblastoma can metastasize to the brain, bones, and lymph nodes. Because the organs to which hepatoblastomas metastasize do not take up ICG, compared to the liver, the contrast achieved between the tumor and the healthy tissue is remarkably good. For this reason, minute metastases can be detected; in our experience a lung metastasis with a diameter of 62 μm was detected and resected during surgery. In contrast to hepatocellular carcinoma, the prognosis of hepatoblastoma can be improved by the surgical resection of metastases in the lungs and other organs [4–8]. This means that the identification and resection of even minute metastases are of great significance. In preparation for this procedure, we intravenously inject 0.5 mg/kg of ICG 24 h before surgery [9, 14, 15].

31.2.2.1 Lung Metastases

While there are cases in which metastases may disappear following presurgical chemotherapy, proactive resection of remaining metastases is effective in improving the prognosis [4–8]. Under normal circumstances, lung metastases often occur in the periphery of the lungs, and issues associated with false-negatives are rare, due to the limit of infrared penetration depth. However, even in cases where lesions are located relatively deep, infrared can easily reach the affected area, as the lung can be collapsed by performing one-lung ventilation, which flattens the lung, especially in children. Our surgical procedure is to perform a thoracotomy under one-lung ventilation and use PDE-neo to identify the tumor, which is generally removed with a wedge resection. Thoracoscopic surgery is not performed for two reasons. Firstly, palpation by the surgeon remains essential. Secondly, staples are used on resections in thoracoscopic surgery, which involve excessive lung tissue, compared with hand-sewn sutures. Staples also appear as artifacts on postoperative computed tomography, making judgment of subsequent recurrence difficult. To date we have performed surgery for lung metastases using this method on ten patients with hepatoblastoma with lung metastases and have resected a total of 250 masses (Fig. 31.1). The median number of resected masses per patient was 13 (range, 1–97), and the median number of lung surgeries per patient was 2.0 (range, 1–11). Of the ten cases, eight went into remission, and two cases are undergoing chemotherapy.

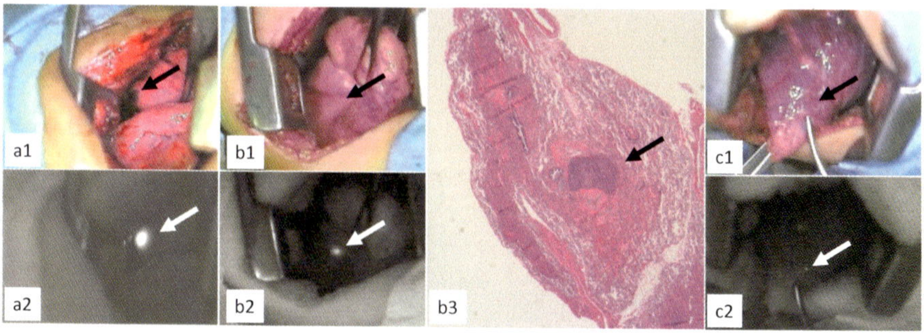

Fig. 31.1 Applications of ICG fluorescence imaging during lung metastasectomy. Metastatic lesions with diameters of 5 mm (**a**), 1 mm (**b**), and 0.07 mm (**c**) were detected by ICG fluorescence imaging. Initial photos (**a1**, **b1**, **c1**) and following photos (**a2**, **b2**, **c2**) indicate the same view of each lesion under room light and ICG fluorescence imaging, respectively. Histopathological finding of b1 lesion appears in b3

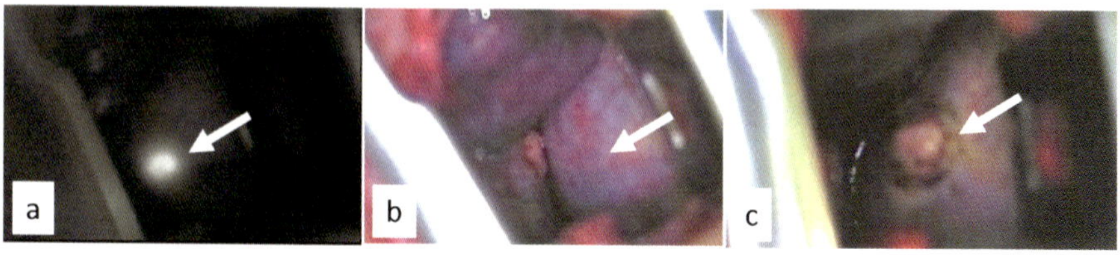

Fig. 31.2 Intraoperative view of a metastatic mediastinal lymph node. (**a**) ICG fluorescence imaging indicates the node. (**b**) Room light view of the lesion. (**c**) After an incision of the mediastinal pleura

31.2.2.2 Lymph Node Metastases

Although infrequent, the ICG method is effective in treating lymph node metastases. Metastatic lymph nodes of the hepatic portal region and mediastinum can be confirmed with satisfactory contrast. This method is particularly effective in cases where the involved lymph node is situated among several other lymph nodes, as the metastatic lymph nodes can be singled out and resected (Fig. 31.2).

31.2.2.3 Peritoneal Metastases

In cases where metastases are suspected in the peritoneum, a laparotomy is performed, and the ICG method is used (Fig. 31.3). In such cases, the timing of ICG administration is approximately 72 h before surgery. The reason for this is that the florescence of the digestive tract is too strong due to excreted bile.

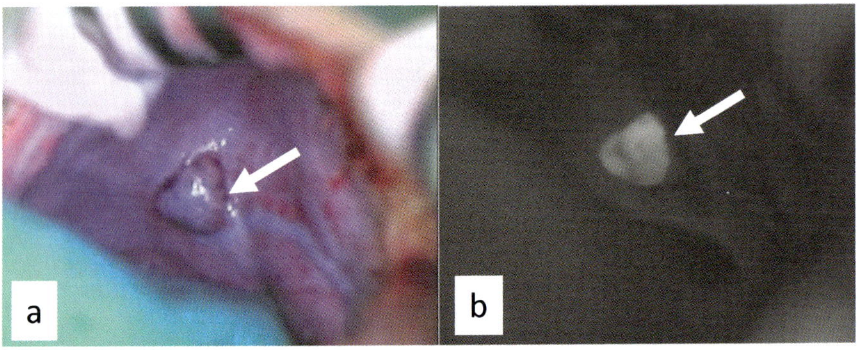

Fig. 31.3 Intraoperative view of a metastatic peritoneal lesion of the right diaphragm. (**a**) Room light view of the lesion. (**b**) ICG fluorescence imaging

31.3 Problems

31.3.1 False-Positive

Of the 250 masses that were identified as positive and resected, tumors could not be histopathologically detected in 29 masses. Interestingly, these false-positives were concentrated in two patients and were not recognized in the remaining eight. The following two reasons may be possible explanations for these false-positives:

1. Fluorescence of tissue other than the tumor. According to observations through a fluorescence microscope within the fluorescence wavelength of ICG, we were able to confirm that thrombi and granuloma were the cause of this non-tumorous fluorescence. While it is unclear why ICG detected these "masses," they consisted of tissue not observed in healthy lungs and may be an alteration after chemotherapy.
2. The possibility that the tumor is too small to be detected. The smallest tumor histopathologically confirmed with the ICG method was 62 μm. On the other hand, paraffin-embedded tissue sections are usually cut out at approximately 20 μm. Therefore, if there are tumors smaller than 20 μm, it is possible that these would not be included in the slice.

31.3.2 False-Negative

We have not experienced any cases of false-negatives, wherein fluorescence is not confirmed with ICG fluorescence, despite the detection of a nodule by imaging or visual inspection and palpation, and the lesion is histopathologically proven to be hepatoblastoma.

31.4 Conclusion

Before the introduction of the present method, intraoperative detection of lung metastases was dependent on visual inspection and palpation, where the entire surface of the lung was carefully searched and then the resection performed. The identification of small lesions depended on the surgeon's experience. The use of the ICG method has increased the ease with which lung metastases can be detected intraoperatively. The variability in detection rates between surgeons has disappeared, and areas to be resected can now be determined objectively. However, whether or not removing every small lesion of this kind improves prognosis is currently unclear and requires further observation in the future.

Acknowledgments I am grateful to Seiji Ohtsubo, DDS, and Mitsuo Kusano, MD, for searching of the false-positive lesions with a special fluorescent microscope. Also I am grateful to Mio Tanaka, MD, and Yukichi Tanaka, MD, for pathological diagnosis.

References

1. von Schweinitz D (2011) Hepatoblastoma: recent developments in research and treatment. Semin Pediatr Surg 21:21–30
2. von Schweinitz D, Hecker H, Harms D et al (1995) Complete resection before development of drug resistance is essential for survival from advanced hepatoblastoma-a report from the German Cooperative Pediatric Liver Tumor Study HB-89. J Pediatr Surg 30:845–852
3. Hishiki T, Matsunaga T, Sasaki F et al (2011) Outcome of hepatoblastomas treated using the Japanese Study Group for Pediatric Liver Tumor (JPLT) protocol-2: report from the JPLT. Pediatr Surg Int 27:1–8
4. Black CT, Luck SR, Musemeche CA et al (1991) Aggressive excision of pulmonary metastases is warranted in the management of childhood hepatic tumors. J Pediatr Surg 26:1082–1085
5. Passmore SJ1, Noblett HR, Wisheart JD, et al (1995) Prolonged survival following multiple thoracotomies for metastatic hepatoblastoma. Med Pediatr Oncol 24: 58–60
6. Meyers RL, Katzenstein HM, Krailo M et al (2007) Surgical resection of pulmonary metastatic lesions in children with hepatoblastoma. J Pediatr Surg 42:2050–2056
7. Zsíros J, Maibach R, Shafford E et al (2010) Successful treatment of childhood high-risk hepatoblastoma with dose-intensive multiagent chemotherapy and surgery: final results of the SIOPEL-3HR study. J Clin Oncol 28:2584–2590
8. Wanaguru D, Shun A, Price N et al (2013) Outcomes of pulmonary metastases in hepatoblastoma-is the prognosis always poor? J Pediatr Surg 48:2474–2478
9. Ishizawa T, Fukushima N, Shibahara J et al (2009) Real-time identification of liver cancers by using indocyanine green fluorescent imaging. Cancer 115:2491–2504
10. Gotoh K, Yamada T, Ishikawa O et al (2009) A novel image-guided surgery of hepatocellular carcinoma by indocyanine green fluorescence imaging navigation. J Surg Oncol 100:75–79
11. Kim S, Lim YT, Soltesz EG et al (2004) Near-infrared fluorescent type II quantum dots for sentinel lymph node mapping. Nat Biotechnol 22:93–97
12. Kaibori M, Ishizaki M, Matsui K et al (2011) Intraoperative indocyanine green fluorescent imaging for prevention of bile leakage after hepatic resection. Surgery 150:91–98

13. Sakaguchi T, Suzuki A, Unno N, et al (2009) Bile leak test by indocyanine green fluorescence images after hepatectomy. Am J Surg 200:e19–23
14. Satou S, Ishizawa T, Masuda K et al (2013) Indocyanine green fluorescent imaging for detecting extrahepatic metastasis of hepatocellular carcinoma. Gastroenterology 48:1136–1143
15. Kitagawa N, Shinkai M, Mochizuki K et al (2015) Navigation using indocyanine green fluorescence imaging for hepatoblastoma pulmonary metastases surgery. Pediatr Surg Int 31:407–411

Chapter 32
Indocyanine Green-Related Transporters in Hepatocellular Carcinoma

Yasushi Shibasaki, Y. Morita, T. Sakaguchi, and H. Konno

Abstract Intraoperative indocyanine green (ICG) fluorescent imaging under near-infrared light is a useful procedure to detect hepatocellular carcinoma (HCC). However, the mechanisms of ICG accumulation in HCC have been unclear. We hypothesized that some transporters on the hepatocytes may be involved in the process of ICG accumulation and examined the expression levels of influx and efflux transporters using resected HCC tissues. Among influx transporter, organic anion-transporting polypeptide 1B3 (OATP1B3) and sodium-taurocholate transport protein (NTCP) are suggested to be responsible for ICG export in HCC. Interestingly, multidrug resistance p-glycoprotein-3 (MDR3), an efflux transporter to canaliculi, is also one of the important ICG transporters and a prognostic factor of HCC. We speculated that ICG is uptaken into hepatocytes through OATP1B3 and accumulated into the blunt-end pseudo-glands or bile canaliculi in HCC tissues through the efflux by MDR3.

Keywords ICG • HCC • Transporter • OATP1B3 • NTCP • MDR3

32.1 Introduction

Indocyanine green (ICG) has been utilized for measurement of the liver function prior to liver resection. Recently, this greenish dye which becomes fluorescent under near-infrared (NIR) light after binding to serum protein is frequently used in various clinical situations: angiography [23, 32], lymphography [31], and cholangiography [19, 25].

Hepatocellular carcinoma (HCC) is the fifth most common cancer worldwide and a leading cause of cancer deaths [14]. Although liver resection without residual cancer component is the most effective treatment for this malignant tumor, it is very

Y. Shibasaki (✉) • Y. Morita • T. Sakaguchi • H. Konno
Second Department of Surgery, Hamamatsu University School of Medicine, 1-20-1 Handayama, Higashi-ku, Hamamatsu, Shizuoka 431-3192, Japan
e-mail: yasushi.shibasaki@gmail.com

M. Kusano et al. (eds.), *ICG Fluorescence Imaging and Navigation Surgery*,
DOI 10.1007/978-4-431-55528-5_32

difficult to detect all of HCCs before hepatectomy albeit recent advances in diagnostic modalities. Ishizawa [12] and Gotoh et al. [8] demonstrated that HCC and metastatic liver tumors with accumulated ICG which administered intravenously before liver resection could be visualized using NIR camera system in real time. They reported that intraoperative ICG fluorography is useful to detect HCCs with high sensitivity and that NIR system enables visualizing small HCCs and precancerous lesions which could not be pointed out by preoperative modalities. We had also reported that 96 % of HCC foci could be observed with ICG fluorography, and some small HCCs were newly distinguished by using NIR camera observations [21]. Thus, this system is thought to be a strong tool for complete resection of HCC. However, the reasons why the ICG, injected preoperatively for the ICG clearance test, accumulated and retained in HCC tissues with several fluorescent patterns are still elusive.

We hypothesized that some transporters on the hepatocytes may be involved in the process of ICG accumulation and examined the expression levels of influx and efflux transporters using resected HCC tissues.

32.2 ICG Fluorescent Pattern

We and Ishizawa et al. [12] classified the ICG fluorescent patterns into three types as follows: uniform (total), uneven (partial), and rim-like fluorescent type (Fig. 32.1a) [21]. Histologically, the low differentiation state was significantly correlated to the low ICG emission pattern. In addition, it is suggested that the morphological characteristics of HCCs contribute to such several patterns of ICG, for instance, pseudo-gland structure encloses ICG into cancer tissue leading to high ICG emission; fibrotic capsule and septal wall compress the ICG fluorescence beneath the tumor border, forming rim-like appearance; and the heterogeneity of HCC component constitutes various fluorescent patterns. These findings suggest that NIR spectroscopy, to some extent, helps us to analyze the property of HCC qualitatively. Since the direct quantitation of the ICG fluorescent signal is presently difficult, we investigated 40 HCC specimens and divided ICG fluorescent patterns into two categories, for further semiquantitative analysis, as follows: ICG high (IH), tumors in which fluorescence was detected on >50 % of the cut surface, and ICG low (IL), tumors in which fluorescence was detected on <50 % of the cut surface (Fig. 32.1b) [27]. Histologically, the frequency of the formation of septal walls and pseudo-gland structures was significantly higher in the IH group [27].

(A)

Fluorescent pattern	Gross appearance	Fluorescent image	Pathological feature
Uniform (Total) fluorescent type	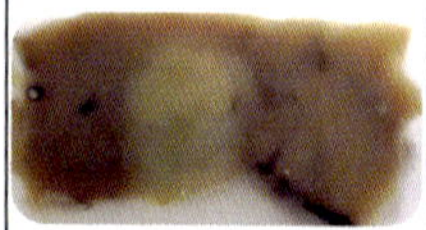	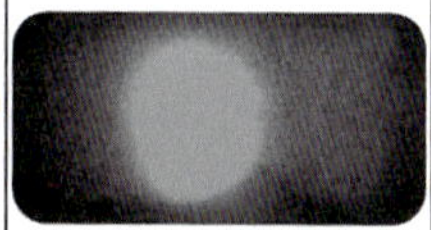	ICG High • Pesudogland (+) • sf (+)
Uneven (Partial) fluorescent type	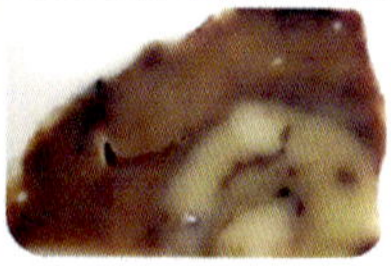	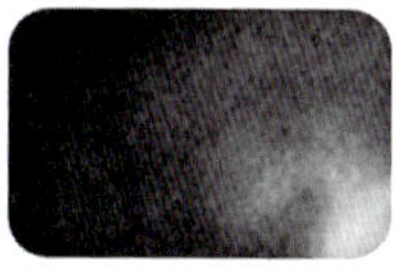	↕
Rim fluorescent type	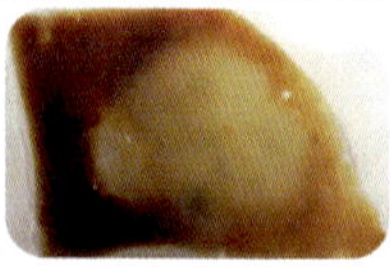	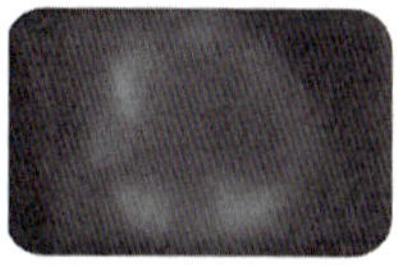	ICG Low • Poor differentiation

(B) ICG High ⟷ ICG Low

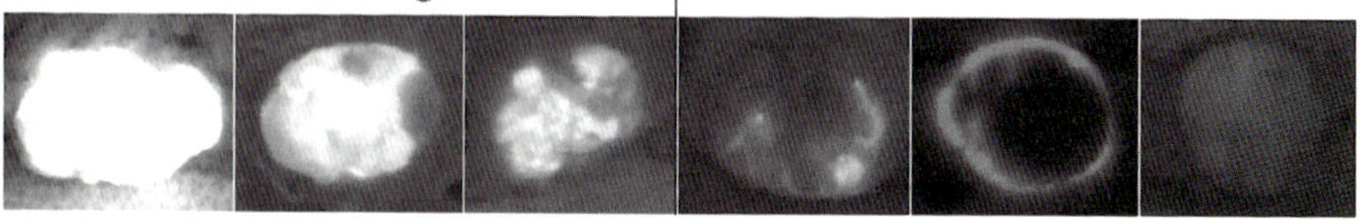

Fig. 32.1 Representative images of ICG fluorescence. (**a**) The center two panels show gross appearance (*left*) and ICG fluorescent image (*right*) of resected HCC specimen. (**b**) Left three panels are ICG-high (IH) group which fluorescence was detected on ≧50 % of the cut surface. The right three panels show ICG low which fluorescence was detected on <50 % of the cut surface

32.3 ICG Pharmacokinetics

Various drugs and substrates are taken into hepatocytes by the influx transporters, metabolized by detoxifying enzymes, and are subsequently excreted to bile canaliculi or blood circulation by the efflux transporters (Fig. 32.2) [6, 26, 34]. ICG is an organic anion, in which molecular formula and molecular weight are $C_{43}H_{47}N_2NaO_6S_2$ and 775 Da, and is taken up exclusively by the liver and rapidly excreted to bile canaliculi without biotransformation [3, 22]. The rate of uptake of ICG is correlated with hepatic blood flow, and its rate of excretion correlates with hepatic function and biliary excretion [4, 28]. In addition, ICG has a characteristic maximum absorption peak of 805 nm in the near-infrared light region, which allows direct measurement of hepatic tissue ICG concentration using NIR [28]. Thus, the reasons why the HCC tissues raise ICG fluorescence visualized by NIR camera may result from some alterations of the hepatic metabolic processes abovementioned.

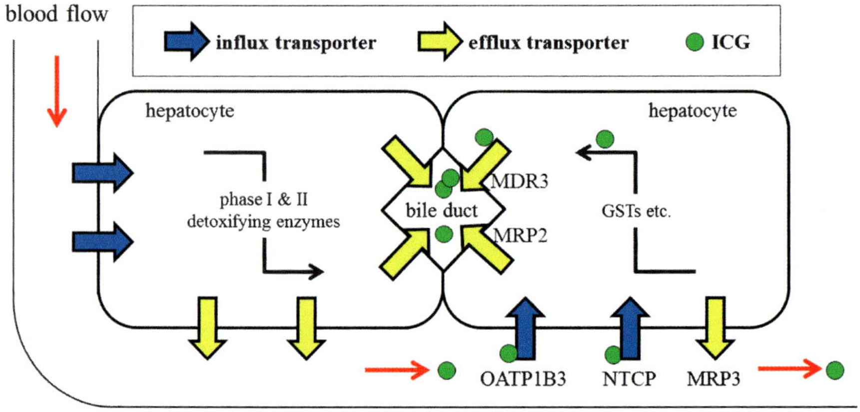

Fig. 32.2 A schema of hepatic metabolism of xenobitics and ICG. *Blue arrows*, influx transporters; *yellow arrows*, efflux transporters; green circle, ICG; ICG, indocyanine green; OATP1B3, organic anion-transporting polypeptide 1B3; NTCP, Na + –taurocholate cotransporting polypeptide; MRP, multidrug resistance-associated protein; MDR3, multidrug resistance p-glycoprotein-3; GST, glutathione S-transferase

32.4 ICG Fluorography and Magnetic Resonance Imaging

Gadolinium ethoxybenzyl diethylenetriamine pentaacetic acid (EOB), a magnetic resonance imaging (MRI) contrast medium, is known to be taken up into hepatocytes but not into typical hepatocellular carcinoma cells. However, some HCCs show higher EOB-MRI intensity levels, at the hepatobiliary phase, compared to adjacent noncancerous parenchyma. It is reported that such phenomena are derived from the expression levels of hepatic influx transporter, organic anion-transporting polypeptide 1B3 (OATP1B3), and efflux transporters including multidrug resistance-associated protein (MRP) 2 and 3 [16, 30]. We incidentally noticed that such high EOB HCCs had high ICG fluorescent levels (Fig. 32.3a). In our study [27], 19 of 22 HCCs (86.4 %) were detected as typical hypointense masses under hepatobiliary phase of EOB-MRI. The other three HCCs were detected as hyperintense masses compared to the surrounding liver parenchyma. All three EOB-accumulated HCCs were categorized into ICG-high (IH) group. Overall, relative intensity (tumor-to-surrounding parenchyma) under hepatobiliary phase of EOB-MRI in IH group was significantly higher than that in ICG-low (IL) group (Fig. 32.3b). Moreover, it is reported recently that EOB-MRI is a useful method to evaluate the liver function correlating with ICG retention test [24]. Therefore, we suspect that EOB dynamics and ICG accumulation pattern may have common mechanisms reflecting transporters' expression in HCC.

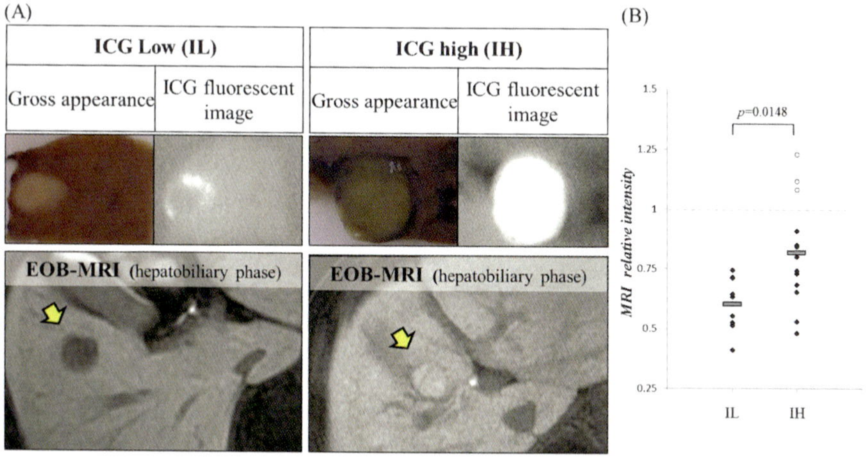

Fig. 32.3 Relationship between ICG fluorescent imaging and EOB-MR imaging. (**a**) The *left panel* shows the typical rim emission pattern HCC which represented low intensity relative to the surrounding parenchyma at hepatobiliary phase of EOB-MRI. The *right panels* show the typical uniform emission pattern HCC which represented high intensity relative to the surrounding parenchyma at hepatobiliary phase of EOB-MRI. Macroscopically, these EOB-high HCCs are usually greenish (so-called green hepatoma). (**b**) Relative MRI intensity of HCC compared to adjacent noncancerous parenchyma in hepatobiliary phase of EOB-MRI was measured in IL (ICG-low) and IH (ICG-high) group

32.5 Expression of Hepatic Transporters in HCC

We analyzed the intratumoral expression levels of transporters using an immunoblot analysis in 20 and immunohistochemistry in 40 resected HCC tissues, with OATP1B3 and sodium-taurocholate transport protein (NTCP) as influx transporters and multidrug resistance p-glycoprotein-3 (MDR3), MRP2, and MRP3 as efflux transporters. OATP1B3 protein levels were significantly higher in the IH group and MDR3 protein levels, an exporter to bile canaliculi, were significantly higher in the IH group [27]. NTCP and MRP2 tended to be higher in IH group, but did not reach the statistical significance. Conversely, MRP3 seemed to diminish in IH HCCs (Fig. 32.4). Ishizawa et al. [13] also reported that OATP1B3 and NTCP are responsible for ICG accumulation in HCC tissues.

32.5.1 Influx Transporter

Hepatic influx transporters export various endogenous and exogenous substrates from the basolateral membrane side into hepatocyte. OATP1B3 is an organic anion transporter, encoded by the solute carrier family 21A8 (*SLC21A8*), localizing in the

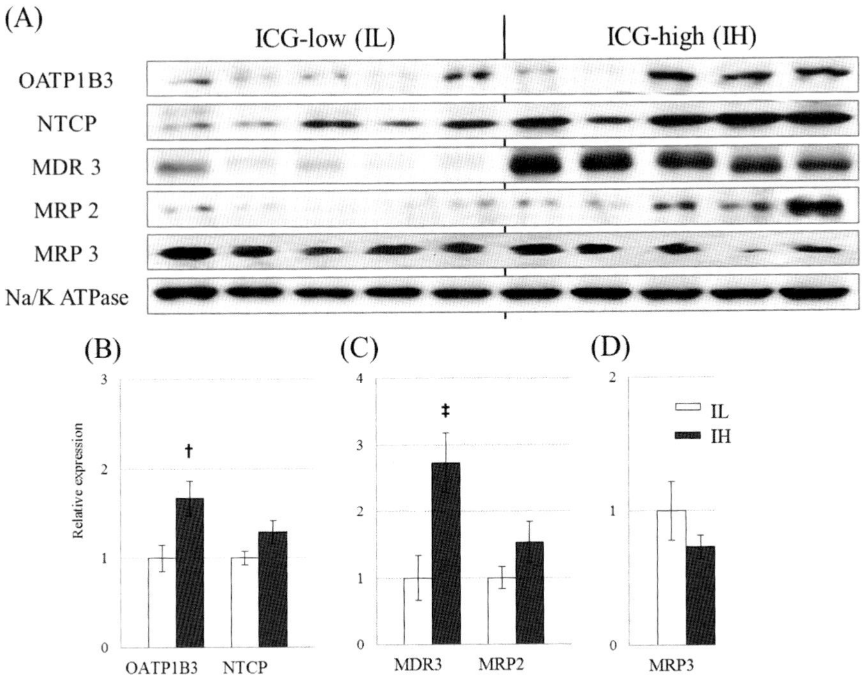

Fig. 32.4 Immunoblot analysis of hepatic transporter expression: Panel (**a**) shows a typical immunoblot analysis of hepatic transporters. Panels (**b**), (**c**), and (**d**) show the densitometric quantification results of influx transporters (OATP1B3 and NTCP), canalicular efflux transporters (MDR3 and MRP2), and the sinusoidal efflux transporter MRP3, using Na+/K+ ATPase as an internal standard, respectively. Statistical analysis was performed using the Mann–Whitney *U* test; †, $p < 0.05$, ‡, $p < 0.01$ significant difference between the IL (*left white bars*) and IH (*right black bars*) groups

sinusoidal side of the plasma membrane. OATP1B3 have broad substrate specificity and accept a number of therapeutic drugs [29] concomitant with transporting of endogenous substrates, including bile acids, thyroid hormones, prostaglandins, and bilirubin glucuronide [9].

We analyzed OATP1B3 immunostaining in 40 HCC specimens and revealed that high OATP1B3 expressions were significantly correlated with high ICG fluorescence [27]. Although OATP1B3 exists predominantly in the liver, several cancers of the other organ origin express this influx transporter [10, 37], indicating the modulation of the sensitivity to anticancer reagents. In some articles, it is reported that OATP1B3 is one of the targets for anticancer therapy and is thought to be a possible prognostic factor of cancers [18] including HCCs [36].

NTCP, sodium-taurocholate cotransporting polypeptide, is a member of the solute carrier family 10 (*SLC10*), the major bile acid transporter in human hepatocytes, that localizes to the basolateral hepatocyte membrane [35]. This has been shown to also transport some xenobiotics in a Na^+-dependent manner [11] and

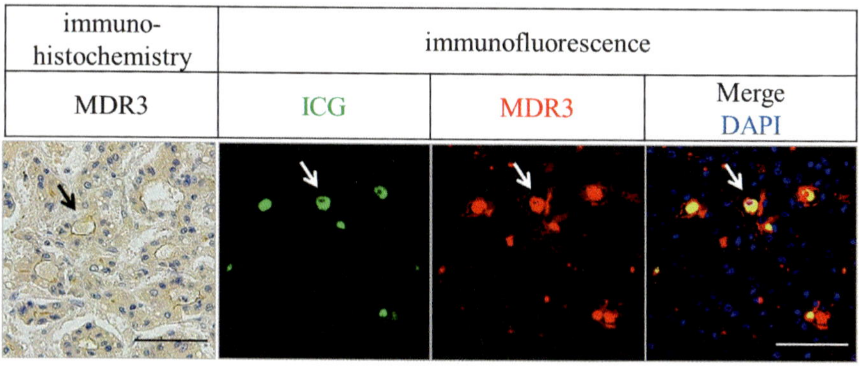

Fig. 32.5 Immunohistochemical and immunofluorescent images of the MDR3 protein and accumulated ICG. *Left panels* show MDR3 immunohistochemical staining image. In the right three panels, green and red colors indicate ICG deposits and MDR3 fluorescent staining, respectively. Nuclei are shown in *blue* with DAPI staining. These panels show representative figures of HCC with pseudo-glandular structures (*arrows*). The scale bar shows 100 μm

transport indocyanine green [3]. Although its expression is known to be reduced in hepatocellular carcinoma [38], some HCC may use this transporter as the ICG export system [13].

It is reasonable to assume that the high expression of these transporters induces abundant intracellular ICG accumulation in a short time after ICG administration. However, the intraoperative fluorography was performed usually several days after intravenous ICG injection, and ICG deposition were scarcely seen in intracellular space but mainly seen in extracellular structures such as pseudo-glands (Fig. 32.5). Thus, high expression of influx transporter is one of the necessary conditions, but the other mechanism is also needed for ICG accumulation in HCCs.

32.5.2 *Efflux Transporter*

Hepatic excretions of the endogenous and exogenous substrates were regulated mainly by ATP-binding cassette (ABC) transporters. Until now, 48 members of the ABC transporter family have been isolated and identified [7]. The ABC transporter efflux activity is driven by the energy derived from the hydrolysis of ATP to adenosine diphosphate (ADP) to transport substrates across the cellular membrane [1]. MDR3, also known as ABCB4, is reported to regulate ICG excretion [17]. We demonstrated that MDR3 expression was positively correlated to ICG deposition in hepatocellular carcinoma tissues.

Generally, efflux transporters facilitate the clearance of intracellular substrate from hepatocyte. In normal hepatocyte with normal bile duct formation, ICG which metabolized in the hepatocyte are exported to apical-sided canaliculi leading to the excretion into the intestine and subsequently ICG disappearance from the liver. Therefore, we thought at first that high MDR3 expression is contradictory to the accumulation of ICG in HCC tissues. To uncover this contradiction, we performed fluorescent microscope analysis. We found that ICG was condensed inside the bile canaliculi and MDR3 high expression was observed around these spaces (Fig. 32.5). It is well known that HCCs frequently have pseudo-glands and anomalous bile canaliculi which do not connect to the main bile duct that is dead end. A conceivable reason for the abovementioned discrepancy is that excreted ICG into the blind-end canaliculi through MDR3 would cause the deposition of ICG.

MDR3 is also known as a flippase and/or floppase of membranous phospholipids [2, 33], and the loss of its mouse homologous gene, MDR2, has been shown to induce hepatocarcinogenesis in mice [15]. Since we speculated that MDR3 expression in HCC tissues would influence the prognosis, we examined MDR3 immunostaining and investigated the relationship to HCC outcomes. To evaluate the expression of transporters with immunohistochemistry, 40 specimens were scored and divided into four categories as follows: score 0, negative or minimal; score 1, positive to a lesser extent than the adjacent liver parenchyma; score 2, positive to the same extent as the adjacent liver parenchyma; and score 3, positive to a higher extent than the adjacent liver parenchyma (Fig. 32.6a). MDR3 immunostaining analysis revealed that eight specimens were negative (score 0) for the expression of MDR3. The tumor size of MDR3-negative HCC was significantly larger than that of MDR3-positive HCC, and serum a-fetoprotein (AFP) levels were significantly higher in MDR3-negative HCC than in MDR3-positive HCC [27]. The MDR3 score correlated with disease-free survival (DFS) and overall survival (OS) rates following hepatectomy. Patients with MDR3-negative HCC (score 0) had significantly worse DFS and slightly worse OS rates than those with MDR3-positive HCC (Fig. 32.6b).

This poor outcome of MDR3-negative HCC may be caused by altered membranous phospholipid compositions, such as phosphatidylcholine species [20]. In our study, MRP2 and MRP3 did not significantly correlate with ICG deposition in HCC. It is reported that the overexpression of some of ABC transporters is able to efflux drugs out of the tumor cell, leading the resistance to chemotherapy [5]. If ICG fluorography can reflect such particular transporter expression state, NIR system may become potent predictor of drug resistance and HCC prognosis. Further investigation is needed to elucidate the complete mechanism of ICG pooling in HCC.

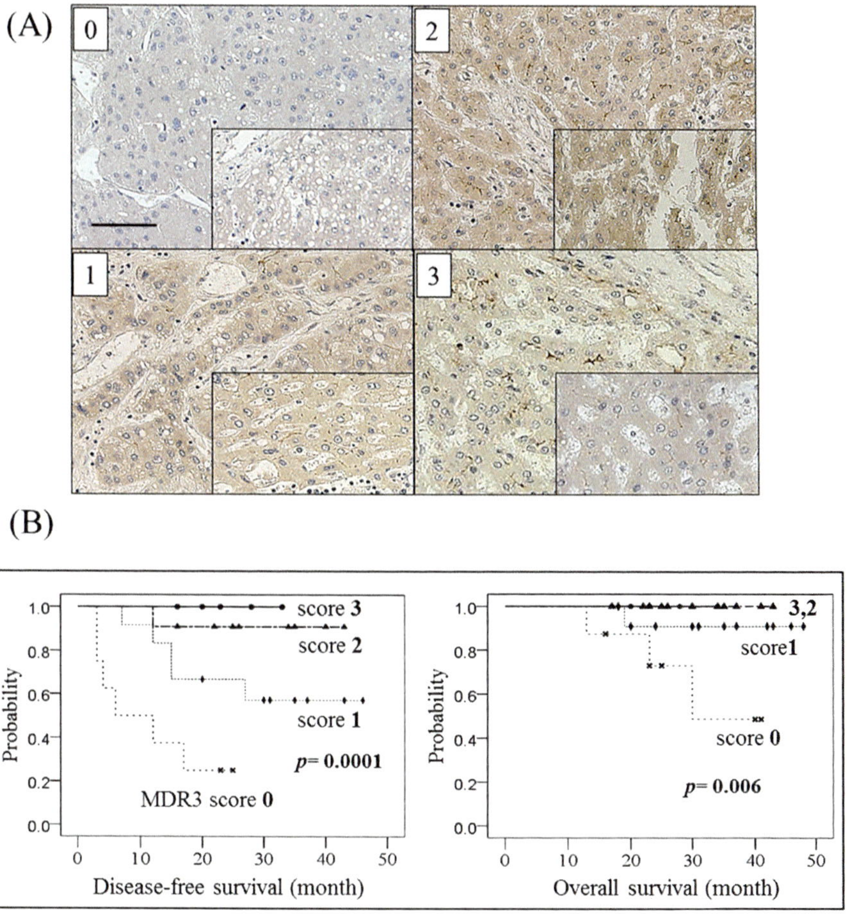

Fig. 32.6 (**a**) Representative figures of MDR3 immunohistochemistry. The scale bars show 100 μm. The main panels show cancer tissues, and the right lower inset shows adjacent noncancerous tissues. A score of 0 indicated the negative expression of MDR3, and scores of 1–3 indicated the positive expression of MDR3 and were divided according to a staining intensity comparison between HCC tissues and adjacent noncancerous tissues. (**b**) Disease-free (*left*) and overall survival (*right*) curves following hepatectomy using the Kaplan-Meier method stratified by MDR3 staining scores

32.6 Conclusion

In HCC tissues, ICG is exported into cancer cells by OATP1B3 and NTCP, being metabolized in intracellular space without biotransformation and secreted to apical membrane of cancer cells by MDR3. If HCCs have normal biliary duct, ICG shall disappear from the liver parenchyma. But if cancer tissues have dead-end canaliculi or pseudo-glands, ICG which has been excreted by MDR3 have to be stagnant in HCC tissues for several days after ICG injection (Fig. 32.7).

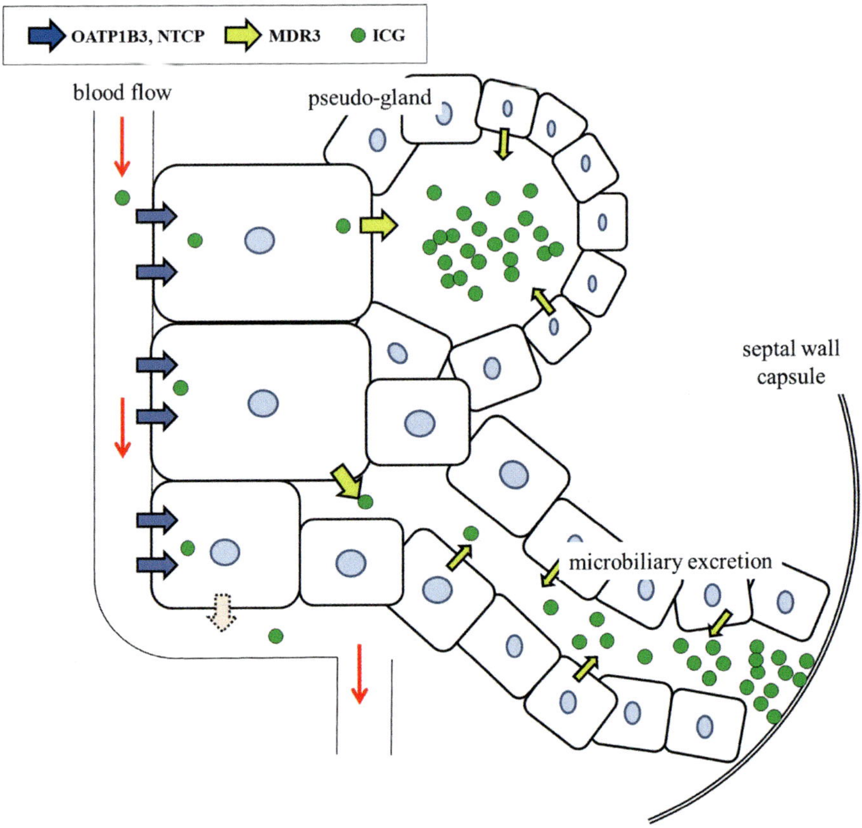

Fig. 32.7 Postulated schema of ICG accumulation mechanism in HCC. First, ICG are taken into hepatocyte by influx transporters (*blue arrows*), OATP1B3 and NTCP, from blood flow (*red arrows*). Second, ICG which underwent intracellular exporting without biotransformation are effluxed to canalicular membrane by MDR3 (*yellow arrows*). Third, excreted ICG are pooling in pseudo-glands and/or micro-canaliculi which are dead-ended

References

1. Anreddy N, Gupta P, Kathawala RJ et al (2014) Tyrosine kinase inhibitors as reversal agents for ABC transporter mediated drug resistance. Molecules (Basel, Switzerland) 19:13848–13877
2. Borst P, Zelcer N, Van Helvoort A (2000) ABC transporters in lipid transport. Biochim Biophys Acta 1486:128–144
3. De Graaf W, Hausler S, Heger M et al (2011) Transporters involved in the hepatic uptake of (99m) Tc-mebrofenin and indocyanine green. J Hepatol 54:738–745
4. El-Desoky A, Seifalian AM, Cope M et al (1999) Experimental study of liver dysfunction evaluated by direct indocyanine green clearance using near infrared spectroscopy. Br J Surg 86:1005–1011
5. Fletcher JI, Haber M, Henderson MJ et al (2010) ABC transporters in cancer: more than just drug efflux pumps. Nat Rev Cancer 10:147–156

6. Giacomini KM, Huang SM, Tweedie DJ et al (2010) Membrane transporters in drug development. Nat Rev Drug Discov 9:215–236
7. Gillet JP, Efferth T, Remacle J (2007) Chemotherapy-induced resistance by ATP-binding cassette transporter genes. Biochim Biophys Acta 1775:237–262
8. Gotoh K, Yamada T, Ishikawa O et al (2009) A novel image-guided surgery of hepatocellular carcinoma by indocyanine green fluorescence imaging navigation. J Surg Oncol 100:75–79
9. Hagenbuch B, Meier PJ (2003) The superfamily of organic anion transporting polypeptides. Biochim Biophys Acta 1609:1–18
10. Han S, Kim K, Thakkar N et al (2013) Role of hypoxia inducible factor-1alpha in the regulation of the cancer-specific variant of organic anion transporting polypeptide 1B3 (OATP1B3), in colon and pancreatic cancer. Biochem Pharmacol 86:816–823
11. Ho RH, Tirona RG, Leake BF et al (2006) Drug and bile acid transporters in rosuvastatin hepatic uptake: function, expression, and pharmacogenetics. Gastroenterology 130:1793–1806
12. Ishizawa T, Fukushima N, Shibahara J et al (2009) Real-time identification of liver cancers by using indocyanine green fluorescent imaging. Cancer 115:2491–2504
13. Ishizawa T, Masuda K, Urano Y et al (2014) Mechanistic background and clinical applications of indocyanine green fluorescence imaging of hepatocellular carcinoma. Ann Surg Oncol 21:440–448
14. Jemel A, Bray F, Center MM et al (2011) Global cancer statistics. CA Cancer J Clin 61:69–90
15. Katzenellenbogen M, Mizrahi L, Pappo O et al (2007) Molecular mechanisms of liver carcinogenesis in the mdr2-knockout mice. Mol Cancer Res 5:1159–1170
16. Kitao A, Zen Y, Matsui O et al (2010) Hepatocellular carcinoma: signal intensity at gadoxetic acid-enhanced MR Imaging–correlation with molecular transporters and histopathologic features. Radiology 256:817–826
17. Kusuhara H, Sugiyama Y (2010) Pharmacokinetic modeling of the hepatobiliary transport mediated by cooperation of uptake and efflux transporters. Drug Metab Rev 42:539–550
18. Lockhart AC, Harris E, Lafleur BJ et al (2008) Organic anion transporting polypeptide 1B3 (OATP1B3) is overexpressed in colorectal tumors and is a predictor of clinical outcome. Clin Exp Gastroenterol 1:1–7
19. Mitsuhashi N, Kimura F, Shimizu H et al (2008) Usefulness of intraoperative fluorescence imaging to evaluate local anatomy in hepatobiliary surgery. J Hepatobiliary Pancreat Surg 15:508–514
20. Morita Y, Sakaguchi T, Ikegami K et al (2013) Lysophosphatidylcholine acyltransferase 1 altered phospholipid composition and regulated hepatoma progression. J Hepatol 59:292–299
21. Morita Y, Sakaguchi T, Unno N et al (2011) Detection of hepatocellular carcinomas with near-infrared fluorescence imaging using indocyanine green: its usefulness and limitation. Int J Clin Oncol 18:232–241
22. Paumgartner G (1975) The handling of indocyanine green by the liver. Schweiz Med Wochenschr 105:1–30
23. Rubens FD, Ruel M, Fremes SE (2002) A new and simplified method for coronary and graft imaging during CABG. Heart Surg Forum 5:141–144
24. Saito K, Ledsam J, Sourbron S et al (2014) Measuring hepatic functional reserve using low temporal resolution Gd-EOB-DTPA dynamic contrast-enhanced MRI: a preliminary study comparing galactosyl human serum albumin scintigraphy with indocyanine green retention. Eur Radiol 24:112–119
25. Sakaguchi T, Suzuki A, Unno N et al (2010) Bile leak test by indocyanine green fluorescence images after hepatectomy. Am J Surg 200:e19–e23
26. Sevior DK, Pelkonen O, Ahokas JT (2012) Hepatocytes: the powerhouse of biotransformation. Int J Biochem Cell Biol 44:257–261
27. Shibasaki Y, Sakaguchi T, Hiraide T et al (2014) Expression of indocyanine green-related transporters in hepatocellular carcinoma. J Surg Res 193:567–576

28. Shinohara H, Tanaka A, Kitai T et al (1996) Direct measurement of hepatic indocyanine green clearance with near-infrared spectroscopy: separate evaluation of uptake and removal. Hepatology 23:137–144
29. Shitara Y, Maeda K, Ikejiri K et al (2013) Clinical significance of organic anion transporting polypeptides (OATPs) in drug disposition: their roles in hepatic clearance and intestinal absorption. Biopharm Drug Dispos 34:45–78
30. Tsuboyama T, Onishi H, Kim T et al (2010) Hepatocellular carcinoma: hepatocyte-selective enhancement at gadoxetic acid-enhanced MR imaging–correlation with expression of sinusoidal and canalicular transporters and bile accumulation. Radiology 255:824–833
31. Unno N, Inuzuka K, Suzuki M et al (2007) Preliminary experience with a novel fluorescence lymphography using indocyanine green in patients with secondary lymphedema. J Vasc Surg 45:1016–1021
32. Unno N, Suzuki M, Yamamoto N et al (2008) Indocyanine green fluorescence angiography for intraoperative assessment of blood flow: a feasibility study. Eur J Vasc Endovasc Surg 35:205–207
33. Van Helvoort A, Smith AJ, Sprong H et al (1996) MDR1 P-glycoprotein is a lipid translocase of broad specificity, while MDR3 P-glycoprotein specifically translocates phosphatidylcholine. Cell 87:507–517
34. Wu KC, Cui JY, Klaassen CD (2012) Effect of graded Nrf2 activation on phase-I and -II drug metabolizing enzymes and transporters in mouse liver. PLoS One 7, e39006
35. Xiao F, Mckeating JA, Baumert TF (2013) A bile acid transporter as a candidate receptor for hepatitis B and D virus entry. J Hepatol 58:1246–1248
36. Yamashita T, Kitao A, Matsui O et al (2014) Gd-EOB-DTPA-enhanced magnetic resonance imaging and alpha-fetoprotein predict prognosis of early-stage hepatocellular carcinoma. Hepatology 60:1674–1685
37. Yuan J, Yi X, Yan F et al (2014) Nearinfrared fluorescence imaging of prostate cancer using heptamethine carbocyanine dyes. Mol Med Rep 11:821–828
38. Zollner G, Wagner M, Fickert P et al (2005) Hepatobiliary transporter expression in human hepatocellular carcinoma. Liver Int 25:367–379

Part XIII
Hepato-Pancreatic-Biliary Surgery: Liver Transplantation

Chapter 33
Liver Transplantation Guided by ICG Fluorescence Imaging: Assessment of Hepatic Vessel Reconstruction

Yoshikuni Kawaguchi, Takeaki Ishizawa, and Norihiro Kokudo

Abstract This chapter covers assessments of hepatic vessel reconstruction using fluorescence imaging techniques with administration of indocyanine green (ICG) during liver transplantation (LT). Recent advancements in surgical techniques, postoperative management, and immunosuppression have improved the safety of LT. The intraoperative modality to survey reconstructed hepatic vessels is limited mainly to ultrasound. We herein describe ICG fluorescence imaging technique to assess reconstruction of hepatic vessels during LT.

Keywords ICG fluorescence imaging • Fluorescence angiography • Veno-occlusive region

Abbreviations

LT	liver transplantation
IOUS	intraoperative ultrasound
ICG	indocyanine green
MHV	middle hepatic vein

33.1 Introduction

Advancements in surgical techniques, postoperative management, and immunosuppression have improved the safety of liver transplantation (LT) [1–5]. However, reoperation rate in patients undergoing LT remains high, ranging from 9.2 to 34 %

Y. Kawaguchi, M.D. • T. Ishizawa, M.D., Ph.D.
Hepato-Biliary-Pancreatic Surgery Division, Department of Surgery, Graduate School of Medicine, University of Tokyo, 7-3-1 Hongo, Bunkyo-ku, Tokyo 113-8655, Japan

N. Kokudo, M.D., Ph.D. (✉)
Hepato-Biliary-Pancreatic Surgery Division, Artificial Organ and Transplantation Division, Department of Surgery, Graduate School of Medicine, University of Tokyo, Tokyo, Japan
e-mail: KOKUDO-2SU@h.u-tokyo.ac.jp

M. Kusano et al. (eds.), *ICG Fluorescence Imaging and Navigation Surgery*,
DOI 10.1007/978-4-431-55528-5_33

[6–10], compared to that for liver resection which ranges from 2.5 to 10.9 % [11–13]. That is most likely due to requirement of reconstruction of hepatic vessels, including the hepatic artery, the portal vein, and the hepatic vein, and enhances the importance of surveillance for hepatic vessel reconstruction to improve the posttransplant outcomes. Intraoperative ultrasound (IOUS) and Doppler IOUS are the simplest and most reliable modalities for the intraoperative evaluation of reconstructed hepatic vessels.

Recently, fluorescence imaging technique using indocyanine green (ICG) has been applied to hepatobiliary surgery for intraoperative visualization of bile ducts [14–16], liver cancers [17, 18], hepatic segments to be resected [19, 20], and evaluation of portal uptake function in veno-occlusive regions [21]. This technique was also utilized for LT to assess the reconstructed hepatic vessels [16, 22, 23]. We herein describe ICG fluorescence imaging technique which visualizes hepatic flows of reconstructed vessels and regions with venous occlusion to improve the safety of LT.

33.2 Fluorescence Angiography During Recipient Surgery

33.2.1 Background

Fluorescence angiography using ICG was originally used to assess coronary artery bypass graft patency during cardiac surgery [24, 25]. This technique was also applied to visualize anastomotic sites of arteries and lymphatic vessels in plastic surgery [26, 27]. Kubota et al. first reported the usefulness of this technique to assess blood flow passing the anastomotic sites of the hepatic artery and portal vein [23]. The authors' group reported fluorescence angiography using the system which overlays fluorescence images on the background color images [16].

33.2.2 Administration of ICG

Intraoperative fluorescence angiography is performed by intravenous injection of 1 mL ICG (2.5 mg).

33.2.3 Visualization of Hepatic Blood Flow After Reconstruction of Hepatic Vessels

After placement of liver grafts and reconstruction of all hepatic vessels, the camera head of the fluorescence imaging system (PDE, Hamamatsu Photonics, Hamamatsu, Japan) was positioned 20 cm above the anastomotic sites of hepatic

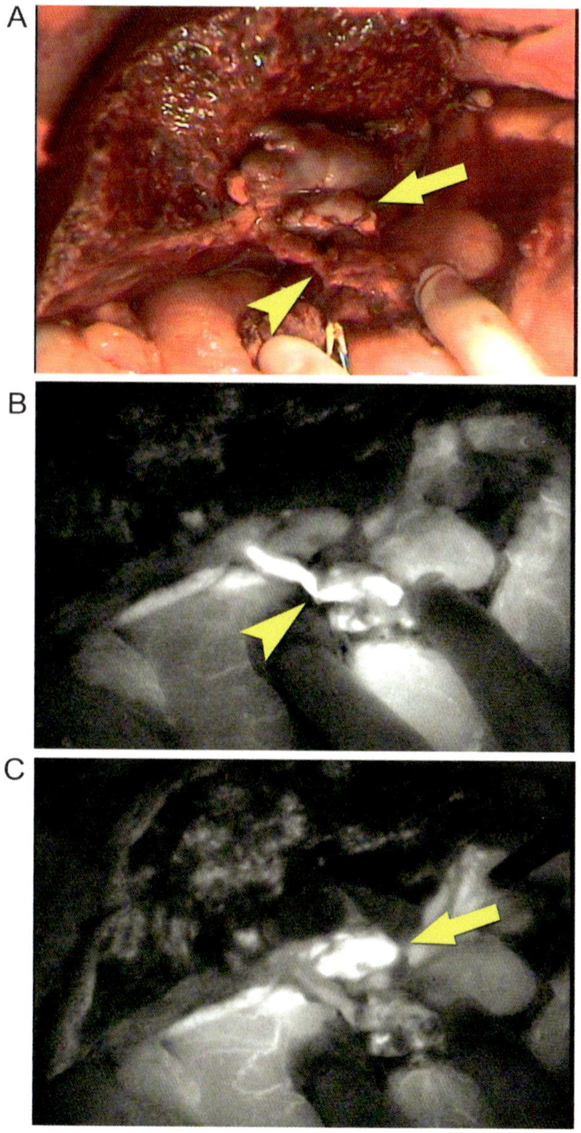

Fig. 33.1 Fluorescence angiography. (**a**) Intraoperative gross appearance of the right liver graft after the reconstruction of the hepatic artery (*arrowhead*) and the portal vein (*arrow*). (**b**) Following the intravenous injection of ICG, fluorescence imaging delineated continuous blood flow through the anastomotic site (arrowhead). (**c**) The portal flow (arrow) was subsequently visualized

vessels. Fluorescence images of continuous arterial blood and portal venous flow were obtained following intravenous injection of ICG. Fluorescence images of hepatic blood flow of the right liver graft were shown in Fig. 33.1. Arterial blood flow through the anastomotic sites was first delineated and portal flow was subsequently visualized.

33.3 Intraoperative Visualization of Veno-occlusive Regions in the Liver Graft

33.3.1 Background

In living-donor liver transplantation using the right liver graft without the middle hepatic vein (MHV), venous occlusion of the MHV tributaries needs to be addressed to avoid adverse events such as necrosis [28], insufficient regeneration [29], and difficulty in postoperative management [30, 31]. The MHV tributaries including V5 draining segment 5 and V8 draining segment 8 were reconstructed or sacrificed based on the institutional criteria. The modality to evaluate success/failure of venous reconstruction and the extent of regions with venous occlusion is limited mainly to intraoperative ultrasound or Doppler ultrasound. Recently, authors' group evaluated portal uptake function in veno-occlusive regions of the remnant liver or the liver graft using fluorescence imaging following intravenous injection of ICG [21]. This technique was applied to visualize the extent of regions with venous occlusion in the liver graft [22].

33.3.2 Administration of ICG

Following procedure of liver transplantation, the camera head of the florescence imaging system (PDE) was positioned 20 cm above the liver surface, and surgical lights were turned off. The output of the light-emitting diodes (760 nm) was set at 0.21 mW per cm^2. ICG (2.5 μg per 1 mL of remnant liver volume calculated based on preoperative computed tomography) was injected intravenously.

33.3.3 Visualization of Regions with Venous Flow After Reconstruction of the Hepatic Venous Tributaries

The FI values on the liver surface increased linearly during first 200 s and then reached a plateau in an average, providing clear demarcation between veno-occlusive regions and non-veno-occlusive regions. [21] Reconstruction of the hepatic veins can be evaluated using ICG fluorescence imaging because FI is lower in veno-occlusive regions than in non-veno-occlusive regions.

Clinical application of this technique is shown in Fig. 33.2. Following placement of a right liver graft and reconstruction of all hepatic vessels, ICG was injected intravenously. FI in regions drained by the right hepatic vein and V8 increased gradually, while FI on the surface of regions drained by V5 was lower than the other regions in the graft. Portal uptake of ICG in the regions drained by V5 was impaired due to sacrifice of the tributaries of V5. By contrast, the drainage area of the right

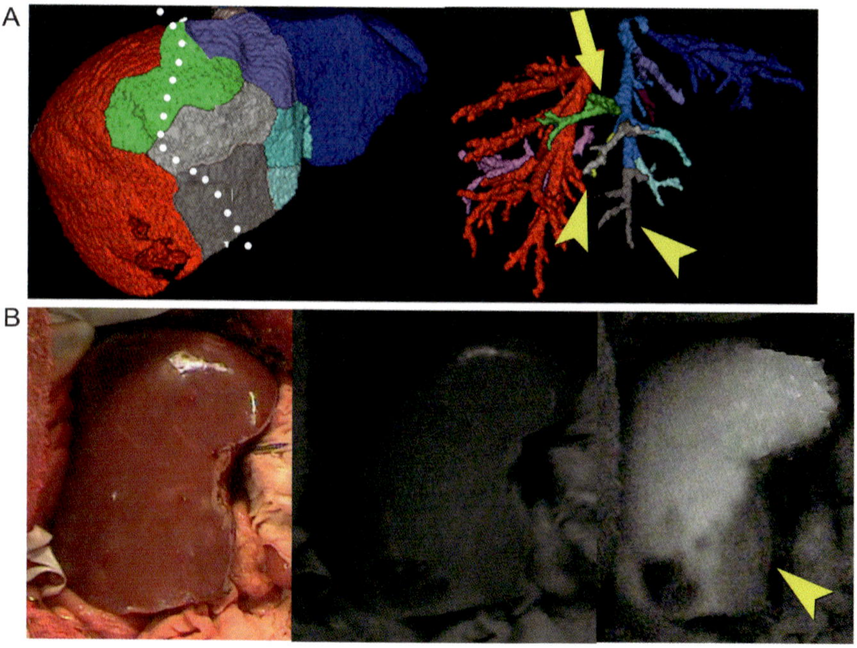

Fig. 33.2 Evaluation of the hepatic vein reconstruction. (**a**) Procurement of the right liver graft without the middle hepatic vein was scheduled along the border between the left and the right liver (*white dotted line*). The volume of regions drained by V8 (*arrow*) was 45 mL (5.3 % of recipient standard liver volume), while the volume of regions drained by two V5s (*arrowheads*) was 40 mL (4.7 % of recipient standard liver volume). Reconstructions of V8 and the right hepatic veins were scheduled because the drainage areas of V5 in the right liver graft were smaller than those of V8 and the graft volume without venous occlusion (475 mL, 56.3 % of recipient standard liver volume) was sufficient for the recipient (**b**) Fluorescence imaging revealed a clear demarcation between the veno-occlusive regions (*arrowhead*) and non-veno-occlusive regions. Reconstruction of the right hepatic vein and V8 was judged to be successful because FI in their drainage areas increased and was higher than veno-occlusive regions in which the corresponding drainage vessels were not reconstructed

hepatic vein and V8 was not impaired due to reconstruction of those drainage veins and preservation of venous outflow. Doppler ultrasound identifies the flow of the reconstructed vessels and help surgeons to decide success/failure of the reconstruction. This technique is useful to identify the regions with or without venous outflow and assess the level of portal uptake in regions as well. This information complements assessment of Doppler ultrasound and is expected to improve the safety of LT.

These evaluations required approximately 10 min in total. One of advantages of these techniques is that they enable visualization of the degree and the extent of the portal uptake in the regions as a result of hepatic vessel reconstruction. These techniques are expected to more accurately estimate the portal uptake in regions with or without venous occlusion, ensuring the safety of liver resection and liver transplantation.

33.4 Conclusion

ICG fluorescence imaging enables real-time assessment of reconstructed hepatic vessels during LT. Anastomotic sites of the hepatic artery and portal vein were visualized after injection of ICG, and the extent and degree of portal uptake were evaluated referring to fluorescence images on the liver surface. These techniques are expected to complement intraoperative ultrasound which is utilized to assess the hepatic flow after reconstruction, enhancing the safety of LT.

Acknowledgment This work was supported by grants from the Takeda Science Foundation, the Kanae Foundation for the Promotion of Medical Science, the Pancreas Research Foundation of Japan, the Canon Foundation in Europe, and the Ministry of Education, Culture, Sports, Science and Technology of Japan (No.23689060).

Financial Disclosure The authors have no relevant affiliations or financial involvement with any organization or entity with a financial interest in or financial conflict with the subject matter or materials discussed in this manuscript. This includes employment, consultancies, honoraria, stock ownership or options, expert testimony, grants or patents received or pending, and royalties. No writing assistance was utilized in the production of this manuscript.

References

1. Starzl TE, Klintmalm GB, Porter KA, Iwatsuki S, Schroter GP (1981) Liver transplantation with use of cyclosporin a and prednisone. N Engl J Med 305:266–269
2. Sugawara Y, Makuuchi M, Kaneko J, Ohkubo T, Imamura H, Kawarasaki H (2002) Correlation between optimal tacrolimus doses and the graft weight in living donor liver transplantation. Clin Transpl 16:102–106
3. Sugawara Y, Makuuchi M, Akamatsu N, Kishi Y, Niiya T, Kaneko J et al (2004) Refinement of venous reconstruction using cryopreserved veins in right liver grafts. Liver Transpl 10:541–547
4. Kokudo N, Sugawara Y, Imamura H, Sano K, Makuuchi M (2005) Tailoring the type of donor hepatectomy for adult living donor liver transplantation. Am J Transplant 5:1694–1703
5. Pomposelli JJ, Verbesey J, Simpson MA, Lewis WD, Gordon FD, Khettry U et al (2006) Improved survival after live donor adult liver transplantation (LDALT) using right lobe grafts: program experience and lessons learned. Am J Transplant 6:589–598
6. Hendriks HG, van der Meer J, de Wolf JT, Peeters PM, Porte RJ, de Jong K et al (2005) Intraoperative blood transfusion requirement is the main determinant of early surgical re-intervention after orthotopic liver transplantation. Transpl Int 17:673–679

7. Freise CE, Gillespie BW, Koffron AJ, Lok AS, Pruett TL, Emond JC et al (2008) Recipient morbidity after living and deceased donor liver transplantation: findings from the A2ALL Retrospective Cohort Study. Am J Transplant 8:2569–2579
8. Kappa SF, Gorden DL, Davidson MA, Wright JK, Guillamondegui OD (2010) Intraoperative blood loss predicts hemorrhage-related reoperation after orthotopic liver transplantation. Am Surg 76:969–973
9. Yoshiya S, Shirabe K, Kimura K, Yoshizumi T, Ikegami T, Kayashima H et al (2012) The causes, risk factors, and outcomes of early relaparotomy after living-donor liver transplantation. Transpl J 94:947–952
10. Kawaguchi Y, Sugawara Y, Akamatsu N, Kaneko J, Hamada T, Tanaka T et al (2014) Impact of early reoperation following living-donor liver transplantation on graft survival. PLoS One 9, e109731
11. Schroeder RA, Marroquin CE, Bute BP, Khuri S, Henderson WG, Kuo PC (2006) Predictive indices of morbidity and mortality after liver resection. Ann Surg 243:373–379
12. Barbas AS, Turley RS, Mallipeddi MK, Lidsky ME, Reddy SK, White RR et al (2013) Examining reoperation and readmission after hepatic surgery. J Am Coll Surg 216:915–923
13. Imamura H, Seyama Y, Kokudo N, Maema A, Sugawara Y, Sano K et al (2003) One thousand fifty-six hepatectomies without mortality in 8 years. Arch Surg 138:1198–1206, discussion 1206
14. Mitsuhashi N, Kimura F, Shimizu H, Imamaki M, Yoshidome H, Ohtsuka M et al (2008) Usefulness of intraoperative fluorescence imaging to evaluate local anatomy in hepatobiliary surgery. J Hepatobiliary Pancreat Surg 15:508–514
15. Ishizawa T, Bandai Y, Ijichi M, Kaneko J, Hasegawa K, Kokudo N (2010) Fluorescent cholangiography illuminating the biliary tree during laparoscopic cholecystectomy. Br J Surg 97:1369–1377
16. Kawaguchi Y, Ishizawa T, Masuda K, Sato S, Kaneko J, Aoki T et al (2011) Hepatobiliary surgery guided by a novel fluorescent imaging technique for visualizing hepatic arteries, bile ducts, and liver cancers on color images. J Am Coll Surg 212:e33–e39
17. Ishizawa T, Fukushima N, Shibahara J, Masuda K, Tamura S, Aoki T et al (2009) Real-time identification of liver cancers by using indocyanine green fluorescent imaging. Cancer 115:2491–2504
18. Gotoh K, Yamada T, Ishikawa O, Takahashi H, Eguchi H, Yano M et al (2009) A novel image-guided surgery of hepatocellular carcinoma by indocyanine green fluorescence imaging navigation. J Surg Oncol 100:75–79
19. Aoki T, Murakami M, Yasuda D, Shimizu Y, Kusano T, Matsuda K et al (2010) Intraoperative fluorescent imaging using indocyanine green for liver mapping and cholangiography. J Hepatobiliary Pancreat Sci 17:590–594
20. Harada N, Ishizawa T, Muraoka A, Ijichi M, Kusaka K, Shibasaki M et al (2010) Fluorescence navigation hepatectomy by visualization of localized cholestasis from bile duct tumor infiltration. J Am Coll Surg 210:e2–e6
21. Kawaguchi Y, Ishizawa T, Miyata Y, Yamashita S, Masuda K, Satou S et al (2013) Portal uptake function in veno-occlusive regions evaluated by real-time fluorescent imaging using indocyanine green. J Hepatol 58:247–253
22. Kawaguchi Y, Sugawara Y, Ishizawa T, Satou S, Kaneko J, Tamura S et al (2013) Identification of veno-occlusive regions in a right liver graft after reconstruction of vein segments 5 and 8: application of indocyanine green fluorescence imaging. Liver Transpl 19:778–779
23. Kubota K, Kita J, Shimoda M, Rokkaku K, Kato M, Iso Y et al (2006) Intraoperative assessment of reconstructed vessels in living-donor liver transplantation, using a novel fluorescence imaging technique. J Hepatobiliary Pancreat Surg 13:100–104
24. Rubens FD, Ruel M, Fremes SE (2002) A new and simplified method for coronary and graft imaging during CABG. Heart Surg Forum 5:141–144
25. Taggart DP, Choudhary B, Anastasiadis K, Abu-Omar Y, Balacumaraswami L, Pigott DW (2003) Preliminary experience with a novel intraoperative fluorescence imaging technique to

evaluate the patency of bypass grafts in total arterial revascularization. Ann Thorac Surg 75:870–873
26. Liu DZ, Mathes DW, Zenn MR, Neligan PC (2011) The application of indocyanine green fluorescence angiography in plastic surgery. J Reconstr Microsurg 27:355–364
27. Yamamoto T, Yamamoto N, Azuma S, Yoshimatsu H, Seki Y, Narushima M et al (2014) Near-infrared illumination system-integrated microscope for supermicrosurgical lymphaticovenular anastomosis. Microsurgery 34:23–27
28. Lee S, Park K, Hwang S, Lee Y, Choi D, Kim K et al (2001) Congestion of right liver graft in living donor liver transplantation. Transplantation 71:812–814
29. Akamatsu N, Sugawara Y, Kaneko J, Sano K, Imamura H, Kokudo N et al (2003) Effects of middle hepatic vein reconstruction on right liver graft regeneration. Transplantation 76:832–837
30. Buell JF, Funaki B, Cronin DC, Yoshida A, Perlman MK, Lorenz J et al (2002) Long-term venous complications after full-size and segmental pediatric liver transplantation. Ann Surg 236:658–666
31. Akamatsu N, Sugawara Y, Kaneko J, Kishi Y, Niiya T, Kokudo N et al (2004) Surgical repair for late-onset hepatic venous outflow block after living-donor liver transplantation. Transplantation 77:1768–1770

Part XIV
Hepato-Pancreatic-Biliary Surgery: Biliary Tract

Chapter 34
Fluorescence Imaging for Intraoperative Identification of Pancreatic Leak

Suguru Yamashita, Takeaki Ishizawa, Mako Kamiya, Yasuteru Urano, and Norihiro Kokudo

Abstract Pancreatic fistula (PF) remains the most serious complication of digestive surgery. The primary reason for PF not being successfully averted is that there are no techniques that identify pancreatic leak from the pancreatic stump during surgery or that rapidly evaluate protease activities in leakage fluid, which can cause severe tissue damage. To improve the safety of pancreatic surgery, the development of a novel technique that would identify pancreatic leak during surgery has been anticipated. We have designed and developed a novel fluorescence probe (glutaryl phenylalanine hydroxymethyl rhodamine green) that is activated by chymotrypsin in pancreatic juice. We evaluated the probe's ability to identify a pancreatic leak and directly sprayed it on the pancreatic stump in an animal experiment; the real-time gross visualization of a pancreatic leak was confirmed.

S. Yamashita, M.D., Ph.D.
Hepato-Biliary-Pancreatic Surgery Division, Department of Surgery, The University of Tokyo, 7-3-1 Hongo, Bunkyo-ku, Tokyo 113-8655, Japan

T. Ishizawa, M.D., Ph.D., F.A.C.S.
Hepato-Biliary-Pancreatic Surgery Division, Department of Surgery, The University of Tokyo, 7-3-1 Hongo, Bunkyo-ku, Tokyo 113-8655, Japan

Department of Gastroenterological Surgery, Cancer Institute Hospital, Japanese Foundation for Cancer Research, Tokyo, Japan

M. Kamiya, Ph.D.
Laboratory of Chemical Biology and Molecular Imaging, Graduate School of Medicine, The University of Tokyo, Tokyo, Japan

Y. Urano, Ph.D.
Laboratory of Chemical Biology and Molecular Imaging, Graduate School of Medicine, The University of Tokyo, Tokyo, Japan

Laboratory of Chemistry and Biology, Graduate School of Pharmaceutical Sciences, The University of Tokyo, Tokyo, Japan

N. Kokudo, M.D., Ph.D., F.A.C.S. (✉)
Hepato-Biliary-Pancreatic Surgery Division, Artificial Organ and Transplantation Division, Department of Surgery, Graduate School of Medicine, University of Tokyo, Tokyo, Japan
e-mail: KOKUDO-2SU@h.u-tokyo.ac.jp

M. Kusano et al. (eds.), *ICG Fluorescence Imaging and Navigation Surgery*,
DOI 10.1007/978-4-431-55528-5_34

Keywords Pancreatic fistula • Pancreatic leak • Glutaryl phenylalanine hydroxymethyl rhodamine green • Chymotrypsin

Abbreviations

PF	pancreatic fistula
ICG	indocyanine green
gPhe-HMRG	glutaryl phenylalanine hydroxymethyl rhodamine green

34.1 Introduction

Pancreatic cancer generally has a poor prognosis, and only 10–15 % of patients are eligible for surgical resection [1], which is at present the only potentially curative treatment option. Despite the development of various operative techniques or perioperative management options, morbidity rates after pancreatic resection have remained essentially unchanged. Pancreatic fistula (PF) in particular is the most common and clinically relevant complication because it results in further complications, including mortality and prolonged hospitalization, which leads to enormous medical expenses. PFs still occur at an incidence of 10–25 % after pancreaticoduodenectomy and 30–50 % after distal pancreatectomy [2–5].

In hepatobiliary surgery, for example, leakage of bile juice can also develop and lead to serious postoperative complications. However, intraoperative identification of leaking bile juice is usually not so difficult by naked eye examinations. In addition, fluorescence imaging using indocyanine green (ICG), which is excreted into bile following intravenous injection, has recently been applied to intraoperative visualization of the bile duct anatomy and bile leak in clinical settings [6–8]. In contrast to bile juice, it is difficult to identify clear pancreatic juice leaking from the pancreatic stump by gross eye examinations during surgery, and even fluorescence imaging using ICG is of no use for visualization of pancreatic juice, which would have made prevention of PF difficult for decades.

In order to visualize pancreatic juice leaking from pancreatic stump during surgery, the authors have developed a novel fluorescence probe (glutaryl phenylalanine hydroxymethyl rhodamine green, gPhe-HMRG) that is activated by chymotrypsin in pancreatic juice. Chymotrypsin is one of the major peptidases derived from chymotrypsinogen, which is synthesized only in the pancreas in humans [9]. The novel probe gPhe-HMRG [10] emits fluorescence only when it is hydrolyzed by chymotrypsin (Fig. 34.1). HMRG is excited by long-wavelength light (approximately 490 nm) and emits a fluorescence signal with a peak wavelength of approximately 520 nm [11]. Because pure pancreatic juice in humans normally contains chymotrypsinogen and not chymotrypsin [9], gPhe-HMRG was used with a small amount of trypsin (chymotrypsin probe) to detect pancreatic juice leakage (Fig. 34.1). This technique was inspired by the report of rapid cancer detection after topically spraying a γ-glutamyl transpeptidase-activated fluorescent probe [11], which is also hydrolyzed

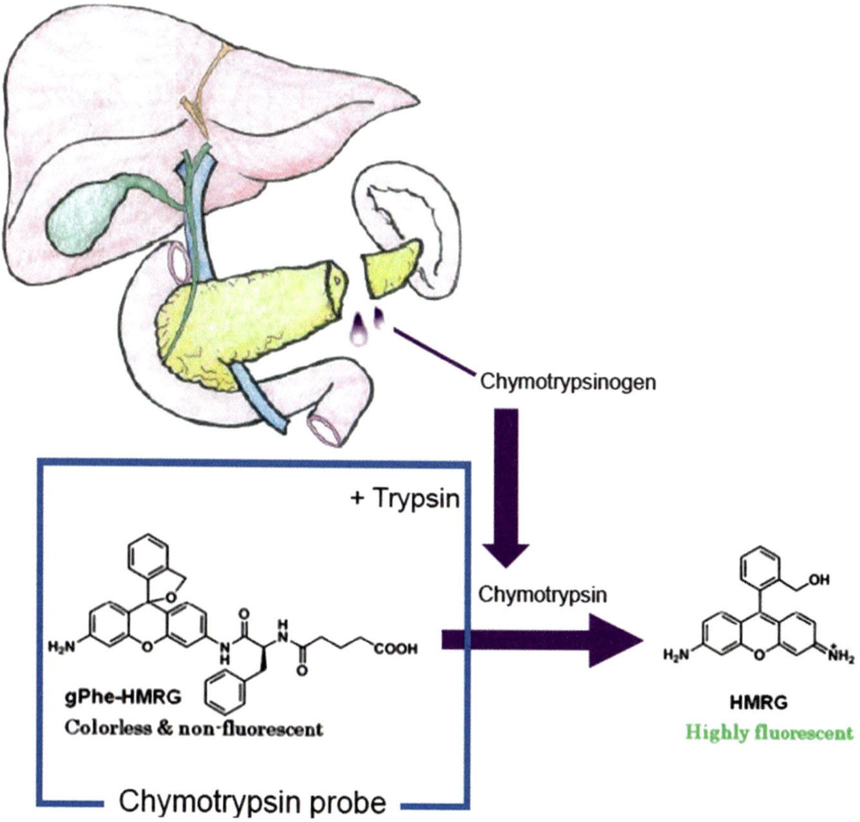

Fig. 34.1 Structure and chemical reaction of glutaryl phenylalanine hydroxymethyl rhodamine green (gPhe-HMRG). gPhe-HMRG was used with a small amount of trypsin (chymotrypsin probe) to detect chymotrypsinogen in pancreatic juice leakage; gPhe-HMRG emits fluorescence when it is hydrolyzed by chymotrypsin

by γ-glutamyl transpeptidase and provides fluorescence. Expression of γ-glutamyl transpeptidase, a cell surface enzyme involved in cellular glutathione homeostasis, is often significantly increased in human tumors [12]. Although the chymotrypsin probe has not been approved for intra-abdominal administrations in clinical settings, mechanistic background and technical details of fluorescence imaging of pancreatic leak are demonstrated in this chapter for future application to pancreatic surgery.

34.2 Pancreatic Chymotrypsin as a Target Substance for Fluorescence Imaging

When increased fluorescence intensity by the novel chymotrypsin probe was calculated in vitro by evaluating fluorescence intensity for the various chymotrypsin concentration samples, we confirmed the possibility of quantitative evaluation

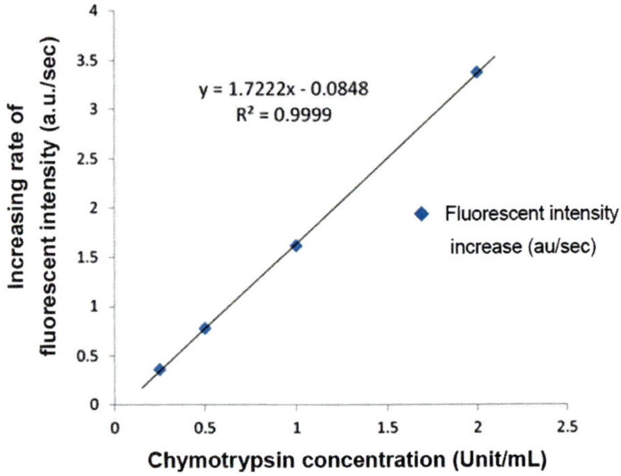

Fig. 34.2 Relationship between the chymotrypsin concentration and the increasing rate of fluorescence intensity. The rate of fluorescence intensity increased with an increase in the concentration of chymotrypsin. We confirmed that the chymotrypsin probe could quantitatively detect the activity of chymotrypsin with sufficient linearity

of chymotrypsin activity with sufficient linearity (Fig. 34.2). Yamashita et al. had previously revealed that this probe could specifically identify pancreatic juice in surgically drained fluids after pancreatic resection [10]. In the same study on patients undergoing pancreaticoduodenectomy, fluorescence imaging, after the chymotrypsin probe was sprayed on filter paper transcribing the pancreatic stump, enabled visualization of a pancreatic leak and accurate estimation of symptomatic postoperative PF [10].

It is also an innovation that the chymotrypsin probe targets the type of protease—not amylase—that can potentially cause severe tissue damage and lead to serious postoperative complications associated with PFs. Postoperative PF is presently diagnosed by evaluating amylase levels [13, 14] using International Study Group on Pancreatic Fistula classification grades [15]. It is unlikely that amylase, which is simply a glycolytic enzyme, directly triggers the complications stemming from postoperative PFs. Some authors have indicated that the current definition of postoperative PF, which is based on amylase levels in drainage fluids, does not always reflect complication severity [16, 17]. Pancreatic protease secretion can result from several factors, such as diet, pancreatic disease, and stimulatory or inhibitory mediators, and may not parallel amylase secretion [18, 19].

34.3 Application of the Chymotrypsin Probe for Pancreatic Resection in a Swine Model

Ideally, the chymotrypsin probe should be sprayed directly onto the pancreatic stump in the patient's abdominal cavity to enable surgeons to accurately suture the pancreatic leak location. However, such usage has not yet been approved in humans (pending completion of safety trials); therefore, this technique was simulated using a swine model. Chymotrypsin probe was sprayed on the pancreatic stump in

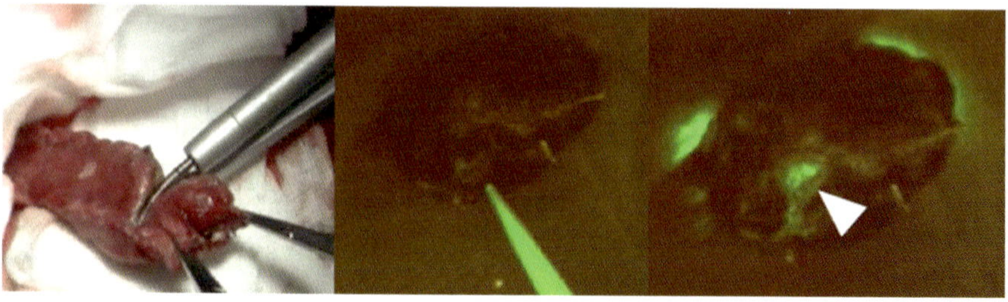

Fig. 34.3 Fluorescence images of pancreatic juice leaking from a pancreatic stump using the chymotrypsin probe in a swine model. After the division of the pancreatic parenchyma with the Harmonic Scalpel (*left*), chymotrypsin probe was sprayed on the pancreatic stump in abdominal cavity (middle). Five minutes after the chymotrypsin probe was sprayed onto the pancreatic stump, fluorescence imaging enabled identification of pancreatic juice leaking point (*right, arrowhead*)

abdominal cavity, following full mobilization and division of the pancreatic parenchyma with the Focus Ultracision Harmonic Scalpel (Ethicon Endo-Surgery Inc., Cincinnati, OH, USA). Five minutes after the chymotrypsin probe was sprayed onto the pancreatic stump, fluorescence imaging using a FluorVivo imaging system (INDEC, Inc., Santa Clara, CA) with a blue-filter setting (excitation, 470–490 nm; emission, 515 nm long pass) enabled identification of pancreatic juice leaking point (Fig. 34.3). Fluorescence of pancreatic juice was also identifiable by naked eye examination through light-blocking glasses (515 nm long pass), which enabled surgeons to apply pinpoint sutures and confirm pancreatic leak arrest. This technique may also enable surgeons to determine whether prophylactic abdominal drainage during pancreatic resection is needed, based on protease activities of pancreatic juice in each patient, as well to determine the presence or absence of pancreatic leak after closure/reconstruction of the pancreatic remnant.

34.4 Conclusion

In this chapter, mechanistic background and potential roles of fluorescence imaging using chymotrypsin probe are demonstrated. Following preclinical safety trials, first-in human study will be conducted in order to evaluate efficacy of intraoperative real-time fluorescence imaging of pancreatic leak in reducing incidence and severity of postoperative PF.

Acknowledgment This work was supported by grants from the Takeda Science Foundation; the Mochida Memorial Foundation for Medical and Pharmaceutical Research; the Ministry of Education, Culture, Sports, Science and Technology of Japan; and the Ministry of Health, Labour and Welfare of Japan.

References

1. Jemal A, Siegel R, Ward E et al (2008) Cancer statistics, 2008. CA Cancer J Clin 58:71–96
2. Yeo CJ, Cameron JL, Sohn TA et al (1997) Six hundred fifty consecutive pancreaticoduodenectomies in the 1990s: pathology, complications, and outcomes. Ann Surg 226:248–257
3. Mckay A, Mackenzie S, Sutherland FR et al (2006) Meta-analysis of pancreaticojejunostomy versus pancreaticogastrostomy reconstruction after pancreaticoduodenectomy. Br J Surg 93:929–936
4. Fuks D, Piessen G, Huet E et al (2009) Life-threatening postoperative pancreatic fistula (grade C) after pancreaticoduodenectomy: incidence, prognosis, and risk factors. Am J Surg 197:702–709
5. Kleeff J, Diener MK, Z'graggen K et al (2007) Distal pancreatectomy: risk factors for surgical failure in 302 consecutive cases. Ann Surg 245:573–582
6. Ishizawa T, Bandai Y, Ijichi M et al (2010) Fluorescent cholangiography illuminating the biliary tree during laparoscopic cholecystectomy. Br J Surg 97:1369–1377
7. Kaibori M, Ishizaki M, Matsui K et al (2011) Intraoperative indocyanine green fluorescent imaging for prevention of bile leakage after hepatic resection. Surgery 150:91–98
8. Sakaguchi T, Suzuki A, Unno N et al (2010) Bile leak test by indocyanine green fluorescence images after hepatectomy. Am J Surg 200:e19–e23
9. Whitcomb DC, Lowe ME (2007) Human pancreatic digestive enzymes. Dig Dis Sci 52:1–17
10. Yamashita S, Sakabe M, Ishizawa T et al (2013) Visualization of the leakage of pancreatic juice using a chymotrypsin-activated fluorescent probe. Br J Surg 100:1220–1228
11. Urano Y, Asanuma D, Hama Y et al (2009) Selective molecular imaging of viable cancer cells with pH-activatable fluorescence probes. Nat Med 15:104–109
12. Pompella A, De Tata V, Paolicchi A et al (2006) Expression of gamma-glutamyltransferase in cancer cells and its significance in drug resistance. Biochem Pharmacol 71:231–238
13. Veillette G, Dominguez I, Ferrone C et al (2008) Implications and management of pancreatic fistulas following pancreaticoduodenectomy: the Massachusetts General Hospital experience. Arch Surg 143:476–481
14. Balcom JH IV, Keck T, Warshaw AL et al (2002) Prevention of pancreatic fistula with a new synthetic, absorbable sealant: evaluation in a dog model. J Am Coll Surg 195:490–496
15. Bassi C, Dervenis C, Butturini G et al (2005) International Study Group on pancreatic fistula definition. Postoperative pancreatic fistula: an international study group (ISGPF) definition. Surgery 138:8–13
16. Gebauer F, Kloth K, Tachezy M et al (2012) Options and limitations in applying the fistula classification by the International Study Group for Pancreatic Fistula. Ann Surg 256:130–138
17. Shyr YM, Su CH, Wu CW et al (2003) Does drainage fluid amylase reflect pancreatic leakage after pancreaticoduodenectomy? World J Surg 27:606–610
18. Wormsley KG, Goldberg DM (1972) The interrelationships of the pancreatic enzymes. Gut 13:398–412
19. Dagorn JC, Sahel J, Sarles H (1977) Nonparallel secretion of enzymes in human duodenal juice and pure pancreatic juice collected by endoscopic retrograde catheterization of the papilla. Gastroenterology 73:42–45

Chapter 35
Intraoperative Indocyanine Green Fluorescent Imaging for Prevention of Bile Leakage After Hepatic Resection

Masaki Kaibori, Kosuke Matsui, Morihiko Ishizaki, Hiroya Iida, and Masanori Kon

Abstract Bile leakage is one of the most common complications after hepatic resection and is associated with postoperative sepsis and liver failure. We present here the use of indocyanine green (ICG) fluorescent cholangiography for preventing postoperative bile leakage. The subjects were 132 patients who underwent hepatic resection without biliary reconstruction. Patients underwent a leakage test using ICG dye, followed by ICG fluorescent cholangiography using the photodynamic eye. Postoperative bile leakage occurred in seven of 132 patients (5 %). The incidence of postoperative bile leakage was 0 % in patients with type A pattern of fluorescence (no fluorescence type; no fluorescence detected on the cut surface of the liver, suggesting absence of bile ducts at the surgical margin; $n = 37$), 2 % in patients with type B pattern (intact bile duct type; fluorescence showed one or more intact bile ducts on the cut surface; $n = 51$), 6 % in patients with type C pattern (injured bile duct type; leakage of dye from one or more bile duct stumps on the cut surface; $n = 31$), and 31 % in patients with type D pattern (unconfirmed type; leakage of dye from the cut surface, but the source was unclear; $n = 13$). ICG fluorescent cholangiography may be useful for preventing bile leakage after hepatic resection, but patients with type D pattern of fluorescence should be carefully monitored for leakage for several weeks.

Keywords Hepatic resection • Intraoperative indocyanine green fluorescent imaging • Postoperative bile leakage • Injured bile duct type • Unconfirmed bile duct type

M. Kaibori (✉) • K. Matsui • M. Ishizaki • H. Iida • M. Kon
Department of Surgery, Hirakata Hospital, Kansai Medical University, 2-5-1 Shinmachi, Hirakata, Osaka 573-1191, Japan
e-mail: kaibori@hirakata.kmu.ac.jp

M. Kusano et al. (eds.), *ICG Fluorescence Imaging and Navigation Surgery*,
DOI 10.1007/978-4-431-55528-5_35

35.1 Introduction

Improvements in surgical techniques and perioperative care have increased the safety of hepatic surgery over recent years, resulting in reduced operative mortality [1–4]. Despite the overall reduction in postoperative complications, the incidence of postoperative bile leakage has not changed and has a reported range of 3.6 to 33 % [5–13], making it one of the most common complications after hepatic surgery. Bile leakage is associated with increased risks of postoperative sepsis, liver failure, and mortality and a longer hospital stay [6]. It is therefore important to minimize the occurrence of this complication. We evaluated that fluorescent cholangiography using ICG would be able to detect minor bile leakage from the cut surface of the remnant liver after hepatic resection.

35.2 Materials and Methods

35.2.1 Patients

All 132 patients who were scheduled for liver resection at Hirakata Hospital of Kansai Medical University (Osaka, Japan) between August 2010 and December 2012 were included in this study. Of these, 72 had hepatocellular carcinoma, 9 had intrahepatic cholangiocellular carcinoma, 47 had colorectal liver metastasis, and 4 had another pathology. The patients were 108 males and 24 females with a mean age of 69.3 years. The operative procedure was extended hemihepatectomy in 14 patients, hemihepatectomy in 35, sectionectomy in 38, segmentectomy in 12, and limited resection in 33.

35.2.2 Surgical Techniques

Transection of the hepatic parenchyma was performed using the cavitron ultrasonic surgical aspirator (CUSA) system (Valleylab, Boulder, CO). After hepatic resection, a disposable cholangiography catheter was inserted into the cystic duct and ligated in place. The common bile duct was clamped below the cystic duct, and 10 ml of dilute ICG solution (Diagnogreen 2.5 mg/ml; Daiichi Sankyo Co., Tokyo, Japan) was injected into the bile duct. Any sites of major dye leakage from the cut surface of the remnant liver were repaired by z-suturing with 6–0 nonabsorbable sutures or by ligation with absorbable sutures, after which the absence of further leakage was confirmed by injecting 5–7 ml of saline. Only one injection of ICG solution was administered to each patient. Fluorescent imaging was performed with a photodynamic eye (PDE) imaging system (Hamamatsu Photonics K.K., Shizuoka, Japan) (Fig. 35.1) after the injection of ICG solution. The PDE system includes a

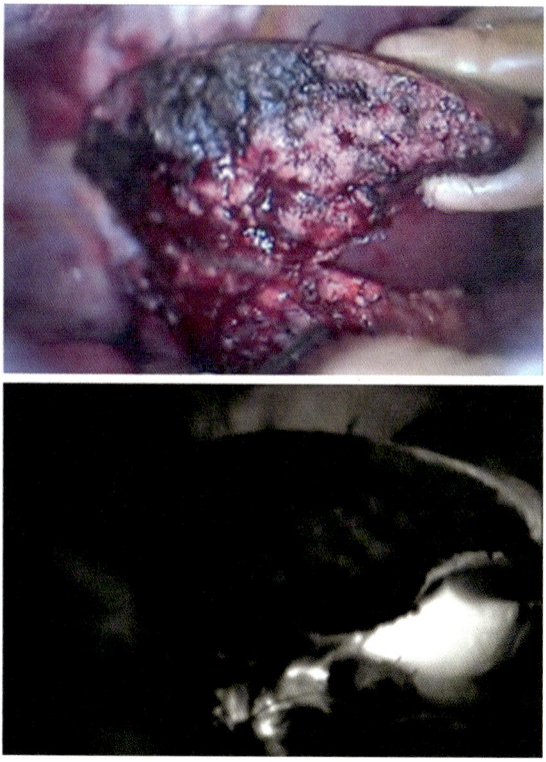

Fig. 35.1 Type A pattern of fluorescence (no fluorescence type). Fluorescent imaging showed no fluorescence detected on the cut surface of the liver, suggesting absence of bile ducts at the surgical margin. The cut surface of the liver under conventional white light illumination (**a**) and fluorescent imaging (**b**)

control unit (322 × 283 × 55 mm, 2.8 kg) and a camera unit (80 × 181 × 80 mm, 0.5 kg). The camera unit contains a charge-coupled device camera that filters out light with a wavelength of less than 820 nm and 36 light-emitting diodes with a wavelength of 760 nm. The camera head was positioned 20 cm above the remnant liver, and the operating lights were turned off (the room lights were left on). The operating field was therefore visible to the surgeons directly and on the television monitor. The fluorescent images of the cut surface of the liver were displayed on the monitor and showed white spots representing potential bile leaks. The areas showing white spots were compressed with gauze, and leakage was tested by additional injection of 3–5 ml of saline (Fig. 35.2). If fluorescence was detected through the gauze, the white spots were considered to indicate minor leaks on the cut surface of the liver, and the presumably injured bile ducts were repaired by z-suturing or ligation.

Postoperative bile leakage was diagnosed by the following findings: detection of bile leakage from the wound or through the drainage tube (total bilirubin level in the drainage fluid >3 times the serum level), intra-abdominal accumulation of bile confirmed by drainage, or demonstration of bile leakage on postoperative cholangiography.

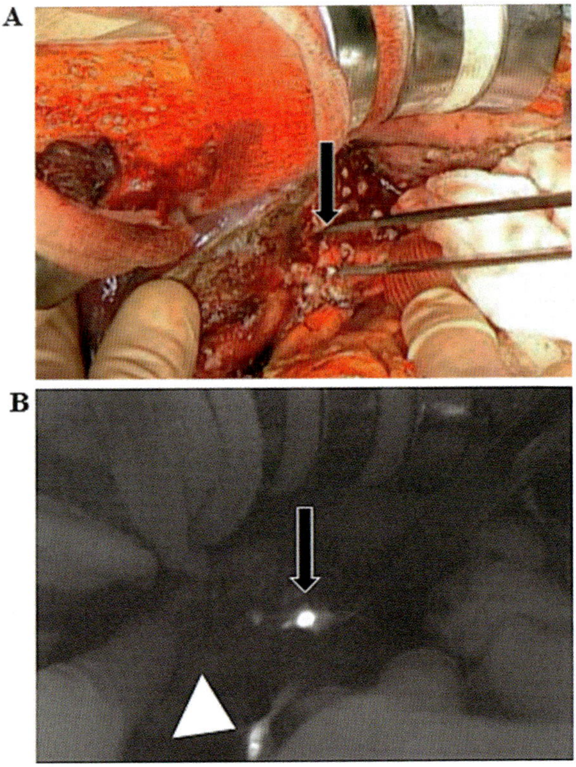

Fig. 35.2 Type B pattern of fluorescence (intact bile duct type). Fluorescent imaging showed one fluorescent duct on the cut surface of the liver (*arrow*). Common bile duct (*arrowhead*). There was an intact bile duct corresponding to the fluorescent area on the cut surface (*arrow*) under conventional white light illumination (**a**) and fluorescent imaging (**b**)

35.3 Results

Thirty-two of the 132 patients (24 %) had major leakage of ICG, defined as leakage of green dye without fluorescent imaging. Repair was performed by z-suturing with 6–0 nonabsorbable sutures in 28 patients and by ligation with 4–0 absorbable sutures in four patients. The leaks were all successfully repaired during surgery and were further tested with fluorescent imaging.

35.3.1 Patterns of Fluorescence

In 37 of the 132 patients (19 %), no fluorescence was detected on the cut surface of the remnant liver on ICG fluorescent cholangiography, suggesting absence of bile ducts at the surgical margin (*type A* pattern of fluorescence) (Fig. 35.1). In the remaining 95 patients, the pattern of fluorescence was classified into the following three types: intact bile duct type (*type B*, fluorescence showed one or more intact bile ducts on the cut surface of the liver; $n = 51$) (Fig. 35.2), injured bile duct type (*type C*, leakage of dye from one or more bile duct stumps on the cut surface;

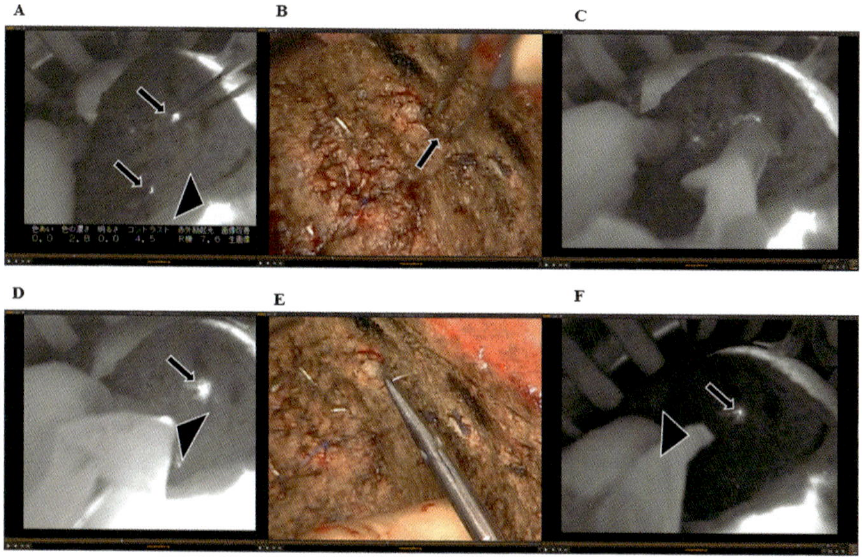

Fig. 35.3 Type C pattern of fluorescence (injured bile duct type). (**a**) Fluorescent imaging showed two areas of fluorescence corresponding to ducts on the cut surface of the liver (*arrows*). The lower bile duct was intact (*lower arrow*). Common bile duct (*arrowhead*). (**b**) The lower area of fluorescence corresponded to a partly closed bile duct stump (*arrow*) under conventional white light illumination. Minor leakage (leaking duct) that is not visible to the surgeons (*arrow*) is compressed with gauze. (**c**, **d**) Fluorescent imaging after the application of gauze shows minor leakage on the cut surface of the liver (*arrow*), as fluorescence is detected through the gauze (*arrowhead*). (**e**) The bile duct stump was repaired by z-suturing with 6–0 nonabsorbable sutures. (**f**) Fluorescent imaging after the treatment for the minor leakage on the cut surface of the liver (*arrow*), as fluorescence is not detected through the gauze (*arrowhead*)

$n = 31$) (Fig. 35.3), and unconfirmed type (*type D*, leakage of dye from the cut surface, but the source was unclear; $n = 13$) (Fig. 35.4). In type D pattern, the minor dye leaks could not be visualized by the surgeon and could only be detected by viewing the fluorescent images on the monitor.

No repair was performed in patients with types A and B patterns of fluorescence. In patients with type C pattern, repair was performed by z-suturing with 6–0 nonabsorbable sutures in 42 patients (1.5 ± 0.8 (mean $\pm$ SD) sutures per patient) and by ligation with 4–0 absorbable sutures in the remaining nine patients (1.0 ± 0.2 ligatures per patient). In the three patients with type D pattern, fibrin sealant was applied to the area showing leakage (two pieces of 2.0×1.5 cm sealant per patient).

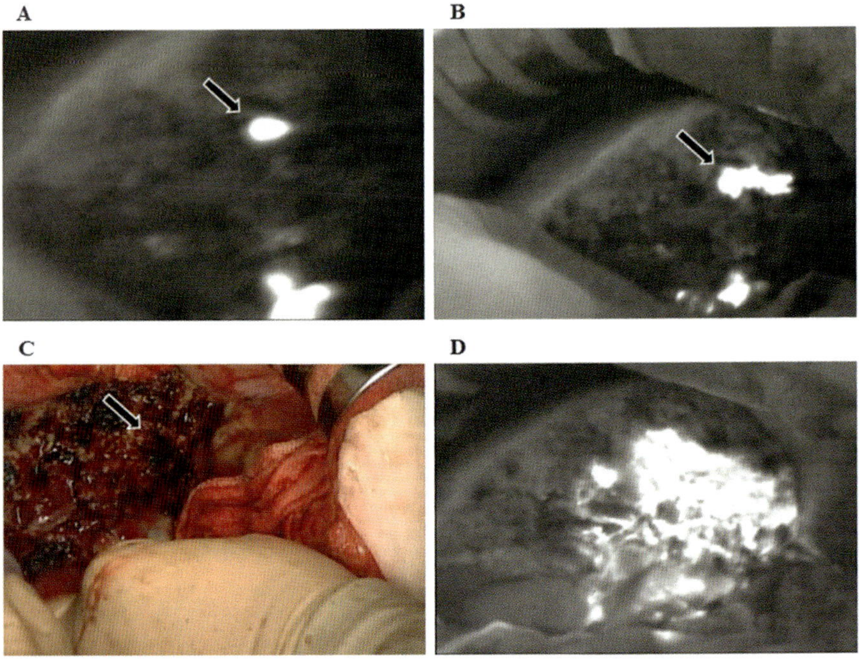

Fig. 35.4 Type D pattern of fluorescence (unconfirmed type). (**a**, **b**) Fluorescent imaging showed an area of fluorescence on the cut surface of the liver (*arrow*). (**c**) Minor leakage of dye is not visible to the surgeons (*arrow*) under conventional white light illumination. (**d**) There is major leakage of dye from the cut surface, but the source was unclear

Table 35.1 Incidence of postoperative bile leakage for each pattern of fluorescence

	Indocyanine green fluorescent imaging	Number of patients	Number with postoperative bile leakage	%
Type A	No fluorescence was detected on the cut surface	37	0	0
Type B	Intact bile duct type	51	1	2
Type C	Injured bile ducts were detected and successfully repaired	31	2	6
Type D	Unconfirmed site of intraoperative bile leakage	13	4	31
Total		132	7	5

35.3.2 Postoperative Bile Leakage

Postoperative bile leakage occurred in seven of the 132 hepatectomy patients (5 %) and persisted for a median period of 6 weeks (range, 2–15 weeks). Table 35.1 shows the incidence of each pattern of fluorescence. The rate of type D pattern differed from the rates of the other three patterns.

35.4 Discussion

Postoperative bile leakage remains a challenging problem in patients undergoing hepatic surgery, especially major hepatectomy, as it is associated with serious complications such as sepsis and liver failure [7]. The objective of the bile leakage test is to detect insufficiently closed bile duct stumps on the cut surface of the liver. However, such a test cannot completely prevent postoperative bile leakage, as leakage may occur from small ducts that are not in communication with the main part of the biliary tree [14]. There is no standard method of preventing postoperative bile leakage. We suspected that small bile duct stumps on the cut surface of the liver might be missed by the usual bile leakage test.

ICG fluorescent cholangiography is safe and feasible. ICG is already used worldwide to evaluate liver function before surgery, and the incidence of adverse reactions after intravenous injection of ICG is very low (approximately 0.003 %) [15]. Intraoperative ICG fluorescent cholangiography showed that 32 of our 132 patients had insufficient closure of bile duct stumps on the cut surface of the liver, and these stumps were treated by z-suturing or ligation. The major limitation of ICG fluorescent cholangiography is that it is not possible to visualize deep intrahepatic bile ducts or extrahepatic bile ducts covered by surrounding organs using this technique, because of the limited tissue penetration of the near-infrared light emitted by the current imaging system. However, the results of this study show that ICG fluorescent cholangiography enables evaluation of the cut surface of the liver. In our previous study, postoperative bile leakage occurred in five of the 50 patients in the control group versus none of the 52 patients in the PDE group [16]. In this study, the incidence of postoperative bile leakage was 0 % in patients with type A pattern of fluorescence, 2 % in patients with type B pattern, 6 % in patients with type C pattern, and 31 % in patients with type D pattern. In type D pattern, visualization of white spots on the whole cut surface of the remnant liver suggested leakage of a high volume of ICG dye from the stumps or leakage of bile from ducts that were not in communication with the main part of the biliary tree. We consider that it is necessary to place intra-abdominal drainage catheters after hepatic resection to treat potential postoperative bike leakage. Patients with type D pattern of fluorescence should be carefully monitored for bile leakage for several weeks after hepatic resection, because late-onset bile leakage can cause serious complications.

In conclusion, ICG fluorescent cholangiography enabled detection of leaking bile duct stumps that were missed by the conventional bile leakage test. ICG fluorescent cholangiography may be useful for the prevention of bile leakage after hepatic resection.

References

1. Imamura H, Seyama Y, Kokudo N, Maema A, Sugawara Y, Sano K et al (2003) One thousand fifty-six hepatectomies without mortality in 8 years. Arch Surg 138:1198–1206
2. Capussotti L, Polastri R (1998) Operative risks of major hepatic resections. Hepatogastroenterology 45:184–190
3. Jarnagin WR, Gonen M, Fong Y, DeMatteo RP, Ben-Porat L, Little S et al (2002) Improvement in perioperative outcome after hepatic resection: analysis of 1,803 consecutive cases over the past decade. Ann Surg 236:397–407
4. Poon RT, Fan ST, Lo CM, Liu CL, Lam CM, Yuen WK et al (2004) Improving perioperative outcome expands the role of hepatectomy in management of benign and malignant hepatobiliary diseases: analysis of 1222 consecutive patients from a prospective database. Ann Surg 240:698–710
5. Lo CM, Fan ST, Liu CL, Lai EC, Wong J (1998) Biliary complications after hepatic resection: risk factors, management, and outcome. Arch Surg 133:156–161
6. Yamashita Y, Hamatsu T, Rikimaru T, Tanaka S, Shirabe K, Shimada M et al (2001) Bile leakage after hepatic resection. Ann Surg 233:45–50
7. Nagano Y, Togo S, Tanaka K, Masui H, Endo I, Sekido H et al (2003) Risk factors and management of bile leakage after hepatic resection. World J Surg 27:695–698
8. Terajima H, Ikai I, Hatano E, Uesugi T, Yamamoto Y, Shimahara Y et al (2004) Effectiveness of endoscopic nasobiliary drainage for postoperative bile leakage after hepatic resection. World J Surg 28:782–786
9. Ijichi M, Takayama T, Toyoda H, Sano K, Kubota K, Makuuchi M (2000) Randomized trial of the usefulness of a bile leakage test during hepatic resection. Arch Surg 135:1395–1400
10. Rudow DL, Brown RS Jr, Emond JC, Marratta D, Bellemare S, Kinkhabwala M (2004) One-year morbidity after donor right hepatectomy. Liver Transpl 10:1428–1431
11. Tanaka S, Hirohashi K, Tanaka H, Shuto T, Lee SH, Kubo S et al (2002) Incidence and management of bile leakage after hepatic resection for malignant hepatic tumors. J Am Coll Surg 195:484–489
12. Nakayama H, Masuda H, Shibata M, Amano S, Fukuzawa M (2003) Incidence of bile leakage after three types of hepatic parenchymal transection. Hepatogastroenterology 50:1517–1520
13. Capussotti L, Ferrero A, Vigano L, Sgotto E, Muratore A, Polastri R (2006) Bile leakage and liver resection: where is the risk? Arch Surg 141:690–695
14. Neuhaus P (1989) Complications of liver surgery and their management. In: Lygidakis NJ, Tytgat GNJ (eds) Hepatobiliary and pancreatic malignancies: diagnosis, medical and surgical management. Thieme-Stratton Inc, New York, pp 254–259
15. Cherrick GR, Stein SW, Leevy CM, Davidson CS (1960) Indocyanine green: observations on its physical properties, plasma decay, and hepatic extraction. J Clin Invest 39:592–600
16. Kaibori M, Ishizaki M, Matsui K, Kwon AH (2011) Intraoperative indocyanine green fluorescent imaging for prevention of bile leakage after hepatic resection. Surgery 150:91–98

Chapter 36
ICG Fluorescence Cholangiography During Laparoscopic Cholecystectomy

Nobumi Tagaya

Abstract We report our experience for an intraoperative exploration of the biliary anatomy using fluorescence imaging with indocyanine green (ICG) for 25 patients who were planned to perform laparoscopic cholecystectomy. They included ten males and 15 females with a mean age of 57 years and body mass index of 24.5 kg/m^2. ICG was administered intravenously 1 h before surgery. We observed the biliary tract under a laparoscope with infrared function, and the cystic artery was also observed after reinjection of ICG. There were no additional ports or conversion to open cholecystectomy. The mean operation time was 83 min. We identified the biliary tract with fluorescence imaging in all patients, and the cystic artery was recognized approximately 10 s after reinjection of ICG. There were no specific perioperative complications related to the intravenous injection of ICG. The median postoperative hospital stay was 3 days. Intraoperative exploration of the biliary anatomy using ICG is a useful and safe navigation modality for identification of the biliary anatomy without cannulation manner into the cystic duct, arrangement of X-ray equipment, or use of radioactive materials. This technique will become routine, offering a lower degree of invasiveness that will help to avoid or minimize bile duct and vessel injuries.

Keywords Fluorescence imaging • Indocyanine green • Intraoperative cholangiography • Navigation surgery • Laparoscopic cholecystectomy

36.1 Introduction

Laparoscopic procedures for the diseases in the abdominal field have been recognized as a standard technique worldwide. Although a large number of laparoscopic cholecystectomies were performed, the occurrence of perioperative complications including bile duct injury (BDI) or bleeding is still remained up to date. In particular, BDI is the most common and complicated problem during

N. Tagaya, M.D. (✉)
Department of Surgery, Dokkyo Medical University Koshigaya Hospital, 2-1-50, Minamikoshigaya, Koshigaya, Saitama 343-8555, Japan
e-mail: tagaya@dokkyomed.ac.jp

M. Kusano et al. (eds.), *ICG Fluorescence Imaging and Navigation Surgery*,
DOI 10.1007/978-4-431-55528-5_36

cholecystectomy, and the occurrence rate distributed from 0.1 to 1.5 % in the literature [1–5]. To prevent or minimize that issue, we introduced a clinical practice to use fluorescence imaging with indocyanine green (ICG; Diagnogreen, Daiichi Sankyo Co., Tokyo, Japan) [6, 7]. ICG has routinely used for the evaluation of liver function before hepatic resection. Recently, it has been introduced into various fields including an identification of sentinel lymph node and tumor location, vascular anatomy, blood flow after organ transplantation, and so on [7]. Here we report our experience for an intraoperative exploration of the biliary anatomy using fluorescence imaging with ICG during laparoscopic cholecystectomy.

36.2 Materials and Methods

During the recent 3 years, we performed laparoscopic cholecystectomy for 25 patients being diagnosed with gallbladder stones or polyps. They were 10 males and 15 females, and their mean age and body mass index were 57 years (range, 31–84 years) and 24.5 kg/m^2 (range, 19.1–49.6 kg/m^2), respectively. Surgical procedures consisted of standard four-port technique in 11 patients and single-incision technique in the other 14 patients. The ethics committee of Dokkyo Medical University Koshigaya Hospital approved this study. All patients were obtained an informed consent preoperatively. ICG (25 mg/vials) was adjusted to 2.5 mg/ml and injected 1.0 ml/body intravenously one h before surgery.

36.2.1 Laparoscopic Approach

Under general anesthesia, we introduced four ports (a 12-mm port at the umbilicus and three 5-mm ports in the subxiphoid and right subcostal regions) or a 2.5-cm vertical skin incision at the umbilicus with a 5.5 surgical glove containing three 5-mm ports attached to a wound retractor into the peritoneal cavity after creating pneumoperitoneum by CO_2 insufflation. Using a 10-mm laparoscope with infrared function (Olympus Medical Systems Corp., Tokyo, Japan; Karl Storz Co., Tuttlingen, Germany), we observed the area from the hepatic hilum to the duodenum at the point of initial insertion of the laparoscope under fluorescence imaging guidance (Fig. 36.1a and b) during the division, after identification and dissection of the cystic duct and artery (Fig. 36.2a and b), and before closure of the wounds (Fig. 36.3a and b), respectively. To observe a blood flow within the cystic artery, 1 ml of ICG (2.5 mg/ml) was readministered intravenously through the venous line after identifying the vessel structure. If the florescent image was unclear due to inflammation around the gallbladder or dense adipose tissue in the hepatoduodenal ligament, an originally manufactured transparent flat plastic device (TFPD) was used to achieve local compression, allowing clearer fluorescence imaging over the biliary tract (Fig. 36.4a and b).

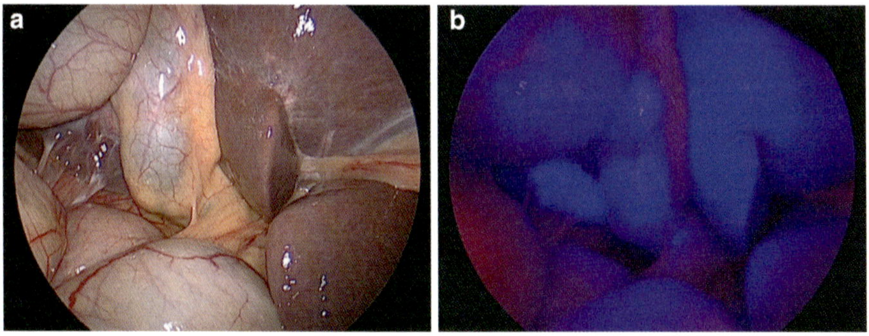

Fig. 36.1 (**a**) and (**b**): Ordinary view and fluorescence image obtained at the time of initial insertion of the infrared laparoscope

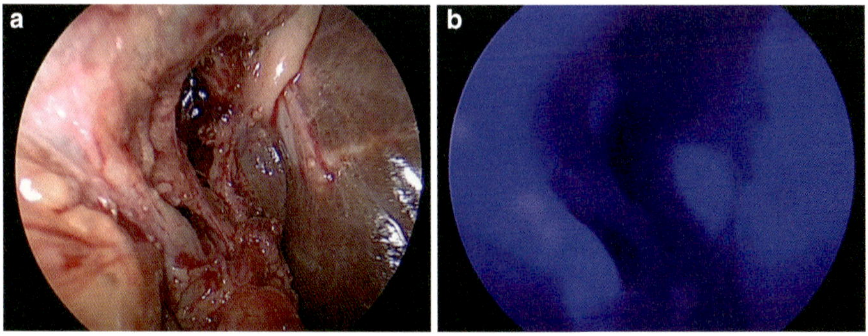

Fig. 36.2 (**a**) and (**b**): Fluorescence imaging after identification of the cystic duct and artery

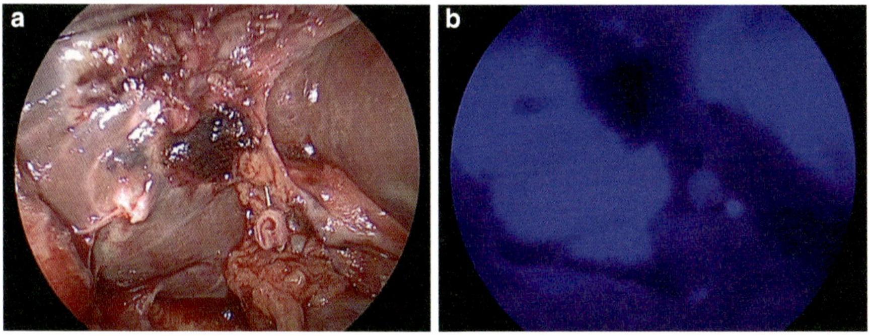

Fig. 36.3 (**a**) and (**b**): We confirmed no bile leakage from the stump of the cystic duct

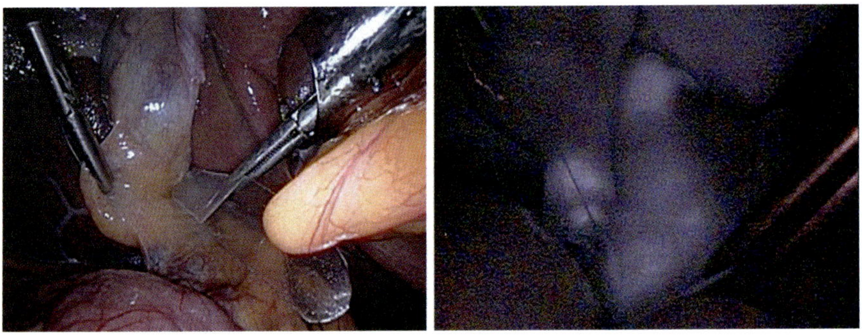

Fig. 36.4 (**a**) and (**b**): Clearer fluorescence imaging over the biliary tract obtained after compression of TFPD

36.3 Results

There were no conversions to open cholecystectomy. The mean operation time was 83 min (range, 46–163 min), and the estimated intraoperative blood loss was minimal. The fluorescence imaging over the biliary tract including common hepatic duct, common bile duct, and cystic duct was clearly obtained through the laparoscope in all patients. However, gallbladder could not be clearly visualized due to inflammation, edema, or an impacted stone in the neck of the gallbladder. Local compression by our original TFPD provided a clearer fluorescence image of the biliary tract against dense adipose tissues. In particular, the identification of the confluence between the cystic duct and the common bile duct was important to perform the safe procedure. The location and blood flow within the cystic artery were identified approximately 10 s after reinjection of ICG (2.5 mg/body) intravenously. However, an identification of cystic artery also depends on the underlying conditions of the patients. There were no adverse events related to the administration of ICG. The mean postoperative hospital stay was 3 days (range, 2–4 days), and there were no postoperative complications during the follow-up period.

36.4 Discussion

ICG is stabilized in plasma protein after intravenous injection, and protein-bounding ICG emits light with a peak fluorescence wavelength of 845 nm when exposed with near-infrared light with a wavelength of 760 nm. ICG is known to be safe at the doses used in routine clinical practice, and the risk of adverse events is quite low (approximately 0.003 %) at doses exceeding 0.5 mg/kg [8]. Indeed we administered ICG at only 1 ml/body (0.04–0.05 mg/kg) at a concentration of 2.5 mg/ml for intraoperative exploration of the biliary tract. In the literature, there are no reports of adverse events related with intravenous injection of ICG in hepatobiliary surgery [6–8, 10–16].

BDI during cholecystectomy is a serious surgical complication that brings poor quality of patient's life. Törnqvist et al. [5] reported that an early detection of BDI during primary surgery improved survival, and the intention to use intraoperative cholangiography (IOC) reduced the risk of death after cholecystectomy. Therefore, an intraoperative modality for the detection of the biliary anatomy is an important factor to obtain a safe outcome. Although IOC via cannulation of the cystic duct during cholecystectomy was a standard and routine method for obtaining the information of the biliary system including bile leakage or common bile duct stone up to date, recently, near-infrared fluorescence imaging with ICG has been penetrated as an intraoperative assessment for an identification of biliary anatomy in several institutions [6, 10–12]. Fluorescence imaging realized a real-time observation, noninvasiveness, and easy performance compared with ordinary intraoperative cholangiography and became an attractive tool for identification of biliary anatomy including biliary tract and hepatic arteries.

To obtain an adequate fluorescence imaging during cholecystectomy, the injection timing of ICG is a very important factor. From the literature, Matsui et al. [17] reported that the time interval between intravenous injection and the recognition of extrahepatic bile duct with florescence imaging was quantified at 90 min in pig models, Aoki et al. [11] reported that satisfactory results were obtained by the administration of ICG 30 min or 1 h before surgery in human study, and Schols et al. [14] reported that ICG was visible in the liver and bile ducts within 20 min after injection. Ishizawa et al. [18] reported that the time interval before dissection of the triangle of Calot ranged from 35 to 75 min. Our time interval using pig models was approximately within 20 min after intravenous injection; however, fluorescence imaging of the gallbladder required further 30 min. Therefore, we have routinely injected ICG 1 h before surgery to observe an adequate fluorescence imaging from the biliary tract including the extrahepatic bile duct, cystic duct, and gallbladder at the insertion of laparoscope [6]. However, the time interval greatly depends on the individual liver function. Recently, Verbeek et al. [16] reported that a prolonged interval (24 h) permitted optimal near-infrared cholangiography with minimal liver background fluorescence. Therefore, we have to consider the ICG injection time (at the time of endotracheal intubation [12] or 10–15 min [8], 20 min [14], 30 min [10, 11], or 1 h [6, 11] before surgery according to the individual conditions).

Regarding the dose of ICG, we adjusted 2.5 mg/ml and administered 1 ml/body intravenously [6], and another institutions reported 0.1–0.5 mg/ml/kg or 2, 5, 10 ml/body of 2.5 mg/ml as a bolus in clinical use [6–19]. These dose differences are not greatly influenced in actual visualization during surgery. Furthermore, the duration of fluorescence (biliary secretion of ICG) was reported to last until 20 h after intravenous injection [19]. Therefore, there is no anxiousness about the duration of adequate fluorescence imaging during open or laparoscopic cholecystectomy.

Although the injection time and dosage of ICG are important factors to obtain a sufficient fluorescence imaging, the penetration depth of infrared light through tissue also relates to an identification of biliary tract. Mitsuhashi et al. [10] reported that the penetration depth was 3–5 mm and the intensity of fluorescence was affected to tissue thickness. Therefore, thc thickness of the gallbladder wall or the volume of adjacent connective tissues is greatly affected by obesity or edema and dense adhesion due to acute or chronic inflammation during cholecystectomy. To resolve this issue, we introduced an originally manufactured transparent flat plastic device (TFPD), and its compression over the biliary tract led to increase the intensity of fluorescence and improved an identification of fluorescence imaging of the biliary tract [6]. It is a useful device to check the biliary anatomy and minimize the intraoperative complications.

The advantages of this modality are no requirement of cannulation into the cystic duct, no special arrangements for X-ray equipment, and no exposure to radioactivity for human body. ICG fluorescence imaging is a simple and convenient tool to obtain the biliary anatomy without any preparation for an additional procedure. In clinical practice, the recognition rates of florescence images in the cystic, common, and hepatic ducts were improved after the dissection of Calot's triangle compared with before that [8, 12, 13]. However, in our experience, TFPD allowed us to recognize the fluorescence images of the biliary tract before dissection of connective tissues in all cases [6]. Anatomical anomalies of the bile duct or hepatic artery are often encountered during hepatobiliary surgery. Ishizawa et al. [12] reported that an accessory bile duct was detected by fluorescence cholangiography in all cases confirming by radiological diagnosis preoperatively. In particular, the location of hepatic arteries including a cystic artery can be visualized in real time repeatedly by reinfusion of 1 ml (2.5 mg) ICG. Furthermore, near-infrared endoscopy offers early recognition of bile leakage, facilitates early treatment, and minimizes BDI owing to having high sensitivity for bile juice during laparoscopic cholecystectomy [6].

We have an issue regarding the detection of common bile duct (CBD) stones during cholecystectomy using ICG fluorescence imaging. Although ordinary intraoperative cholangiography via the cystic duct with cannulation can detect stones in CBD as defects during procedure, our experience using fluorescence imaging even in open cholecystectomy showed no recognition of CBD stones that had been diagnosed preoperatively by computed tomography or magnetic resonance imaging. The presence of fluorescing bile around stones in CBD may mask the existence of stone itself nnn. Therefore, preoperative evaluation using interventional radiology is still mandatory for the treatment of CBD stones.

In conclusion, intraoperative exploration of the biliary tract using ICG is a useful and safe navigation modality for identification of the biliary anatomy without the need for cannulation into the cystic duct, X-ray equipment, or use of radioactive materials. We expect that this method will become routine, offering a lower degree of invasiveness that will help avoid or minimize bile duct or vessel injuries.

References

1. Sicklick JK, Camp MS, Lillemoe KD et al (2005) Surgical management of bile duct injuries sustained during laparoscopic cholecystectomy. Ann Surg 241:786–792; discussion 793–795
2. Connor S, Garden OJ (2006) Bile duct injury in the era of laparoscopic cholecystectomy. Br J Surg 93:158–168. doi:10.1002/bjs.5266
3. Hogan AM, Hoti E, Winter DC et al (2009) Quality of life after iatrogenic bile duct injury: a case control study. Ann Surg 249:292–295. doi:10.1097/SLA.0b013e318195c50c
4. Buddingh KT, Nieuwenhuijs VB, van Buuren L et al (2011) Intraoperative assessment of biliary anatomy for prevention of bile duct injury: a review of current and future patient safety interventions. Surg Endosc 25:2449–2461. doi:10.1007/s00464-011-1639-8
5. Törnqvist B, Stromberg C, Persson G et al (2012) Effect of intended intraoperative cholangiography and early detection of bile duct injury on survival after cholecystectomy: population based cohort study. BMJ 345:e6457. doi:10.1136/bjm.e6457
6. Tagaya N, Shimoda M, Kato M et al (2010) Intraoperative exploration of biliary anatomy using fluorescence imaging of indocyanine green in experimental and clinical cholecystectomies. J Hepatobiliary Pancreat Sci 17:595–600. doi:10.1007/s00534-009-0195-2
7. Tagaya N, Sugamata Y, Makino N et al (2013) Frontiers of gastrointestinal research. Fluorescent imaging: treatment of hepatobiliary and pancreatic diseases. In: Kokudo N, Ishizawa T (eds) Clinical application of indocyanine green fluorescence imaging. Fluorescent cholangiography in laparoscopic cholecystectomy: experience in Japan. Karger, Basel, pp 73–79. doi:10.1159/000348615
8. Boni L, David G, Mangano A et al (2014) Clinical applications of indocyanine green (ICG) enhanced fluorescence in laparoscopic surgery. Surg Endosc. doi:10.1007/s00464-014-3895-x
9. Speich R, Saesseli B, Hoffmann U et al (1988) Anaphylactoid reaction after indocyanine-green administration. Ann Intern Med 109:345–346
10. Mitsuhashi N, Kimura F, Shimizu H et al (2008) Usefulness of intraoperative fluorescence imaging to evaluate local anatomy in hepatobiliary surgery. J Hepatobilary Pancreat Surg 15:508–514. doi:10.1007/s00534-007-1307-5
11. Aoki T, Murakami M, Yasuda D et al (2010) Intraoperative fluorescent imaging using indocyanine green for liver mapping and cholangiography. J Hepatobiliary Pancreat Sci 17:590–594. doi:10.1007/s00534-009-0197-0
12. Ishizawa T, Bandai Y, Ijichi M et al (2010) Fluorescent cholangiography illuminating the biliary tree during laparoscopic cholecystectomy. Br J Surg 97:1369–1377. doi:10.1002/bjs.7125
13. Buchs NC, Hagen ME, Pugin F et al (2012) Intra-operative fluorescent cholangiography using indocyanine green during robotic single site cholecystectomy. Int J Med Robotics Comput Assist Surg. doi:10.1002/rcs.1437
14. Schols RM, Bouvy ND, van Dam RM et al (2013) Combined vascular and biliary fluorescence imaging in laparoscopic cholecystectomy. Surg Endosc 27:4511–4517. doi:10.1007/s00464-013-3100-7
15. Scroggie DL, Jones C (2014) Fluorescence imaging of the biliary tract during laparoscopic cholecystectomy. Ann Surg Innov Res 8:5. http://www.asir-journal.com/contents/8/1/5
16. Verbeek FPR, Schaafsma BE, Tummers QRJG et al (2014) Optimization of near-infrared fluorescence cholangiography for open and laparoscopic surgery. Surg Endosc 28:1076–1082. doi:10.1007/s00464.013.3305-9
17. Matsui A, Tanaka E, Choi HS et al (2010) Real-time intraoperative near-infrared fluorescence identification of the extrahepatic bile ducts using clinically available contrast agents. Surgery 148:87–95. doi:10.1016/j.surg.2009.12.004

18. Ishizawa T, Kaneko J, Inoue Y et al (2011) Application of fluorescence cholangiography to single-incision laparoscopic cholecystectomy. Surg Endosc 25:2631–2636. doi:10.1007/s00464-011-1616-2
19. Ishizawa T, Tamura S, Masuda K et al (2008) Intraoperative fluorescent cholangiography using indocyanine green: a biliary load map for safe surgery. J Am Coll Surg 208:e1–e4. doi:10.1016/j-jamcollsurg.2008.09.024

Chapter 37
Usefulness of ICG Fluorescence Imaging in Laparoscopic Liver Resection

Yuichiro Otsuka and Hironori Kaneko

Abstract Laparoscopic liver resection (LLR) is now widely used as a minimally invasive surgical option for benign and malignant liver disease. Recent advances in LLR technique and instrumentation have enabled various procedures, including anatomic resection in liver surgery. However, the endoscopic approach is limited by its two-dimensional view, the absence of tactile sense, and the difficulty in establishing anatomic orientation, due to the use of a magnified view. Indocyanine green (ICG) fluorescence imaging is a tool for real-time surgical navigation in hepatobiliary surgery. It is useful in identifying anatomic portal parenchymal territory, localizing liver tumors, and detecting bile leakage during open liver surgery. With the development of laparoscopic fluorescence imaging systems, this technology can now be used for LLR. As LLR is increasingly adopted for treatment of liver disease, uptake of intraoperative real-time image guidance systems is likely to accelerate. The ICG fluorescence imaging system will be helpful as a surgical "third eye" in ensuring safe and precise LLR.

Keywords Laparoscopic liver resection • Indocyanine green • Fluorescence imaging • Navigation surgery

37.1 Introduction

Liver resection is the preferred treatment for patients with locally resectable liver disease. During the last two decades, improvements in patient evaluation, surgical techniques, and perioperative care have significantly decreased mortality and morbidity from liver resection. New perioperative diagnostic imaging modalities such as ultrasound, magnetic resonance imaging, and multidimensional computed tomography have greatly improved navigation during liver surgery [1–4].

Laparoscopic liver resection (LLR) was first described, in 1991, by Reich et al. [5] and is now widely used as a surgical option that is both minimally invasive

Y. Otsuka • H. Kaneko (✉)
Division of General and Gastroenterological Surgery, Department of Surgery, Toho University Faculty of Medicine, 6-11-1 Omorinishi, Ota-ku, Tokyo 143-8541, Japan
e-mail: hironori@med.toho-u.ac.jp

M. Kusano et al. (eds.), *ICG Fluorescence Imaging and Navigation Surgery*,
DOI 10.1007/978-4-431-55528-5_37

and effective for patients with benign or malignant liver disease. We previously reported that LLR safely improved postoperative quality of life, with no reduction in disease curability for liver tumors, in selected patients [6, 7]. In addition, major advances in LLR technique and instrumentation now permit anatomic liver resection, including major hepatectomy, in pure laparoscopic procedures. However, the endoscopic approach is restricted to a two-dimensional view, allows no tactile sense, and may hinder understanding of anatomic orientation, due to the use of a magnified view.

Indocyanine green (ICG) has unique pharmacodynamic characteristics—it is taken up by the liver and excreted into bile—and has thus been widely used in evaluating functional hepatic reserve in modern liver surgery. Furthermore, ICG binds plasma proteins (α1-lipoproteins) that are excited with near-infrared energy (at 805 nm) and emits light at 835 nm, which is detectable by special telescopes equipped with a photodynamic eye. This has been demonstrated in intraoperative real-time navigation, including the mapping of sentinel lymph nodes [8, 9] and evaluation of blood flow patency during intraoperative angiography [10, 11]. This technology has also been used to detect anatomic portal parenchymal territory [12], localization of liver tumors [13], and the presence of bile leakage [14, 15] during open liver surgery. Because of recent improvements in laparoscopic fluorescence imaging systems, this technology can now be used during laparoscopic surgery. We review the literature and describe our experience regarding the usefulness of ICG fluorescence imaging in LLR.

37.2 Materials

A laparoscopic system (Karl Storz GmbH & Co. KG, Tuttlingen, Germany) with a xenon light source (D-LIGHT P SCB, Karl Storz) was used. Images were generated by a high-end full high-definition camera system (IMAGE 1 SPIESTM, Karl Storz) connected to a laparoscope (HOPKINS®II ICG telescope, Karl Storz) with a 30° field of view and a diameter of 10 mm equipped with integrated filters for optimal detection of near-infrared fluorescence and white light. These modes can be alternated with a foot pedal controlled by the surgeon (Fig. 37.1).

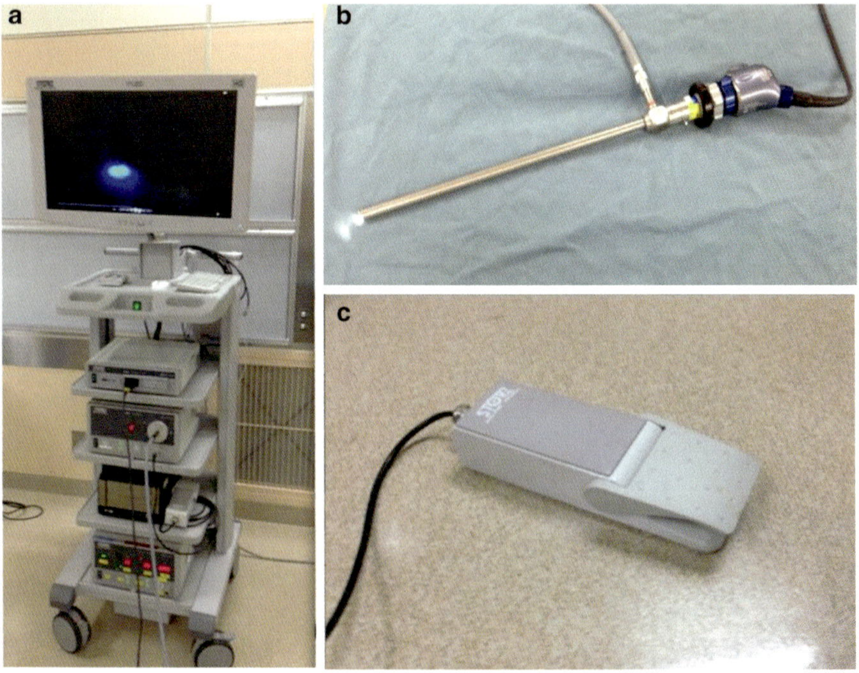

Fig. 37.1 The laparoscopic ICG fluorescent imaging system (Karl Storz GmbH & Co. KG, Tuttlingen, Germany)
(**a**) High-end full high-definition camera system (IMAGE 1 SPIESTM, Karl Storz)
(**b**) Laparoscope (HOPKINS®II ICG telescope, Karl Storz)
(**c**) Foot switch

37.3 Role of ICG Fluorescence Imaging in Laparoscopic Liver Resection

37.3.1 Identification of Anatomic Domain in the Liver

37.3.1.1 Background

Systemic removal of a segment-oriented territory confined by tumor-bearing portal tributaries was reported to be essential in radical resection of hepatocellular carcinoma (HCC) [16]. Parenchymal-sparing anatomic liver resection is often selected for patients with chronic liver impairment. Identification of the boundaries of hepatic sections or segments is usually done by means of ischemic demarcation followed by selective occlusion of the hepatic portal pedicle, with or without mapping with blue dye staining-guided intraoperative ultrasound [1, 17]. However, these strategies sometimes result in inadequate visualization of the stained domain, especially in cirrhotic liver. Aoki et al. [18] reported that ICG fluorescent mapping identified the stained hepatic domain in more than 90 % of patients undergoing open anatomic liver resection and that the techniques was successful even against the background of liver cirrhosis. A recent report by Sakoda et al. [19] indicated that this technology was useful during LLR.

37.3.1.2 Mechanism

Liver parenchyma fluoresces due to uptake by Kupffer cells within 2–3 min after intravenous injection of 0.5 mg/kg dilute ICG solution, the same dose used for preoperative evaluation of hepatic functional reserve.

37.3.1.3 Method

In anatomically oriented liver resection, the fundamental technique involves selective occlusion of the portal pedicles of the liver parenchyma, using a Glissonean approach or individual isolation of hepatic inflow vessels before hepatic parenchymal transection [1, 20]. ICG is administered intravenously after selective vascular occlusion is achieved. Consequently, the inflow-preserved liver area is fluorescent, and ischemic area is discolored as counterstaining fashion.

37.3.1.4 Case Presentation

Case description: Hepatocellular carcinoma and liver cirrhosis in segment 6 in a 56-year-old male. The patient underwent LLR of segment 6. The Glissonean sheath to segment 6 was isolated and ligated before liver parenchymal transection. After administration of ICG, the fluorescent imaging system allowed clear identification of the territory of the Glissonean sheath to segment 6 as an ischemic area (Fig. 37.2a–b). Liver resection was performed along the fluorescence boundary on the liver surface and parenchyma (Fig. 37.2c). After hepatic parenchymal transection, the entire resection plane was visualized as a fluorescence-emitting plane (Fig. 37.2d).

37.3.1.5 Assessment

The inflow-occluded area usually appears as an ischemic demarcation on the liver surface but is not always clearly visible during surgery, especially in cases of liver cirrhosis associated with portal hypertension, which leads to turbulent portal flow [21]. Similarly, the inflow-occluded area on the liver surface may also be indistinct after adhesiolysis. In our experience, these trends are obvious when visible white light is used during conventional endoscopy. Thus, ICG fluorescent imaging may be beneficial and sensitive in identifying anatomic segmentation in the liver surface

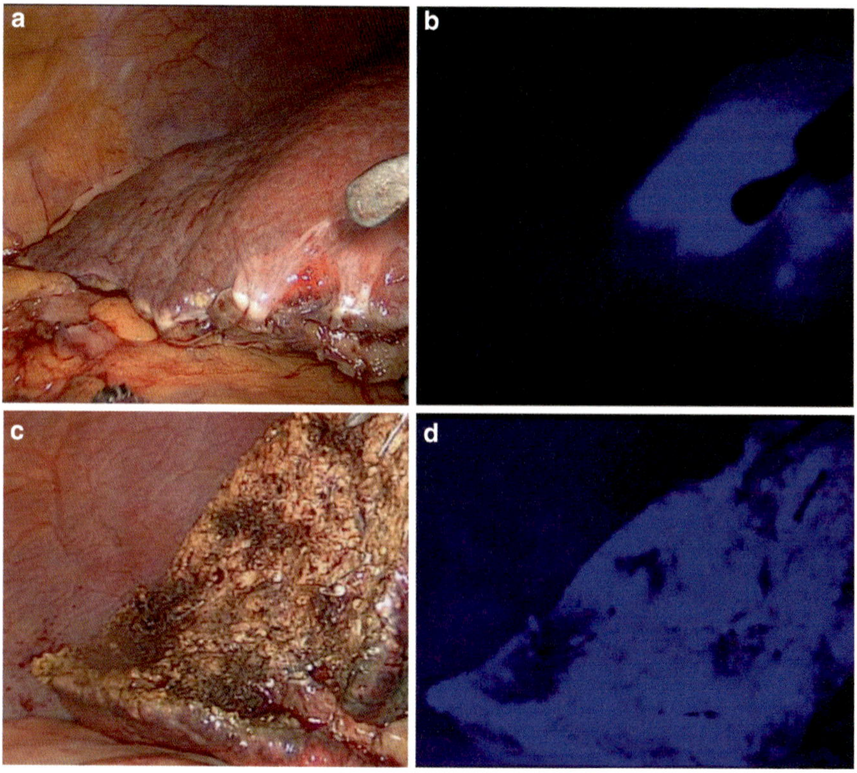

Fig. 37.2 Identification of anatomic domain in the liver
(**a**) After ligation of the Glissonean sheath to segment 6, the demarcation area is observed under white light
(**b**) After ICG administration, the territory of the Glissonean sheath of segment 6 is clearly visualized, after counterstaining, by the fluorescent imaging system
(**c**) LLR of segment 6 was performed along the fluorescence boundary on the liver surface and interior
(**d**) After hepatic parenchymal transection, the entire plane of resection is visualized as a fluorescence-emitting plane

achieved by a control portal pedicle in the laparoscopic setting. The distribution of ICG fluorescence can be identified even inside the liver. In our experience, navigation using the ICG system would make easier to reveal the orientation of anatomic boundaries within the liver parenchyma, compared with observation of ischemic discoloration or dye staining. Thus, ICG fluorescence staining could help address the main limitation of LLR—its difficulty in determining anatomic orientation due to its reliance on a two-dimensional magnified view.

37.3.2 Detection of Liver Tumors

37.3.2.1 Background

In open liver surgery, the location and extent of tumors are usually determined by visualization and surgical palpation, with ultrasound assistance. However, macroscopically unidentifiable, small, subcapsular lesions might be missed even in open procedures. Ishizawa et al. reported that ICG fluorescent imaging, with preoperative ICG administration, enables highly sensitive detection of small and grossly unidentifiable liver cancers near the liver surface, through visualization of uptake and abnormalities in biliary excretion of ICG in cancer and noncancerous liver tissues. They concluded that this technology enhanced the accuracy of liver resection and operative staging [13].

A disadvantage of laparoscopic surgery is the limited ability to palpate the tumor. The recent development of laparoscopic ICG fluorescence imaging may compensate for this limitation in the diagnosis of hepatic malignancy during LLR. Satou et al. [22] reported that extrahepatic metastases from HCC emitted fluorescence on ICG fluorescent imaging. As compared with open procedures, inspection of the whole abdomen is often easier when done laparoscopically. Therefore, ICG fluorescence imaging should be more often utilized in laparoscopic surgery.

37.3.2.2 Mechanism

Although the precise mechanism of ICG accumulation in liver tumors is unknown, Ishizawa et al. found that well-differentiated HCC tissues take up ICG during preoperative administration, although biliary excretion of ICG is impaired in HCC because of morphologic or functional abnormalities. In contrast, poorly differentiated HCC and metastatic liver cancers do not take up ICG. However, such tumors can be visualized as rings of fluorescence, which result from impaired bile excretion in surrounding nontumorous tissues that are compressed by tumors [13, 23]. Using a fluorescence microscope, they also noted ICG fluorescence in the cytoplasm and pseudoglands of well-differentiated HCCs. Fluorescence was also seen in nontumorous liver tissue compressed by tumors in cases of poorly differentiated HCC and colorectal cancer metastases, as in the abovementioned macroscopic findings [24]. This variation in enhancement pattern may be caused by varied expression of organic anion-transporting polypeptide 8 [25].

37.3.2.3 Method

Within the 2 weeks before surgery, 0.5 mg/kg of ICG (Diagnogreen; Daiichi Sankyo, Tokyo, Japan) is administered intravenously for preoperative evaluation

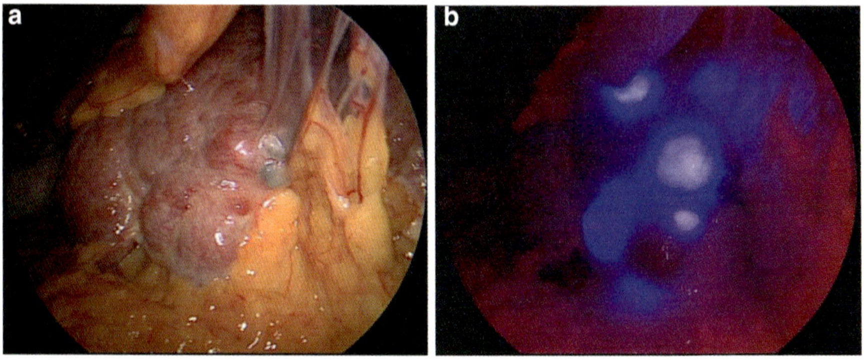

Fig. 37.3 Detection of liver tumors
(**a**) Macroscopic cirrhosis with multiple regenerative nodules as visualized in visible white light mode. The tumors are not clearly visible from the liver surface
(**b**) Fluorescence imaging reveals multiple subcapsular tumors, which were later resected

of hepatic functional reserve. The entire abdomen, including the liver, is inspected with the ICG fluorescence imaging system during surgery.

37.3.2.4 Case Presentation

Case description: Multiple recurrent HCC in the left lateral section, 3 years after partial resection of segment 3 for initial HCC, in a 79-year-old female with Child B liver cirrhosis. Macroscopic cirrhosis with multiple regenerative nodules was observed with the visible white light mode of the laparoscope; however, no tumors were clearly visible on the liver surface (Fig. 37.3a). After introduction of the fluorescence imaging, multiple subcapsular tumors were resected (Fig. 37.3b). No other emission-suspected extrahepatic metastasis was seen in the abdomen. Laparoscopic left lateral sectionectomy was performed. Pathologic analysis of the specimen showed well-differentiated HCC.

37.3.2.5 Assessment

Kudo et al. [26] described the sensitivity of laparoscopic ICG fluorescence imaging in 12 HCCs (75 %) and 11 liver metastases (69 %) on the liver surface, which were distributed over Couinaud segments 1–8, including tumors unidentifiable by white light. However, inability to visualize tumors $\geq$8 mm from the liver surface is a major limitation of ICG fluorescence imaging in open and laparoscopic procedures [13]. Therefore, intraoperative ultrasound remains an indispensable diagnostic tool for assessment of liver tumor, including deep lesions.

False-positive emission is another concern in the detection of liver malignancies. Morita et al. reported and noted very small emission spots on the liver surface and cut plane. Pathologic examination showed that these emissions were derived from a dysplastic nodule, liver parenchyma, bile plug, and cyst [27]. Tanaka et al. suggested that ICG might accumulate in regenerative nodules [28]. The many false-positive emissions are believed to be due to severe liver function disorder and biliary excretion disorders [13, 28–30], which are frequently seen in cirrhotic liver.

Ishizawa et al. demonstrated that the signal intensity of noncancerous liver parenchyma was higher in patients with an unfavorable ICG retention rate and in patients who had received an ICG injection within the 24 h before surgery [13]. They proposed that an interval longer than 2 days might be necessary in order to obtain good lesion-to-liver contrast, especially in patients with advanced cirrhosis [31].

37.3.3 Visualization of Biliary Leakage

37.3.3.1 Background

Postoperative bile leak is a common complication (up to 10 % of cases) [32–34] and can worsen outcomes after liver surgery, even in the modern era [32, 33]. For the best outcome, bile leakage should be detected intraoperatively; however, a randomized trial found that use of a bile leak test requiring injection of saline solution through the cystic duct offered no advantage [34], probably because of the transparency of saline. Intrabiliary injection of dyes such as methylene blue [35] and ICG [33, 36] has also been attempted, but these dyes can densely stain tissue and complicate repeat inspection. A randomized control trial [14] found that ICG fluorescent cholangiography was useful in detecting bile leakage not detected on a leak test using saline. Sakaguchi et al. [15] reported that ICG fluorescent cholangiography was sufficiently sensitive to identify bile leakage.

37.3.3.2 Mechanism

Human bile juice contains proteins that bind ICG [37]; therefore, fluorescent images of the biliary tract can be obtained after intrabiliary injection of ICG [38].

37.3.3.3 Method

After completion of hepatic resection, a catheter is cannulated into the common bile duct through the cystic duct, and 5–10 ml of dilute ICG solution blended with bile juice (0.05 mg/ml) is injected into the bile duct, while the common bile duct is distally occluded to the cystic duct. Emitted leakage from the cut surface of the liver or intrahepatic bile duct is repaired by suture or clip.

a b

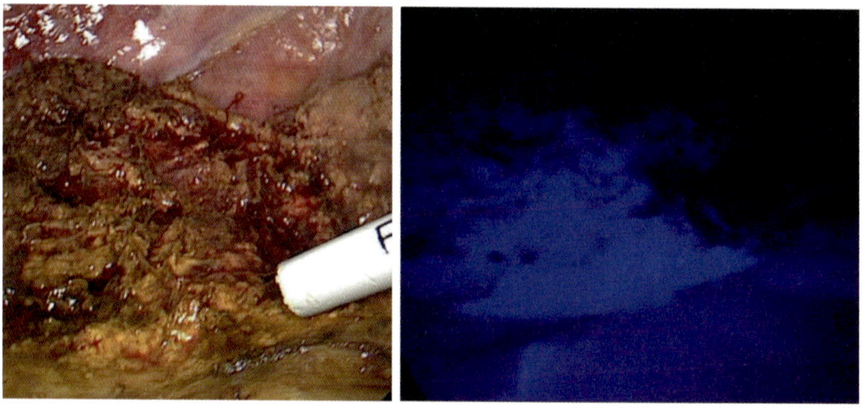

Fig. 37.4 Visualization of biliary leakage
(**a**) Bile leakage was suspected on the hepatic hilum. However, the site of leakage could not be clearly identified with the visible white light mode of the laparoscope
(**b**) Fluorescence imaging allowed detection and elimination of bile leakage from the left hepatic duct

37.3.3.4 Case Presentation

Case description: HCC (size, 8 cm) in segments 4–8 in a 73-year-old female. Pure laparoscopic anatomic liver resection of the medial section with the ventral area of the anterior section was performed. After hepatectomy was completed, bile leakage was suspected on the hepatic hilum. However, the leakage site could not be clearly identified using the visible white light mode of the laparoscope (Fig. 37.4a). The fluorescence mode was activated, and bile leakage from the left hepatic duct was detected and repaired by suturing (Fig. 37.4b).

37.3.3.5 Assessment

A limitation of ICG fluorescent cholangiography is that it cannot adequately visualize the intrahepatic and extrahepatic bile ducts, which are covered by surrounding tissue, due to the limited tissue penetration of near-infrared light.

37.4 Conclusion

We conclude that LLR will be increasingly used for treatment of liver disease, as it is minimally invasive, preserves postoperative quality of life of patients, and is effective in curing disease. Intraoperative real-time image guidance systems will become indispensable tools for hepatobiliary surgery and in laparoscopic settings.

ICG is a safe agent: the incidence of adverse reactions after intravenous injection is rare, approximately 0.003 % [39]. An advantage of laparoscopic ICG fluorescence imaging is that surgeons can use a foot pedal to instantly change the mode from visible white light to fluorescence, using the same monitor. The ICG fluorescence imaging system will certainly prove useful as a surgical "third eye" in the safe and precise performance of LLR.

References

1. Makuuchi M, Hasegawa H, Yamazaki S (1985) Ultrasonically guided subsegmentectomy. Surg Gynecol Obstet 161:346–350
2. Lamade W, Vetter M, Hassenpflug P, Thorn M, Meinzer HP, Herfarth C (2002) Navigation and image-guided HBP surgery: a review and preview. J Hepatobiliary Pancreat Surg 9:592–599
3. Wigmore SJ, Redhead DN, Yan XJ et al (2001) Virtual hepatic resection using three-dimensional reconstruction of helical computed tomography angioportograms. Ann Surg 233:221–226
4. Beller S, Hunerbein M, Eulenstein S, Lange T, Schlag PM (2007) Feasibility of navigated resection of liver tumors using multiplanar visualization of intraoperative 3-dimensional ultrasound data. Ann Surg 246:288–294
5. Reich H, McGlynn F, DeCaprio J, Budin R (1991) Laparoscopic excision of benign liver lesions. Obstet Gynecol 78:956–958
6. Kaneko H, Takagi S, Shiba T (1996) Laparoscopic partial hepatectomy and left lateral segmentectomy: technique and results of a clinical series. Surgery 120:468–475
7. Kaneko H, Takagi S, Otsuka Y, Tsuchiya M, Tamura A, Katagiri T et al (2005) Laparoscopic liver resection of hepatocellular carcinoma. Am J Surg 189:190–194
8. Troyan SL, Kianzad V, Gibbs-Strauss SL, Gioux S, Matsui A, Oketokoun R, Ngo L, Khamene A, Azar F, Frangioni JV (2009) The FLARE intraoperative near-infrared fluorescence imaging system: a first-in-human clinical trial in breast cancer sentinel lymph node mapping. Ann Surg Oncol 16:2943–2952
9. Tajima Y, Yamazaki K, Masuda Y, Kato M, Yasuda D, Aoki T, Kato T, Murakami M, Miwa M, Kusano M (2009) Sentinel node mapping guided by indocyanine green fluorescence imaging in gastric cancer. Ann Surg 249:58–62
10. Rubens FD, Ruel M, Fremes SE (2002) A new and simplified method for coronary and graft imaging during CABG. Heart Surg Forum 5:141–144
11. Unno N, Suzuki M, Yamamoto N et al (2008) Indocyanine green fluorescence angiography for intraoperative assessment of blood flow: a feasibility study. Eur J Vasc Endovasc Surg 35:205–207
12. Aoki T, Yasuda D, Shimizu Y, Odaira M, Niiya T, Kusano T, Mitamura K, Hayashi K, Murai N, Koizumi T, Kato H, Enami Y, Kusano M (2008) Image-guided liver mapping using fluorescence navigation system with indocyanine green for anatomical hepatic resection. World J Surg 32:1763–1767

13. Ishizawa T, Fukushima N, Shibahara J, Masuda K, Tamura S, Aoki T et al (2009) Real-time identification of liver cancers by using indocyanine green fluorescent imaging. Cancer 115:2491–2504
14. Kaibori M, Ishizaki M, Matsui K, Kwon AH (2011) Intraoperative indocyanine green fluorescent imaging for prevention of bile leakage after hepatic resection. Surgery 150:91–98
15. Sakaguchi T, Suzuki A, Unno N, Morita Y, Oishi K, Fukumoto K, Inaba K, Suzuki M, Tanaka H, Sagara D, Suzuki S, Nakamura S, Konno H (2010) Bile leak test by indocyanine green fluorescence images after hepatectomy. Am J Surg 200(1):e19–e23
16. Hasegawa K, Kokudo N, Imamura H, Matsuyama Y, Aoki T, Minagawa M, Sano K, Sugawara Y, Takayama T, Makuuchi M (2005) Prognostic impact of anatomic resection for hepatocellular carcinoma. Ann Surg 242:252–259
17. Takayama T, Makuuchi M, Watanabe K, Kosuge T, Takayasu K, Yamazaki S et al (1991) A new method for mapping hepatic subsegment: counterstaining identification technique. Surgery 109:226–229
18. Aoki T, Murakami M, Yasuda D, Shimizu Y, Kusano T, Matsuda K, Niiya T, Kato H, Murai N, Otsuka K, Kusano M, Kato T (2010) Intraoperative fluorescent imaging using indocyanine green for liver mapping and cholangiography. J Hepatobiliary Pancreat Sci 17:590–594
19. Sakoda M, Ueno S, Iino S, Hiwatashi K, Minami K, Kawasaki Y, Kurahara H, Mataki Y, Maemura K, Uenosono Y, Shinchi H, Natsugoe S (2014) Anatomical laparoscopic hepatectomy for hepatocellular carcinoma using indocyanine green fluorescence imaging. J Laparoendosc Adv Surg Tech A 24(12):878–882
20. Yamamoto M, Takasaki K, Ohtsubo T, Katsuragawa H, Fukuda C, Katagiri S (2001) Effectiveness of systematized hepatectomy with Glisson's pedicle transection at the hepatic hilus for small nodular hepatocellular carcinoma: retrospective analysis. Surgery 130:443–448
21. Uchiyama K, Ueno M, Ozawa S, Kiriyama S, Shigekawa Y, Hirono S, Kawai M, Tani M, Yamaue H (2011) Combined intraoperative use of contrast-enhanced ultrasonography imaging using a sonazoid and fluorescence navigation system with indocyanine green during anatomical hepatectomy. Langenbecks Arch Surg 396:1101–1107
22. Satou S, Ishizawa T, Masuda K, Kaneko J, Aoki T, Sakamoto Y, Hasegawa K, Sugawara Y, Kokudo N (2013) Indocyanine green fluorescent imaging for detecting extrahepatic metastasis of hepatocellular carcinoma. J Gastroenterol 48:1136–1143
23. van der Vorst JR, Schaafsma BE, Hutteman M, Verbeek FP, Liefers GJ, Hartgrink HH et al (2013) Near-infrared fluorescence-guided resection of colorectal liver metastases. Cancer 119:3411–3418
24. Ishizawa T, Harada N, Muraoka A et al (2010) Scientific basis and clinical application of ICG fluorescence imaging: hepatobiliary cancer. Open Surg Oncol J 2:31–36
25. Kitao A, Zen Y, Matsui O et al (2010) Hepatocellular carcinoma: signal intensity at gadoxetic acid-enhanced MR Imaging–correlation with molecular transporters and histopathologic features. Radiology 256:817–826
26. Kudo H, Ishizawa T, Tani K, Harada N, Ichida A, Shimizu A, Kaneko J, Aoki T, Sakamoto Y, Sugawara Y, Hasegawa K, Kokudo N (2014) Visualization of subcapsular hepatic malignancy by indocyanine-green fluorescence imaging during laparoscopic hepatectomy. Surg Endosc 28:2504–2508
27. Morita Y, Sakaguchi Y, Unno N, Shibasaki Y, Suzuki A, Fukumoto K, Inaba K, Konno H (2013) Detection of hepatocellular carcinomas with near-infrared fluorescence imaging using indocyanine green: its usefulness and limitation. Int J Clin Oncol 18:232–241
28. Lin WR, Lim SN, Macdonald SA, Graham T, Wright VL, Peplow CL et al (2010) The histogenesis of regenerative nodules in human liver cirrhosis. Hepatology 51:1017–1026
29. Nakanuma Y (1995) Non-neoplastic nodular lesions in the liver. Pathol Int 45:7013–7714
30. Sathirakul K, Suzuki H, Yasuda K, Hanano M, Tagaya O, Horie T et al (1993) Kinetic analysis of hepatobiliary transport of organic anions in Eisai hyperbilirubinemic mutant rats. J Pharmacol Exp Ther 265:1301–1312

31. Tanaka T, Takatsuki M, Hidaka M, Hara T, Muraoka I, Soyama A, Adachi T, Kuroki T, Eguchi S (2014) Is a fluorescence navigation system with indocyanine green effective enough to detect liver malignancies? J Hepatobiliary Pancreat Sci 21:199–204
32. Lo CM, Fan ST, Liu CL et al (1998) Biliary complications after hepatic resection: risk factors, management, and outcome. Arch Surg 133:156–161
33. Yamashita Y, Hamatsu T, Rikimaru T et al (2001) Bile leakage after hepatic resection. Ann Surg 233:45–50
34. Ijichi M, Takayama T, Toyoda H et al (2000) Randomized trial of the usefulness of a bile leakage test during hepatic resection. Arch Surg 135:1395–1400
35. Lam CM, Lo CM, Liu CL et al (2001) Biliary complications during liver resection. World J Surg 25:1273–1276
36. Suehiro T, Shimada M, Kishikawa K et al (2005) In situ dye injection bile leakage test of the graft in living donor liver transplantation. Transplantation 80:1398–1401
37. Mulllock BM, Shaw LJ, Fitzharris B, Peppard J, Hamilton MJ, Simpson MT et al (1985) Sources of proteins in human bile. Gut 26:500–509
38. Ishizawa T, Tamura S, Masuda K, Aoki T, Hasegawa K, Imamura H et al (2009) Intraoperative fluorescent cholangiography using indocyanine green: a biliary road map for safe surgery. J Am Coll Surg 208:e1–e4
39. Cherrick GR, Stein SW, Leevy CM, Davidson CS (1960) Indocyanine green: observations on its physical properties, plasma decay, and hepatic extraction. J Clin Invest 39:592–600

Part XV
Hepato-Pancreatic-Biliary Surgery: Pancreas

Chapter 38
Detection of Hepatic Micrometastases from Pancreatic Cancer

Naoyuki Yokoyama, Hideki Hashidate, and Tetsuya Otani

Abstract The detection of hepatic metastases is critical in the treatment of pancreatic cancer, because their presence suggests systemic disease with poor prognosis. Although recent advances in high-resolution imaging have allowed physicians to delineate small hepatic tumors, some of those might still be missed owing to their location and miniscule size. Such micrometastases may result in early-term hepatic relapse after radical surgery for pancreatic cancer. We utilize indocyanine green (ICG) near-infrared (NIR) fluorescence imaging which better detects extremely small hepatic lesions to identify hepatic micrometastases intraoperatively. Our experience demonstrates that ICG-NIR imaging successfully detects hepatic micrometastases in approximately one sixth of pancreatic cancer patients without suspicion of hepatic disease before surgery. The hepatic micrometastases detected microscopically originate from the tumor thrombi at the intrahepatic portal triad, and their local invasion results in focal obstructive jaundice that might fluoresce under ICG-NIR. Patients with hepatic micrometastases frequently experience overt hepatic relapse within 6 months after surgery; therefore, such hepatic micrometastases seem to be clinically evident as distant metastases. ICG-NIR fluorescence examination contributes to real-time cancer staging and the elucidation of pancreatic cancer biology.

Keywords Neoplasm micrometastasis • Pancreatic ductal carcinoma • Liver neoplasms • Optical imaging

---

N. Yokoyama, M.D. (✉) • T. Otani, M.D.
Department of Digestive Surgery, Niigata City General Hospital, 463-7 Shumoku, Chuo-ku, Niigata, Japan
e-mail: yokonao@hosp.niigata.niigata.jp

H. Hashidate, M.D.
Department of Pathology, Niigata City General Hospital, 463-7 Shumoku, Chuo-ku, Niigata, Japan

M. Kusano et al. (eds.), *ICG Fluorescence Imaging and Navigation Surgery*,
DOI 10.1007/978-4-431-55528-5_38

38.1 Rationale for the Detection of Hepatic Micrometastases from Pancreatic Cancer

Clinical oncologists are enthusiastic about imaging modalities that specifically detect neoplastic lesion. Recent advances in clinical imaging including magnetic resonance imaging and multidetector computed tomography (MDCT) allow for the precise detection of considerably small tumors. Moreover, examinations such as positron emission tomography CT and indocyanine green (ICG) or aminolevulinic acid fluorescence imaging which can discriminate neoplasms from normal tissue based on cancer-specific metabolic processes have also been developed [1–4].

ICG near-infrared (NIR) fluorescence imaging has been used for real-time visualization of blood or lymphatic flow in various fields [5–9]. In 2009, Ishizawa et al. reported that hepatic tumors could be detected with high sensitivity using this technique [2]. They also demonstrated that the examination was feasible in not only primary but also metastatic liver tumors regardless of their origin. We have accordingly applied the concept to pancreatic cancer surgery for real-time detection of hepatic micrometastases [10, 11]. In pancreatic cancer, hepatic metastases suggest systemic disease with poor prognosis; therefore, their precise detection for accurate cancer staging is clinically very important [12, 13]. In this chapter, we review the pathological and clinical results of ICG-NIR examination for the detection of hepatic micrometastases from pancreatic cancer.

38.2 Procedures

We defined hepatic micrometastases as histologically confirmed cancer metastases that are not identified during preoperative imaging or intraoperative gross examination but could be detected on fluorescence imaging. The detailed procedures for the examination have been previously described [10, 11]. We generally inject 25 mg of ICG per body the day before surgery with further dose adjustment according to patients' age and the body size. Allergic reactions such as a drop in blood pressure, nausea, or local pain with ICG injection have been reported in 0.17 % of the patients and should be carefully monitored. Patients are also informed about the benefits and risks of the examination.

Several types of NIR fluorescence equipment are commercially available. We use photodynamic eye system (Hamamatsu Photonics, Japan) for open surgery and a laparoscopic examination system (Olympus, Japan) for laparoscopic surgery to detect hepatic micrometastases from pancreatic cancer. Both systems have their own technical advantages and disadvantages. During an open surgery, the clinician can use tactile sensation to help with fluorescent examinations; however, surgical light in the operating room must be turned off for NIR observation. On the other hand, the laparoscopic fluorescence system can be switched from normal vision to fluorescent imaging with "one push of a button" at the fiberscope, and the location of an abnormal hepatic lesion can be easily recognized with close laparoscopic observation. Furthermore, the less invasive laparoscopic examination allows patients to avoid major laparotomy procedures. Thus, it might become the mainstream for detecting hepatic micrometastases from pancreatic cancer in the near future [14–16].

Abnormal hepatic foci that fluoresce under NIR are suspected to be micrometastases. Small nodules could be palpated or observed via gross examination in certain cases under the guide of fluorescent imaging, and they could be biopsied eventually. If no other lesions are observed, the liver tissue around the fluorescent area is then excised for histological examination. The biopsied specimens are frozen and sectioned for initial pathological evaluation and subsequently processed into permanent for highly detailed histological examination. "False-positive fluorescence" cases are registered when hepatic metastases could not be detected in the biopsied specimens.

38.3 Detection of Hepatic Micrometastases

In our experience treating 102 patients with invasive pancreatic cancer, abnormal hepatic lesions were detected in 26 (25.5 %) by using intraoperative fluorescence examination (Fig. 38.1). Most of these lesions exhibited spotty pattern and measured 2–5 mm in diameter, but the fluorescent area exceeded 3 cm^2 in some cases. Subsequently, hepatic metastases were histologically confirmed in those 18 patients (17.6 %). The numbers of hepatic micrometastases were purulent in all of the 18 patients.

The gallbladder and extrahepatic bile ducts which contain biliary juice with physiologically secreted ICG showed fluorescence. Additionally, simple biliary cysts could also be positive for NIR examination. When those benign foci were excluded, the false-positive fluorescence rate was 7.8 % (8/102 patients) in our experience. Both the false-positive samples and those with histologically confirmed micrometastases via frozen section examination were submitted for further histological evaluation.

38.4 Histopathological Features of Hepatic Micrometastases

Our histopathological examination revealed that the hepatic micrometastases from pancreatic cancer detected by using fluorescence imaging were mainly located at the portal triad (Fig. 38.2). Most of them seemed to be derived from the tumor thrombi of the portal vein in the intrahepatic portal triads, and their extravenous invasion caused desmoplastic reaction around the foci. Such a reaction then resulted in obstruction and stasis of local biliary flow and bile stasis at the peripheral liver

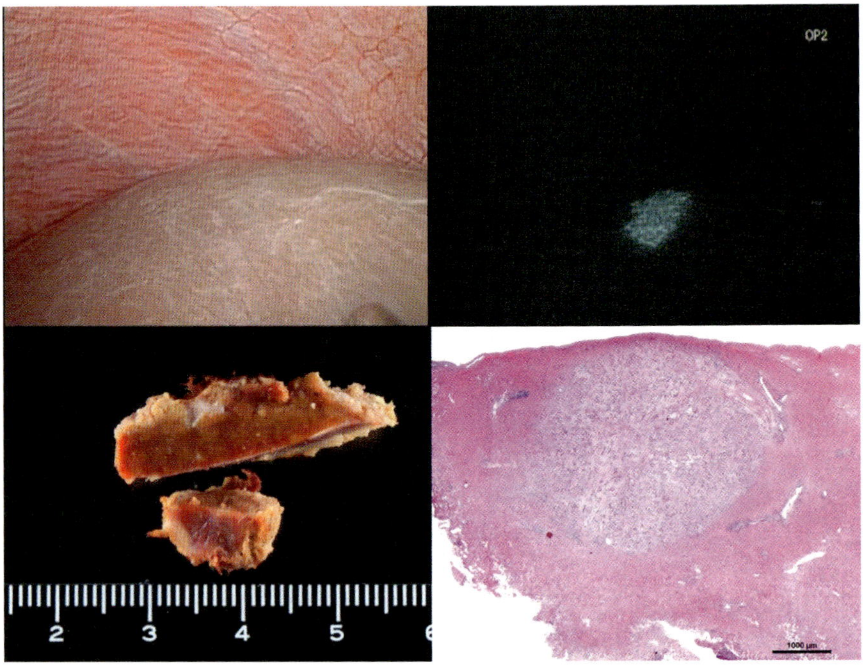

Fig. 38.1 Hepatic micrometastases detected by using an indocyanine green fluorescent system are demonstrated. Although a hepatic tumor was not readily observable via macroscopic inspection, a fluorescent lesion was delineated using near-infrared imaging, and metastatic adenocarcinoma was confirmed via histological examination of the collected specimen

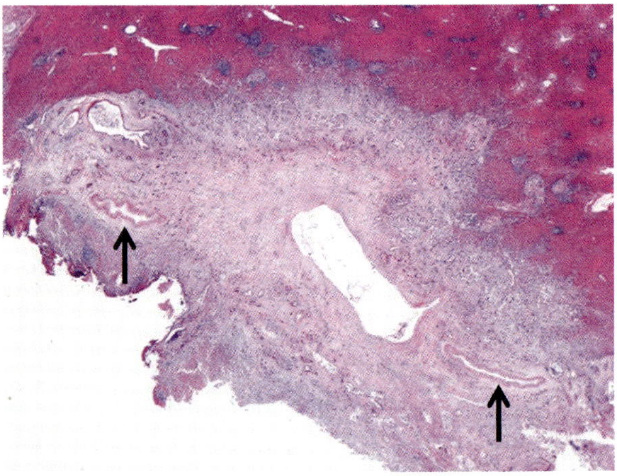

Fig. 38.2 Histopathological findings of hepatic micrometastases from pancreatic cancer are shown. Metastatic adenocarcinoma originating from the portal thrombi invaded toward the parenchyma of the portal triad. Desmoplastic reaction due to tumor invasion caused local biliary obstruction and resulted in dilation of the peripheral bile ducts (*arrows*)

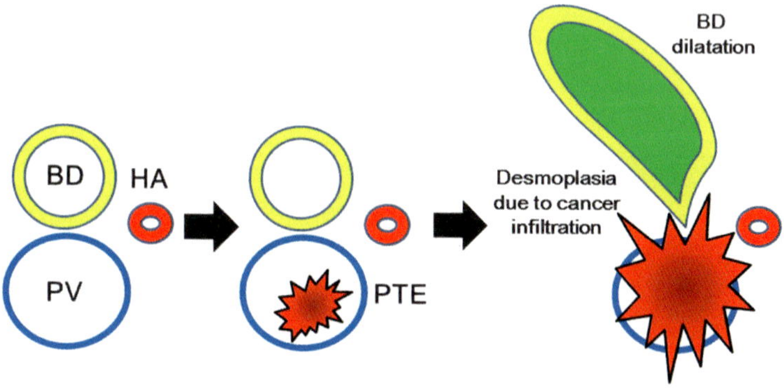

Fig. 38.3 Schematic diagrams of hepatic micrometastases and their fluorescence mechanism are shown. Micrometastases do not fluoresce, but indocyanine green-contained stagnant bile caused by cancer development at the portal triad does under near-infrared examination

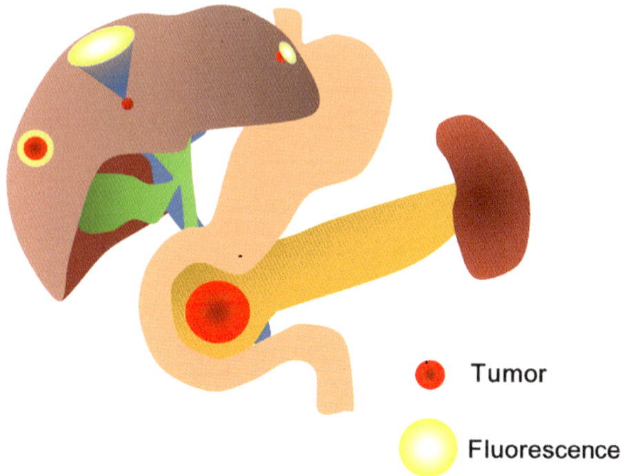

Fig. 38.4 The site and area of fluorescence observed on the liver surface were not in accord with those of the actual hepatic micrometastases

(Fig. 38.3). Thereafter, focal dilation of the biliary ducts was frequently observed in the specimens with hepatic micrometastases.

We observed eight cases of false-positive fluorescence in which benign foci were not distinguishable from micrometastases during intraoperative gross examination. Histological examination of the permanent specimens from those cases revealed different biliary congestive conditions including biliary hamartoma, focal steatohepatitis, and cholangiectasis of unknown origin [17]. Thus, some types of bile stasis were found in all cases with abnormal hepatic fluorescence regardless of the histological confirmation of micrometastases. We therefore hypothesize that the ICG-containing stagnant bile is the reason for fluorescence, and hepatic micrometastases themselves do not fluoresce [10, 17]. As a result, the size and location of the fluorescence are not in accord with those of the actual micrometastases (Fig. 38.4). Moreover, diffuse fluorescence was observed in the

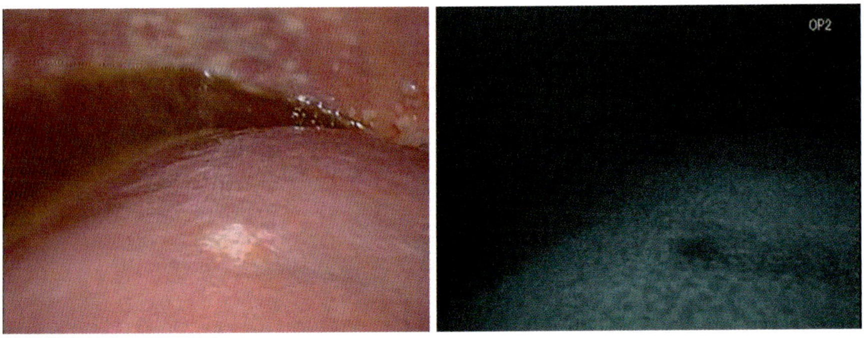

Fig. 38.5 Macroscopic features of hepatic micrometastases from pancreatic cancer detected in a patient with obstructive jaundice are shown. The liver fluoresced diffusely on indocyanine green near-infrared examination, but the metastatic focus observable via gross inspection did not

entire liver of patients with obstructive jaundice, owing to biliary stasis, which supports our hypothesis. In contrast, metastatic foci showed negative fluorescence in those patients (Fig. 38.5). This finding of false-positive results might be associated with inadequate sample collection.

38.5 Clinical Impact of Hepatic Micrometastases

The most important issue regarding hepatic micrometastases from pancreatic cancer is whether they have the same clinical significance as the overt distant metastases. To date, we have treated the two conditions similarly [10]. In cases of histologically confirmed hepatic micrometastases, even if the disease is considered as loco-regionally resectable stage, systemic chemotherapy is administrated after exploratory surgery or palliative bypass operation. On the other hand, patients without hepatic micrometastases (including those with false-positive findings) undergo radical or palliative surgery according to other staging factors. All patients are periodically followed up with MDCT regardless of curative or palliative surgery.

Hepatic overt metastases were more frequently observed in patients with micrometastases (14/18, 77.8 %) within 6 months after the surgery than in those without (7/84, 8.3 %) (Fig. 38.6). The short-term hepatic relapse often developed in multiple lesions and widespread hepatic area. Therefore, the micrometastases detected during surgery seem to have similar clinical impact to that of overt hepatic metastases. Resection of hepatic micrometastases has little clinical validity even when the number of lesions is limited. In addition, systemic chemotherapy is often unable to control the liver disease; therefore, some liver-targeted therapies (i.e.,

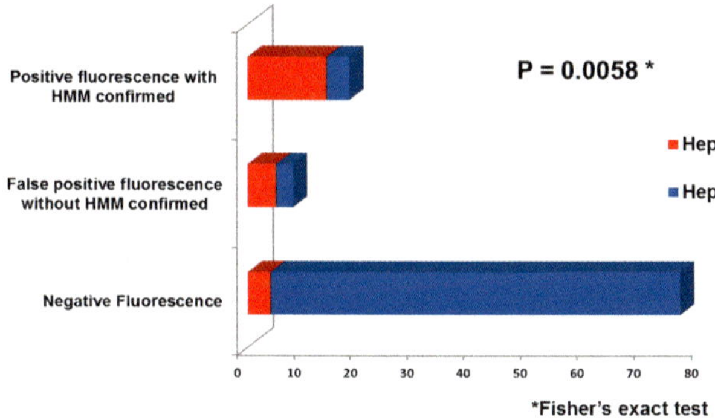

Fig. 38.6 Probability of overt hepatic relapse within 6 months after surgery for pancreatic cancer stratified by near-infrared fluorescence examination

perfusion chemotherapy, radiation) may be needed for patients with hepatic micrometastases [18, 19]. On the contrary, as the probability of hepatic relapse in patients without hepatic micrometastases is significantly lower, loco-regionally curative therapies may play an important role in those patients.

We observed overt hepatic relapse in 62.5 % (5/8) of the patients with false-positive fluorescence findings (Fig. 38.6). The probability was comparable to that of patients with histologically confirmed hepatic micrometastases. Such a phenomenon might be explained by the presence of hepatic micrometastases adjacent to the biopsied specimens, owing to the discrepancies in fluorescence signals and actual tumor foci. Alternatively, the metastases might be too small to be detected even on microscopic examination. In our experience, the positive predictive value of abnormal hepatic fluorescence (including true and false-positive cases) for hepatic relapse was high (73.1 %, 19/26), and the negative predictive value was extremely high (94.7 %, 72/76). Regardless of histological confirmation, fluorescence imaging seems to be a highly sensitive and specific examination for predicting hepatic relapse in pancreatic cancer.

There are several technical limitations of fluorescence imaging examination. The permeation depth of NIR is up to 1 cm; therefore, false-negative results might be expected in cases of deep hepatic foci [2, 8, 9]. On the other hand, the issues of false-positive fluorescence described above should be resolved with careful histological analysis. Future clinical and histopathological studies with a larger number of samples are warranted to address such issues.

38.6 Future Perspectives

ICG-NIR fluorescence imaging enables the detection of hepatic micrometastases from pancreatic cancer that are not identified by using other examination modalities. Their detection contributes to the precise staging and accurate planning of treatment strategy. Moreover, unnecessary radical surgery can be avoided in patients with hepatic micrometastases. Additionally, histopathological information on hepatic micrometastases might increase the oncologic knowledge of pancreatic cancer. In the field of clinical imaging, the altered local circulation caused by hepatic micrometastases at the portal triad might be detected by using dynamic imaging modalities [20]. Their early detection allows for proper treatment of the disease. Thus, the detection of hepatic micrometastases may improve the outcome of the "highly malignant" pancreatic cancer.

References

1. Tajima Y, Yamazaki K, Masuda Y et al (2009) Sentinel node mapping guided by indocyanine green fluorescence imaging in gastric cancer. Ann Surg 249:58–62
2. Ishizawa T, Fukushima N, Shibahara J et al (2009) Real-time identification of liver cancers by using indocyanine green fluorescent imaging. Cancer 115:2491–2504
3. Koizumi N, Harada Y, Murayama Y et al (2013) Detection of metastatic lymph nodes using 5-aminolevulinic acid in patients with gastric cancer. Ann Surg Oncol 20:3541–3548
4. Frei KA, Bonel HM, Frick H et al (2004) Photodynamic detection of diseased axillary sentinel lymph node after oral application of aminolevulinic acid in patients with breast cancer. Br J Cancer 90:805–809
5. Oliveila JG, Beck J, Seifert V et al (2007) Assessment of flow in perforating arteries during intracranial aneurysm surgery using intraoperative near-infrared indocyanine green videoangiogaphy. Neurosurgery 61:63–73
6. Aoki T, Yasuda D, Shimizu Y et al (2008) Image-guided liver mapping using fluorescence navigation system with indocyanine green for anatomical hepatic resection. World J Surg 32:1763–1767
7. Ishizawa T, Bandai Y, Ijichi M et al (2010) Fluorescent cholangiography illuminating the biliary tree during laparoscopic cholecystectomy. Br J Surg 97:1369–1377
8. Kim S, Lim YT, Soltesz EG et al (2004) Near-infrared fluorescent type II quantum dots for sentinel lymph node mapping. Nat Biotechnol 22:93–97
9. Mitsuhashi N, Kimura F, Shimizu H et al (2008) Usefulness of intraoperative fluorescence imaging to evaluate local anatomy in hepatobiliary surgery. J Hepatobiliary Pancreat Surg 15:508–514
10. Yokoyama N, Otani T, Hashidate H et al (2012) Real-time detection of hepatic micrometastases from pancreatic cancer by intraoperative fluorescence imaging: preliminary results of a prospective study. Cancer 118:2813–2819
11. Yokoyama N, Otani T (2013) Identification of occult liver metastases. In: Kokudo N, Ishizawa T (eds) Fluorescent imaging: treatment of hepatobiliary and pancreatic diseases, frontiers of gastrointestinal research, vol 31. Karger, Basel, pp 25–33
12. Shrikhande SV, Kleeff J, Reiser C et al (2007) Pancreatic resection for M1 pancreatic ductal adenocarcinoma. Ann Surg Oncol 14:118–127
13. Seelig S, Burkert B, Chromik A et al (2010) Pancreatic resections for advanced M1-pancreatic carcinoma: the value of synchronous metastasectomy. HPB Surg. doi: 10.1155/2010/579672
14. Bouvet M, Hoffman R (2013) Laparoscopic fluorescence imaging for identification and resection of pancreatic and hepatobiliary cancer. In: Kokudo N, Ishizawa T (eds) Fluorescent imaging. Treatment of hepatobiliary and pancreatic diseases, frontiers of gastrointestinal research, vol 31. Karger, Basel, pp 92–99
15. Miyashiro I, Kishi K, Yano M et al (2011) Laparoscopic detection of sentinel node in gastric cancer by indocyanine green imaging. Surg Endosc 25:1672–1676

16. Kudo H, Ishizawa T, Harada N et al (2014) Visualization of subcapsular hepatic malignancy by indocyanine-green fluorescence imaging during laparoscopic hepatectomy. Surg Endosc 28:2504–2508
17. Katada T, Hashidate H, Yokoyama N et al (submitted) Histopathological features of hepatic micrometastases from pancreatic cancer detected by real-time fluorescent imaging
18. Hishinuma S, Ogata Y, Tomikawa M et al (2005) Prophylactic hepatic irradiation following curative resection of pancreatic cancer. J Hepatobiliary Pancreat Surg 12:235–242
19. Kurosaki I, Kawachi Y, Nihei K et al (2009) Liver perfusion chemotherapy with 5-fluorouracil followed by systemic gemcitabine administration for resected pancreatic cancer: preliminary results of a prospective phase 2 study. Pancreas 38:161–167
20. Gabata T, Matsui O, Terayama N et al (2008) Imaging diagnosis of hepatic metastases of pancreatic carcinomas: significance of transient wedge-shaped contrast enhancement mimicking arterioportal shunt. Abdom Imaging 33:437–443

Part XVI
Surgery for Lymphedema

Chapter 39
Superficial Lymph Flow of the Upper Limbs Observed by an Indocyanine Green Fluorescence Method: Lymph Flow in Healthy Persons and Patients with Breast Cancer-Related Lymphedema

Seiji Ohtsubo, Mitsuo Kusano, and Miyoko Mori

Abstract *Objectives*: Reports of evaluations of normal superficial lymph flow using indocyanine green (ICG) fluorescence lymphography are rare. Here we investigated the normal superficial ICG fluorescence (IF) lymph flows and the characteristic IF images of lymphedema. We also evaluated the effect of complete decongestive physiotherapy (CDP) as a rehabilitation approach for lymphedema in the upper limbs, using IF imaging.

Methods: Five normal volunteers and three patients with breast cancer-related lymphedema (BCRL) were the subjects. ICG solution (0.4 mL) was injected subcutaneously at three points between the bases of the fingers, and we then observed the superficial IF lymph flow of the upper limbs using a near-infrared camera system.

Results: In the observation of normal superficial lymph flows of the upper limb, there were two major lymph flows, one to the radial side and the other to the ulnar side, which were clearly recognized by the IF lymphography. Those lymph flows were building a network along with the lymphatic flow. Many of the lymphatic back flow images of the upper arms of the BCRL patients showed "dermal backflow (DB)." In one patient, the DB decreased sharply after she underwent CDP for 1 year.

S. Ohtsubo (✉)
Department of Oral and Maxillofacial Surgery, Japan Labor Health & Welfare Organization, Kushiro Rosai Hospital, 13-23 Nakazono-cho, Kushiro, Hokkaido 085-8533, Japan
e-mail: s-ohtsubo@kushiroh.rofuku.go.jp

M. Kusano
Department of Surgery, Seiwa Memorial Hospital, 1-5-1-1, Kotoni, Nishi-ku, Sapporo, Hokkaido 063-0811, Japan

M. Mori
Department of Nursing, Japan Labor Health & Welfare Organization, Kushiro Rosai Hospital, 13-23 Nakazono-cho, Kushiro, Hokkaido 085-8533, Japan

M. Kusano et al. (eds.), *ICG Fluorescence Imaging and Navigation Surgery*,
DOI 10.1007/978-4-431-55528-5_39

Conclusions: We evaluated the normal and abnormal superficial lymphatic flows in the upper limbs in real time by an IF method. We expect that these characteristic images will not only help elucidate the anatomy of the lymph system but also be used in therapeutic procedures for lymphedema of the upper limbs in patients with BCRL.

Keywords Indocyanine green • Fluorescence imaging • Lymphedema • Complete decongestive physiotherapy • Breast cancer-related lymphedema

39.1 Introduction

Breast cancer-related lymphedema (BCRL) is one of the unsolved complications for patients who have undergone a radical mastectomy. Patients with BCRL in an upper limb suffer from not only disfigurement of their limbs but also functional and psychological stress. Complete decongestive physiotherapy (CDP) is recommended for these patients [1, 2]. In our hospital, CDP has been carried out for 240 lymphedema patients since April 2009. We have obtained relatively good results with the CDP; however, we could not assess its efficacy precisely due to the shortage of useful methods to evaluate the effects of the CDP. Evaluations of the anatomy and the lymph dynamic physiology of normal lymph flow are the first step toward developing more effective lymphedema treatments.

In recent years, the ICG fluorescence (IF) imaging method has been used for the detection of the sentinel lymph nodes in breast cancer [3, 4] and for evaluations of lymphedema after an axillary lymph node dissection [5]. The evaluation of abnormal images of lymph flow in lymphedema with the IF imaging method has been reported [6–8], but reports of the normal superficial lymph flow using the IF imaging method are very rare.

The primary purpose of the present study was to observe the normal superficial lymph flow by the IF imaging method, and the secondary purpose was to evaluate the characteristic IF images of lymphedema. The third purpose was to clarify the effectiveness of CDP in the upper limbs using the IF imaging method.

39.2 Materials and Methods

Five healthy adult volunteers and three BCRL patients participated in this study. Their ages ranged from 26 to 65 years (mean age 48 years). ICG solution was injected subcutaneously at three points between the bases of the fingers and thumb (Fig. 39.1), and we then observed the superficial ICG fluorescence images of lymph flow of each subject's upper limbs using a near-infrared (photodynamic eye; Hamamatsu Photonics, Hamamatsu, Japan) system (Fig. 39.2).

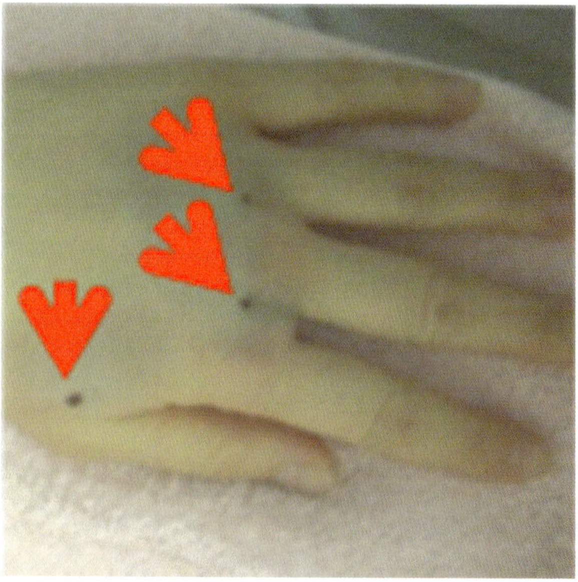

Fig. 39.1 Injection points of ICG solution

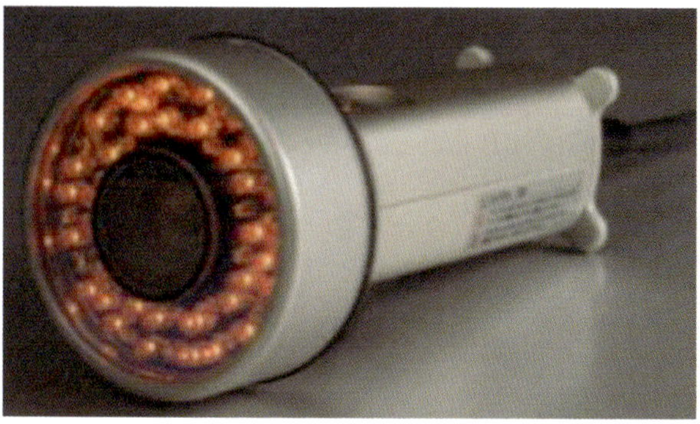

Fig. 39.2 PDE camera (PDE-neo)

We observed the normal and abnormal lymph flows in real time, but it was difficult to observe the entire images of lymph flows in the upper limbs (Fig. 39.3) due to the wide observation field. Therefore, we traced the IF images directly on the skin of the subjects' arm with a black felt pen (Fig. 39.4).

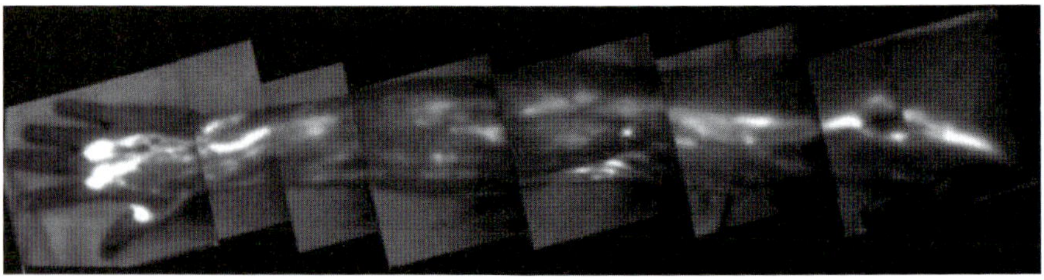

Fig. 39.3 Entire images of lymph flow of upper limb

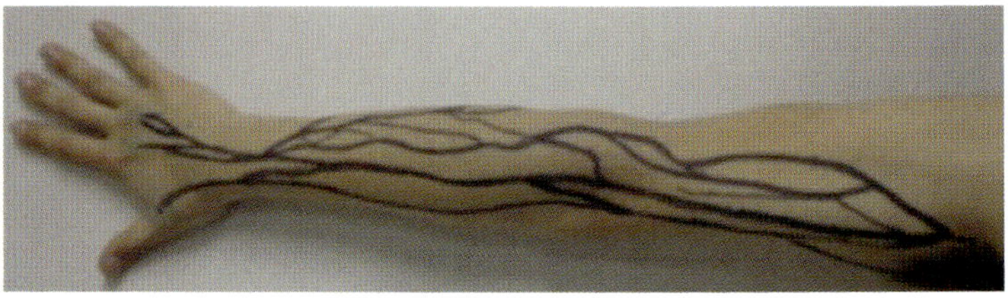

Fig. 39.4 Tracing of IF images by black felt pen

39.3 Results

39.3.1 The Normal IF Lymphography of Superficial Lymph Flows

We were able to observe several IF images in which the ICG solution ran from the forearm to the upper arm immediately after the injection of the solution in all five healthy volunteers. We also observed that the IF images reached the axilla area within 4–5 min after the injection of ICG in the normal arms. When the ICG solution was injected at the base of the thumb and forefinger, the lymph vessels were observed to run nearly straight to the deltoid muscle area. When the ICG solution was injected at the root of the third finger, the lymph vessel's lines ran toward the axilla region after surrounding the elbow. The networks are demonstrated in an upper arm and forearm in Fig. 39.5.

39.3.2 Characteristic ICG Fluorescence Images of BCRL Patients

The speed of the IFG lymphatic flow became extremely slow compared to the normal arms. The normal IFG lymph flows were observed as a linear pattern (Fig. 39.6a). Abnormal IF images of lymphedema were classified into three

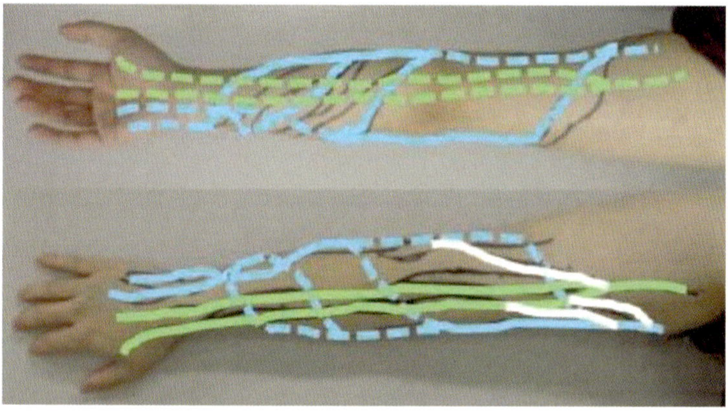

Fig. 39.5 *Green lines*: the lymph flows on the radial side. *Blue lines*: the lymph flows on the ulnar side. *White lines*: these networks in an upper arm and forearm

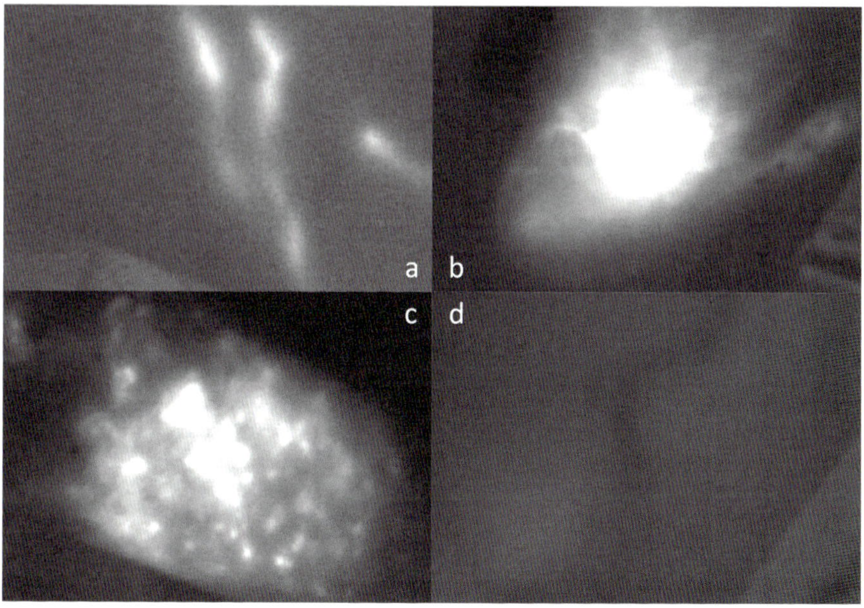

Fig. 39.6 Characteristic patterns of ICG fluorescence images. (**a**): Linear (normal lymph flow), (**b**): splash, (**c**): stardust, and (**d**): diffuse. Panels (**b–d**) show an abnormal pattern of BCRL called dermal backflow (DB)

characteristic patterns called "dermal backflow (DB)": the splash (Fig. 39.6b), stardust (Fig. 39.6c), and diffuse (Fig. 39.6d) patterns. In the present study, these patterns were confirmed in the BCRL patients with lymphedema of the limbs.

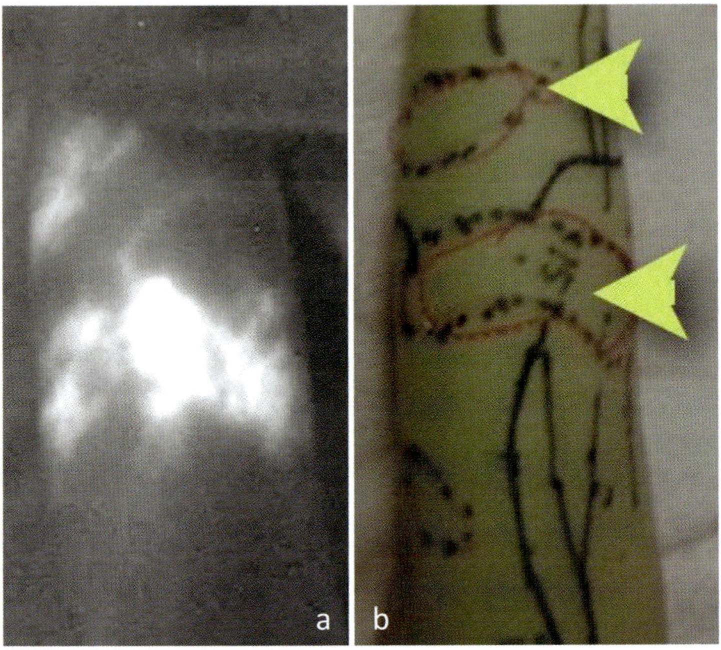

Fig. 39.7 IF image (**a**) and marking image (**b**) before CDP. *Arrowheads*: the splash pattern

39.3.3 Evaluation of the Effect of CDP for the Upper Limbs Using the IF Method

A case was reported in which the lymphedema of the upper limb was dramatically improved by CDP (Figs. 39.7 and 39.8). We observed many instances of DB (the splash pattern) in the IF images of the superficial lymph flow in the BCRL patients' forearms before CDP (Fig. 39.7a). We marked the lymphedema points for the IF imaging (Fig. 39.7b). The splash pattern decreased and the linear pattern appeared on the forearm in one patient after 1 year of CDP treatment (Fig. 39.8a, b).

39.4 Discussion

The incidence of BCRL has a strong correlation with axillary dissection and radiotherapy [9–12]. BCRL is major complication that interferes with a patient's quality of life, and it induces psychological stress. The effectiveness of CDP for BCRL patients has been shown [1, 2].

At our hospital, CDP has been carried out in 240 patients with lymphedema since April 2009, and we have obtained rather good results with the CDP (data not

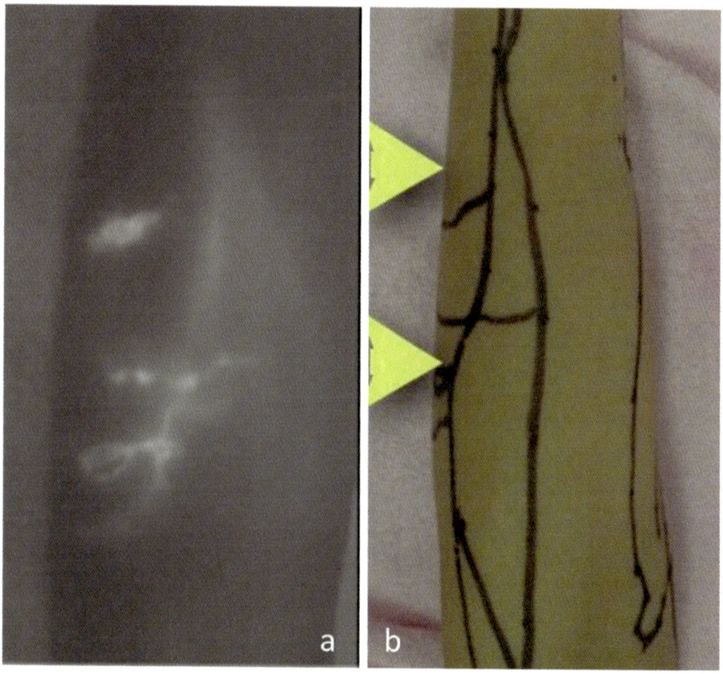

Fig. 39.8 IFG image (**a**) and marking image (**b**) after CDP. *Arrowheads*: the improved points

shown). Although lymphoscintigraphy [13, 14], computed tomography (CT) [15, 16], and magnetic resonance imaging (MRI) [17] have been used for the assessment of lymphedema and CDP's effects, they do not provide enough information about the dynamic images of lymph flow in real time.

A method using IF and near-infrared observation has been used to map the sentinel nodes [3, 4], and ICG has been used as the contrast medium for angiography. When the ICG solution is irradiated with near-infrared light at ~760 nm, it discharges the fluorescence at ~845 nm [18]. The fluorescence cannot be seen by the naked eye because it is a light wave in the near-infrared region. We therefore used a near-infrared camera system (Fig. 39.2) when we observed the fluorescence images.

Although the observation of lymphedema using the IF method has been reported [6–8], there are few reports that mention the real-time detection of the normal superficial lymph flows of the upper limb. We emphasize that the clarification of the normal lymph flows is essential when we seek to understand the pathophysiology of lymphedema.

Here we observed the normal lymph flows as reliable linear images (Fig. 39.6a; the linear pattern), and we observed other two major lymph flows in the upper limbs (Figs. 39.4 and 39.5). The lymph flows on the arm's radial side run approximately straight toward the deltoid muscle area. The lymph flows on the arm's ulnar side run toward the axilla region after surrounding the elbow. These lymph flows were building a network along the way (Figs. 39.4 and 39.5). The drainage into the two main flows is an advantage for the enhancement of the effectiveness of CDP. We also found that in the normal arms, the ICG reached the axilla area within 4–5 min after the injection of ICG solution.

Our observation of three BCRL patients by the IF method revealed that the speed of lymphatic flow became extremely slow, and we saw that many of the lymph back flow images showed dermal backflow in its characteristic splash, stardust, and diffuse patterns. These patterns are useful for the assessment of the severity of lymphedema [6–8]. The ICG diffuse pattern indicates the most severe lymphedema. The BCRL patients showed a high degree of DB in the images of their upper limbs.

Few studies have examined superficial IFIs of the upper limb in real time prior to and after CDP in BCRL patients, and we thus focused on the changes of lymph flow due to CDP. The DB observed in one patient's arms before CDP (Fig. 39.7) decreased sharply after 1 year of CDP treatment, and then it changed to the normal linear-pattern lymphatic flow (Fig. 39.8), which strongly supports the usefulness of CDP for BCRL.

It is necessary to preserve normal lymph flow as much as possible in order to decrease the rate of the occurrence of BCRL. It is also important for breast surgeons to know the normal superficial lymphatic flow of the upper limbs.

BCRL requires treatment from the early stage. However, it is difficult to diagnose the early state of edema in real time. Observations of lymphatic flows in BCRL patients by the IF imaging method will be useful for the detection of lymphedema in the early postoperative period.

We propose that images of the normal superficial lymph flows and the characteristic abnormal images of lymphedema detected by the IF imaging method provide important anatomical maps of the lymph flow of the upper arm, which is essential not only for breast surgery but also for the application of therapy for lymphedema of the upper limbs.

References

1. Liao SF, Li SH, Huang HY et al (2013) The efficacy of complex decongestive physiotherapy (CDP) and predictive factors of lymphedema severity and response to CDP in breast cancer-related lymphedema (BCRL). Breast 22(5):703–706. doi: 10.1016/j.breast.2012.12.018. Epub 2013 Jan 12
2. Szolnoky G, Lakatos B, Keskeny T et al (2009) Intermittent pneumatic compression acts synergistically with manual lymphatic drainage in complex decongestive physiotherapy for breast cancer treatment-related lymphedema. Lymphology 42(4):188–194
3. Sugie T, Kassim KA, Takeuchi M et al (2010) A novel method for sentinel lymph node biopsy by indocyanine green fluorescence technique in breast cancer. Cancers (Basel) 2(2):713–720. doi: 10.3390/cancers2020713
4. Murawa D, Hirche C, Dresel S et al (2009) Sentinel lymph node biopsy in breast cancer guided by indocyanine green fluorescence. Br J Surg 96(11):1289–94. doi:10.1002/bjs.6721

5. Yamamoto T, Narushima M, Yoshimatsu H et al (2014) Dynamic indocyanine green (ICG) lymphography for breast cancer-related arm lymphedema. Ann Plast Surg 73(6):706–709. doi: 10.1097/SAP.0b013e318285875f
6. Yamamoto T, Matsuda N, Doi K et al (2011) The earliest finding of indocyanine green lymphography in asymptomatic limbs of lower extremity lymphedema patients secondary to cancer treatment: the modified dermal backflow stage and concept of subclinical lymphedema. Plast Reconstr Surg 128(4):314e–321e. doi: 10.1097/PRS.0b013e3182268da8
7. Yamamoto T, Iida T, Matsuda N et al (2011) Indocyanine green (ICG)-enhanced lymphography for evaluation of facial lymphoedema. J Plast Reconstr Aesthet Surg 64(11):1541–1544. doi: 10.1016/j.bjps.2011.05.025. Epub 2011 Jun 17
8. Yamamoto T, Matsuda N, Todokoro T et al (2011) Lower extremity lymphedema index: a simple method for severity evaluation of lower extremity lymphedema. Ann Plast Surg 67 (6):637–640. doi: 10.1097/SAP.0b013e318208fd75
9. DiSipio T, Rye S, Newman B et al (2013) Incidence of unilateral arm lymphedema after breast cancer: a systematic review and meta-analysis. Lancet Oncol 14(6):500–515. doi: 10.1016/S1470-2045(13)70076-7. Epub 2013 Mar 27
10. Kim M, Kim SW, Lee SU et al (2013) A model to estimate the risk of breast cancer-related lymphedema: combinations of treatment-related factors of the number of dissected axillary nodes, adjuvant chemotherapy, and radiation therapy. Int J Radiat Oncol Biol Phys 86 (3):498–503. doi: 10.1016/j.ijrobp.2013.02.018. Epub 2013 Mar 28
11. Meric F, Buchholz TA, Mirza NQ et al (2002) Long-term complications associated with breast-conservation surgery and radiotherapy. Ann Surg Oncol 9(6):543–549
12. Warren LE, Miller CL, Horick N et al (2014) The impact of radiation therapy on the risk of lymphedema after treatment for breast cancer: a prospective cohort study. Int J Radiat Oncol Biol Phys 88(3):565–571. doi: 10.1016/j.ijrobp.2013.11.232. Epub 2014 Jan 7
13. Pelosi E, Arena V, Baudino B et al (2003) Pre-operative lymphatic mapping and intra-operative sentinel lymph node detection in early stage endometrial cancer. Nucl Med Commun 24(9):971–5
14. Izawa J, Kedar D, Wong F et al (2005) Sentinel lymph node biopsy in penile cancer: evolution and insights. Can J Urol 12 (Suppl 1):24–29
15. Shin SU, Lee W, Park EA et al (2013) Comparison of characteristic CT findings of lymphedema, cellulitis, and generalized edema in lower leg swelling. Int J Cardiovasc Imaging 29 (Suppl 2):135–143. doi: 10.1007/s10554-013-0332-5. Epub 2013 Nov 30
16. Shin SU, Lee W, Park EA et al (2013) Comparison of characteristic CT findings of lymphedema, cellulitis, and generalized edema in lower leg swelling. Int J Cardiovasc Imaging 29 (Suppl 2):135–143. doi: 10.1007/s10554-013-0332-5. Epub 2013 Nov 30
17. Liu NF, Lu Q, Liu PA et al (2010) Comparison of radionuclide lymphoscintigraphy and dynamic magnetic resonance lymphangiography for investigating extremity lymphoedema. Br J Surg 97(3):359–65. doi:10.1002/bjs.6893
18. Benson, RC, Kunes HA (1978) Fluorescence properties of indocyanine green as related to angiography. Phys Med Biol 23(1):159–163

Chapter 40
Indocyanine Green Fluorescent Lymphography and Microsurgical Lymphaticovenous Anastomosis

Akira Shinaoka, Kiyoshi Yamada, and Yoshihiro Kimata

Abstract A variety of lymphatic imaging techniques have been developed, but no technique can provide real-time imaging except for indocyanine green fluorescent lymphography (ICG-LG). The real-time images of ICG-LG make lymphaticovenous anastomosis (LVA) easy to perform. In this chapter, history and methods of ICG-LG for LVA are described in detail.

Keywords Indocyanine green fluorescent lymphography • Lymphaticovenous anastomosis • Lymphedema

40.1 Introduction: History of Lymphatic Imaging Techniques

Lymphedema cases are classified as primary or secondary. Primary lymphedema is a congenital hypoplasia of the lymphatic system, although its essential pathogenesis has not yet been clarified. Secondary lymphedema is acquired damage to the lymphatic system caused by operations, radiotherapy, and infections that lead to inadequate lymph function. These disturbances cause abnormal types of lymph flow that are not seen in healthy individuals.

In order to visualize the abnormal lymph flow, several lymph imaging techniques involving tracers have been developed. However, it is impossible to inject the tracer from the proximal side. Therefore, all lymphatic imaging techniques inject tracer from the peripheral side and represent only part of the lymphatic system.

Direct lymphography is the oldest lymph imaging technique. In this technique lymphatic vessels are directly cannulated and injected with iodinated oil [1]. In

A. Shinaoka, M.D.
Department of Plastic Surgery, Kagawa Prefectural Central Hospital, Kagawa, Japan

K. Yamada, M.D. • Y. Kimata, M.D. (✉)
Department of Plastic and Reconstructive Surgery, Okayama University Hospital, 2-5-1 Shikata-cho, Kita-ku, Okayama 700-0914, Japan
e-mail: ykimata@cc.okayama-u.ac.jp

M. Kusano et al. (eds.), *ICG Fluorescence Imaging and Navigation Surgery*,
DOI 10.1007/978-4-431-55528-5_40

other techniques a tracer is injected into the dermis or subcutaneous tissue and is translocated into the lymphatic vessels prior to imaging. Indirect lymphography utilizes the fact that large-molecular-weight materials (in this case, 5000 kDa~) are primarily taken into the lymphatic system. Although there are various tracers and techniques, the gold standard for the diagnosis of lymphedema is lymphoscintigraphy using 99mTc, first introduced by Sherman in 1953 [2]. A gamma camera is used to obtain images of the limbs and can reveal deep collecting lymphatic vessels and lymph nodes. The sensitivity of lymphoscintigraphy is 73–97 % and the specificity is 100 % [3–5]. Evaluation of lymphatic function is also possible. Quantitation of the accumulation of radiolabeled tracers at regional lymph nodes, clearance from the injection site, and quantitation of disappearance rates from the injection site have been attempted [6–8].

Lymphoscintigraphy is a useful method, but it has three weak points. First is the patient's exposure to radiation. Second is the time-consuming examination. A detailed protocol for lymphoscintigraphy has not yet been established, but the common scan time points are 30 and 120 min after injection. However, more delayed scanning, such as time points of 6 or 24 h, may be needed for very early-stage patients if they show normal lymphatic transport at 120 min. In one series, 32 % of patients would have had normal lymphoscintigraphy results if the scan time had been limited to 60 min [9, 10]. The third weakness is poor anatomical information. Because lymphoscintigraphy is two-dimensional and low resolution, it is not suitable for anatomical evaluation.

40.2 Indocyanine Green Fluorescent Lymphography

Currently, some new lymph imaging techniques for lymphedema have emerged. These include indocyanine green fluorescent lymphography (ICG-LG) [11], magnetic resonance lymphography (MR-LG) [12], and lymphoscintigraphy using a hybrid SPECT/CT system (SPECT-LG). All of the techniques have improved the issue of anatomical evaluation. MR-LG and SPECT-LG are three-dimensional imaging techniques and have better resolution than lymphoscintigraphy. Although ICG-LG is two-dimensional, it has better resolution in real time than lymphoscintigraphy (Fig. 40.1) and is safer and easier than any of the other techniques.

ICG has primarily been used as tracer for angiography. However, in 2007, Unno et al. introduced ICG-LG [11]. By using indocyanine green injection and a portable and easy-to-use infrared camera, real-time imaging of the lymphatic system was obtained. ICG is intradermally injected into the web space between the fingers, binds to albumin, and drains into the lymphatic vessels. The albumin-bound ICG is excited using a 760-nm infrared ray and emits an 840-nm infrared ray. The fluorescence of ICG in near-infrared wavelengths can deeply penetrate living tissue and is advantageous for obtaining noninvasive visual information about the lymphatic systems.

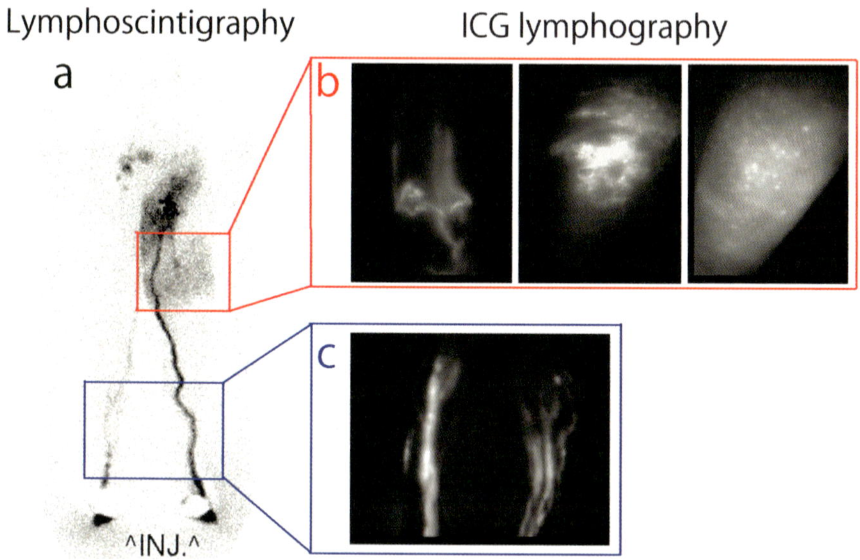

Fig. 40.1 Comparison of lymphoscintigraphy with ICG lymphography
Several patterns of dermal backflow can be recognized in ICG lymphography (**b**), but in lymphoscintigraphy no such pattern is observed (**a**). Each of the lymphatic vessels in the artero-medial bundle can be recognized in ICG lymphography (**c**), but in lymphoscintigraphy, only the artero-medial bundle can be observed (**a**)

ICG-LG has been studied as not only a real-time imaging technique but also a method of diagnosing lymphedema. In 2008, Unno et al. measured the velocity of lymphatic flow with ICG-LG and reported that the decubitus position, exercise loading, and massage promoted lymphatic flow [13]. In 2011, Yamamoto et al. reported three types of dermal backflow (DB) patterns seen in lymphedema patients with ICG-LG: splash, stardust, and diffusion; they also reported relationships between the distribution of these DB patterns and clinical staging [14]. In 2012, Akita et al. reported the possibility that the splash type can serve as an early sign of lymphedema [15]. Nowadays, ICG-LG is gradually gaining acceptance as a screening examination for early-stage lymphedema.

40.3 Surgical Operations for Lymphedema and ICG Lymphography

Various surgical operations for lymphedema have been performed. There are mainly two categories of surgical operations: volume-reduction methods and reconstructions of lymph flow. Volume-reduction methods such as the Kondoleon procedure [16], Charles procedure [17], and liposuction [18] simply attempt to ablate the offending tissue, mainly fatty tissue. Reconstruction of lymph flow attempts to augment lymph flow or egress from the lymphedematous extremity by establishing communication between the congested lymphatic system and a competent drainage system such as deep lymphatic vessels or venulae. There are some classical reconstructions of lymph flow like the Degni procedure [19] and O'Brien [20] procedure, which involve anastomosis to the saphenous vein, but nowadays the mainstream procedure is lymphaticovenous anastomosis (LVA), which involves anastomosis to a venula [21]. All reconstructions of lymph flow first need to discover the thin, transparent lymphatic vessels within the adipose tissues. ICG-LG visualizes the lymphatic vessels clearly in real time without using radiation, resulting in an improved discovery rate of lymphatic vessels.

40.4 Protocol of ICG-LG

ICG lymphography appeared in the 2000s and is a relatively new method. Therefore, the protocol of ICG-LG has not been fully established in detail. Typical methods are shown.

40.4.1 Preparation of Examination

40.4.1.1 Examination Reagent

ICG has been produced as Diagnogreen® for injection (Daiichi Sankyo Company, Ltd., Tokyo). First, 25 mg of Diagnogreen powder is dissolved in 2 ml pure water. Second, the solution of Diagnogreen is added to 2 ml of 1 % Xylocaine® injection. The addition of Xylocaine relieves the pain of the injection of ICG solution. However, it is important not to add Xylocaine to the vial of Diagnogreen first because it cannot dissolve the powder; only water (2–10 ml) can.

40.4.1.2 Pain Control

As the pain of the injection of ICG is extreme, controlling the pain is important. Not only the addition of Xylocaine in solution but also the application of EMLA® cream is effective at reducing pain. Intradermal injection is more painful than subcutaneous injection.

40.4.1.3 Setup of Examination Room

The examination needs to be conducted in a dark room. Even the glimmer of a liquid crystal screen or infrared heater will disturb the observation of the deep lymphatic systems.

40.4.2 Ladder of Examination and Operation

40.4.2.1 Injections

Injections of ICG are performed in the intradermal or subcutaneous layer. It is necessary to consider the differences in lymphatic velocity and lymphatic uptake in ICG-LG.

Our group injects both layers with 30-gauge needle: the intradermal layer receives 0.04 ml and subcutaneous layer receives 0.06 ml for a total of 0.1 ml for one injection point. In the lower extremity, ICG is injected into three points (Fig. 40.2a). In the upper extremity, ICG is injected into five points (Fig. 40.2b and c).

This method does not represent all of subcutaneous lymphatic systems because ICG is injected from the peripheral side. Therefore, it is necessary to consider how to inject ICG further.

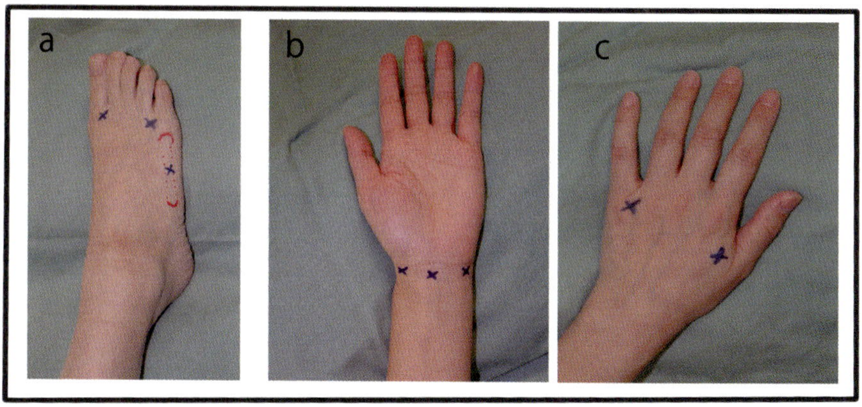

Fig. 40.2 Injection points of extremities in ICG lymphography
In the lower extremity, ICG is injected into three points: the first and fourth web space and the middle of the fifth metatarsal (**a**). In the upper extremity, the palm side is injected at the radial, the ulnar, and the middle of the wrist (**b**), and the dorsal side is injected at the first and fourth web space (**c**)

40.4.2.2 Observations and Selection of Lymphatic Vessels for LVA

One of the most important functions of preoperative ICG-LG is to detect lymphatic vessels without fibrosis, but with high flow for anastomosis. Sometimes the point where dermal backflow (DB) originates can be observed. If there is no DB, it is very easy to detect good lymphatic vessels by ICG-LG. But if DB widespread, the lymphatic vessels will be hidden behind it. It is important to note that physical activity during the examination makes the lymphatic flow increase and, often, the DB area to spread (Fig. 40.3). Therefore, our group observes patients at rest. If lymphatic vessels cannot be observed, a soft massage to the puncture area is added. Lymphatic vessels are mapped as soon as they are observed.

40.4.3 Skin Incision, Preparation, and Anastomosis of Lymphatic Vessels

Small skin incisions are performed above the lymphatic vessel. Most of the lymphatic vessels observed by PDE camera are located under the superficial fascia. Microsurgical lymphovenous anastomoses are performed between lymphatic vessels and venulae (Fig. 40.4). The most commonly performed techniques are direct end-to-end, end-to-side, or side-to-end microsurgical anastomoses. After anastomosis, a PDE camera can check the patency and lymphatic flow in the venula (Fig. 40.5).

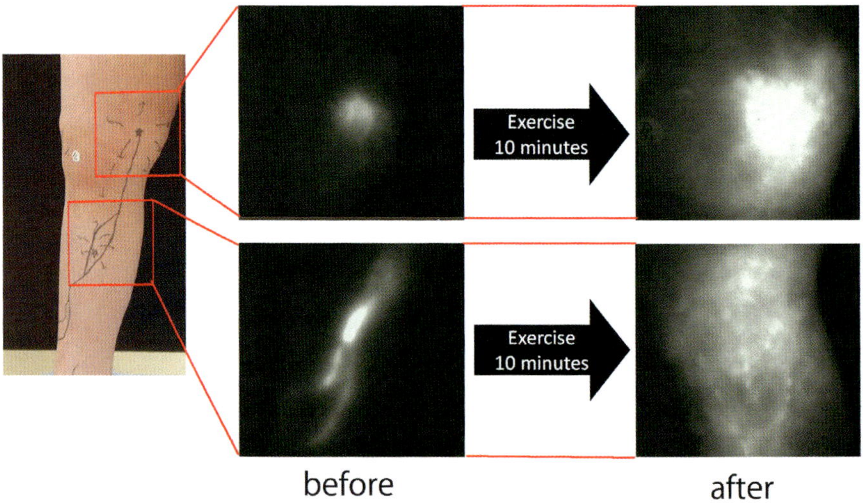

Fig. 40.3 Effects of exercise in ICG lymphography
Before exercise, lymphatic vessels can be observed clearly. But exercise makes dermal backflow appear and become widespread, hiding the lymphatic vessels

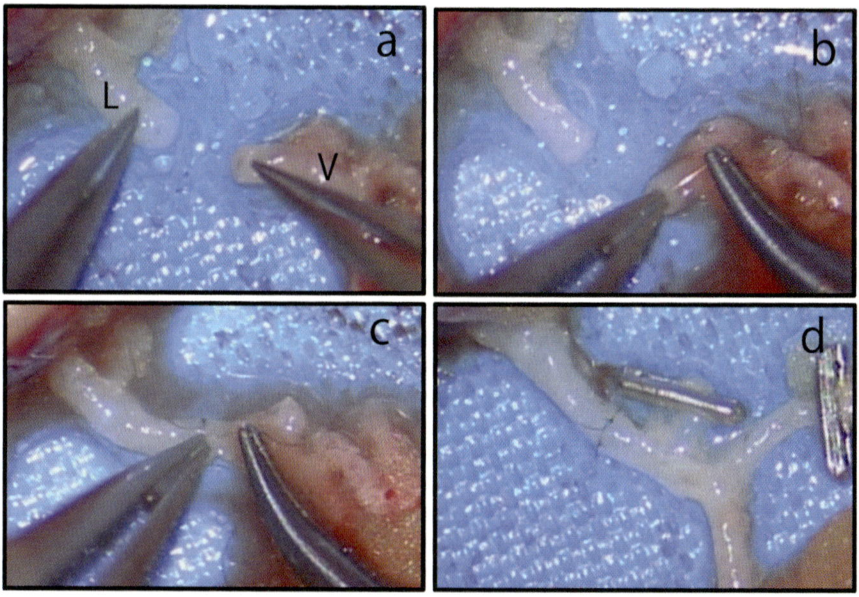

Fig. 40.4 Operative photographs of LVA
Operative photographs (a → b) show the lymphaticovenous end-to-end anastomosis technique. Lymphatic vessel (*L*) is anastomosed to a venula (*V*) using 12-0 nylon sutures. In general, the diameter of lymphatic vessels is 0.3–1.0 mm and the diameter of venulae appropriate for anastomosis is 0.5–1.0 mm

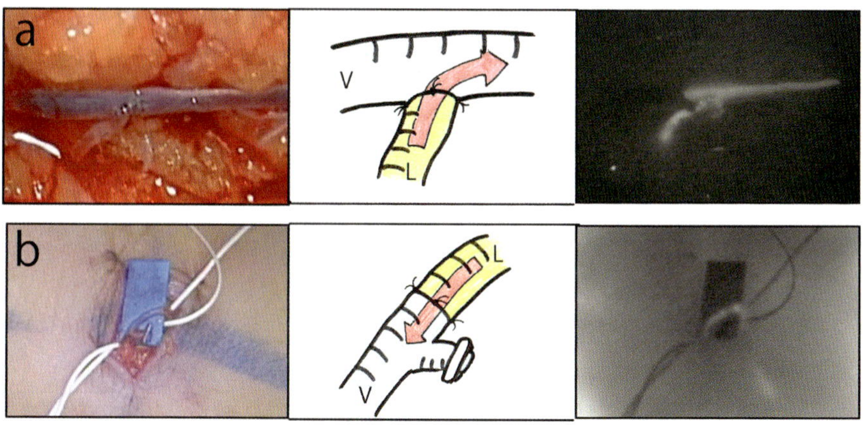

Fig. 40.5 Lymphatic flow to venula in LVA
Lymphaticovenous end-to-side (**a**) and end-to-end (**b**) anastomoses are shown. The *left* pictures are normal viewing and *right* pictures are fluorescent viewing. The *middle* illustrations are figures. Lymphatic flow (*red arrow*) from lymphatic vessel (*L*) to the venula (*V*) can be observed

40.5 Outcomes of LVA

There are some reports about outcomes of microsurgical lymphovenous anastomosis. Campisi, in Italy, reported results in more than 1800 patients [22]. At a mean follow-up of more than 10 years, volume changes showed significant improvement in more than 83 % of the patients. There was an 87 % reduction in the incidence of cellulitis after microsurgery.

Koshima, in Japan, reported results in the unilateral upper extremity in a total of 27 females [21]. The average follow-up after surgery was 2.2 years, and the average decrease in circumference was 4.1 cm (47.3 % of the preoperative excess).

Maegawa, in Japan, published results of 472 lymphaticovenous side-to-end anastomoses in 107 patients with lymphedema [23]. They attempted to assess function at 6 months or later in 57 patients who underwent 223 anastomoses; 48 of the anastomoses were close to the skin and were suitable for lymphoscintigraphic evaluation. An excellent cumulative patency rate of 75 % of the lymphovenous anastomoses was observed at 12 months and 36 % at 24 months.

40.6 Conclusion

Among lymphatic imaging techniques, ICG lymphography is most valuable for its real-time imaging. This feature has made LVA widely used and has simplified the diagnosis of lymphedema. However, the standard protocol and the analytic technique of ICG lymphography are not yet established. The most important challenge in ICG lymphography is to establish a unified global standard protocol and analytic technique to collect reproducible data on lymphatic function that can meaningfully evaluate the results of various therapeutic techniques for lymphedema.

References

1. Weissleder H, Weissleder R (1989) Interstitial lymphangiography: initial clinical experience with a dimeric nonionic contrast agent. Radiology 170:371–374
2. Sherman AI, Ter-Pogossian M (1953) Lymph-node concentration of radioactive colloidal gold following interstitial injection. Cancer 6:1238–1240
3. Gloviczki P, Calcagno D et al (1989) Noninvasive evaluation of the swollen extremity: experiences with 190 lymphoscintigraphic examinations. J Vasc Surg 9:683–689
4. Stewart G, Gaunt JI et al (1985) Isotope lymphography: a new method of investigating the role of the lymphatics in chronic limb oedema. Br J Surg 72:906–909
5. Ter SE, Alavi A et al (1993) Lymphoscintigraphy. A reliable test for the diagnosis of lymphedema. Clin Nucl Med 18:646–654
6. Proby CM, Gane JN et al (1990) Investigation of the swollen limb with isotope lymphography. Br J Dermatol 123:29–37

7. Baulieu F, Baulieu JL et al (1990) The potential usefulness of condensed image processing of sequential lymphoscintigrams in patients with lymphedema. Lymphology 23:15–22
8. Modi S, Stanton AW et al (2007) Human lymphatic pumping measured in healthy and lymphoedematous arms by lymphatic congestion lymphoscintigraphy. J Physiol 583:271–285
9. Tiwari A, Cheng KS et al (2003) Differential diagnosis, investigation, and current treatment of lower limb lymphedema. Arch Surg 138:152–161
10. Larcos G, Foster DR (1995) Interpretation of lymphoscintigrams in suspected lymphoedema: contribution of delayed images. Nucl Med Commun 16:683–686
11. Unno N, Inuzuka K et al (2007) Preliminary experience with a novel fluorescence lymphography using indocyanine green in patients with secondary lymphedema. J Vasc Surg 45:1016–1021
12. Lohrmann C, Foeldi E et al (2006) Indirect magnetic resonance lymphangiography in patients with lymphedema preliminary results in humans. Eur J Radiol 59:401–406
13. Unno N, Nishiyama M et al (2008) Quantitative lymph imaging for assessment of lymph function using indocyanine green fluorescence lymphography. Eur J Vasc Endovasc Surg 36:230–236
14. Yamamoto T, Narushima M et al (2011) Characteristic indocyanine green lymphography findings in lower extremity lymphedema: the generation of a novel lymphedema severity staging system using dermal backflow patterns. Plast Reconstr Surg 127:1979–1986
15. Akita S, Mitsukawa N et al (2013) Early diagnosis and risk factors for lymphedema following lymph node dissection for gynecologic cancer. Plast Reconstr Surg 131:283–290
16. Green TM (1920) Elephantiasis and the Kondoleon Operation. Ann Surg 71:28–31
17. Tilley AR, Douglas LG (1974) Staged treatment of lymphedema praecox. Can Med Assoc J 110:309–312
18. Nava VM1, Lawrence WT (1988). Liposuction on a lymphedematous arm. Ann Plast Surg 21:366–368
19. Degni M (1974) New technique of drainage of the subcutaneous tissue of the limbs with nylon net for the treatment of lymphedema. Vasa 3:329–341
20. O'Brien BM (1977) Microlymphaticovenous surgery for obstructive lymphedema. Aust N Z J Surg 47:284–291
21. Koshima I, Inagawa K et al (2000) Supermicrosurgical lymphaticovenular anastomosis for the treatment of lymphedema in the upper extremities. J Reconstr Microsurg 16:437–442
22. Campisi C, Bellini C et al (2010) Microsurgery for lymphedema: clinical research and long-term results. Microsurgery 30:256–260
23. Maegawa J, Yabuki Y et al (2012) Outcomes of lymphaticovenous side-to-end anastomosis in peripheral lymphedema. J Vasc Surg 55:753–760

Chapter 41
Comprehensive Lymphedema Evaluation Using Dynamic ICG Lymphography

Takumi Yamamoto

Abstract Indocyanine green (ICG) lymphography is becoming popular in lymphedema management, since it can visualize superficial lymph flows in real time without radiation exposure. With lymphedema progression, ICG lymphography pattern changes from normal linear pattern to abnormal dermal backflow (DB) patterns (splash, stardust, and diffuse patterns). Splash represents mild DB and reversible change; on the other hand, stardust/diffuse represents moderate/severe DB and irreversible change. DB stages [leg DB (LDB) stage, arm DB (ADB) stage, genital DB (GDB) stage, and facial DB (FDB) stage] allow pathophysiological lymphedema severity staging based on ICG lymphography findings. ICG velocity, lymph pump function, decreases as lymphedema progresses. ICG lymphography is also used as pre- and intraoperative navigation for lymphatic supermicrosurgery such as lymphaticovenular anastomosis. A surgeon can easily find lymphatic vessels in linear pattern. Progression of ICG lymphography pattern represents progression of lymphosclerosis; the more severe DB pattern is detected on ICG lymphography, the more sclerotic lymphatic vessels are. Dynamic ICG lymphography, dual-phase lymphography, allows pathophysiological severity staging, evaluation of lymph transportation capacity, and navigation for lymphatic surgery with one ICG injection. Dynamic ICG lymphography is useful for evaluation of lymphedema prognosis and therapeutic interventions.

Keywords Lymphedema • Indocyanine green • Lymphography • Microsurgery • Anastomosis • Navigation

T. Yamamoto (✉)
Department of Plastic and Reconstructive Surgery, The University of Tokyo, 7-3-1 Hongo, Bunkyo-ku, Tokyo 113-8655, Japan
e-mail: tyamamoto-tky@umin.ac.jp

M. Kusano et al. (eds.), *ICG Fluorescence Imaging and Navigation Surgery*,
DOI 10.1007/978-4-431-55528-5_41

41.1 ICG Lymphography for Lymphedema Evaluation

There are several modalities to visualize lymph flows for lymphedema evaluation. Among them, lymphoscintigraphy is considered a gold standard, but its image is obscure and it has a risk of radiation exposure [1]. Near-infrared fluorescence lymphography using indocyanine green (ICG), ICG lymphography, has been reported for lymphedema evaluation in 2007, and then, this new modality is becoming popular because it can visualize superficial lymph flows far more clearly than lymphoscintigraphy in real time without radiation exposure [2, 3]. ICG lymphography has been applied in evaluation of arm, leg, genital, and facial lymphedema and used for pre- and intraoperative navigation for lymphatic surgeries and for postoperative evaluation [3–11]. Dynamic ICG lymphography has been developed to allow all of the abovementioned evaluations with one ICG injection (Fig. 41.1) [12, 13].

41.2 Dynamic ICG Lymphography

Dynamic ICG lymphography consists of 2 phase observations: early transient phase for evaluation of lymph pump function, and late plateau phase for evaluation of lymph circulation and for navigation of lymphatic surgery [4, 5, 8, 11–13]. Dynamic ICG lymphography is performed as follows: An examinee is kept still for 15 min, and 0.05–0.2 ml of ICG (Diagnogreen 0.25 %; Daiichi Pharmaceutical, Tokyo, Japan) is subdermally injected (at the 2nd web space for extremity and genital lymphedema, and at the glabella and the philtrum for facial lymphedema). Immediately after ICG injection, fluorescent lymph flow images are obtained using an infrared camera system (transient phase). Examinees are kept still in supine position during lymph pump function measurement. After completion of the measurement (5 min after injection), examinees are allowed to move freely [12, 13].

Approximately 12–18 h after ICG injection, ICG movement reaches a plateau (plateau phase). In a plateau phase, lymph circulation is assessed based on ICG lymphography findings as mentioned in Sect. 43.2.2, which allows pathophysiological severity staging and pre- and intraoperative navigation for lymphatic surgery [3–11, 14–16]. For more rapid and convenient assessment, patients are better

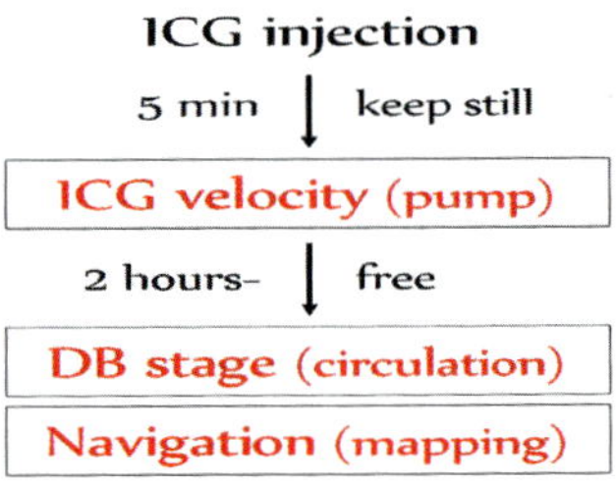

Fig. 41.1 Dynamic indocyanine green lymphography

to be instructed to move their extremity rigorously. When patients move their extremity rigorously, ICG can reach a plateau 2 h after ICG injection. Plateau phase continues until 72 h after ICG injection; evaluation of abnormal lymph circulation is possible between 2 and 72 h after ICG injection.

41.2.1 Assessment of Lymph Pump Function

A major strength of ICG lymphography is real-time evaluation. Lymph pump function can be easily and directly measured by observing ICG movement at an early transient phase. Several methods have been reported to evaluate lymph transportation capacity, and ICG velocity is the most practical one; unlike other measurements that sometimes require 1 h for lymphedema evaluation, measurement of ICG velocity can be completed within 5 min after ICG injection [12, 13]. The distance between the injection point and the farthest point where ICG is observed is measured 5 min after ICG injection. ICG velocity is calculated as follows:

$$\text{ICG Velocity} = \frac{\text{Distance}}{\text{Time}}(\text{cm/min})$$

When ICG reaches the groin/axilla in extremity lymphedema cases within 5 min, ICG velocity is calculated by dividing the distance between the groin/axilla and the injection point by the time required for transition. ICG velocity decreases with lymphedema progression and increases after successful treatments. As ICG velocity is a quantitative measurement, it is quite easy to evaluate lymph transportation capacity before and after treatments.

41.2.2 Assessment of Lymph Circulation

With progression of obstructive lymphedema, ICG lymphography pattern changes from normal linear pattern to abnormal dermal backflow (DB) patterns. DB patterns include splash (mild DB), stardust (moderate DB), and diffuse (severe DB) patterns (Fig. 41.2) [3]. Lymph flow is obstructed after dissection and/or radiation of lymph nodes, which leads to lymphatic hypertension, dilatation of lymphatic vessels, lymphatic valve insufficiency, lymphosclerosis, and lymph backflow. Lymph backflow is visualized as DB patterns on ICG lymphography [3–7, 17, 18]. Splash pattern represents dilated superficial lymphatic precollectors and capillaries that can work as collateral lymph pathways. Lymph extravasation takes place when the collateral fails to compensate lymph overload, which is visualized as spots on ICG lymphography, stardust pattern. With progression of lymph extravasation, the number of spots on ICG lymphography increases the point where spots cannot be

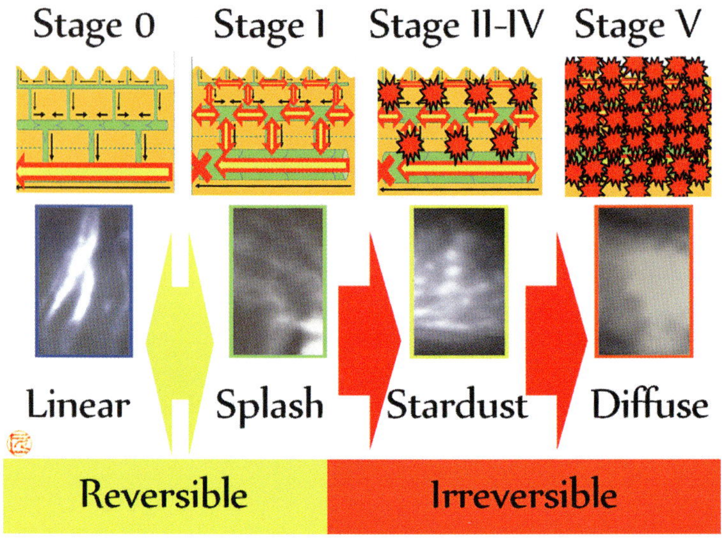

Fig. 41.2 Indocyanine green lymphography findings and lymph circulation

distinguished from each other, diffuse pattern. In obstructive lymphedema, DB patterns usually extend from proximal to distal region. Assessment of abnormal lymph circulation using ICG lymphography allows pathophysiological severity staging and prediction of lymphatic vessels before lymphatic surgery.

41.2.2.1 Pathophysiological Severity Staging Systems for Secondary Lymphedema (Dermal Backflow Stages)

Pathophysiological severity staging system for obstructive lymphedema, DB stage, is determined based on ICG lymphography findings. There are 4 DB stages: leg DB (LDB) stage for leg lymphedema, arm DB (ADB) stage for arm lymphedema, genital DB (GDB) stage for genital and lower abdominal lymphedema, and facial DB (FDB) stage for head and neck lymphedema [4–7, 19].

LDB stage is a severity staging system for obstructive lower extremity lymphedema (Fig. 41.3) [3, 4, 11, 20]. In LDB stage 0, no DB pattern is observed. In LDB stage I, splash pattern is observed around the groin. In LDB stage II through V, stardust pattern is observed. In LDB stage II, stardust pattern is limited proximal to the patella. In LDB stage III, stardust pattern exceeds the patella. In LDB stage IV, stardust pattern is detected throughout the lower extremity. In LDB stage V, diffuse pattern is observed with background of stardust pattern.

ADB stage is a severity staging system for obstructive arm lymphedema (Fig. 41.4) [5, 11, 20]. In ADB stage 0, no DB pattern is observed. In ADB stage I, splash pattern is observed around the axilla. In ADB stage II through V, stardust

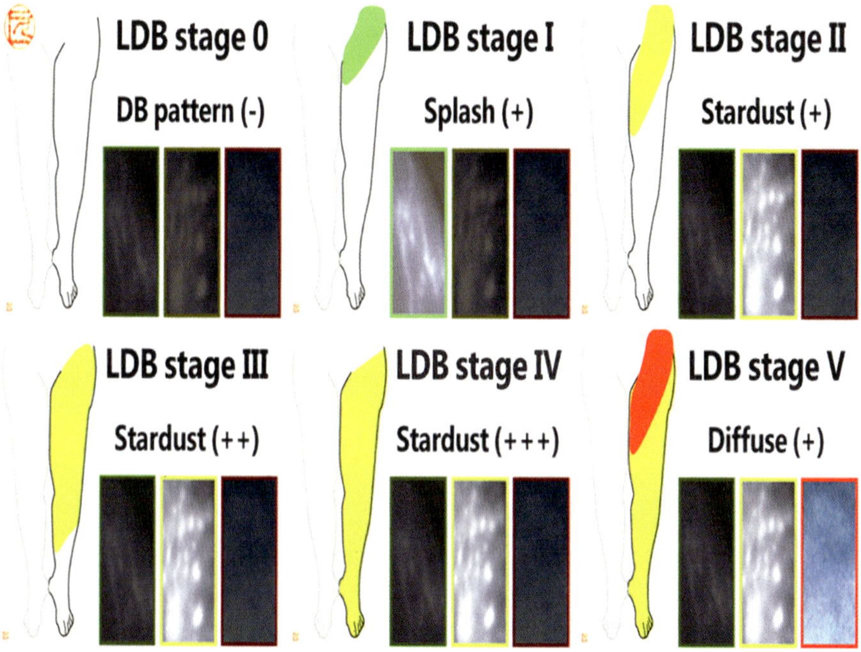

Fig. 41.3 Leg dermal backflow (LDB) stage for pathophysiological severity staging of leg lymphedema using indocyanine green lymphography

pattern is observed. In ADB stage II, stardust pattern is limited proximal to the olecranon. In ADB stage III, stardust pattern exceeds the olecranon. In ADB stage IV, stardust pattern is detected throughout the upper extremity. In ADB stage V, diffuse pattern is observed with background of stardust pattern.

GDB stage is a severity staging system for obstructive lower abdominal and genital lymphedema [6, 11, 20, 21]. In GDB stage 0, no DB pattern is observed. In GDB stage I, splash pattern is observed around the groin and/or lower abdominal region. In GDB stage II, stardust pattern is seen around the groin and/or lower abdominal region. In GDB stage III, stardust pattern is observed around the groin, the lower abdominal, and the genital region. In GDB stage IV, diffuse pattern is observed with background of stardust pattern.

FDB stage is a severity staging system for obstructive head and neck lymphedema [7, 11, 20]. In FDB stage 0, no DB pattern is observed. In FDB stage I, splash pattern is observed around the neck. In FDB stage II through V, stardust pattern is observed. In FDB stage II, stardust pattern is observed in the neck. In FDB stage III, stardust pattern is seen in the face and neck. In FDB stage IV, stardust pattern is detected throughout the head and neck region. In ADB stage V, diffuse pattern is observed with background of stardust pattern.

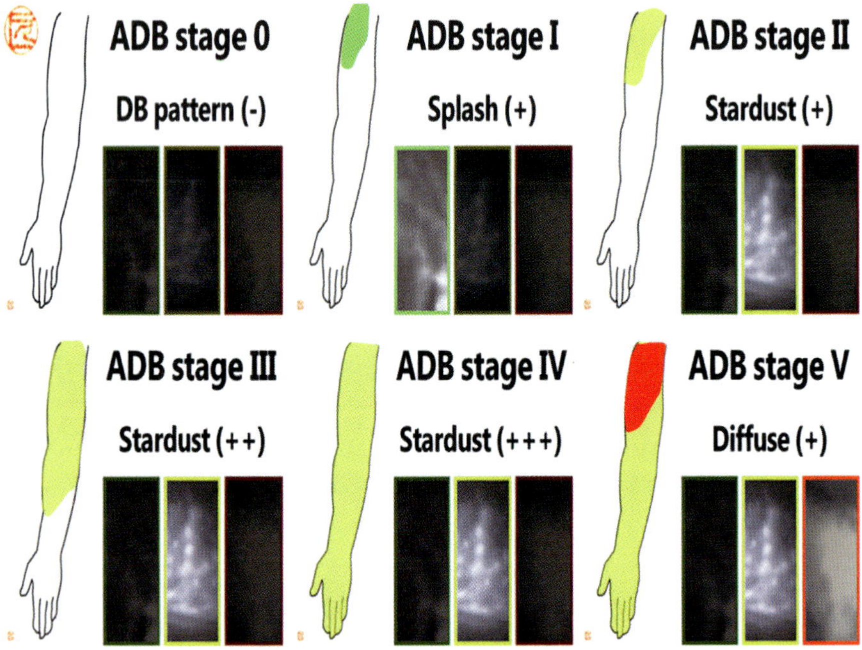

Fig. 41.4 Arm dermal backflow (ADB) stage for pathophysiological severity staging of arm lymphedema using indocyanine green lymphography

41.2.2.2 ICG Lymphography Classification for Primary Lymphedema

Since primary lymphedema has a wide variety of etiologies, it is important to visualize abnormalities in lymphatic systems for evaluation and diagnosis. Although ICG lymphography can visualize only superficial lymph flows, ICG lymphography has been reported to be useful to evaluate and classify primary lymphedema [22]. The ICG lymphography primary lymphedema classification includes four patterns: proximal DB (PDB), distal DB (DDB), less enhancement (LE), and no enhancement (NE) patterns (Fig. 41.5).

In PDB pattern, DB pattern extends from proximal to distal region like DB stages for obstructive lymphedema. Patients with PDB pattern should undergo work-up to rule out malignancy because the findings are very similar to that of cancer-related lymphedema. Lymphatic malformation in the trunk is suspected. Therapeutic strategy is also similar to that of cancer-related obstructive lymphedema. Earlier interventions work better to improve lymph circulation [23].

In DDB pattern, DB pattern is observed in the distal part but not in the proximal part, and the remaining region shows linear pattern or no enhanced images. Localized distal malformation or lymphatic valve malformation is suspected. Patients with DDB pattern usually have past history of cellulitis, and lymphatic vessels are likely to be affected by inflammation.

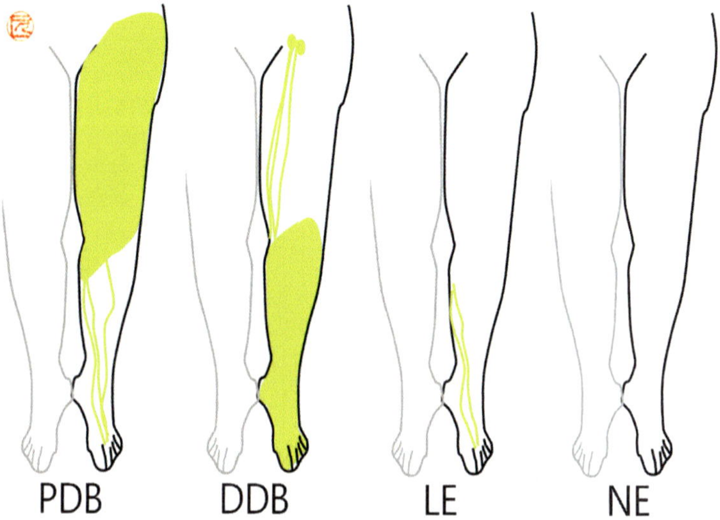

Fig. 41.5 Indocyanine green lymphography classification for primary lymphedema. Proximal dermal backflow (*PDB*) pattern, distal dermal backflow (*DDB*) pattern, less enhancement (*LE*) pattern, and no enhancement (*NE*) pattern

In LE pattern, linear pattern is observed only in the distal part, and the remaining proximal part shows no enhanced image; no DB pattern is detected. Relative hypoplasia of superficial lymphatic system is suspected, and aging-related pump dysfunction may affect development of symptomatic lymphedema. Patients with LE pattern usually find themselves prone to physiologic temporary leg swelling before onset of pathologic and progressive leg edema.

In NE pattern, no lymphatic is enhanced other than injected sites; there is neither linear pattern nor DB pattern. Segmental lymphatic aplasia, severe hypoplasia, or severe lymph malabsorption is suspected. Most patients with NE pattern developed lymphedema at birth and suffer from more severe lymphedema compared with those with other ICG lymphography patterns. Lympho-venous shunt operations rarely work to improve the disease.

41.2.3 Navigation for Lymphatic Supermicrosurgery

ICG lymphography is useful for preoperative guidance of supermicrosurgical lymphaticovenular anastomosis (LVA) [8–10, 14–16, 24–28]. As mentioned above, different ICG lymphography pattern represents different condition of lymph circulation. With progression of ICG lymphography pattern (linear to splash, to stardust, and, finally, to diffuse pattern), the lymphatic vessel changes to more sclerotic with less lymph flow [3, 11, 17, 18, 29]. The diameter of the lymphatic vessel is approximately 0.5 mm in linear/splash/stardust pattern regions and 0.3 mm in diffuse pattern region. Diffuse region should be avoided for LVA surgical field because detection rate of lymphatic vessel is insufficient and efficacy of LVA is considered to be low [11, 19, 30, 31].

ICG lymphography is also useful for intraoperative navigation and assessment of LVA [8–10, 15, 16, 26, 28]. For a surgeon with less experience of LVA, it is difficult to find the lymphatic vessel because the lymphatic vessel is small and translucent surrounded with yellow fat tissue. Intraoperative usage of ICG lymphography significantly reduces time for dissection of lymphatic vessel and skin incision length, and allows precise evaluation of LVA patency intraoperatively [8, 9, 16]. When anastomosis patency is not good, a surgeon can immediately decide to revise the anastomosis.

41.3 Lymphedema Management Using ICG Lymphography

A prospective observational cohort study in which 100 consecutive pelvic cancer patients were followed using ICG lymphography revealed that splash pattern is a reversible lymph circulatory change whereas stardust pattern is an irreversible change [32]. Thirty-one patients showed splash pattern (LDB stage I) after cancer treatments, of which 5 improved to linear pattern (LDB stage 0), 17 stayed in splash pattern (LDB stage I), and 9 progressed to stardust pattern (LDB stage II). Once stardust pattern is observed on ICG lymphography, it never improves to splash or linear pattern even with conservative treatments. Patients with splash pattern (DB stage I) should be closely followed as "subclinical" lymphedema to prevent lymphedema development and overtreatment [4, 31]. On the other hand, a patient with stardust pattern (DB stage II) should undergo LVA or other physiological lymphedema surgery because conservative treatment cannot improve lymph circulation [11, 17, 18, 32].

When lymphedema treatments are indicated, conservative therapies should be applied first; conservative treatments should also be performed before lymphedema surgery as perioperative management [11, 14, 23]. When lymphedema progresses despite conservative treatments, lymphatic surgeries are indicated. For DB stage I (subclinical lymphedema) or DB stage II (early-stage lymphedema) patients, LVA would be the choice of treatment due to its effectiveness and minimal invasiveness; LVA can be performed via a small skin incision under local infiltration anesthesia [11, 16, 31]. LVA can be performed also for DB stage III (progressed lymphedema) patients, but treatment efficacy is sometimes not enough to improve the disease. It is difficult to reduce lymphedematous volume with LVA in DB stage V patients [4, 14, 23, 33–36]. When lymphedema is refractory to LVA, vascularized lymphatic tissue transfer with or without debulking procedure such as liposuction is indicated [11, 18, 31]. Before decision making of lymphedema management, ICG

Table 41.1 Lymphedema management according to ICG lymphography findings

DB stage	ICG pattern	Clinical condition	Management
Stage I	Splash (+)	Subclinical	Follow or CT or LVA
Stage II	Stardust (+)	Early	LVA
Stage III	Stardust (++)	Progressed	LVA ± LNT ± LS
Stage IV	Stardust (+++)		
Stage V	Diffuse (+)		

ICG indocyanine green, *DB* dermal backflow, *CT* conservative treatment, *LVA* lymphaticovenular anastomosis, *LNT* lymph node transfer, *LS* liposuction

lymphography should be performed to maximize treatment efficacy and to minimize a risk of overtreatment (Table 41.1).

References

1. Zhibin Y, Quanyong L, Libo C et al (2006) The role of radionuclide lymphoscintigraphy in extremity lymphedema. Ann Nucl Med 20:341–344
2. Unno N, Inuzuka K, Suzuki M et al (2007) Preliminary experience with a novel fluorescence lymphography using indocyanine green in patients with secondary lymphedema. J Vasc Surg 45:1016–1021
3. Yamamoto T, Narushima M, Doi K et al (2011) Characteristic indocyanine green lymphography findings in lower extremity lymphedema: the generation of a novel lymphedema severity staging system using dermal backflow patterns. Plast Reconstr Surg 127(5):1979–1986
4. Yamamoto T, Matsuda N, Doi K et al (2011) The earliest finding of indocyanine green (ICG) lymphography in asymptomatic limbs of lower extremity lymphedema patients secondary to cancer treatment: the modified dermal backflow (DB) stage and concept of subclinical lymphedema. Plast Reconstr Surg 128(4):314e–321e
5. Yamamoto T, Yamamoto N, Doi K et al (2011) Indocyanine green (ICG)-enhanced lymphography for upper extremity lymphedema: a novel severity staging system using dermal backflow (DB) patterns. Plast Reconstr Surg 128(4):941–947
6. Yamamoto T, Yamamoto N, Yoshimatsu H et al (2013) Indocyanine green lymphography for evaluation of genital lymphedema in secondary lower extremity lymphedema patients. J Vasc Surg 1(4):400–405
7. Yamamoto T, Iida T, Matsuda N et al (2011) Indocyanine green (ICG)-enhanced lymphography for evaluation of facial lymphoedema. J Plast Reconstr Aesthet Surg 64(11):1541–1544
8. Yamamoto T, Yamamoto N, Azuma S et al (2013) Near-infrared illumination system-integrated microscope for supermicrosurgical lymphaticovenular anastomosis. Microsurgery 34(1):23–27
9. Yamamoto T, Yamamoto N, Numahata T et al (2014) Navigation lymphatic supermicrosurgery for the treatment of cancer-related peripheral lymphedema. Vasc Endovasc Surg 48(2):139–143
10. Yamamoto T, Yoshimatsu H, Koshima I (2014) Navigation lymphatic supermicrosurgery for iatrogenic lymphorrhea: supermicrosurgical lymphaticolymphatic anastomosis and lymphaticovenular anastomosis under indocyanine green lymphography navigation. J Plast Reconstr Aesthet Surg [epub ahead of print]
11. Yamamoto T, Yamamoto N, Narushima M (2012) Lymphaticovenular anastomosis with guidance of ICG lymphography. J Jpn Coll Angiol 52:327–331

12. Yamamoto T, Narushima M, Yoshimatsu H et al (2013) Indocyanine green velocity: lymph transportation capacity deterioration with progression of lymphedema. Ann Plast Surg 71 (5):59–594
13. Yamamoto T, Narushima M, Yoshimatsu H et al (2013) Dynamic indocyanine green lymphography for breast cancer-related arm lymphedema. Ann Plast Surg [Epub ahead of print]
14. Yamamoto T, Narushima M, Kikuchi K et al (2011) Lambda-shaped anastomosis with intravascular stenting method for safe and effective lymphaticovenular anastomosis. Plast Reconstr Surg 127(5):1987–1992
15. Yamamoto T, Yoshimatsu H, Narushima M et al (2013) A modified side-to-end lymphaticovenular anastomosis. Microsurgery 33(2):130–133
16. Yamamoto T, Narushima M, Yoshimatsu H et al (2014) Minimally invasive lymphatic supermicrosurgery (MILS): indocyanine green lymphography-guided simultaneous multi-site lymphaticovenular anastomoses via millimeter skin incisions. Ann Plast Surg 72(1):67–70
17. Yamamoto T, Narushima M, Koshima I (2012) ICG lymphography and lymphaticovenular anastomosis for diagnosis and treatment of lymphedema, fascicular turnover flap for nerve reconstruction. Jpn J Orthop Traumatol 55(4):357–364
18. Yamamoto T, Yamamoto N, Narushima M et al (2012) Lymphaticovenular anastomosis with guidance of ICG lymphography. J Jpn Coll Angiol 52:327–331
19. Yamamoto T, Yamamoto N, Narushima M et al (2013) Evaluation of peripheral lymphedema using ICG lymphography. Jpn J Phlebol 24(1):57–62
20. Lee BB, Antignani P, Baroncelli TA et al (2014) IUA-ISVI consensus for diagnosis guideline of chronic lymphedema of the limbs. Int Angiol [Epub ahead of print]
21. Yamamoto T, Yamamoto N, Furuya M et al (in press) Genital lymphedema score: genital lymphedema severity scoring system based on subjective symptoms. Ann Plast Surg
22. Yamamoto T, Yoshimatsu H, Narushima M et al (2014) Indocyanine green lymphography findings in primary leg lymphedema. Eur J Vasc Endovasc Surg [Epub ahead of print]
23. Yamamoto T, Koshima I, Yoshimatsu H et al (2011) Simultaneous multi-site lymphaticovenular anastomoses for primary lower extremity and genital lymphoedema complicated with severe lymphorrhea. J Plast Reconstr Aesthet Surg 64(6):812–815
24. Yamamoto T, Yoshimatsu H, Yamamoto N et al (2013) Side-to-end lymphaticovenular anastomosis through temporary lymphatic expansion. PLoS ONE 8(3):e59523
25. Yamamoto T, Yamamoto N, Yamashita M et al (2014) Efferent lymphatic vessel anastomosis (ELVA): supermicrosurgical efferent lymphatic vessel-to-venous anastomosis for the prophylactic treatment of subclinical lymphedema. Ann Plast Surg [Epub ahead of print]
26. Yamamoto T, Chen WF, Yamamoto N et al (2014) Technical simplification of the supermicrosurgical side-to-end lymphaticovenular anastomosis using the parachute technique. Microsurgery [epub ahead of print]
27. Yamamoto T, Yoshimatsu H, Narushima M et al (2013) Split intravascular stents for side-to-end lymphaticovenular anastomosis. Ann Plast Surg 71(5):538–540
28. Yamamoto T, Yoshimatsu H, Narushima M et al (2014) Sequential anastomosis for lymphatic supermicrosurgery: multiple lymphaticovenular anastomoses on one venule. Ann Plast Surg 73(1):46–49
29. Yamamoto T, Koshima I (2014) Supermicrosugical anastomosis of superficial lymphatic vessel to deep lymphatic vessel for a patient with cellulitis-induced chronic localized leg lymphedema. Microsurgery [epub ahead of print]
30. Yamamoto T, Yoshimatsu H, Yamamoto N et al (2014) Modified lambda-shaped lymphaticovenular anastomosis with supermicrosurgical lymphoplasty technique for a cancer-related lymphedema patient. Microsurgery 34(4):308–310
31. Yamamoto T, Koshima I (2013) Subclinical lymphedema: understanding is the clue to decision making. Plast Reconstr Surg 132(3):472e–473e
32. Akita S, Mitsukawa N, Rikihisa N et al (2013) Early diagnosis and risk factors for lymphedema following lymph node dissection for gynecologic cancer. Plast Reconstr Surg 131(2):283–289

33. Yamamoto T, Matsuda N, Todokoro T et al (2011) Lower extremity lymphedema index: a simple method for severity evaluation of lower extremity lymphedema. Ann Plast Surg 67 (6):637–640
34. Yamamoto T, Yamamoto N, Hara H et al (2013) Upper Extremity Lymphedema (UEL) index: a simple method for severity evaluation of upper extremity lymphedema. Ann Plast Surg 70 (1):47–49
35. Yamamoto N, Yamamoto T, Hayashi N et al (2014) Arm volumetry versus upper extremity lymphedema index: validity of upper extremity lymphedema index for body-type corrected arm volume evaluation. Ann Plast Surg [Epub ahead of print]
36. Yamamoto T, Yamamoto N, Hayashi N et al (in press) Practicality of lower extremity lymphedema index: lymphedema index versus volumetry-based evaluations for body-type corrected lower extremity volume evaluation. Ann Plast Surg

Chapter 42
Lymphatic Pumping Pressure in the Legs and Its Association with Aging, Edema, and Quality of Life

Naoki Unno

Abstract Lymph is transported in part by intrinsic contraction of the lymphatic vessels. The failure of the transporting system may be associated with lymphedema. Using indocyanine green (ICG) fluorescence lymphography and a transparent sphygmomanometer calf, we invented a novel method of measuring the pumping pressure of lymph propulsion (lymphatic pumping pressure; $P_{lymph\ pump}$) in human legs. With this method, we recruited healthy volunteers and measured the leg $P_{lymph\ pump}$ in the participants. The results demonstrated a progressive decrease in $P_{lymph\ pump}$ with advancing age in both sexes. Next, we investigated the association of decreased $P_{lymph\ pump}$ with edema occurrence and their quality of life (QOL) using Short Form 36 (SF-36) in healthy volunteers. The survey revealed that the poor $P_{lymph\ pump}$ group ($P_{lymph\ pump} < 20$ mmHg in both legs) had a significantly lower PF (physical function) and GH (general health) scores than the good $P_{lymph\ pump}$ group ($P_{lymph\ pump} > 40$ mmHg in both legs). These results suggested that the value of $P_{lymph\ pump}$ may reflect the degenerative changes of lymph vessels due to lymphosclerosis and affect human QOL.

Keywords Lymphatic pumping pressure • Lymphosclerosis • Quality of life • Edema • Aging

42.1 Background

The lymphatic transport system plays an important role in the maintenance of body fluid and macromolecular balances, lipid absorption, and immune reactions. Among the systems, lymphatic pumping or the intrinsic contractions of the lymphatics have been proposed as one of the major mechanisms that propel lymph to the central lymphatic systems (Fig. 42.1). Decreased activity of the lymphatic pumping may cause lymph stasis, or lymphedema [1–4]. However, the mechanisms

N. Unno, M.D., Ph.D. (✉)
Second Department of Surgery, Hamamatsu University School of Medicine, 1-20-1 Handayama, Higashi-ku, Hamamatsu, Shizuoka 431-3192, Japan
e-mail: unno@hama-med.ac.jp

M. Kusano et al. (eds.), *ICG Fluorescence Imaging and Navigation Surgery*,
DOI 10.1007/978-4-431-55528-5_42

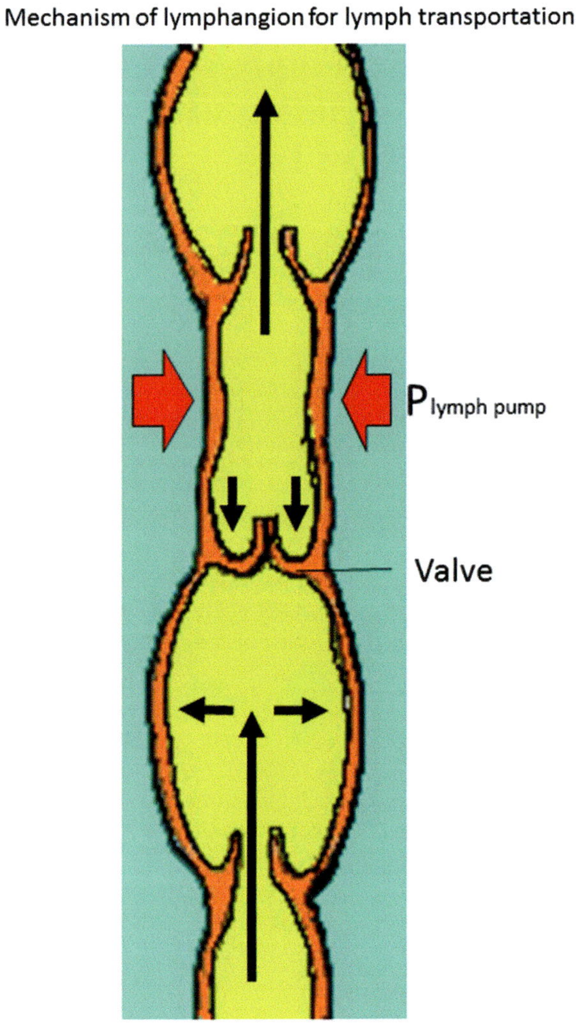

Fig. 42.1 Mechanisms of lymphangion for lymph transportation

underline contraction, and the association between failed pumping and disease development has not been clarified. In 1979, Olzewski et al. was the first to measure lymphatic pressure in the human subcutaneous collecting lymph vessel of the leg [5]. They cannulated a pressure transducer directly into the lumen of lymph vessels and measured the lymphatic pressure at 2–5 postoperative days after the cannulation, and they reported that the pressure ranged from 1 to 40 mmHg. However, since this method is invasive, it cannot be used to measure the lymphatic pressure of healthy people. The lack of a noninvasive method for measuring lymphatic pumping has prevented physicians from studying the role of lymphatic pumping. Recently, we introduced indocyanine green (ICG) fluorescence lymphography as a novel imaging test for visualizing real-time lymph flow and reported that the new imaging technique is useful to assess lymphatic flow both morphologically and functionally [6, 7]. Recently, we have developed a novel method of measuring lymph pumping in human legs using a custom-made transparent sphygmomanometer cuff and indocyanine green (ICG) fluorescence lymphography [8]. Since no study has investigated the normal ranges of human lymph pumping pressure ($P_{lymph\ pump}$) in healthy people, we studied the leg lymph pumping pressure in healthy volunteers to determine the ranges to simultaneously assess the effects of aging and the quality of life (QOL) on $P_{lymph\ pump}$. Similarly, we surveyed the occurrence of leg edema and participants QOL using the Medical Outcome Study Short Form 36 (SF-36) to investigate the association of P lymph pump with leg edema and QOL.

42.2 Methods

42.2.1 Measuring the Human Lymph Pumping Pressure

All the studies described herein were approved by the Ethical Committee of Hamamatsu University School of Medicine, and informed consent was obtained from all the participants.

The measurement was performed as previously reported [9]. Briefly, using a 27-gauge needle, we subcutaneously injected 0.3 mL of ICG (Diagnogreen 0.5 %; Daiichi-Sankyo Pharmaceutical, Tokyo, Japan) at the dorsum of each participant's foot. Immediately after the injection, fluorescence images of the subcutaneous lymphatic drainage were obtained using an infrared camera system (PDE™, Hamamatsu Photonics K.K. Hamamatsu, Japan), which activates ICG with light emitted at a wavelength of 760 nm and filters out light at a wavelength <820 nm. The light source for the emission of ICG consisted of 760-nm light-emitting diodes, and the detector was a charge-coupled device camera. The fluorescence images were continuously observed on the monitor of a laptop (VAIO, Type T; SONY Co., Tokyo, Japan).

Before the injection of ICG, a custom-made transparent sphygmomanometer cuff was wrapped around the lower leg just below the popliteal fossa. The cuff was connected to a standard mercury sphygmomanometer. Lymphatic pumping was measured with the participants in the sitting position. Immediately after the subcutaneous injection of ICG, the transparent cuff was inflated to 70 mmHg, and then, it was gradually deflated to lower the pressure by increments of 5 mmHg every 2 min. This was performed until the fluorescence dye exceeded the upper border of the cuff, indicating that the lymphatic contraction had overcome the cuff pressure. The value of the cuff pressure at this point was used to measure P lymph pump (Fig. 42.2).

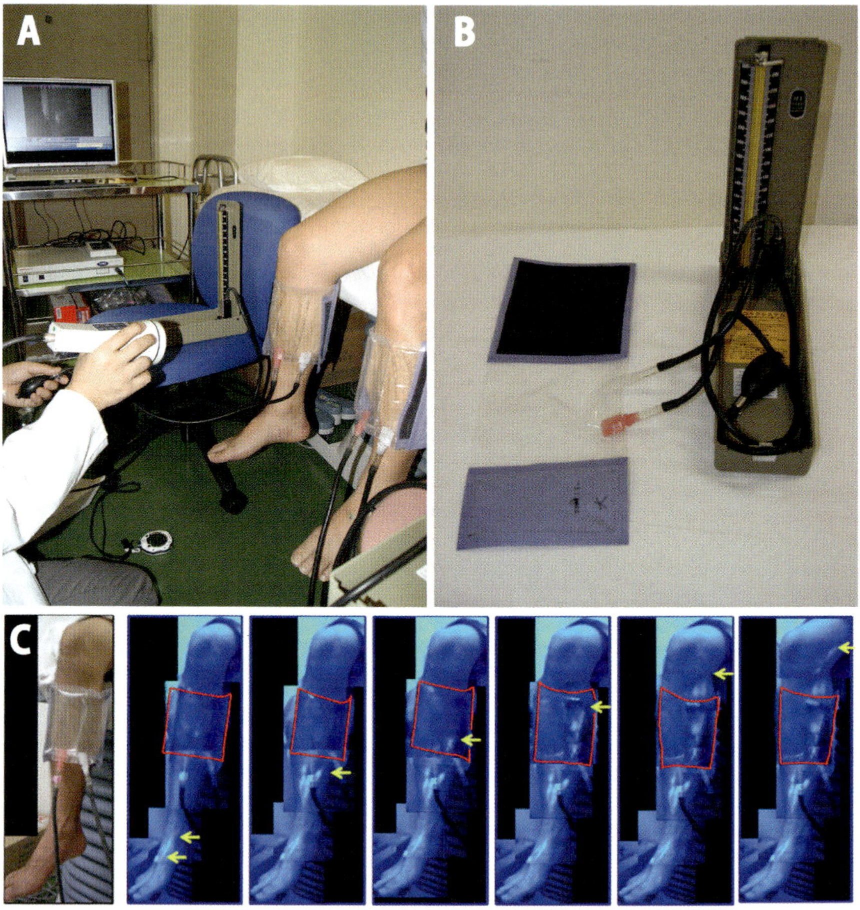

Fig. 42.2 (**a**) The measurement of lymphatic pumping pressure in the sitting position using PDE™ (Hamamatsu Photonics K.K. Hamamatsu, Japan)
(**b**) A custom-made transparent sphygmomanometer cuff and a standard mercury sphygmomanometer
(**c**) Real-time images of indocyanine green fluorescence lymphography after subcutaneous injection at the dorsum of the foot. The *arrows* (*yellow*) indicate the most advanced indocyanine *green* contrast agent in the lymph vessel; the solid *line* (*red*) outlines the transparent cuff (Cited from Ref. [9])

This method was confirmed by comparing data with the values obtained with a dynamic lymphoscintigram using the same cuff technique. We found that there was a significant correlation between the values with ICG fluorescence lymphography and dynamic lymphoscintigraphy [8].

42.2.2 *The Effect of Aging on Human Lymph Pumping Pressure*

Three hundred and ninety-nine participants (199 men and 200 women) were recruited from the Hamamatsu University School of Medicine. The subjects medical history was screened preliminarily, and those with no serious allergy and no history of leg injury or surgery were included. Those with an iodine allergy were excluded according to the industry's recommendation because ICG contains iodine. In addition, subjects with varicose vein in the leg (i.e., C3, 4, and 5 according to the Clinical Etiology Anatomy Pathophysiology (CEAP) classification) were excluded. P lymph pump was measured as previously described.

Figure 42.3 shows that there was a significant correlation between the leg lymphatic pumping and age: $r = -0.34$ ($p < 0.0001$). Both sexes showed a significant correlation between leg lymphatic pumping and age (male: $r = -0.32$, $p < 0.0001$; female: $r = -0.37$, $p < 0.0001$).

Aging affects the arteries and causes arteriosclerosis. However, venous stasis syndrome causes phlebosclerosis. Based on this study's findings, aging may affect the lymph vessels and cause lymphosclerosis. This concept was proposed by Rabinovits et al. almost half century ago [10]. They performed a histological study on the human thoracic duct in elderly humans and reported changes in the distribution of smooth muscle cells and fibrosis. Our novel method of measuring enabled to demonstrate that "lymphosclerosis" may change the lymphatic vessels functionally. The mechanisms of contraction/relaxation in lymph vessels are yet to be fully understood. Similar to blood vessels, lymphatic endothelial cells have an ability to produce nitric oxide (NO) [11]. The endothelium-dependent modulation via NO production is considered to be a key mechanism of lymph pumping. In an animal study, endothelial NO synthase expression in the thoracic duct was markedly decreased, and flow-dependent modulation of the lymph pumping was

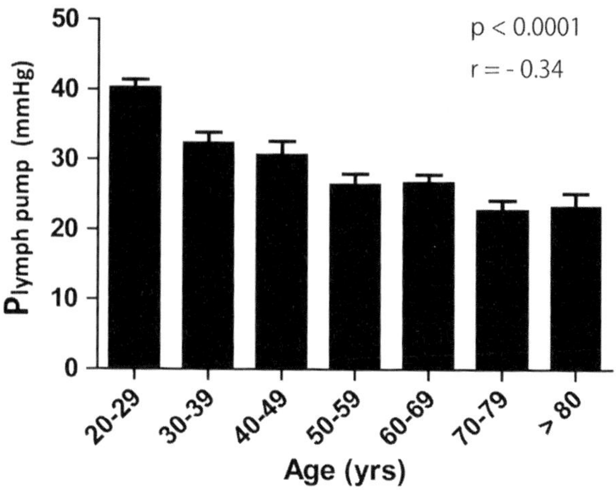

Fig. 42.3 The influence of age and sex on leg lymphatic pumping pressure ($P_{lymph\ pump}$) (Cited from Ref. [12])

completely abolished, suggesting that aging may disturb NO-dependent regulatory mechanisms of the lymphatic vessels [12].

Our study demonstrated the effect of aging on lymphatic vessels, which may begin a new era of lymphatic research regarding antiaging, lifestyle, and new drug developments [9].

42.2.3 Value of Human Lymphatic Pumping Pressure in Association with Leg Edema and Quality of Life

42.2.3.1 Methods

Four hundred and sixty-five healthy volunteers (78 men and 387 women; aged 30–85 years) participated in the study. A standard questionnaire was administered to obtain complaints of leg edema, body weight and height to calculate the body mass index (BMI), smoking status, and comorbid diseases (e.g., hypertension, diabetes mellitus, and hyperlipidemia). Complaints of leg edema were defined as a feeling of edema for at least 5 days per week even before noon. Subjects with varicose veins in the legs (C3, 4, and 5 according to the CEAP classification) or a medical history of lymphedema, deep vein thrombosis, radiation therapy, prescribed cancer agents, current pregnancy, or leg trauma were excluded.

The SF-36 was used to assess the participants subjective health conditions and their QOL. The SF-36 is a well-validated instrument that provides estimates for the following eight health concepts: physical functioning (PF); role functioning-physical (RP); bodily pain (BP); general health (GH); vitality (VT); social functioning (SF); role functioning-emotional (RE); and mental health (MH). Responses to the 36 questions represent these health concepts on a scale from 0 (worst possible health) to 100 (best possible health). $P_{lymph\ pump}$ was measured as described above.

42.2.3.2 Quality of Life with or Without Leg Edema

Approximately, 10 % of the participants complained of leg edema. There were no significant differences between those with and without edema with regard to BMI, smoking status, or comorbidities. The mean leg $P_{lymph\ pump}$ in the edema + and edema − groups were 20.4 ± 12.7 mmHg and 23.3 ± 15.6 mmHg, respectively ($p = 0.23$). There was no significant difference in the leg $P_{lymph\ pump}$ between the two groups, and there was no significant difference in age between the groups.

With regard to the QOL, the SF-36 showed that participants who complained of edema in the lower legs had a significantly lower PF, RP, BP, and VT scores than participants who did not complain of edema in the lower legs ($p = 0.022$, 0.0012, 0.0046, and 0.0076, respectively) (Fig. 42.4). Therefore, leg edema was clearly associated with a lower QOL. However, there were no significant differences in the $P_{lymph\ pump}$ between the two groups, suggesting that $P_{lymph\ pump}$ is not necessarily a

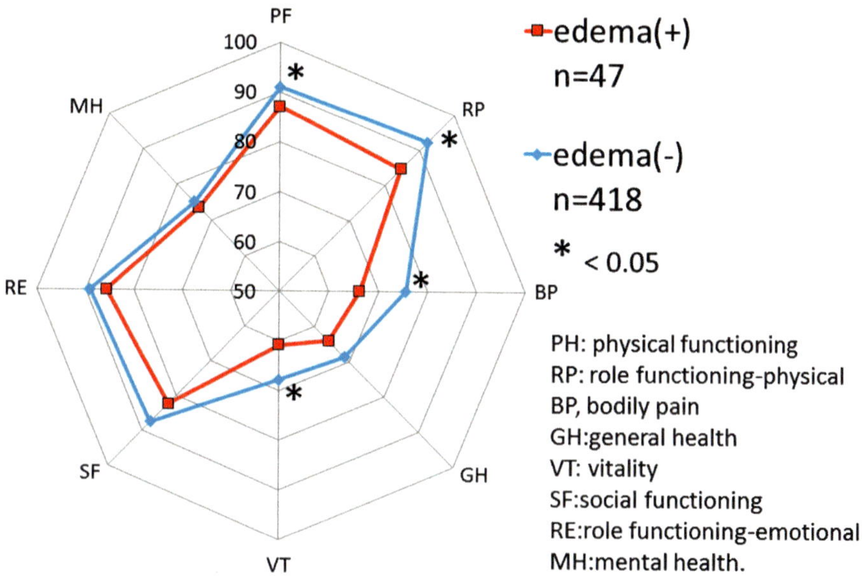

Fig. 42.4 Means of the Short Form Health Survey subscales scores with/without leg edema (Cited from Ref. [12])

decisive factor that causes edema. Among healthy people, other factors such as exercise, occupation, or mild venous insufficiency (i.e., C1 and 2 according to the CEAP classification) may affect the occurrence of edema [13]. [14],

42.2.3.3 Quality of Life and Leg $P_{lymph\ pump}$

The participants were divided into three groups according to their leg $P_{lymph\ pump}$. Participants with a $P_{lymph\ pump} < 20$ mmHg in both legs, 20–49 mmHg in either leg, and > 40 mmHg in both legs were classified into the poor, moderate, and good $P_{lymph\ pump}$ group, respectively. The mean $P_{lymph\ pump}$ of both legs in the good, moderate, and poor $P_{lymph\ pump}$ groups was 44.0 ± 7.4 mmHg, 19.3 ± 10.8 mmHg, and 4.2 ± 5.2 mmHg, respectively (Table 42.1). There were no significant differences among the three groups with regard to sex, smoking status, BMI, or comorbidities. However, the occurrence of leg edema was significantly higher in the poor $P_{lymph\ pump}$ group than in the good $P_{lymph\ pump}$ groups (15.7 % vs. 4 %) (Table 42.1). The SF-36 revealed that the poor $P_{lymph\ pump}$ group had a significantly lower PF score than the good $P_{lymph\ pump}$ group. The poor $P_{lymph\ pump}$ group also had a significantly lower GH score than both the moderate and good $P_{lymph\ pump}$ groups (Fig. 42.5). Therefore, the low $P_{lymph\ pump}$ may affect people's QOL unfavorably by causing leg edema [14].

Table 42.1 Participant characteristics according to $P_{lymph\ pump}$

	Good $P_{lymph\ pump}$ group	Moderate $P_{lymph\ pump}$ group	Poor $P_{lymph\ pump}$ group	
	$n = 100$ (21.5 %)	$n = 314$ (67.5 %)	$n = 51$ (11.0 %)	*p*-value
Age (years)	51.2 ± 12.8	52.9 ± 12.8	55.0 ± 13.8	0.2
Sex (male/female)	16/84	55/259	7/44	0.78
BMI (kg/m^2; mean ± SD)	21.6 ± 3.0	21.5 ± 3.0	22.3 ± 4.3	0.39
Previous smoking	7 (7.0 %)	33 (10.5 %)	4 (7.8 %)	0.53
Current smoking	4 (4.0 %)	20 (6.4 %)	5 (9.8 %)	0.37
Hypertension (%)	12 (12.0 %)	51 (16.2 %)	8 (15.7 %)	0.59
Diabetes mellitus (%)	4 (4.0 %)	10 (3.2 %)	3 (5.9 %)	0.62
Hyperlipidemia (%)	19 (19.0 %)	58 (18.5 %)	11 (21.6 %)	0.87
Edema complaints (%)	4 (4.0 %)	35 (11.1 %)	8 (15.7 %)*	0.044
$P_{lymph\ pump}$ (mmHg)	44.0 ± 7.4	19.3 ± 10.8	4.2 ± 5.2*	<0.001

∗Statistically significant
*Significant at $p < 0.05$
BMI body mass index, *SD* standard deviation, $P_{lymph\ pump}$ Human lymph pumping pressure

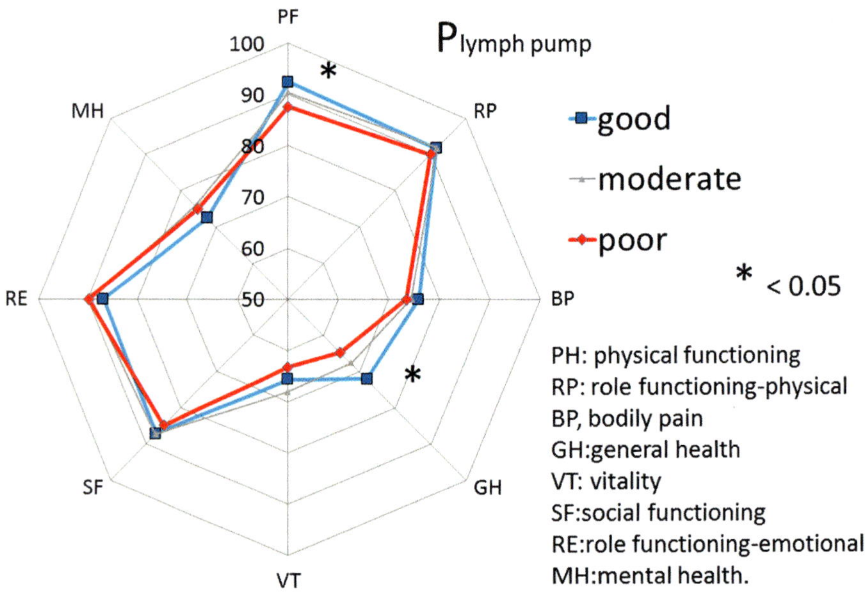

Fig. 42.5 The means of the Short Form Health Survey subscales scores. A comparison among the three groups classified by the leg lymphatic pumping pressure with $P_{lymph\ pump}$ (Cited from Ref. [12])

42.3 Conclusions

This novel method for measuring $P_{lymph\ pump}$ using ICG lymphography with an occlusion cuff offers minimally invasive screening of lymphatic function in a large population study. In our study, this method demonstrated that poor $P_{lymph\ pump}$ may be responsible for leg edema in a substantial proportion of healthy people and for worsening their QOL. Currently, no study has been performed to improve the lymphatic pumping function of humans. Therefore, such a study is needed to prevent leg edema and to improve QOL in individuals.

Acknowledgments We wish to thank all the staff of the Second Department of Surgery at the Hamamatsu University School of Medicine and Angiology Laboratory of Hamamatsu University School Hospital for their assistance and support in this study. The contents of this chapter summarize previous publications (reference nos. 8, 9, and 14). These studies were supported by a Grant-in-Aid for Scientific Research (C) (22591400) and (B) (20291958) to Naoki Unno from the Japan Society for the Promotion of Science. The Hamamatsu University School of Medicine has a patent for the lymphatic pressure-measuring system and the method for controlling the same (PCT /JP2010/051706), and Naoki Unno invented in the patent.

References

1. Williams WH, Witte CL, Witte MH, McNeill GC (2000) Radionuclide lymphangioscintigraphy in the evaluation of peripheral lymphedema. Clin Nucl Med 25:451–464
2. Stanton AW, Modi S, Mellor RH, Peters AM, Svenson WE, Levick JR, Mortimer PS (2006) A quantitative lymphoscintigraphic evaluation of lymphatic function in the swollen hands of women with lymphoedema following breast cancer treatment. Clin Sci 110:553–561
3. Modi S, Stanton AWB, Svensson WE, Peters AM, Mortimer PS, Levick JR (2007) Human lymphatic pumping measured in healthy and lymphoedematous arms by lymphatic congestion lymphoscintigraphy. J Physiol 583:271–285
4. Stanton AW, Modi S, Mellor RH, Levick JR, Mortimer PS (2009) Recent advances in breast cancer-related lymphedema of the arm: lymphatic pump failure and predisposing factors. Lymphat Res Biol 7:29–45
5. Olszewski WL, Engeset A (1979) Lymphatic contractions. New Engl J Med 300:316
6. Unno N, Inuzuka K, Suzuki M, Yamamoto N, Sagara D, Nishiyama M, Konno H (2007) Preliminary experience with a novel fluorescence lymphography using indocyanine green in patients with secondary lymphedema. J Vasc Surg 45:1016–1021
7. Unno N, Nishiyama M, Suzuki M, Yamamoto N, Inuzuka K, Sagara D, Tanaka H, Konno H (2008) Quantitative lymph imaging for assessment of lymph function using indocyanine greenfluorescence lymphography. Eur J Vasc Endovasc Surg 36:230–236
8. Unno N, Nishiyama M, Suzuki M, Tanaka H, Yamamoto N, Sagara D, Mano Y, Konno H (2010) A novel method of measuring human lymphatic pumping using indocyanine green fluorescence lymphography. J Vasc Surg 52:946–952
9. Unno N, Tanaka H, Suzuki M, Yamamoto N, Mano M, Sano M, Saito T, Konno H (2011) Influence of age and gender on human lymphatic pumping pressure in the leg. Lymphology 44:113–120
10. Rabinovitz AJ, Saphir O (1965) The thoracic duct; significance of age-related changes and of lipid in the wall. Circulation 31:899–905

11. Ohhashi T, Takahashi N (1991) Acetylcholine-induced release of endothelium-derived relaxing factor from lymphatic endothelial cells. Am J Physiol 260:H1172–H1178
12. Gasheva OY, Knippa K, Nepiushchikh ZV, Muthuchamy M, Gashev AA (2007) Age-related alterations of active pumping mechanisms in rat thoracic duct. Microcirculation 14:827–839
13. Suzuki M, Unno N, Yamamoto N, Nishiyama M, Sagara D, Tanaka H, Mano Y, Konno H (2009) Impaired lymphatic function recovered after great saphenous vein stripping in patients with varicose vein: venodynamic and lymphodynamic results. J Vasc Surg 50:1085–1091
14. Saito T, Unno N, Yamamoto N, Inuzuka K, Tanaka H, Sano M, Sugisawda R, Katahashi K, Konno H (2015) Low lymphatic pumping pressure in the legs is associated with leg edema and lower quality of life in healthy volunteers. Lymph Res Biol 13(2):154–159

Chapter 43
ICG Fluorescence Lymphography for Confirming Mid- to Long-term Patency of Lymphatic Venous Side-to-End Anastomosis in the Treatment of Peripheral Lymphedema

Jiro Maegawa

Abstract Since indocyanine green (ICG) fluorescence lymphography was introduced in 2007, lymphatic venous anastomosis has been widely adopted for the treatment of chronic lymphedema. However, the results and other features remain unclear. In this chapter, I demonstrate the primary outcomes of ICG fluorescence lymphography to evaluate the patency of lymphatic venous anastomosis (LVA), particularly lymphaticovenous side-to-end anastomosis (LVSEA), peri- and postoperatively. The cumulative patency rate of LVSEA decreased over time, but I observed long-term patency (>5 years after surgery) and good clinical results in microsurgical treatment of peripheral lymphedema. Through this study, I recognized the usefulness, importance, and limitations of ICG fluorescence lymphography to evaluate superficial lymph flow and patency of LVSEA in patients with peripheral lymphedema.

Keywords Long-term result • Mid-term result • Postoperative patency • Lymphatic venous anastomosis

43.1 Lymphatic Venous Side-to-End Anastomosis

Lymphatic venous anastomosis has been reported for the treatment of chronic lymphedema [1, 2], but several modes are available for the anastomotic technique, and the results, particularly in terms of patency, are not clear. Campisi's group [3] reported clinical experiences and results of LVA using invagination techniques at proximal sites such as groin regions. Recently, with advances in optic devices and microsurgical goods, intima-intima approximation techniques have been used for

---

J. Maegawa (✉)
Department of Plastic and Reconstructive Surgery, School of Medicine, Yokohama City University, 3-9 Fukuura, Kanazawa-ku, Yokohama, Kanagawa 236-0004, Japan
e-mail: jrmaegawa@gmail.com

M. Kusano et al. (eds.), *ICG Fluorescence Imaging and Navigation Surgery*,
DOI 10.1007/978-4-431-55528-5_43

multiple configuration anastomosis [4, 5]. In this technique, an end-to-end mode seems most common, but I have adopted lymphaticovenous side-to-end anastomosis (LVSEA) [6–8] because if the anastomosis becomes closed, original lymph flow in the lymph vessels can still be maintained. Since indocyanine green (ICG) fluorescence lymphography was introduced in 2007 [9, 10], I have confirmed the patency of LVSEA using this new modality.

43.1.1 Indications for LVSEA

Lymphoscintigraphy is the standard method for evaluating the severity of lymph edema and dysfunction of the lymphatic system. Several reports have investigated evaluation of the lymphatic system by lymphoscintigraphy [6, 11–14]. Decisions on the surgical indications for LVSEA can be made mainly by lymphoscintigraphy because proximal obstruction of lymph flow is one of the main indications for lymphatic venous anastomosis. Dermal backflow (DBF) on lymphoscintigraphic images, local spread of the radiotracer in the dermal and subdermal layers, is a phenomenon involving reverse flow of lymph from the collector vessels into the lymph capillaries due to obstruction and/or dysfunction of the collectors. We can find collectors for lymphatic venous anastomosis distal to or within the area of DBF. The discovery of lines on anteroposterior or posteroanterior images carries a high possibility of indicating the presence of collectors.

Near-infrared ICG fluorescence lymphography can show real-time images of the lymphatic system [9, 10]. Classification of the severity of lymphedema based on fluorescence lymphographic images has been reported [15]. This is also a good modality to decide the indications for LVA or LVSEA. Visualization of linear fluorescence on images enables easy determination of functional lymph vessels, but if the patient has thick skin or fibrous subcutaneous tissue, locating functional vessels by lymphography is not easy. I consider this as a limitation of ICG fluorescence lymphography in detecting lymph vessels during surgery and evaluating whether the anastomosis has remained patent postoperatively.

43.1.2 Perioperatively Locating Sites for Anastomosis

ICG fluorescence lymphography using a near-infrared camera system is helpful to pinpoint sites for anastomosis because lymph vessels can be detected as linear fluorescence and subcutaneous veins as black lines due to non-fluorescence. Areas where linear fluorescences and black lines cross can be considered as potential sites for anastomosis. However, using this method, lymphatics cannot be detected in the thigh area or in cases with thickened skin because the maximum depth that near-infrared rays can reach is 1–2 cm. Lines can be marked on the skin along the linear fluorescence, to highlight the lymphatics.

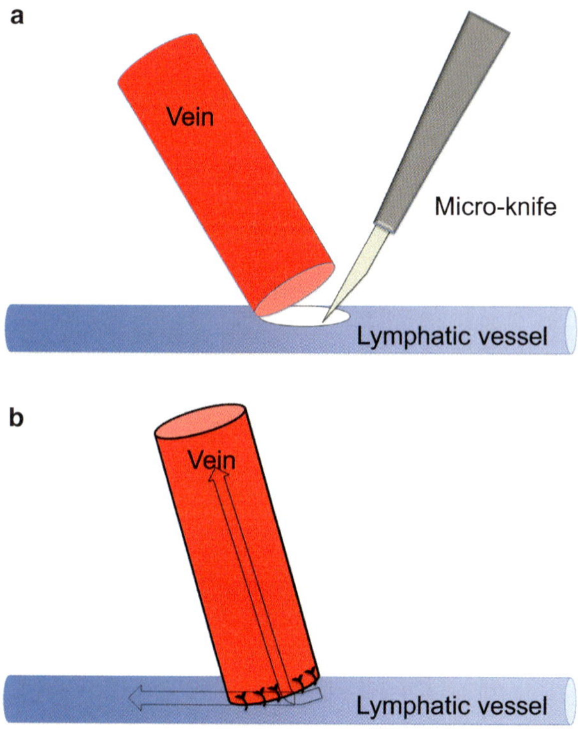

Fig. 43.1 Schema of LVSEA
(**a**) Sidewall of the lymph vessel is incised with a micro-knife. The incision should be no wider than the outer diameter of the venous stump
(**b**) Lymph passes (*open arrows*) from the lymph vessel to the vein and flows proximally

43.1.3 Side-to-End Anastomosis (Fig. 43.1)

Skin incisions 2–3 cm in length are made at each selected anastomotic site. For side-to-end anastomosis, the side of the lymphatic vessel is incised with a micro-knife. When the tip of the knife reaches the lumen of the lymphatic vessel, lymph flows out through the incision. The incision on the lymphatic vessel should be no longer than the outer diameter of the vein (Fig. 43.1a). Stents (6-0 nylon stitch, 3 mm in length) are inserted to secure the lumen of the lymph vessel [16, 17]. Several stitches should be placed to secure a watertight junction between the lymphatic vessel and vein (Fig. 43.1b). Otherwise, the blood from the vein will reach the anastomosis and may become a cause of obstruction of the anastomosis.

43.1.4 Intraoperative Confirmation of Patency

After completion of the anastomosis, patency can be confirmed by direct visualization through the microscope and by ICG fluorescence lymphography (Fig. 43.2a, b). If the anastomosis is technically well done, lymph will pass from the lymph

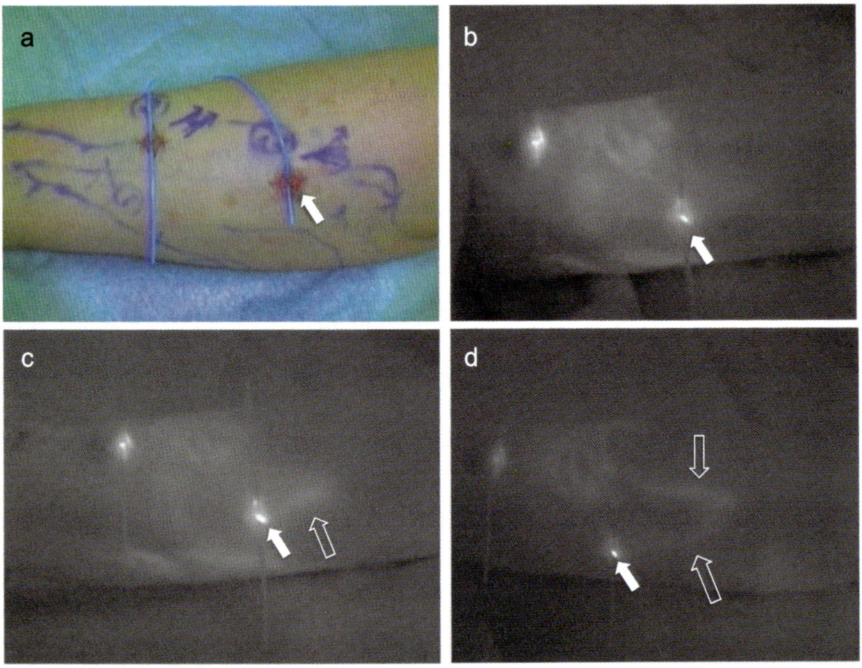

Fig. 43.2 Positive "runoff test" in a 58-year-old woman with chronic lymphedema of the left arm after breast cancer treatment
(**a**) Two anastomoses were performed in the forearm
(**b**) ICG fluorescence lymphangiography shows patency of anastomoses in the forearm
(**c**) Positive "runoff test" of lymph is confirmed by ICG fluorescence lymphangiography (on the *right side*). *Open arrow* shows a vein in which ICG is flowing from the lymphatic vessel
(**d**) The anastomosed vein is observed for longer than in C following manual massage

vessel to the vein, and the vein will become engorged by massage. In cases with good flow of lymph to the vein, the vein can be observed through the skin, representing a good "runoff test" (Fig. 43.2c, d). In my experience, postoperative patency rates seem high in such cases.

43.2 Postoperative Evaluations

The primary surgical outcome for lymphatic venous anastomosis is patency of the anastomosis, with volume reduction of the affected limb and improvements in the patient's activities of daily living (ADL) as secondary and tertiary outcomes, respectively [8]. Patency can be assessed by ICG fluorescence lymphography.

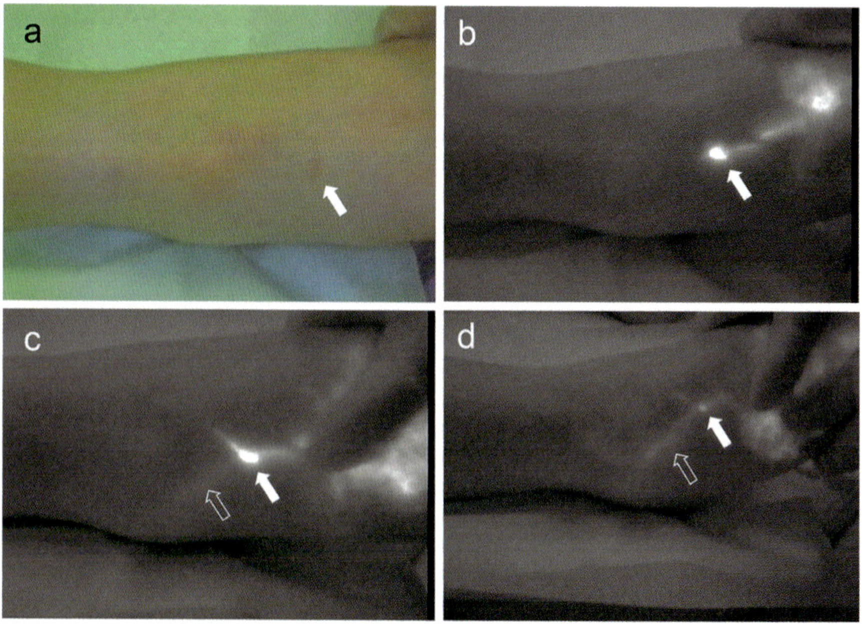

Fig. 43.3 Short-term (6 months after surgery) patency of LVSEA in a 44-year-old woman with right lower-limb lymphedema after treatment for uterine cancer
(**a**) *Closed arrow* shows the site of LVSEA in the dorsum of the right foot
(**b**) ICG fluorescence lymphography shows the lymphatic vessel (linear fluorescence) and anastomosis site (*closed arrow*)
(**c**) The anastomosed vein (*open arrow*) is observed by fluorescence
(**d**) The anastomosed vein (*open arrow*) is observed for longer than that in C following massage

43.2.1 Postoperative Patency

Evaluation by ICG fluorescence lymphography is performed about 6 months after surgery. In my protocol for the treatment of lymphedema, physiotherapy is continued postoperatively for about 6 months, roughly equivalent to the period of preoperative physiotherapy, the content of which is attempted to be reduced thereafter. If the content can be reduced, ADL of the patient increases. Evaluation of patency should therefore be performed at about 6 months after surgery (Fig. 43.3a–d). Through this evaluation, we can clarify the short-term patency. In cases with a patent LVSEA, postoperative ICG fluorescence lymphography shows a Y-shaped pattern of fluorescence (Fig. 43.3c), and branches of the vein also fluoresce (Fig. 43.3d).

As described in this chapter, ICG fluorescence lymphography is limited in its ability to detect the lymphatics and veins selected for anastomosis. If the anastomoses are performed in a relatively superficial layer of subcutaneous tissue, this method can evaluate the patency of the anastomoses. In my study, among 223 anastomoses in the lower limb, only 79 (35 %) could be evaluated by ICG lymphography. The remaining 144 anastomoses could not be evaluated because the subcutaneous layer was too thick to allow detection of the lymph vessels. In the 79 anastomoses that could be evaluated, cumulative patency rates of LVSEA were 75 ± 7.1 % at 12 months and 36 ± 9.4 % at 24 months after surgery [8]. Patency rates thus showed a gradual decrease over time, but we have seen some patients who have shown relatively long-term patency (Fig. 43.5).

43.2.2 Other Findings in Postoperative ICG Fluorescence Lymphography

In my clinical experience of postoperative ICG lymphography, I sometimes observe new pathways of superficial lymph flow created near the site of anastomosis where obvious patency could not be observed (Fig. 43.4a, b). This indicates that it may be possible to create new lymph pathways via surgical stimulation. On the other hand, the status of anastomosis at sites that cannot be evaluated due to thickness of the skin and subcutaneous fat or masking by DBF remains unclear.

43.3 Case Presentation

43.3.1 Mid-term Results (Fig. 43.5)

A 56-year-old woman with left upper-limb lymphedema after breast cancer treatment was referred for lymphatic microsurgery. This patient received complex decongestive physiotherapy for 3 years, but edema in the forearm (volume, 1880 ml) had not improved (Fig. 43.5a). LVSEA was planned and three anastomoses in the upper limb were performed (Fig. 43.5b). Volume of the left upper limb was decreased immediately after surgery and good condition was maintained with a volume of 1646 ml at 2 years and 10 months after surgery (Fig. 43.5c). ICG fluorescence lymphography showed one anastomosis was patent, one was undetectable, and one was non-patent at both 6 months (Fig. 43.5d) and 2 years 10 months (Fig. 43.5e) after surgery.

43.3.2 Long-term Results

A 52-year-old woman with primary lymphedema of the right lower limb had been treated by combined decongestive physiotherapy for several years, but edema of the limb remained unimproved. She came to my hospital for lymphatic microsurgery

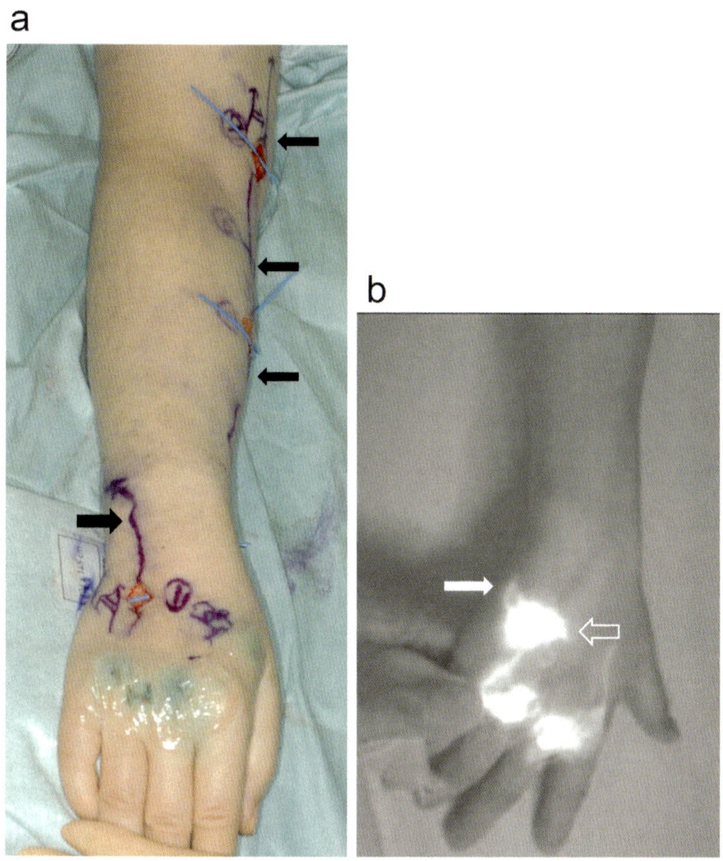

Fig. 43.4 ICG fluorescence lymphography in the right arm of a 47-year-old woman with breast cancer-related lymphedema
(**a**) Perioperative ICG fluorescence lymphography shows linear fluorescence (*closed arrows*) in the hand and arm. Five LVSEAs were performed in the upper limb
(**b**) Postoperative ICG fluorescence lymphography performed 7 months after surgery. Dermal backflow (*open arrow*) that was not observed at the operation has developed at the site of LVSEA in the hand. Linear fluorescence (*closed arrow*) that was likewise not apparent at the operation is observed from dermal backflow to the forearm

(Fig. 43.6a). Volume of the right lower limb was 5437 ml at the first visit. She underwent 7 LVSEAs at the first operation (Fig. 43.6b) and 2 at a second operation. The patient became freed from any complex decongestive physiotherapy, and volume of the right lower limb was decreased to 3784 ml at 5 years 6 months after the first operation (Fig. 43.6c). LVSEA above the ankle remained patent (*n*).

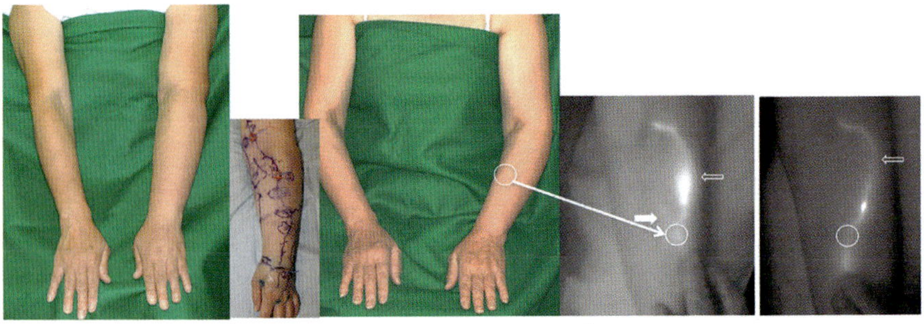

a b c d e

Fig. 43.5 Mid-term patency of LVSEA in a 56-year-old-woman with breast-related lymphedema on the left upper limb
(**a**) Clinical photo before surgery
(**b**) Operative photo. Three anastomoses were performed
(**c**) Clinical photo 2 years 10 months after surgery. Volume of the affected arm has decreased to 1646 ml (on the *left*). One LVSEA in the left arm (*open circle*) remains patent
(**d**) ICG fluorescence lymphography 6 months after surgery. The LVSEA is patent (*open circle*). The vein (*open arrow*) and lymphatic vessel (*closed arrow*) show fluorescence proximal to the LVSEA
(**e**) ICG fluorescence lymphography 2 years 10 months after surgery. The same LVSEA (*open circle*) is still patent and the same vein (*open arrow*) shows fluorescence

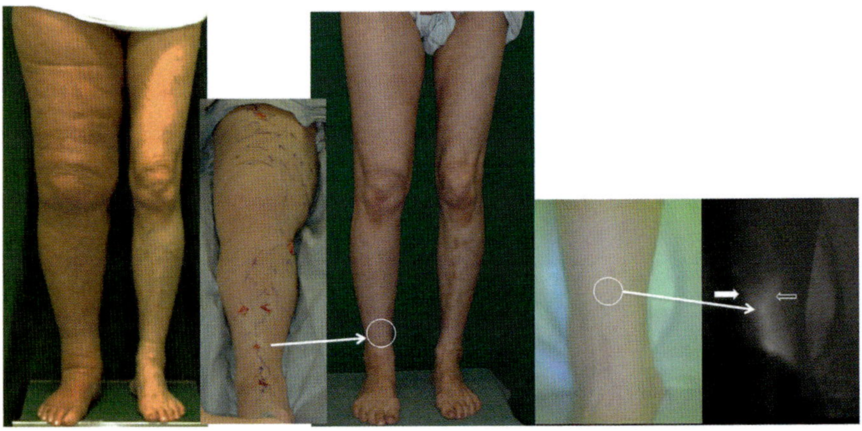

a b c d e

Fig. 43.6 Long-term patency of LVSEA in a 52-year-old woman with primary lymphedema of the right lower limb
(**a**) Clinical photo before surgery
(**b**) Clinical photo 5 years 6 months after surgery. The patient does not need any compressive therapy
(**c**) The operation scar (*open circle*) above the ankle on the affected side (*left*) and ICG fluorescence lymphography 5 years and 6 months after surgery show lymph drainage from the lymph vessel to the vein (*open arrow*)

43.4 Conclusions

ICG fluorescence lymphography is important to evaluate patency of LVA or LVSEA, which can physiologically improve lymphedema and offers a less invasive technique than other surgical methods to treat lymphedema. While some limitations exist to the detection of lymph vessels, mid- and long-term results of patency can be confirmed using ICG fluorescence lymphography. We can also clarify superficial lymph flow before and after surgery, providing useful information to decide on plans to treat lymphedema at each stage of lymphedema.

References

1. O'Brien BM, Sykes P, Threlfall GN, Browning FS (1977) Microlymphaticovenous anastomoses for obstructive lymphedema. Plast Reconstr Surg 60:197–211
2. Huang GK, Hu RQ, Liu ZZ, Shen YL, Lan TD, Pan GP (1985) Microlymphaticovenous anastomosis in the treatment of lower limb obstructive lymphedema: analysis of 91 cases. Plast Reconstr Surg 76:671–685
3. Campisi C, Boccardo F, Zilli A, Macciò A, Napoli F (2001) Long-term results after lymphatic-venous anastomoses for the treatment of obstructive lymphedema. Microsurgery 21:135–139
4. Koshima I, Nanba Y, Tsutsui T, Takahashi Y, Itoh S (2003) Long-term follow-up after lymphaticovenular anastomosis for lymphedema in the leg. J Reconstr Microsurg 19:209–215
5. O'Brien BM, Mellow CG, Khazanchi RK, Dvir E, Kumar V, Pederson WC (1990) Long-term results after microlymphaticovenous anastomoses for the treatment of obstructive lymphedema. Plast Reconstr Surg 85:562–572
6. Maegawa J, Mikami T, Yamamoto Y, Satake T, Kobayashi S (2010) Types of lymphoscintigraphy and indications for lymphaticovenous anastomosis. Microsurgery 30:437–442
7. Maegawa J, Hosono M, Tomoeda H, Tosaki A, Kobayashi S, Iwai T (2012) Net effect of lymphaticovenous anastomosis on volume reduction of peripheral lymphoedema after complex decongestive physiotherapy. Eur J Vasc Endovasc Surg 43:602–608
8. Maegawa J, Yabuki Y, Tomoeda H, Hosono M, Yasumura K (2012) Outcomes of lymphaticovenous side-to-end anastomosis in peripheral lymphedema. J Vasc Surg 55:753–760
9. Ogata F, Narushima M, Mihara M, Azuma R, Morimoto Y, Koshima I (2007) Intraoperative lymphography using indocyanine green dye for near- infrared fluorescence labeling in lymphedema. Ann Plast Surg 59:180–184
10. Unno N, Inuzuka K, Suzuki M, Yamamoto N, Sagara D, Nishiyama M et al (2007) Preliminary experience with a novel fluorescence lymphography using indocyanine green in patients with secondary lymphedema. J Vasc Surg 45:1016–1021
11. Szuba A, Strauss W, Sirsikar SP, Rockson SG (2002) Quantitative radionuclide lymphoscintigraphy predicts outcome of manual lymphatic therapy in breast cancer-related lymphedema of the upper extremity. Nucl Med Commun 23:1171–1175
12. Pecking AP, Albérini JL, Wartski M, Edeline V, Cluzan RV (2008) Relationship between lymphoscintigraphy and clinical findings in lower limb lymphedema (LO): toward a comprehensive staging. Lymphology 41:1–10
13. Vaqueiro M, Gloviczki P, Fisher J, Hollier LH, Schirger A, Wahner HW (1986) Lymphoscintigraphy in lymphedema: an aid to microsurgery. J Nucl Med 27:1125–1130
14. Mikami T, Hosono M, Yabuki Y, Yamamoto Y, Yasumura K, Sawada H et al (2011) Classification of lymphoscintigraphy and relevance to surgical indication for lymphaticovenous anastomosis in upper limb lymphedema. Lymphology 44:155–167

15. Yamamoto T, Narushima M, Doi K, Oshima A, Ogata F, Mihara M et al (2011) Characteristic indocyanine green lymphography findings in lower extremity lymphedema: the generation of a novel lymphedema severity staging system using dermal backflow patterns. Plast Reconstr Surg 127:1979–1986
16. Shaper NJ, Rutt DR, Browse NL (1992) Use of Teflon stents for lymphovenous anastomosis. Br J Surg 79:633–636
17. Narushima M, Mihara M, Yamamoto Y, Iida T, Koshima I, Mundinger GS (2010) The intravascular stenting method for treatment of extremity lymphedema with multiconfiguration lymphaticovenous anastomoses. Plast Reconstr Surg 125:935–943

Printed by Printforce, the Netherlands